Principles of anatomy and physiology for nursing and healthcare students in Australia

FIRST EDITION

Ian Peate

Suzanne Evans

Amy-Louise Byrne

William Deasy

Michele Dowlman

Pauline Gillan

Sivaraman Purushothuman

Dan Wadsworth

WILEY

First edition published 2022 by
John Wiley & Sons Australia, Ltd
42 McDougall Street, Milton Qld 4064

Typeset in 10/12pt Times LT Std

A catalogue record for this book is available from the National Library of Australia.

Wiley acknowledges the Traditional Custodians of the land on which we operate, live and gather as employees, and recognise their continuing connection to land, water and community. We pay respect to Elders past, present and emerging.

Creators/contributors
Ian Peate (Editor), Suzanne Evans (Editor), Carl Clare (Contributor), Noleen Jones (Contributor), Jacinta Hope Martin (Contributor), Karen Mate (Contributor), Louise McErlean (Contributor), Janet G. Migliozzi (Contributor), Karen Nagalingam (Contributor), Jessie Maree Sutherland (Contributor), Jude Weidenhofer (Contributor), Anthony Wheeldon (Contributor), Amy-Louise Byrne (Adapting author), William Deasy (Adapting author), Michele Dowlman (Adapting author), Pauline Gillan (Adapting author), Sivaraman Purushothuman (Adapting author), Dan Wadsworth (Adapting author)

Wiley
Mark Levings (Publishing Manager, Tertiary and Professional), David Hobson (Product Manager), Kylie Challenor (Senior Manager, Education Content Management), Emily Brain (Production Editor), Tara Seeto (Publishing Coordinator), Delia Sala (Cover Design)

Cover image: © SEBASTIAN KAULITZKI / Getty Images

Typeset in India by diacriTech

Printed in Singapore
M115561_060721

BRIEF CONTENTS

Preface *x*
About the editors *xii*
About the adapting authors *xiii*
Prefixes, suffixes *xv*
How to use your textbook *xxvi*

Chapter 1: Basic scientific principles of physiology 1
Chapter 2: Cells, cellular compartments, transport systems, fluid movement between compartments 23
Chapter 3: Genetics 45
Chapter 4: Tissue 79
Chapter 5: Embryology 101
Chapter 6: The muscular system 125
Chapter 7: The skeletal system 157
Chapter 8: The circulatory system 187
Chapter 9: The cardiac system 221
Chapter 10: The digestive system 253
Chapter 11: The renal system 287
Chapter 12: The respiratory system 317
Chapter 13: The reproductive systems 349
Chapter 14: The nervous system 377
Chapter 15: The senses 411
Chapter 16: The endocrine system 451
Chapter 17: The immune system 481
Chapter 18: The skin 517

Answers *541*
Normal values *543*
Index *547*

CONTENTS

Preface x
About the editors xii
About the adapting authors xiii
Prefixes, suffixes xv
How to use your textbook xxvi

CHAPTER 1

Basic scientific principles of physiology 1

Introduction 2
1.1 Levels of organisation 2
1.2 Characteristics of life 3
Bodily requirements 3
1.3 Life at the chemical level 4
The elements 4
The smallest unit of matter: the atom 4
Chemical reactions and chemical bonds 6
1.4 Acids and bases 10
Blood and pH values 11
Representing chemical reactions in written form: chemical equations 11
1.5 Organic molecules 12
Examples of organic substances 13
1.6 Homeostasis 15
Units of measurement 17
Summary 20
Key terms 20
Activities 21
Test your learning 21
Find out more 21
Reference 22
Acknowledgements 22

CHAPTER 2

Cells, cellular compartments, transport systems, fluid movement between compartments 23

Introduction 24
2.1 Inside the cell 24
2.2 Structure of the cell membrane 25
2.3 Transport of substances across the cell membrane 26
Passive transport 27
Osmosis: a special case of simple diffusion 28
Facilitated diffusion 30
Active transport 30
The energy to power active transport comes from the cell's mitochondria 31
How do cells communicate? 32
Fluid compartments in the body 32
Bulk transport across the cell membrane 33
2.4 The composition of body fluids 34
Electrolyte and water balance 34
2.5 Fluid movement between compartments 37
Summary 41
Key terms 41
Activities 42
Find out more 42
Chemical symbols 42
Conditions 42
References 43
Further reading 43
Acknowledgements 43

CHAPTER 3

Genetics 45

Cellular anatomical map 46
Introduction 46
3.1 Deoxyribonucleic acid (DNA) and ribonucleic acid (RNA) 46
3.2 The DNA double helix 49
Chromosomes 50
3.3 Gene expression: from DNA to proteins 52
Protein synthesis 52
Summary of relationship between DNA, RNA and protein 56
3.4 The transference of genes — the cell cycle 56
Mitosis 58
Meiosis 58
3.5 Inheritance 60
Mendelian inheritance 61
Autosomal dominant inheritance 63
Autosomal recessive inheritance 63
Morbidity and mortality of dominant versus recessive disorders 67
X-linked recessive disorders 67
3.6 Non-Mendelian (complex) inheritance 69
Spontaneous mutation 70
Disorders of chromosomes 72
Summary 74
Key terms 74
Activities 76
Conditions 76
References 76
Further reading 77
Acknowledgements 78

CHAPTER 4

Tissue 79

Introduction 80
4.1 Epithelial tissue 80
Simple epithelium 81
Stratified epithelium 84
Glandular epithelia 85
4.2 Connective tissue 87
Ground substance 88
Fibres 88
Connective tissue proper 89
Cartilage 90
Bone 91
Liquid connective tissue 91
Membranes 92
4.3 Muscle tissue 94
4.4 Nervous tissue 94
4.5 Tissue repair 94
Summary 99
Key terms 99
References 100
Further reading 100
Acknowledgements 100

CHAPTER 5

Embryology 101

Introduction 102
A note on timings 102
5.1 Final maturation of the oocyte and sperm 102
Oocyte maturation and ovulation 102
Sperm maturation 103
Day 1: Fertilisation 104
5.2 Days 2–5: Pre-implantation development 105
5.3 Day 6: Implantation 106
Week 2: Early placental formation 106
5.4 Weeks 3–8: Post-implantation embryonic development 109
Differentiation of embryonic or germ layers 109
Week 3 110
Week 4 111
Week 5 111
Week 6 111
Weeks 7 and 8 111
Late gestation and birth: gestational weeks 13–40 (embryonic weeks 11–38) 113
5.5 Complications of pregnancy 116
Ectopic pregnancies 116
Pregnancy loss/miscarriage and stillbirth 116
Summary 121
Key terms 121
References 121
Further reading 122
Acknowledgements 123

CHAPTER 6

The muscular system 125

Body map 125
Introduction 126
6.1 Types of muscle tissue 126
Smooth or visceral muscle 126
Cardiac 126
Skeletal 126
Functions of the muscular system 126
Composition of skeletal muscle tissue 127
Gross anatomy of skeletal muscles 128
Microanatomy of skeletal muscle fibre 129
6.2 Skeletal muscle contraction and relaxation 132
6.3 Energy sources for muscle contraction 136
Aerobic respiration 136
6.4 Organisation of the skeletal muscular system 139
Skeletal muscle movement 150
The effects of ageing 152
Summary 153
Key terms 153
Find out more 153
Conditions 153
References 154
Further reading 155
Acknowledgements 155

CHAPTER 7

The skeletal system 157

Body map 157
Introduction 158
7.1 The functions of the skeletal system 158
7.2 Bone as a tissue 160
Osteoblasts 161
Osteoclasts 161
Osteocytes 161
7.3 Other connective tissues closely associated with the skeletal system 162
Cartilage 162
Ligaments 163
Tendons 163
Bone formation 164
Bone growth 165
Bone remodelling 168
Bone fractures 170
7.4 The axial and appendicular skeleton 172
Bone shapes 174
Joints 178
Summary 182
Key terms 182
Activities 183
Match each bone to its correct shape 183
Find out more 183
Conditions 184
References 184

Further reading 185
Acknowledgements 185

CHAPTER 8
The circulatory system 187
Body map 187
Introduction 188
8.1 Components of blood 188
Properties of blood 189
Plasma 190
8.2 Functions of blood 191
Formation of blood cells 192
Red blood cells 193
Haemoglobin 193
White blood cells 197
Platelets 200
Haemostasis 200
Blood groups 204
8.3 Blood vessels 206
Structure and function of arteries and veins 207
Capillaries 209
Blood pressure 210
8.4 Lymphatic system 212
Lymph 212
Lymph capillaries and large lymph vessels 214
Lymph nodes 214
Lymphatic organs 217
Summary 218
Key terms 218
Find out more 219
Conditions 219
References 219
Further reading 220
Acknowledgements 220

CHAPTER 9
The cardiac system 221
Body map 221
Introduction 222
9.1 Size and location of the heart 222
The structures of the heart 223
9.2 The cardiac action potential 226
Endocardium 226
The heart chambers 226
9.3 The blood supply to the heart 230
Blood flow through the heart 235
9.4 The electrical pathways of the heart 237
9.5 The cardiac cycle 240
Factors affecting cardiac output 244
Regulation of stroke volume 244
Regulation of heart rate 245
Summary 248
Key terms 248
Conditions 250
References 250
Further reading 251
Acknowledgements 251

CHAPTER 10
The digestive system 253
Body map 253
Introduction 254
10.1 The activity of the digestive system 254
The organisation of the digestive system 255
The digestive system organs 255
The structure of the digestive system 259
10.2 Accessory organs of the digestive system 268
Teeth 268
Salivary glands 268
The pancreas 270
The liver and production of bile 272
The gall bladder 274
10.3 Digestive hormones 274
Chemical digestion 275
10.4 Nutrition, chemical digestion and metabolism 275
Nutrients 275
Balanced diet 275
Nutrient groups 277
Summary 282
Key terms 282
Activities 284
Find out more 284
Test your learning 285
Conditions 285
References 285
Further reading 286
Acknowledgements 286

CHAPTER 11
The renal system 287
Body map 287
Introduction 288
11.1 Functions of the kidney 288
11.2 Kidneys: external and internal structures 289
External structures 289
Blood supply of the kidney 290
Internal structures 294
11.3 Nephrons 296
Bowman's capsule 296
Proximal convoluted tubule 297
Loop of Henle 297
Distal convoluted tubule 298
Collecting ducts 298
11.4 Filtration 299
Selective reabsorption 299
Hormonal control of tubular reabsorption and secretion 301

11.5 Composition of urine 303
Characteristics of normal urine 303
Ureters 307
Urinary bladder 308
Urethra 310
Micturition 312
Summary 313
Key terms 313
Conditions 313
References 314
Further reading 315
Acknowledgements 315

CHAPTER 12

The respiratory system 317

Body map 317
Introduction 318
12.1 Organisation of the respiratory system 318
The upper respiratory tract 319
The lower respiratory tract 320
Blood supply 326
Respiration 327
12.2 Pulmonary ventilation 327
The mechanics of breathing 327
Work of breathing 329
Volumes and capacities 331
12.3 Control of breathing 334
12.4 External respiration 335
Gaseous exchange 335
Factors influencing diffusion 335
Ventilation and perfusion 338
12.5 Transport of gases 338
Transport of oxygen 338
Transport of carbon dioxide 340
Acid–base balance 341
Internal respiration 341
Summary 343
Key terms 343
Conditions 345
References 346
Further reading 347
Acknowledgements 347

CHAPTER 13

The reproductive systems 349

Body map 349
Introduction 350
13.1 The male reproductive system 350
The scrotum 351
The testes 352
Spermatogenesis 353
Sperm 355
Epididymis 355
The vas deferens, spermatic cord and ejaculatory duct 356
The seminal vesicles and prostate gland 356
The penis 356
13.2 Hormonal control of male reproduction 357
13.3 The female reproductive system 359
The ovaries 359
Oogenesis and follicular development 360
Corpus luteum 362
13.4 The role of the female sex hormones 362
The internal organs 363
The external genitalia 367
The breasts 368
13.5 The uterine cycle 369
Summary 372
Key terms 372
Find out more 373
Conditions 373
References 374
Further reading 375
Acknowledgements 375

CHAPTER 14

The nervous system 377

Body map 377
Introduction 378
14.1 Organisation of the nervous system 378
Sensory division of the peripheral nervous system 378
Central nervous system 379
Motor division of the peripheral nervous system 379
14.2 The action potential 382
Simple propagation of nerve impulses 382
Saltatory conduction 382
The refractory period 382
Neurotransmitters 385
Neuroglia 386
The meninges 387
Cerebrospinal fluid 388
14.3 The brain 389
Cerebrum 390
Diencephalon 392
Brainstem 393
Cerebellum 393
The limbic system and the reticular formation 393
14.4 The peripheral nervous system 395
Cranial nerves 395
The spinal cord 397
Functions of the spinal cord 398
Spinal nerves 398
14.5 The autonomic nervous system 401
Sympathetic division (fight or flight) 402
Parasympathetic division (rest and digest) 403
Summary 405
Key terms 405
Find out more 406

Conditions 406
References 407
Further reading 408
Acknowledgements 409

CHAPTER 15

The senses 411

Introduction 412
15.1 The chemical senses 412
The sense of smell (olfaction) 412
Olfactory receptors 413
15.2 The sense of taste 416
Tastebuds 418
The taste receptor 418
The gustatory pathway 419
15.3 The sense of hearing and sense of balance 421
The structure of the ear 421
15.4 Equilibrium 426
Pathways for the equilibrium sensations 428
15.5 The hearing perception — discrimination and interpretation of sound energy 430
The hearing process 432
The hearing reflex 432
15.6 The eye and the sense of sight 434
The structure of the eye 434
15.7 Organisation of the retina 438
15.8 Focusing images onto the retina 441
Refraction 441
Myopia, hyperopia and presbyopia 444
Summary 447
Key terms 447
Conditions 448
References 449
Further reading 450
Acknowledgements 450

CHAPTER 16

The endocrine system 451

Body map 451
Introduction 452
16.1 The endocrine organs 452
16.2 Hormones 454
The transportation of hormones 455
Effects of hormones 455
16.3 Control of hormone release 456
Destruction and removal of hormones 456
The physiology of the endocrine organs 456
The thyroid gland 462
Adrenal cortex 468
16.4 Insulin 473
Glucagon 475
Somatostatin 476
Summary 477
Key terms 477
Conditions 478
References 478
Further reading 479
Acknowledgements 479

CHAPTER 17

The immune system 481

Body map 481
Introduction 482
17.1 Blood cell development 482
17.2 Organs of the immune system 483
The thymus 483
The lymphatic system 484
Lymphoid tissue 488
Types of immunity 488
The innate immune system 489
Blood cells 489
17.3 Phagocytosis 490
Cytotoxicity 493
Inflammation 493
17.4 The acquired immune system 498
Cell-mediated immunity (T-cell lymphocytes) 498
Humoral immunity (B-cell lymphocytes) 500
Immunoglobulins (antibodies) 501
Role of immunoglobulins 503
Natural killer cells 506
17.5 Primary and secondary response to infection 506
Primary immune response 506
Secondary immune response 507
Hypersensitivity 509
Anaphylaxis 510
Immunisations 510
Summary 511
Key terms 511
Activities 513
Find out more 513
Conditions 513
References 514
Further reading 515
Acknowledgements 515

CHAPTER 18

The skin 517

Body map 517
Introduction 518
18.1 The structure of skin 519
The epidermis 519
Layers of the epidermis 523
The dermis 527
The papillary and reticular aspects 527

18.2 The accessory skin structures 528
The hair 528
Sweat glands 529
Nails 530
18.3 The functions of the skin 532
Sensation 532
Protection 534
Excretion and absorption 535
Synthesis of vitamin D 536
Summary 537
Key terms 537
Find out more 538
Conditions 538
References 538
Further reading 539
Acknowledgements 539

Answers 541
Normal values 543
Index 547

PREFACE

The adapting authors for this first Australian edition are committed to the provision of high-quality, safe and effective care to a range of communities. They are all experienced academics working in higher education, with many years of clinical and educational experience, knowledge and skills, teaching multidisciplinary student groups at various academic levels. After you have gained a sound understanding of anatomy and physiology, we are confident you will better understand the needs of those you care for in your career. Each of us should strive to provide high-quality, safe and effective care; however, this will be challenging if we do not fully understand and acknowledge the person in a holistic manner. Those who offer people care and support must consider the anatomical and physiological elements of care; they must also, however, take into consideration the psychosocial aspects of the person and their family, addressing the needs of the whole being, the whole person and, where appropriate, the whole community. This text is designed to encourage learning, understanding and integration. We hope that you enjoy reading it and, importantly, that you are keen to learn more and delve deeper as you grow and develop into a world-class provider of safe and effective healthcare.

We have learnt much from reader feedback as we have adapted this new edition. We have listened to readers' comments and responded by making changes and retaining those features that are most popular.

Within any program of study related to the provision of care, it is important that you are confident and competent with regard to pathophysiology and anatomy and physiology. It is not enough to remember all of the facts (of which there are many) that are related to anatomy and physiology; you must also relate these to the people you offer care and support to. Some of those people may be vulnerable and at risk of harm, and it is your responsibility to ensure that you are well informed and appreciate the complexities of care provision. This new edition of *Principles of Anatomy and Physiology for Nursing and Healthcare Students in Australia* can help you.

Registration with professional bodies, such as the Australian Health Practitioner Regulation Agency (AHPRA), requires that you demonstrate competence and proficiency in a number of areas, including anatomy and physiology.

The human body is as beautiful on the inside as it is on the outside; when synchronised, the mind and body is an astonishing mechanism that has the amazing ability to perform a multitude of complex things. Healthcare students practise and study in a variety of healthcare settings: in the hospital, the primary-care setting/pre-hospital care setting and in a person's own home, where they are certain to meet and care for people who will have a variety of anatomical and physiological problems. By using a fundamental approach with a sound anatomical and physiological understanding, healthcare students can grow in confidence and competence.

Anatomy and physiology

In its simplest form, anatomy can be defined as the science related to the study of the structure of biological organisms; there are dictionaries that use such a definition. *Principles of Anatomy and Physiology for Nursing and Healthcare Students in Australia* focuses on human anatomy, which is defined for the purposes of this text as the study of the structure of the human body. This acknowledges function and also structure; in all biological organisms, structure and function are closely interrelated. The human body will only perform effectively through the cooperation of interrelated systems.

The term 'anatomy' is Greek in origin, meaning 'to cut up' or 'to dissect'. The first scientifically based anatomical studies (attributed to Vesalius, the sixteenth-century Flemish anatomist, doctor and artist) were based on observations of cadavers (dead bodies). More up-to-date approaches to human anatomy differ, however, as they include other means of observation; such as microscopy and other complex and technologically advanced imaging tools. Subdivisions are now associated within the broader field of anatomy, with the word anatomy often preceded with an adjective identifying the method of observation; for example, gross anatomy (the study of body parts that are visible to the naked eye, such as the heart or the bones) or microanatomy (where body parts such as cells or tissues are only visible with the use of a microscope).

Living systems can be defined from a number of perspectives.

- At the smallest of levels, the chemical level, atoms, molecules and the chemical bonds connecting atoms provide the structure on which living activity is grounded.

- The cell is the smallest unit of life. Specialised bodies — organelles — within the cell undertake specific cellular functions. Cells can be specialised, such as bone cells and muscle cells. Tissue is a group of cells that are alike, performing a common function. Muscle tissue, for example, is made up of muscle cells.
- Organs are groups of different types of tissues that work together to perform a specific activity. The stomach is an organ that is made up of muscle, nerve and tissues.
- A system is two or more organs working in unison to carry out a particular activity. The digestive system is an example; it comprises the coordinated activities of a number of organs — these include the stomach, intestines, pancreas and liver.
- Another system having the characteristics of living things is an organism; this has the capacity to obtain and process energy, the ability to react to changes in the environment and the ability to reproduce.

Anatomy is associated with the function of a living organism and is therefore almost always inseparable from physiology. Physiology can be described as the science that deals with the study of the function of cells, tissues, organs and organisms. Physiology is involved with how an organism carries out its various activities, considering how it moves, how it is nourished, how it adapts to environments that change — human and animal, hostile and friendly. It is in principle the study of life.

Physiology is the foundation upon which we build our knowledge of what life is; it can assist us in deciding how to treat disease as well as helping us to adapt and manage changes that are imposed on our bodies by new and changing surroundings — internal and external. Studying physiology assists in understanding disease (pathophysiology) arising from this; physiologists working with others can develop new ways to treat diseases.

There are a number of branches of anatomical study. Similarly, there are several physiological branches that can be studied, such as endocrinology, neurology and cardiology.

There are 18 chapters in this text. The chapters use simple and generously sized full-colour artwork to assist you in your understanding and comprehension of the complexities that are associated with the human body from an anatomical and physiological perspective. There are several features contained within each chapter that will assist you to build upon and develop your knowledge base.

The text takes the reader from the microscopic to macroscopic level in the study of anatomy and physiology. The contents demonstrate the movement from cells and tissues through to systems. This approach to learning and teaching is a tried-and-tested approach, especially when helping a learner understand a topic area that may sometimes be seen as complex.

This book has been written with these key principles in mind, to help inform your practice and also to help with your academic work.

ABOUT THE EDITORS

Ian Peate OBE FRCN

Visiting Professor of Nursing St George's University of London and Kingston University, London, and Visiting Professor Northumbria University. Visiting Senior Clinical Fellow University of Hertfordshire, Head of School, School of Health Studies, Gibraltar. Editor in Chief British Journal of Nursing.

Ian began his nursing a career at Central Middlesex Hospital, becoming an Enrolled Nurse practising in an intensive care unit. He later undertook three years of student nurse training at Central Middlesex and Northwick Park Hospitals, becoming a Staff Nurse then a Charge Nurse. He has worked in nurse education since 1989. His key areas of interest are nursing practice and theory. Ian has published widely. He was awarded an OBE in the Queen's 90th Birthday Honours List for his services to Nursing and Nurse Education and was bestowed a Fellowship from the Royal College of Nursing in 2017.

Suzanne Evans PhD

Director of Teaching and Learning and Deputy Head, School of Biomedical Sciences and Pharmacy, Faculty of Health and Medicine, University of Newcastle, New South Wales, Australia.

Suzanne gained her PhD in neuroscience at the University of Wales in 1989 and has been researching and teaching in universities in the UK, USA, the Caribbean, New Zealand and Australia ever since, receiving numerous teaching awards along the way. She has taught human physiology, pathophysiology and pharmacology at undergraduate and postgraduate level for many years and her special interest is teaching and assessing these subjects in health professional degrees.

ABOUT THE ADAPTING AUTHORS

Amy-Louise Byrne

Amy-Louise gained her Bachelor of Nursing from the University of Newcastle in 2008. She worked in the Hunter New England and North Coast areas of New South Wales before moving to South West Queensland. Amy-Louise's clinical experience spans across emergency nursing, rural and remote nursing, child health and management, education and research. Since 2018, Amy-Louise has lived and worked in Townsville, North Queensland, where she works as an Associate Lecturer with Central Queensland University. Her key areas of interests are in long-term health conditions, nurse-led models of care, social justice, care equity, as well as person-centred care.

William Deasy

William began his teaching career in 2009 at James Cook University, teaching anatomy, physiology and microbiology to students studying nursing, medicine, biomedical sciences and allied health. For his PhD he investigated the effects of the 5:2 intermittent fasting diet and sprint interval training on weight loss and markers of cardiovascular and metabolic health. William is currently a Lecturer at Central Queensland University and is interested in the effects of fasting on indices relating to major depressive disorder and anxiety and the effects of the gut microbiome on general health and wellbeing.

Michele Dowlman

Michele achieved a Bachelor of Nursing in 2005 and a Graduate Certificate in Acute Care in 2011. She has 13 years of experience in acute healthcare. In 2010, she was invited to tutor bioscience for nursing students at the University of Tasmania, and was promoted to Lecturer in Bioscience and Nursing in 2018. Her passion is teaching science to nursing students and doing so within the framework of the Clinical Reasoning Cycle (Levett-Jones 2013). This framework enables students to understand the interface between bioscience and clinical practice. Michele's teaching philosophy is asking students to use the science they have learned to explain their patient's presentation ('Why are you seeing what you are seeing?'), and explain their rationale for care ('Why are you doing what you are doing?'). Her other passion is working with clinical facilitators to encourage them to use the Clinical Reasoning Cycle framework in the practice setting, for continuity of student learning. She also works with a nurse practitioner providing free, drop-in healthcare to people in her community who are experiencing homelessness and/or poverty. They partner with a local not-for-profit organisation to deliver this nurse-led care to vulnerable people.

Pauline Gillan

Pauline is an experienced nursing lecturer with 13 years of tertiary teaching experience at various universities including the Queensland University of Technology, University of New England and University of Newcastle. Most of Pauline's teaching is in the areas of acute care nursing, health assessment and physical examination, aged care, palliative care and cancer nursing. Pauline's research interests are in palliative care and end of life care, and nursing and interprofessional simulation.

Pauline is an experienced Registered Nurse with over 30 years experience in many clinical areas of nursing, including acute care, surgical and medical care, midwifery, early childhood nursing and palliative care nursing within community and inpatient contexts. Pauline is a member of Palliative Care Queensland, Palliative Care Nurses Association and Sigma Theta Tau International Honour Society.

Sivaraman Purushothuman

Sivaraman's interest in neurobiology began early as he studied psychology and medical sciences before undertaking research in neurodegeneration. He is a current NHMRC/ARC Research Fellow and lecturer at Brain and Mind Centre. His passion for education led him to teach physiology and anatomy subjects under medical and nursing courses at the University of Sydney and the University of Tasmania. His main research focuses on the pathology, therapeutics and diagnostics within ageing and neurodegenerative disorders of the brain and retina. Previously, he undertook research in traumatic brain injury and cerebrovascular disease. He has attained competitive research funding, several publications in international peer-reviewed journals and delivered several lectures in conferences and public forums about his research interests. He also engages in strategies and programs aimed at improving education, research and pedagogy in the higher education sector.

Dan Wadsworth

Dan has an extensive history of teaching health science across a range of healthcare professional programs in New Zealand and Australia, specialising in anatomy and physiology and human bioscience, and is currently a Lecturer in Applied Science within the School of Nursing, Midwifery and Paramedicine at the University of the Sunshine Coast (Australia). Grounded in his own experiences as a learner, he aims to make health science as simple and accessible as possible by drawing on real-world foundations and experiences to empower students with the knowledge, skills and confidence to succeed in their chosen field. Dan has a strong research interest in clinical exercise, exploring the many roles that accessible exercise can play in healthy ageing and mental wellbeing, in addition to an ongoing portfolio of educational research looking at best practice in tertiary health science education and the application of knowledge into practice. Dan supervises research students in both fields of enquiry, reviews for various international journals and has engaged in numerous research collaborations resulting in journal articles, book chapters and conference presentations.

PREFIXES, SUFFIXES

Prefix: A prefix is positioned at the beginning of a word to modify or change its meaning. Pre means 'before'. Prefixes may also indicate a location, number or time.

Suffix: The ending part of a word that changes the meaning of the word.

Prefix or suffix	Meaning	Example(s)
a-, an-	not, without	analgesic, apathy
ab-	from; away from	abduction
abdomin(o)-	of or relating to the abdomen	abdomen
acous(io)-	of or relating to hearing	acoumeter, acoustician
acr(o)-	extremity, topmost	acrocrany, acromegaly, acroosteolysis, acroposthia
ad-	at, increase, on, towards	adduction
aden(o)-, aden(i)-	of or relating to a gland	adenocarcinoma, adenology, adenotome, adenotyphus
adip(o)-	of or relating to fat or fatty tissue	adipocyte
adren(o)-	of or relating to adrenal glands	adrenal artery
-aemia	blood condition	anaemia
aer(o)-	air, gas	aerosinusitis
-aesthesi(o)-	sensation	anaesthesia
alb-	denoting a white or pale colour	albino
-alge(si)-	pain	analgesic
-algia, -alg(i)o-	pain	myalgia
all(o-)	denoting something as different, or as an addition	alloantigen, allopathy
ambi-	denoting something as positioned on both sides	ambidextrous
amni-	pertaining to the membranous foetal sac (amnion)	amniocentesis
ana-	back, again, up	anaplasia
andr(o)-	pertaining to a man	android, andrology
angi(o)-	blood vessel	angiogram
ankyl(o)-, ancyl(o)-	denoting something as crooked or bent	ankylosis
ante-	describing something as positioned in front of another thing	antepartum
anti-	describing something as 'against' or 'opposed to' another	antibody, antipsychotic
arteri(o)-	of or pertaining to an artery	arteriole, arterial
arthr(o)-	of or pertaining to the joints, limbs	arthritis

(continued)

Prefix or suffix	Meaning	Example(s)
articul(o)-	joint	articulation
-ase	enzyme	lactase
-asthenia	weakness	myasthenia gravis
ather(o)-	fatty deposit, soft gruel-like deposit	atherosclerosis
atri(o)-	an atrium (especially heart atrium)	atrioventricular
aur(i)-	of or pertaining to the ear	aural
aut(o)-	self	autoimmune
axill-	of or pertaining to the armpit (uncommon as a prefix)	axilla
bi-	twice, double	binary
bio-	life	biology
blephar(o)-	of or pertaining to the eyelid	blepharoplast
brachi(o)-	of or relating to the arm	brachium of inferior colliculus
brady-	'slow'	bradycardia
bronch(i)-	bronchus	bronchiolitis obliterans
bucc(o)-	of or pertaining to the cheek	buccolabial
burs(o)-	bursa (fluid sac between the bones)	bursitis
carcin(o)-	cancer	carcinoma
cardi(o)-	of or pertaining to the heart	cardiology
carp(o)-	of or pertaining to the wrist	carpal tunnel
-cele	pouching, hernia	hydrocele, varicocele
-centesis	surgical puncture for aspiration	amniocentesis
cephal(o)-	of or pertaining to the head (as a whole)	cephalalgy
cerebell(o)-	of or pertaining to the cerebellum	cerebellum
cerebr(o)-	of or pertaining to the brain	cerebrology
chem(o)-	chemistry, drug	chemotherapy
chol(e)-	of or pertaining to bile	cholecystitis
cholecyst(o)-	of or pertaining to the gallbladder	cholecystectomy
chondr(i)o-	cartilage, gristle, granule, granular	chondrocalcinosis
chrom(ato)-	colour	haemochromatosis
-cidal, -cide	killing, destroying	bacteriocidal
cili-	of or pertaining to the cilia, the eyelashes	ciliary
circum-	denoting something as 'around' another	circumcision
col(o)-, colono-	colon	colonoscopy
colp(o)-	of or pertaining to the vagina	colposcopy
contra-	against	contraindicate
coron(o)-	crown	coronary

cost(o)-	of or pertaining to the ribs	costochondral
crani(o)-	belonging or relating to the cranium	craniology
-crine, -crin(o)-	to secrete	endocrine
cry(o)-	cold	cryoablation
cutane-	skin	subcutaneous
cyan(o)-	denotes a blue colour	cyanosis
cyst(o)-, cyst(i)-	of or pertaining to the urinary bladder	cystotomy
cyt(o)-	cell	cytokine
-cyte	cell	leukocyte
-dactyl(o)-	of or pertaining to a finger, toe	dactylology, polydactyly
dent-	of or pertaining to teeth	dentist
dermat(o)-, derm(o)-	of or pertaining to the skin	dermatology
-desis	binding	arthrodesis
dextr(o)-	right, on the right side	dextrocardia
di-	two	diplopia
dia-	through, during, across	dialysis
dif-	apart, separation	different
digit-	of or pertaining to the finger (rare as a root)	digit
-dipsia	suffix meaning '(condition of) thirst'	polydipsia, hydroadipsia, oligodipsia
dors(o)-, dors(i)-	of or pertaining to the back	dorsal, dorsocephalad
duodeno-	duodenum	duodenal atresia
dynam(o)-	force, energy, power	hand strength dynamometer
-dynia	pain	vulvodynia
dys-	bad, difficult, defective, abnormal	dysphagia, dysphasia
ec-	out, away	ectopia, ectopic pregnancy
-ectasia, -ectasis	expansion, dilation	bronchiectasis, telangiectasia
ect(o)-	outer, outside	ectoblast, ectoderm
-ectomy	denotes a surgical operation or removal of a body part; resection, excision	mastectomy
-emesis	vomiting condition	haematemesis
encephal(o)-	of or pertaining to the brain; also see cerebr(o)-	encephalogram
endo-	denotes something as 'inside' or 'within'	endocrinology, endospore
enter(o)-	of or pertaining to the intestine	gastroenterology
eosin(o)-	red	eosinophil granulocyte
epi-	on, upon	epicardium, epidermis, epidural, episclera, epistaxis
erythr(o)-	denotes a red colour	erythrocyte

(continued)

Prefix or suffix	Meaning	Example(s)
ex-	out of, away from	excision, exophthalmos
exo-	denotes something as 'outside' another	exoskeleton
extra-	outside	extradural haematoma
faci(o)-	of or pertaining to the face	facioplegic
fibr(o)	fibre	fibroblast
fore-	before or ahead	forehead
fossa	a hollow or depressed area; trench or channel	fossa ovalis
front-	of or pertaining to the forehead	frontonasal
galact(o)-	milk	galactorrhoea
gastr(o)-	of or pertaining to the stomach	gastric bypass
-genic	formative, pertaining to producing	cardiogenic shock
gingiv-	of or pertaining to the gums	gingivitis
glauc(o)-	denoting a grey or bluish-grey colour	glaucoma
gloss(o)-, glott(o)-	of or pertaining to the tongue	glossology
gluco-	sweet	glucocorticoid
glyc(o)-	sugar	glycolysis
-gnosis	knowledge	diagnosis, prognosis
gon(o)-	seed, semen; also, reproductive	gonorrhoea
-gram, -gramme	record or picture	angiogram
-graph	instrument used to record data or picture	electrocardiograph
-graphy	process of recording	angiography
gyn(aec)o-	woman	gynaecomastia
haemangi(o)-	blood vessels	haemangioma
haemat(o)-, haem-	of or pertaining to blood	haematology
halluc-	to wander in mind	hallucinosis
hemi-	one-half	cerebral hemisphere
hepat- (hepatic-)	of or pertaining to the liver	hepatology
heter(o)-	denotes something as 'the other' (of two), as an addition, or different	heterogeneous
hist(o)-, histio-	tissue	histology
home(o)-	similar	homeopathy
hom(o)-	denotes something as 'the same' as another or common	homosexuality
hydr(o)-	water	hydrophobe
hyper-	denotes something as 'extreme' or 'beyond normal'	hypertension
hyp(o)-	denotes something as 'below normal'	hypovolaemia
hyster(o)-	of or pertaining to the womb, the uterus	hysterectomy

iatr(o)-	of or pertaining to medicine, or a physician	iatrogenic
-iatry	denotes a field in medicine of a certain body component	podiatry, psychiatry
-ics	organised knowledge, treatment	obstetrics
ileo-	ileum	ileocaecal valve
infra-	below	infrahyoid muscles
inter-	between, among	interarticular ligament
intra-	within	intramural
ipsi-	same	ipsilateral hemiparesis
ischio-	of or pertaining to the ischium, the hip joint	ischioanal fossa
-ismus	spasm, contraction	hemiballismus
iso-	denoting something as being 'equal'	isotonic
-ist	one who specialises in	pathologist
-itis	inflammation	tonsillitis
-ium	structure, tissue	pericardium
juxta- (iuxta-)	near to, alongside or next to	juxtaglomerular apparatus
karyo-	nucleus	eukaryote
kerat(o)-	cornea (eye or skin)	keratoscope
kin(e)-, kin(o)-, kinesi(o)-	movement	kinaesthesia
kyph(o)-	humped	kyphoscoliosis
labi(o)-	of or pertaining to the lip	labiodental
lacrim(o)-	tear	lacrimal canaliculi
lact(i)-, lact(o)	milk	lactation
lapar(o)-	of or pertaining to the abdomen wall, flank	laparotomy
laryng(o)-	of or pertaining to the larynx, the lower throat cavity where the voice box is	larynx
latero-	lateral	lateral pectoral nerve
-lepsis, -lepsy	attack, seizure	epilepsy, narcolepsy
lept(o)-	light, slender	leptomeningeal
leuc(o)-, leuk(o)-	denoting a white colour	leukocyte
lingu(a)-, lingu(o)-	of or pertaining to the tongue	linguistics
lip(o)-	fat	liposuction
lith(o)-	stone, calculus	lithotripsy
-logist	denotes someone who studies a certain field	oncologist, pathologist
log(o)-	speech	logopaedics

(continued)

Prefix or suffix	Meaning	Example(s)
-logy	denotes the academic study or practice of a certain field	haematology, urology
lymph(o)-	lymph	lymphoedema
lys(o)-, -lytic	dissolution	lysosome
-lysis	destruction, separation	paralysis
macr(o)-	large, long	macrophage
-malacia	softening	osteomalacia
mammill(o)-	of or pertaining to the nipple	mammillitis
mamm(o)-	of or pertaining to the breast	mammogram
manu-	of or pertaining to the hand	manufacture
mast(o)-	of or pertaining to the breast	mastectomy
meg(a)-, megal(o)-, -megaly	enlargement, million	splenomegaly, megameter
melan(o)-	black colour	melanin
mening(o)-	membrane	meningitis
meta-	after, behind	metacarpus
-meter	instrument used to measure or count	sphygmomanometer
metr(o)-	pertaining to conditions of the uterus	metrorrhagia
-metry	process of measuring	optometry
micro-	denoting something as small, or relating to smallness	microscope
milli-	thousandth	millilitre
mon(o)-	single	infectious mononucleosis
morph(o)-	form, shape	morphology
muscul(o)-	muscle	musculoskeletal system
my(o)-	of or relating to muscle	myoblast
myc(o)-	fungus	onychomycosis
myel(o)-	of or relating to bone marrow or spinal cord	myeloblast
myri-	ten thousand	myriad
myring(o)-	eardrum	myringotomy
narc(o)-	numb, sleep	narcolepsy
nas(o)-	of or pertaining to the nose	nasal
necr(o)-	death	necrosis, necrotising fasciitis
neo-	new	neoplasm
nephr(o)-	of or pertaining to the kidney	nephrology
neur(i)-, neur(o)-	of or pertaining to nerves and the nervous system	neurofibromatosis
normo-	normal	normocapnia

ocul(o)-	of or pertaining to the eye	oculist
odont(o)-	of or pertaining to teeth	orthodontist
odyn(o)-	pain	stomatodynia
-oesophageal, oesophag(o)-	gullet	gastro-oesophageal reflux
-oid	resemblance to	sarcoidosis
-ole	small or little	arteriole
olig(o)-	denoting something as 'having little, having few'	oliguria
-oma (sing.), -omata (pl.)	tumour, mass, collection	sarcoma, teratoma
onco-	tumour, bulk, volume	oncology
onych(o)-	of or pertaining to the nail (of a finger or toe)	onychophagy
oo-	of or pertaining to an egg, a woman's egg, the ovum	oogenesis
oophor(o)-	of or pertaining to the woman's ovary	oophorectomy
ophthalm(o)-	of or pertaining to the eye	ophthalmology
optic(o)-	of or relating to chemical properties of the eye	opticochemical
orchi(o)-, orchid(o)-, orch(o)-	testis	orchiectomy, orchidectomy
-osis	a condition, disease or increase	ichthyosis, psychosis, osteoporosis
osseo-	bony	osseous
ossi-	bone	peripheral ossifying fibroma
ost(e)-, oste(o)-	bone	osteoporosis
ot(o)-	of or pertaining to the ear	otology
ovo-, ovi-, ov-	of or pertaining to the eggs, the ovum	ovogenesis
pachy-	thick	pachyderma
paed-, paedo-	of or pertaining to the child	paediatrics
palpebr-	of or pertaining to the eyelid (uncommon as a root)	palpebra
pan-, pant(o)-	denoting something as 'complete' or containing 'everything'	panophobia, panopticon
papill-	of or pertaining to the nipple (of the chest/breast)	papillitis
papul(o)-	indicates papulosity, a small elevation or swelling in the skin, a pimple, swelling	papulation
para-	alongside of, abnormal	paracyesis
-paresis	slight paralysis	hemiparesis
parvo-	small	parvovirus
path(o)-	disease	pathology

(continued)

Prefix or suffix	Meaning	Example(s)
-pathy	denotes (with a negative sense) a disease, or disorder	sociopathy, neuropathy
pector-	breast	pectoralgia, pectoriloquy, pectorophony
ped-, -ped-, -pes	of or pertaining to the foot; -footed	pedoscope
pelv(i)-, pelv(o)-	hip bone	pelvis
-penia	deficiency	osteopenia
-pepsia	denotes something relating to digestion, or the digestive tract	dyspepsia
peri-	denoting something with a position 'surrounding' or 'around' another	periodontal
-pexy	fixation	nephropexy
phaco-	lens-shaped	phacolysis, phacometer, phacoscotoma
-phage, -phagia	forms terms denoting conditions relating to eating or ingestion	sarcophagia
-phago-	eating, devouring	phagocyte
-phagy	forms nouns that denotes 'feeding on' the first element or part of the word	haematophagy
pharmaco-	drug, medication	pharmacology
pharyng(o)-	of or pertaining to the pharynx, the upper throat cavity	pharyngitis, pharyngoscopy
phleb(o)-	of or pertaining to the (blood) veins, a vein	phlebography, phlebotomy
-phobia	exaggerated fear, sensitivity	arachnophobia
phon(o)-	sound	phonograph, symphony
phot(o)-	of or pertaining to light	photopathy
phren(i)-, phren(o)-, phrenico	the mind	phrenic nerve, schizophrenia
-plasia	formation, development	achondroplasia
-plasty	surgical repair, reconstruction	rhinoplasty
-plegia	paralysis	paraplegia
pleio-	more, excessive, multiple	pleiomorphism
pleur(o)-, pleur(a)	of or pertaining to the ribs	pleurogenous
-plexy	stroke or seizure	cataplexy
pneumat(o)-	air, lung	pneumatocele
pneum(o)-	of or pertaining to the lungs	pneumonocyte, pneumonia
-poiesis	production	haematopoiesis
poly-	denotes a 'plurality' of something	polymyositis
post-	denotes something as 'after' or 'behind' another	post-operation, post-mortem
pre-	denotes something as 'before' another (in [physical] position or time)	premature birth
presby(o)-	old age	presbyopia

prim-	denotes something as 'first' or 'most important'	primary
proct(o)-	anus, rectum	proctology
prot(o)-	denotes something as 'first' or 'most important'	protoneuron
pseud(o)-	denotes something false or fake	pseudoephedrine
psor-	itching	psoriasis
psych(e)-, psych(o)	of or pertaining to the mind	psychology, psychiatry
-ptosis	falling, drooping, downward placement, prolapse	apoptosis, nephroptosis
-ptysis	(a spitting), spitting, haemoptysis, the spitting of blood derived from the lungs or bronchial tubes	haemoptysis
pulmon-, pulmo-	of or relating to the lungs	pulmonary
pyel(o)-	pelvis	pyelonephritis
py(o)-	pus	pyometra
pyr(o)-	fever	antipyretic
quadr(i)-	four	quadriceps
radio-	radiation	radiowave
ren(o)-	of or pertaining to the kidney	renal
retro-	backward, behind	retroversion, retroverted
rhin(o)-	of or pertaining to the nose	rhinoplasty
rhod(o)-	denoting a rose-red colour	rhodophyte
-rrhage	burst forth	haemorrhage
-rrhagia	rapid flow of blood	menorrhagia
-rrhaphy	surgical suturing	nephrorrhaphy
-rrhexis	rupture	karyorrhexis
-rrhoea	flowing, discharge	diarrhoea
-rupt	break or burst	erupt, interrupt
salping(o)-	of or pertaining to tubes, e.g. Fallopian tubes	salpingectomy, salpingopharyngeus muscle
sangui-, sanguine-	of or pertaining to blood	exsanguination
sarco-	muscular, flesh-like	sarcoma
scler(o)-	hard	scleroderma
-sclerosis	hardening	atherosclerosis, multiple sclerosis
scoli(o)-	twisted	scoliosis
-scope	instrument for viewing	otoscope
-scopy	use of instrument for viewing	endoscopy
semi-	one-half, partly	semiconscious
sial(o)-	saliva, salivary gland	sialagogue

(continued)

Prefix or suffix	Meaning	Example(s)
sigmoid(o)-	sigmoid, S-shaped curvature	sigmoid colon
sinistr(o)-	left, left side	sinistrocardia
sinus-	of or pertaining to the sinus	sinusitis
somat(o)-, somatico-	body, bodily	somatic
-spadias	slit, fissure	hypospadias, epispadias
spasmo-	spasm	spasmodic dysphonia
sperma(to)-, spermo-	semen, spermatozoa	spermatogenesis
splen(o)-	spleen	splenectomy
spondyl(o)-	of or pertaining to the spine, the vertebra	spondylitis
squamos(o)-	denoting something as 'full of scales' or 'scaly'	squamous cell
-stalsis	contraction	peristalsis
-stasis	stopping, standing	cytostasis, homeostasis
-staxis	dripping, trickling	epistaxis
sten(o)-	denoting something as 'narrow in shape'	stenography
-stenosis	abnormal narrowing in a blood vessel or other tubular organ or structure	restenosis, stenosis
stomat(o)-	of or pertaining to the mouth	stomatogastric, stomatognathic system
-stomy	creation of an opening	colostomy
sub-	beneath	subcutaneous tissue
super-	in excess, above, superior	superior vena cava
supra-	above, excessive	supraorbital vein
tachy-	denoting something as fast, irregularly fast	tachycardia
-tension, -tensive	pressure	hypertension
tetan-	rigid, tense	tetanus
thec-	case, sheath	intrathecal
therap-	treatment	hydrotherapy, therapeutic
therm(o)-	heat	thermometer
thorac(i)-, thorac(o)-, thoracico-	of or pertaining to the upper chest, chest; the area above the breast and under the neck	thorax
thromb(o)-	of or relating to a blood clot, clotting of blood	thrombus, thrombocytopenia
thyr(o)-	thyroid	thyrocele
thym-	emotions	dysthymia
-tome	cutting instrument	osteotome
-tomy	act of cutting; incising, incision	gastrotomy
tono-	tone, tension, pressure	tonometer

-tony	tension	
top(o)-	place, topical	topical anaesthetic
tort(i)-	twisted	torticollis
tox(i)-, tox(o)-, toxic(o)-	toxin, poison	toxoplasmosis
trache(a)-	trachea	tracheotomy
trachel(o)-	of or pertaining to the neck	tracheloplasty
trans-	denoting something as moving or situated 'across' or 'through'	transfusion
tri-	three	triangle
trich(i)-, trichia, trich(o)-	of or pertaining to hair, hair-like structure	trichocyst
-tripsy	crushing	lithotripsy
-trophy	nourishment, development	pseudohypertrophy
tympan(o)-	eardrum	tympanocentesis
-ula, -ule	small	nodule
ultra-	beyond, excessive	ultrasound
un(i)-	one	unilateral hearing loss
ur(o)-	of or pertaining to urine, the urinary system; (specifically) pertaining to the physiological chemistry of urine	urology
uter(o)-	of or pertaining to the uterus or womb	uterus
vagin-	of or pertaining to the vagina	vagina
varic(o)-	swollen or twisted vein	varicose
vasculo-	blood vessel	vasculotoxicity
vas(o)-	duct, blood vessel	vasoconstriction
ven-	of or pertaining to the (blood) veins, a vein (used in terms pertaining to the vascular system)	vein, venospasm
ventricul(o)-	of or pertaining to the ventricles; any hollow region inside an organ	cardiac ventriculography
ventr(o)-	of or pertaining to the belly; the stomach cavities	ventrodorsal
-version	turning	anteversion, retroversion
vesic(o)-	of or pertaining to the bladder	vesical arteries
viscer(o)-	of or pertaining to the internal organs, the viscera	viscera
xanth(o)-	denoting a yellow colour, an abnormally yellow colour	xanthopathy
xen(o)-	foreign, different	xenograft
xer(o)-	dry, desert-like	xerostomia
zo(o)-	animal, animal life	zoology
zym(o)-	fermentation	enzyme, lysozyme

HOW TO USE YOUR TEXTBOOK

Features contained within your textbook

Learning outcomes provide a summary of the topics covered in a chapter.

LEARNING OUTCOMES

After reading this chapter you will be able to:

1.1 outline the levels of organisation of the body
1.2 describe the characteristics and the requirements of all living things
1.3 interpret chemical symbols and equations and understand the ways in which atoms can bind together
1.4 describe the pH scale and its importance to life
1.5 list the differences between organic and inorganic substances
1.6 outline the regulation of homeostasis in the body.

Your textbook is full of **illustrations** and **tables**.

FIGURE 6.1 Gross anatomy of a skeletal muscle

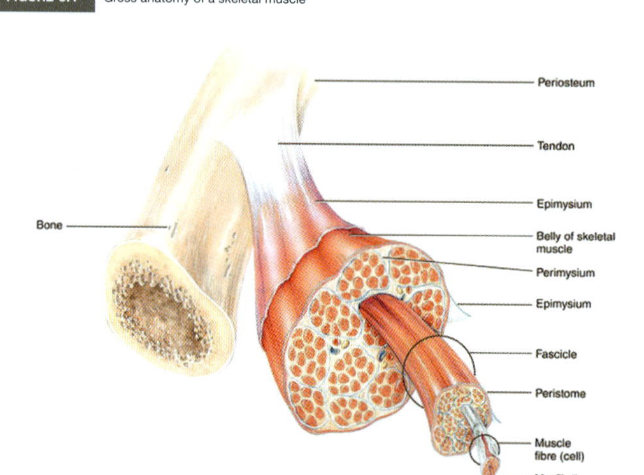

Source: Tortora and Derrickson (2009). Reproduced with permission of John Wiley & Sons.

Microanatomy of skeletal muscle fibre

When examined microscopically, skeletal muscle cells appear cylindrical in shape, have a distinctive banded appearance of alternate light and dark stripes and lie parallel to each other (see figure 6.2). Table 6.2 provides a summary of the cellular components of a muscle fibre.

TABLE 6.2 Cellular components of a muscle fibre

Name	Function
Sarcolemma	Plasma membrane of a muscle fibre that forms T tubules
Sarcoplasm	Cytoplasm of the muscle fibre that contains myofibrils
Myofibril	Consists of bundles of myofilaments and plays a key role in muscle contraction
Myofilament	Consists of thick and thin filaments that give muscle tissue its striated appearance and plays a role in muscle contraction
Myoglobin	A reddish-brown pigment (gives muscle tissue its dark-red colour) that stores oxygen for muscle contraction
T tubule	Fluid-filled tubular structure that releases calcium from the sarcoplasmic reticulum
Sarcoplasmic reticulum	Storage site for calcium ions

Clinical considerations demonstrate the application to your learning, citing specific care issues that you could come across when working with people in care settings.

CLINICAL CONSIDERATIONS

Knee reconstruction

The knee joint bears a lot of weight and often degenerates in the later years oflife, particularly in people who have been active in sports or trade. As a hinge joint, the knee is damaged by twisting actions such as those that can often occur when playing football, when forcing the knee joint to twist can tear the ligaments which hold it in place and the fibrocartilage pads in the joint (the menisci). Over time and use, the articular cartilage at the ends of the femur and tibia can wear away, the menisci (cartilage within the knee) can tear, and one or more of the ligaments that stabilise the joint (the collateral ligaments and the anterior and posterior cruciate ligaments) can tear. There are now surgical options to repair the joint and its associated ligaments and cartilage.

- The articulating surfaces of the femur and tibia can be replaced with metal, or some other hardwearing material, in a procedure known as knee replacement surgery.
- Meniscal injuries, if not too severe, may heal on their own, but bigger tears, particularly in the inner portion of the meniscus without a blood supply, can be surgically trimmed or repaired.
- Injury to the cruciate ligaments of the knee can be surgically repaired by taking a graft from the tendon of nearby muscle. These knee reconstruction procedures are performed by keyhole surgery in the joint, known as arthroscopy, and can be done quite quickly. The post-surgical recovery, however, may be prolonged, due to the slow healing rate of cartilage, tendons and ligaments.

Medicines management boxes discuss the administration of medicines and medicine management issues. This can help you appreciate the importance of understanding anatomy and physiology with the intention of administering medicines safely and effectively.

MEDICINES MANAGEMENT

Iron deficiency anaemia

Anaemia occurs when the body does not have enough red, oxygen-carrying blood cells, which means the body's tissues and cells are not getting enough oxygen. It affects approximately 10 per cent of non-pregnant young women, and is estimated to be highly prevalent in Indigenous communities. Other at-risk groups include the very young and the very old, as well as those with restricted diets such as vegetarians and vegans.

Treatment for iron deficiency anaemia usually involves taking iron supplements and changing the diet to increase the iron levels, as well as treating the underlying cause. Iron supplements may be prescribed to restore the iron missing from the body; iron can also be restored via intravenous iron preparations. The most commonly prescribed supplement is ferrous sulphate which is taken as a tablet two or three times a day, often in tandem with appropriate dietary changes. Nurses need to be aware that patients receiving iron tablets may experience:

- abdominal pain
- constipation or diarrhoea
- heartburn
- feeling sick
- black stools (faeces).

Black stools may also result from an upper gastrointestinal bleed. If these symptoms persist, advise the patient to see their GP so that prompt action can be taken to alleviate the side effects.

See Baird-Gunning and Bromley (2016).

Clinically reasoned episodes of care are case studies that follow the Clinical Reasoning Cycle process for understanding a patient situation, to help you appreciate how the study of anatomy and physiology applies in a clinical setting. The clinical reasoning cycle is a way of reconciling the information and clues collected in a clinical situation to form a logical and accurate conclusion and plan of action. Effective use of the model is dependent on the stages of the cyclic process illustrated below.

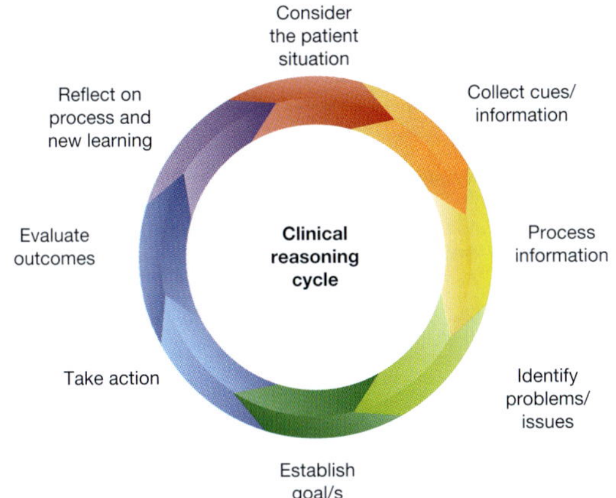

Source: Levett-Jones, T., Hoffman, K., Dempsey, Y., Jeong, S., Noble, D., Norton, C., Roche, J. and Hickey, N. (2010). The 'five rights' of clinical reasoning: An educational model to enhance nursing students' ability to identify and manage clinically 'at risk' patients. *Nurse Education Today*. 30(6): 515–20.

CLINICALLY REASONED EPISODE OF CARE

Hypertropiccardiomyopathy

Consider the patient situation

Stephen is a 14-year-old boy who is reporting increasing shortness of breath when playing sports at school. His mother has hypertrophic cardiomyopathy. Stephen is referred for an echocardiogram.

Collect cues and information

The echocardiogram shows development of hypertrophy of the ventricular **septum** (the wall between the ventricles), which is causing some obstruction of blood flow into the **aorta**.

Stephen reports no problems in everyday life, but when exercising the reduction in blood flow out of the heart leads to a reduction of blood flow to the tissues and the shortness of breath he has been experiencing when playing sports.

Stephen has further testing including 24-hour ECG monitoring, which shows no evidence of cardiac arrhythmias, and an echocardiography while exercising (stress echo).

Process information

Hypertrophic cardiomyopathy (HCM) is the most common inherited cardiac condition (about 1:500 live births), and for many, it causes no symptoms. HCM is a condition that leads to the muscles of the heart (the myocardium) becoming thickened and stiff.

In cases like Stephen's, the thickening of the muscles of the septum between the ventricles can lead to the obstruction of blood flow out of the heart into the aorta – this is known as hypertrophic obstructive cardiomyopathy (HOCM). HCM nearly always affects the left ventricle, but occasionally it will affect the right ventricle as well.

Nursing actions

1. Provide reassurance, support and education for Stephen and his mother prior to and during the procedures.
   Rationale:
   - Quality patient education and support reduces patient anxiety.
2. Provide education around prescribed beta blockers.
   Rationale:
   - Commonly used medications are beta blockers and calcium channel blockers. If there is evidence of arrhythmias (disturbance of the heart rhythm) then anti-arrhythmic medications (such as amiodarone) will be prescribed. In severe cases an implantable cardioverter-defibrillator (ICD) will be implanted into the patient's chest. Severe cases of HCM may require surgical reduction of the heart muscle thickness, or in very severe cases heart transplant.
   - Patient education supports concordance with recommended therapies which will promote good outcomes for the person.
3. Provide education around lifestyle changes.
   Rationale:
   - Recommendations include minimising alcohol, stopping smoking, reducing salt intake, maintaining a healthy weight and reducing caffeine intake. While patients with HCM can (and should) exercise, the levels of exercise recommended differ from patient to patient and should be discussed with a doctor before a new exercise regimen is started.
   - Making lifestyle adjustments will help to reduce the impact of HCM on the life of the person.

Evaluate outcomes

Stephen will have regular medical reviews to check progression of the condition so that therapeutic management can be adjusted.

For more information on HCM (and other cardiomyopathies) see the Cardiomyopathy Association of Australia, www.cmaa.org.au.

Source: Based on the Clinical Reasoning Cycle, Levett-Jones (2013).

Skills in practice help you understand a clinical process that healthcare professionals fulfill in relation to that topic.

SKILLS IN PRACTICE

Mouth care

Patients who are ill can also be dehydrated and therefore their production of saliva is reduced. This can lead to an increased risk of oral infections, as wear and tear within the oral cavity increases. Reduced amounts of saliva leads to less washing away of pathogens to the acid environment of the stomach where they may be destroyed. The oral cavity provides a route for pathogens to enter the respiratory tract, and therefore good oral hygiene practices may help prevent respiratory infections, particularly in patients who are vulnerable due to acute illness, cancer treatments or immobility.

When patients are ill, a sufficient dietary intake is essential for tissue repair and healing; however, a lack of saliva will lead to the food not tasting as it should. The food will not easily form into the required bolus size for ease of swallowing. This may put the patient off eating and drinking and may lead to the patient losing their appetite and potentially delay healing.

Ill health can lead to neglect of hygiene standards for individuals. Mouth care is easy for patients to ignore when they are feeling poorly. However, it is an essential consideration for nursing.

Homeostatic imbalance boxes help you understand what happens to the human body in terms of the pathophysiology.

HOMEOSTATIC IMBALANCE

Cholelithiasis

Cholelithiasis, or gallstones, occurs when cholesterol or bile pigments solidify or crystallise within the gall bladder. These gallstones can then lodge in the bile ducts, causing inflammation and the impairment or blockage of bile flow into the duodenum.

Cholelithiasis is a very common condition and can range from being completely asymptomatic to causing symptoms such as nausea, jaundice, abdominal pain and vomiting. Treatment options range from dietary changes to surgical removal of the gallstones or complete removal of the gall bladder (cholecystectomy) (Health Direct 2020).

At the end of the chapters is a glossary of **key terms**, presented to enable the learning of difficult words or phrases; understanding these words and phrases is important to your success as a health-care student. When you have mastered the words, your medical vocabulary will have grown and you will be in a better position to develop it further.

KEY TERMS

abdominopelvic cavity Body cavity that encompasses the abdominal and pelvic cavities. The abdominal cavity contains the stomach, intestines, spleen, liver and other associated digestive organs. The pelvic cavity contains the bladder and some reproductive organs.
apical surface Surface of body organ that faces outwards, towards the surface.
basal surface Surface that forms the base of a body organ.
cartilage Strong form of connective tissue that contains a dense network of collagen and elastic fibres.
chyme A fluid substance consisting of partially digested food and digestive enzymes, which is found travelling through the digestive tract.
connective tissue Tissue that binds, reinforces, insulates, protects and supports structures.
diffusion The movement of particles from areas of high concentration to low concentration.
endocrine glands Glands that release hormones.
epithelial tissue Tissue that lines or covers body surfaces.
exocrine glands Glands that secrete their products externally (i.e. mucus, sweat).
extracellular matrix A collection oflargely non-living substances that separate the living cells of connective tissue.
glands Structures that manufacture a product (e.g. hormones, mucus, sweat).
glycoproteins Special proteins that contain simple sugar chains. Glycoproteins play an important role in cell-to-cell communication.
hormones Regulatory chemicals released by endocrine glands for use elsewhere in the body (e.g. thyroxine, insulin).
innervated Stimulated by nerve cells.
interstitial fluid The fluid that bathes cells.
keratin A special tough fibrous protein found in skin.
lymph nodes Small lymphatic structures that filter lymphatic fluid.
macrophages White blood cells that specialise in the destruction and consumption of invading pathogens.
membrane A sheet of tissue that covers or lines an area of the body.
mitosis The division and replication of cells.
neuroglia Cells of the nervous system that support and nourish neurones.
neurones A nerve fibre.
oocytes Female reproductive cell.
parenchyma The cells that constitute the function part of an organ.
prophylactic antibiotics Antibiotics prescribed to prevent infection.
spleen Large lymph organ, responsible for production oflymphocytes, immune response and the cleansing of blood.
stroma The internal framework of an organ.
subcutaneous Underneath the skin.
vertebrae The disc-shaped bones that make up the spinal column.

The **conditions** feature located at the end of the most chapters provides you with a list of conditions associated with the topics that have been discussed. You are encouraged to take some time to write notes about each of the conditions listed; this can help you relate theory to practice.

CONDITIONS

The following is a list of common genetic conditions. Take some time and write notes about each of the conditions. You may make the notes taken from textbooks or other resources (e.g. people you work with in a clinical area), or you may make the notes as a result of people you have cared for. If you are making notes about people you have cared for, you must ensure that you adhere to the rules of confidentiality.

Motor neurone disease

Prader–Willi syndrome

Alzheimer's disease, early onset

Neurofibromatosis

Down syndrome

Turner syndrome

Features contained within your interactive eBook

Students who purchase a new print copy of *Principles of Anatomy and Physiology for Nursing and Healthcare Students in Australia*, 1st edition, will have access to the interactive eBook version (a code is provided on the inside of the front cover). The eBook integrates the following media and interactive elements into the narrative content of each chapter.

- **Practitioner videos** provide insights into the application of anatomy and physiology concepts to the provision of healthcare.
- **Interactive questions** provide you with the scaffolding to attempt and solve problems.
- **Lightboard videos** by Australian educators are mini lectures on key topics in the chapter.

CHAPTER 1

Basic scientific principles of physiology

TEST YOUR PRIOR KNOWLEDGE

- What is the difference between anatomy and physiology?
- What are atoms, ions and electrolytes?
- What is an element?
- How do we distinguish living things from non-living things?
- What is homeostasis?

LEARNING OUTCOMES

After reading this chapter you will be able to:

1.1 outline the levels of organisation of the body
1.2 describe the characteristics and the requirements of all living things
1.3 interpret chemical symbols and equations and understand the ways in which atoms can bind together
1.4 describe the pH scale and its importance to life
1.5 list the differences between organic and inorganic substances
1.6 outline the regulation of homeostasis in the body.

Introduction

Learning about the **physiology** of the body is very much like learning a foreign language — there are new vocabulary, grammar and concepts to learn and understand. This first chapter introduces you to this new language so that you can then use your knowledge to understand the physiology of the different parts of the body that are discussed in all the other chapters of this book.

First of all there are two fundamental terms to learn and understand:

- **anatomy** — the study of structure (i.e. 'what is it?')
- physiology — the study of function (i.e. 'how does it work/what does it do?').

However, the two terms are always related. The structure determines the function, which in turn determines how the body/organ, and so on, is structured — the two are interdependent. For example, a sperm is a specific cell designed to prioritise fuel and movement (structure) to enable it to deliver a male's DNA to a female's ova (function).

1.1 Levels of organisation

LEARNING OBJECTIVE 1.1 Outline the levels of organisation of the body.

The body is a very complex organism that consists of many components, starting with the smallest of them — the **atom** — and concluding with the organism itself (figure 1.1).

FIGURE 1.1 Levels of organisation of the body

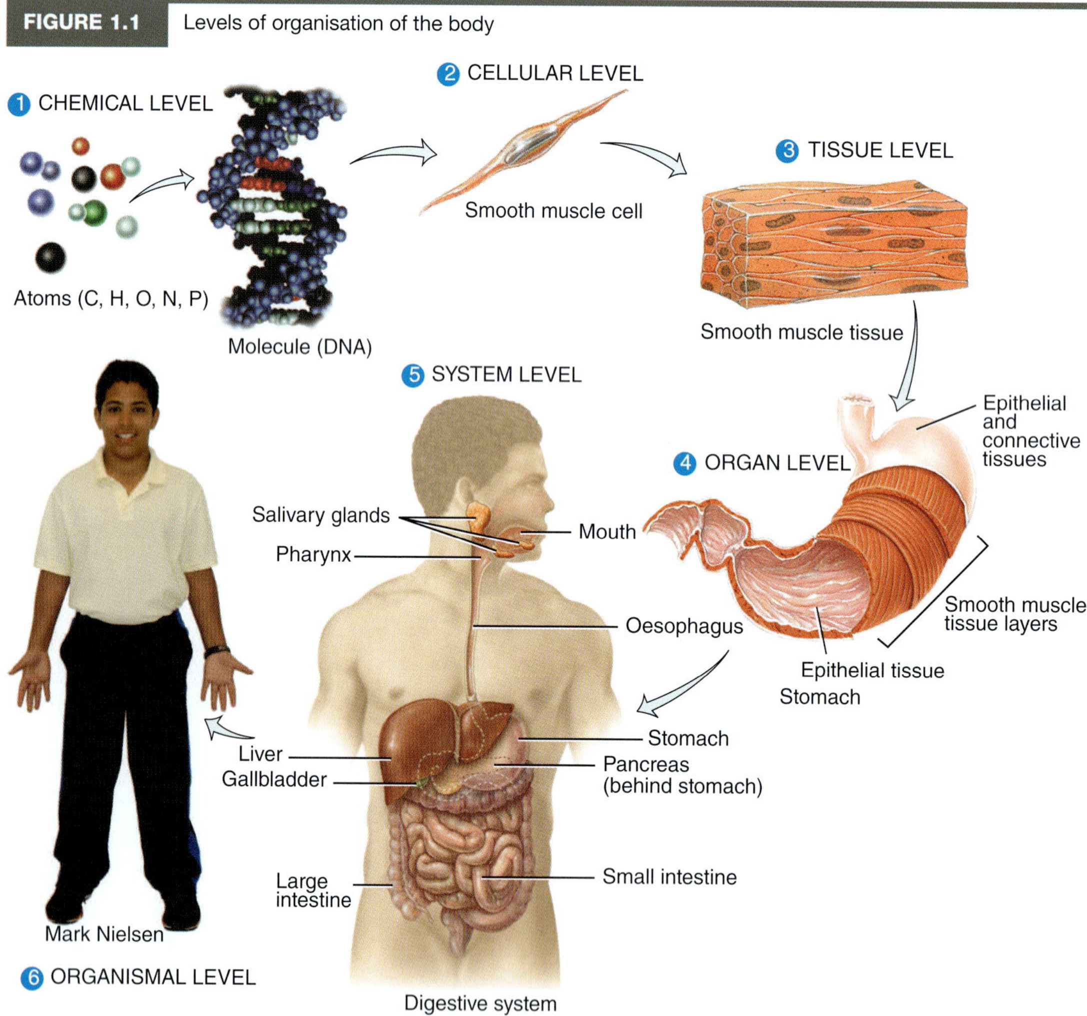

Source: Tortora and Derrickson (2014). Reproduced with permission of John Wiley & Sons.

Starting from the smallest component and working towards the largest, the body operates, and can be studied, on the following levels.

1. Chemical level: the atoms, **molecules** and macromolecules that we are made of.
2. Cellular level: the smallest living functional units in our bodies.
3. Tissue level: the groups of cells specialised to perform specific functions (e.g. nerve or muscle tissue).
4. Organ level: a structure, consisting of many tissues, specialised to perform a specific function (e.g. the heart).
5. System level: a system, consisting of more than one organ, specialised to perform a range of functions (e.g. the cardiovascular system).
6. Organism level: the whole individual.

1.2 Characteristics of life

LEARNING OBJECTIVE 1.2 Describe the characteristics and requirements of all living things.

All living organisms have the following characteristics in common, which are considered essential for the maintenance of life.

- *Sensitivity*. Organisms need to be able to sense and respond to changes in their environment, such as changes in light levels, temperature, chemical composition and the presence of threats.
- *Nutrition*. Seeking out, ingesting and using food to supply energy and the raw materials for growth and development is a very basic requirement.
- *Respiration*. This is the means by which an organism obtains and uses oxygen to release energy from food to power the other activities listed here.
- *Movement*. The ability to change position is essential if an organism is to be able to escape threats, and to find food and other members of the species.
- *Growth*. This is essential for the development of an organism from birth to adulthood, and also for the renewal and repair of body parts during the life of an organism.
- *Reproduction*. This is an essential process, not only for the survival of the individual, but also for the survival of the species. Sexual reproduction has the added bonus of continually mixing and re-mixing genetic material to produce genetically unique individuals each time, which increases the ability of a species to adapt and survive over the very long term.
- *Excretion*. The removal of waste substances produced by metabolic processes from the body, to prevent them from building up to harmful levels.

Bodily requirements

There are four essential requirements that all organisms, including humans, require to thrive and survive.

1. *Water.* Water is the most abundant substance found in the body. At birth, our bodies are approximately 78 per cent water. This reduces to 65 per cent at 1 year of age, and to 55–60 per cent in adulthood. Our biochemistry evolved to operate in a watery (aqueous) environment, and our cells are filled with a watery, salty solution, in which our cellular processes are carried out; those cells are also bathed in a watery, salty solution. While it may not look like it, blood is also mainly water; this makes water important for the transport of substances around our large and complex bodies.

   Additionally, as sweating is an important mechanism for evaporative cooling, body water helps to regulate body temperature, and is also involved in the removal of various wastes (e.g. via urine, faeces and sweat).
2. *Food.* Food supplies the energy and raw materials for the organism to fulfil all of the essential activities of life. In humans, these activities are not only key to our growth and development, but also our everyday functioning, such as allowing our nerves to fire and our muscles to contract/relax.
3. *Oxygen.* Oxygen is required for the release of energy from food, through the oxidation of high-energy food substances. Oxygen is one of the gases that exist naturally in the air (oxygen makes up approximately 20 per cent of the air).
4. *Sunlight.* All life on Earth ultimately depends on sunlight; plants need it to grow, and other organisms depend directly or indirectly on plants for food.

1.3 Life at the chemical level

LEARNING OBJECTIVE 1.3 Interpret chemical symbols and equations and understand the ways in which atoms can bind together.

Studying living things at a chemical level reveals a world of 'chemical machinery' — millions of **chemical reactions** being carried out within our cells every minute to keep us alive, functioning and growing. The continued survival of a living body depends on select simple atoms and molecules, and also some large and very complex molecules (macromolecules), to carry on the business of living, growing and reproducing. We will cover some of the most biologically important chemicals here, and you will find them appearing throughout the rest of this book.

The elements

All matter on Earth is made up of a range of approximately 100 chemical **elements**. A chemical element is a pure chemical substance that cannot be broken down into anything simpler by chemical means.

More than 100 elements are thought to exist, but only 98 are known to occur naturally on Earth. All the elements are shown in the periodic table of the elements, which sets out the elements in terms of their unique atomic structures and their physical (colour, hardness, density, melting and boiling points) and chemical (the ways in which the element reacts chemically) properties. Understanding the properties of an element is important, as it lets us predict how it will behave in different situations. Based on physical and chemical properties, elements are classified as either metals, metalloids or non-metals.

Those classed as metals share the following properties.

- They are solids at room temperature (apart from mercury, which is liquid!).
- They conduct heat and electricity.
- They donate **electrons** when forming **bonds** (see the section on chemical reactions and **chemical bonds**).

Metalloids are elements that share some of the properties of metals and some of non-metals. Non-metals share the following properties.

- They may exist as a solid, a liquid or a gas.
- They are poor conductors of heat and electricity.
- They accept electrons from other atoms when forming bonds (see the section on chemical reactions and chemical bonds).

Below are some examples of metals and non-metals that are very important in biology.

Metals	Non-metals
Calcium (Ca)	Chlorine (Cl)
Potassium (K)	Nitrogen (N)
Sodium (Na)	Oxygen (O)
Iron (Fe)	Carbon (C)
	Sulphur (S)
	Phosphorus (P)

The smallest unit of matter: the atom

As we saw in figure 1.1, atoms are the building blocks of all matter. Each element in the periodic table consists of its own, unique atoms. The word 'atom' comes from a Greek word meaning 'incapable of being divided'. However, we now know that an atom consists of subatomic particles: electrons, **neutrons** and **protons**.

Protons carry a positive electrical charge (think 'p for positive') and electrons carry a negative electrical charge, while the neutron, as its name implies, carries no electrical charge (it is **neutral**).

Figure 1.2 shows how the protons and neutrons cluster together at the centre of the atom (forming the nucleus), while the electrons (which have virtually no weight) orbit constantly around the nucleus, and are kept in orbit by the electromagnetic force exerted by the nucleus (i.e. the positively charged nucleus attracts the negatively charged electrons).

FIGURE 1.2 Schematic diagram of an atom

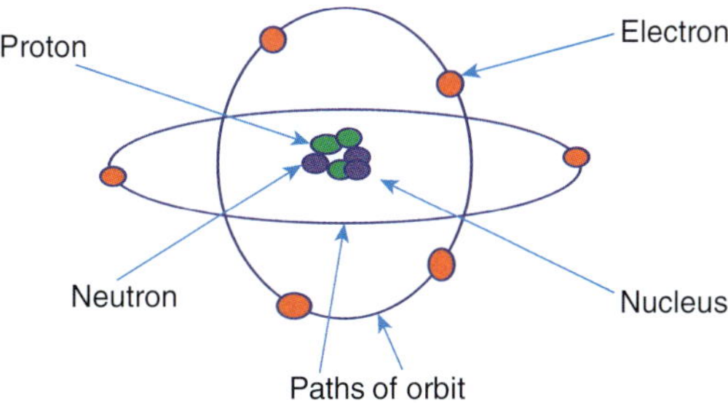

Source: Tortora and Derrickson (2014). Reproduced with permission of John Wiley & Sons.

There are many different types of atoms, differing in the numbers of protons, neutrons and electrons they possess. It is these differences between the various types of atoms that give us the array of chemical elements you will see in the periodic table of the elements.

Regardless of the type of atom, the atomic structures all obey the following rules.

- The nucleus is always central.
- The number of protons an atom possesses in its nucleus is known as the **atomic number** of that atom.
- The total number of particles in the nucleus of an atom (i.e. the number of protons and neutrons added together) is the atomic mass number. The mass of an atom is almost all in its nucleus — remember that the electrons orbiting around the nucleus have virtually no weight. Electrons are really just electrical charges in motion, but they are extremely important to the behaviour of the atom, as you will see.
- As the number of electrons an atom possesses increases, the electrons form layers of orbits, or **shells**, which get larger and further from the nucleus. The inner shell can contain a maximum of two electrons and the second and third shells shell can contain a maximum of eight electrons — much like the number of spaces on each level of a multistorey car park. The electrons in the outermost shell of an atom determine whether and how the atom forms bonds with other atoms to make new chemicals.

  The electrons in the outermost shell are known as the valence electrons, as they are able to take part in bonding reactions with other atoms (see the section on chemical reactions and chemical bonds).

Figure 1.3 shows the atomic structure of some of the most biologically important substances, or elements, with their atomic numbers and mass numbers.

FIGURE 1.3 The structure of some biologically important atoms

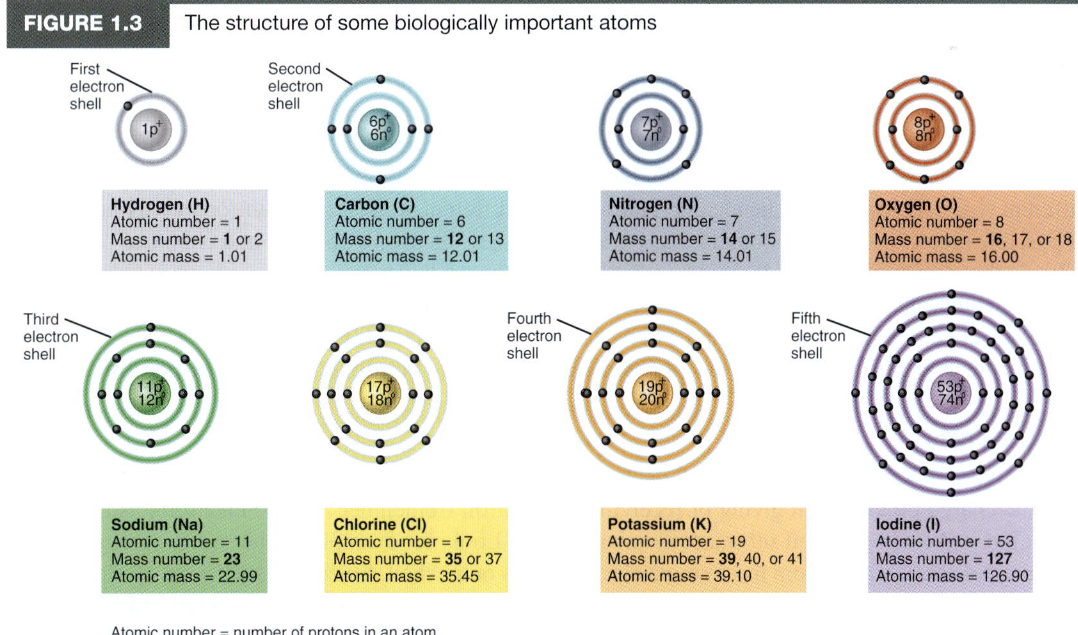

Source: Tortora and Derrickson (2014). Reproduced with permission of John Wiley & Sons.

If you look closely at the number of electrons in the various atoms shown in figure 1.3, you will see that in each atom, the number of electrons is equal to the number of protons. Since each proton carries a positive charge and each electron carries a negative charge, having an equal number of each will mean that the atom has an overall neutral charge. For example, the carbon atom has six electrons, six protons and six neutrons. The equal and opposite electrical charges of the electrons and protons cancel each other out, so that the atom is electrically neutral and it is said to be in a state of equilibrium.

When referring to these different elements, we use symbols to represent each one, rather than writing out their names each time. For example, the symbol for sodium is Na (after its Latin name *natrium*), the symbol for potassium is K (after its Latin name *kalium*), chlorine is Cl, and the symbol of carbon is C.

CLINICAL CONSIDERATIONS

Magnetic resonance imaging (MRI)

Health professional students often question what relevance subatomic particles have to the practice of healthcare. Magnetic resonance imaging, a widely used diagnostic imaging technique, is one example of how the behaviour of subatomic particles is harnessed for medical purposes. MRI, unlike CT or PET scans, does not involve exposing a patient to ionising radiation, and it is able to produce 3D images of all body structures, including soft tissue. It is an extremely versatile diagnostic imaging system, and it works by detecting the spin of protons in water molecules. Patients are placed into a powerful magnetic field, which forces the protons contained in the molecules of body water to align with the field (protons have a positive charge, so they will spin round and align when they find themselves in a charge field such as that of water). When the magnetic field is turned off, those protons all return to their original alignment, but at different speeds, depending on what environment they are in. Capturing these signals released from protons as they realign in various different tissues allows the different tissues to be detected and visualised. Because of the very strong magnetic field, however, metal cannot be placed inside the MRI scanner, so patients with any implants that contain metal cannot be scanned.

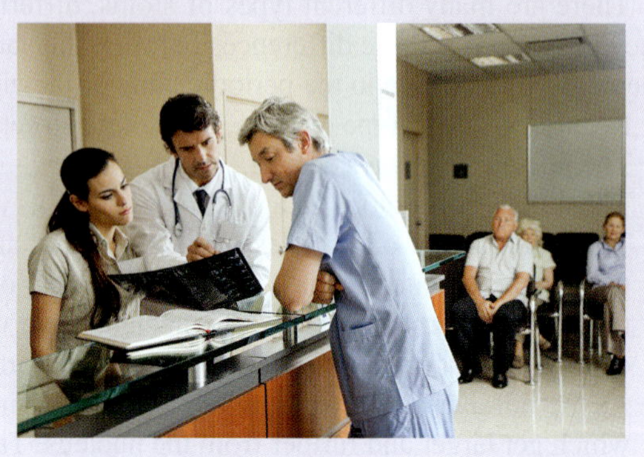

Chemical reactions and chemical bonds

If atoms remained in their neutral state of equilibrium, then the world might be very different — it might contain only the 100 or so species of atom that are known to exist on Earth. However, when the conditions are right, atoms react with other atoms to form molecules and **compounds**. A molecule is formed when two or more of the same atoms bond chemically to each other, while a compound is formed when two or more different types of atoms bond chemically. This ability of different atoms to combine creates a huge variety of possible molecules and compounds, each of which possess their own physical and chemical properties. Why do these reactions occur? Remember that atoms achieve a lower energy, more stable state when they have a full outer shell of electrons. Accordingly, a joining together of two or more atoms that results in a more stable, lower energy state for all of them will be a reaction that will readily occur.

There are a couple of different types of chemical bonds: **ionic bonding** and **covalent bonding**.

Ionic bonds

Ionic bonding involves the exchange of electrons from one atom to another. Because this exchange will alter the charge on any atom giving or receiving an electron (remember that the electron has a negative charge), it will create charged substances known as **ions**. Look, for example, at the sodium atom depicted in figure 1.4. The sodium atom has a single electron in its outer shell. Since that shell needs 8 electrons to be full, then it must pick up another 7 electrons to achieve a lower energy state — a tall order! It could, however, lose that one electron, leaving the full second shell as the outer shell, thus achieving a full outer shell by 'donating' an electron to any atom that might be in need of an extra one. Of course, having donated one electron, the number of protons in the sodium atom will exceed the number of electrons by one, giving the atom a net positive charge. At that point, it becomes known as a sodium ion (Na^+), and since it has a net positive charge, it is a positive ion, also known as a **cation**.

FIGURE 1.4 The single electron in the outer shell of the sodium atom can be donated during a chemical reaction, leaving a positively charged, sodium ion.

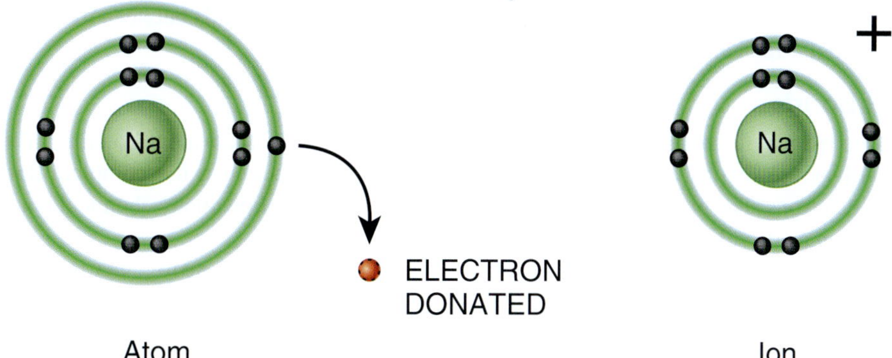

Source: Tortora and Derrickson (2014). Reproduced with permission of John Wiley & Sons.

You don't have to look far to find a suitable electron acceptor; chlorine has an outer shell containing 7 electrons, so accepting an extra electron would allow it to achieve a lower energy state (much easier than donating 7 electrons!).

By the same token, though, the chlorine atom now has one more electron than it has protons, and so gains a net negative charge, and is now known as a chloride ion (Cl^-), and is a negative ion, also known as an **anion** (figure 1.5).

FIGURE 1.5 A chlorine atom needs only one electron to complete its outer shell, so will readily react with electron donors like sodium, and accept the donated electron. This creates a negatively charged, chloride ion.

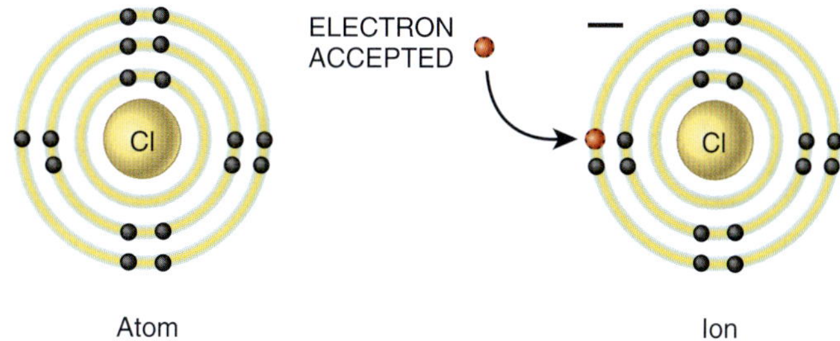

Source: Tortora and Derrickson (2014). Reproduced with permission of John Wiley & Sons.

Having exchanged electrons, the newly formed sodium and chloride ions are now oppositely charged. Opposite charges attract one another, while similar charges repel. The attractive forces between the two ions therefore 'bond' them together, since together, they form an overall neutral molecule, sodium chloride (NaCl) (figure 1.6).

FIGURE 1.6 The ionic bonding between a sodium and a chloride ion results in a neutral molecule, sodium chloride. Sodium chloride molecules pack together to form a regular, lattice, crystalline structure.

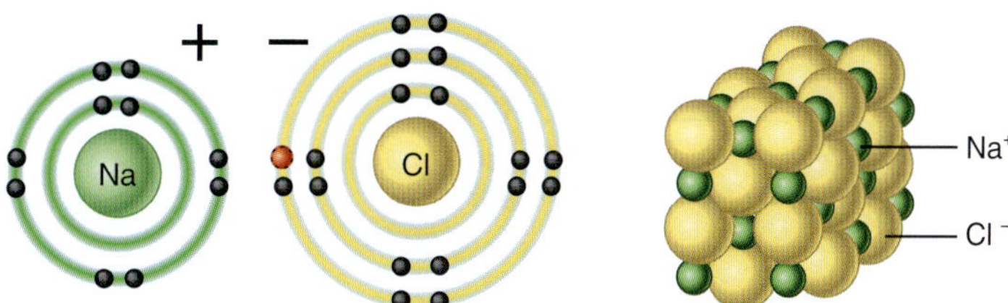

Source: Tortora and Derrickson (2014). Reproduced with permission of John Wiley & Sons.

Since the chemical bond is the result of the attractive force between the two ions, this bond is known as an ionic bond. Ionic bonds, therefore, are those that form between ions because of the attraction between opposite charges. These are not the strongest of chemical bonds because, in the presence of other ions, the individual components of an ionically bonded molecule may be more strongly attracted to other charged substances around them, thus breaking the ionic bond and freeing the two ions from each other. This often happens when ionically bonded substances are placed in water, since the water molecule, while not an ion, is a polar molecule, which can set up weak ionic bonds known as **polar bonds** between itself and ions (see the section on polar molecules).

Covalent bonds

There is a second way in which atoms can bond, and this is known as covalent bonding. This form of bonding involves the sharing of valence (outer shell) electrons rather than the complete donation and accepting of electrons. The number of outer shell electrons determines how many chemical bonds an atom can form, known as its **valency**.

Electrons rapidly orbit the nucleus of an atom, and if two atoms are so close together that their electron outer shells overlap at the closest point, one electron can orbit both atomic nuclei (figure 1.7).

FIGURE 1.7 (a–e) Some covalently bonded substances, showing the sharing of electrons between the atoms

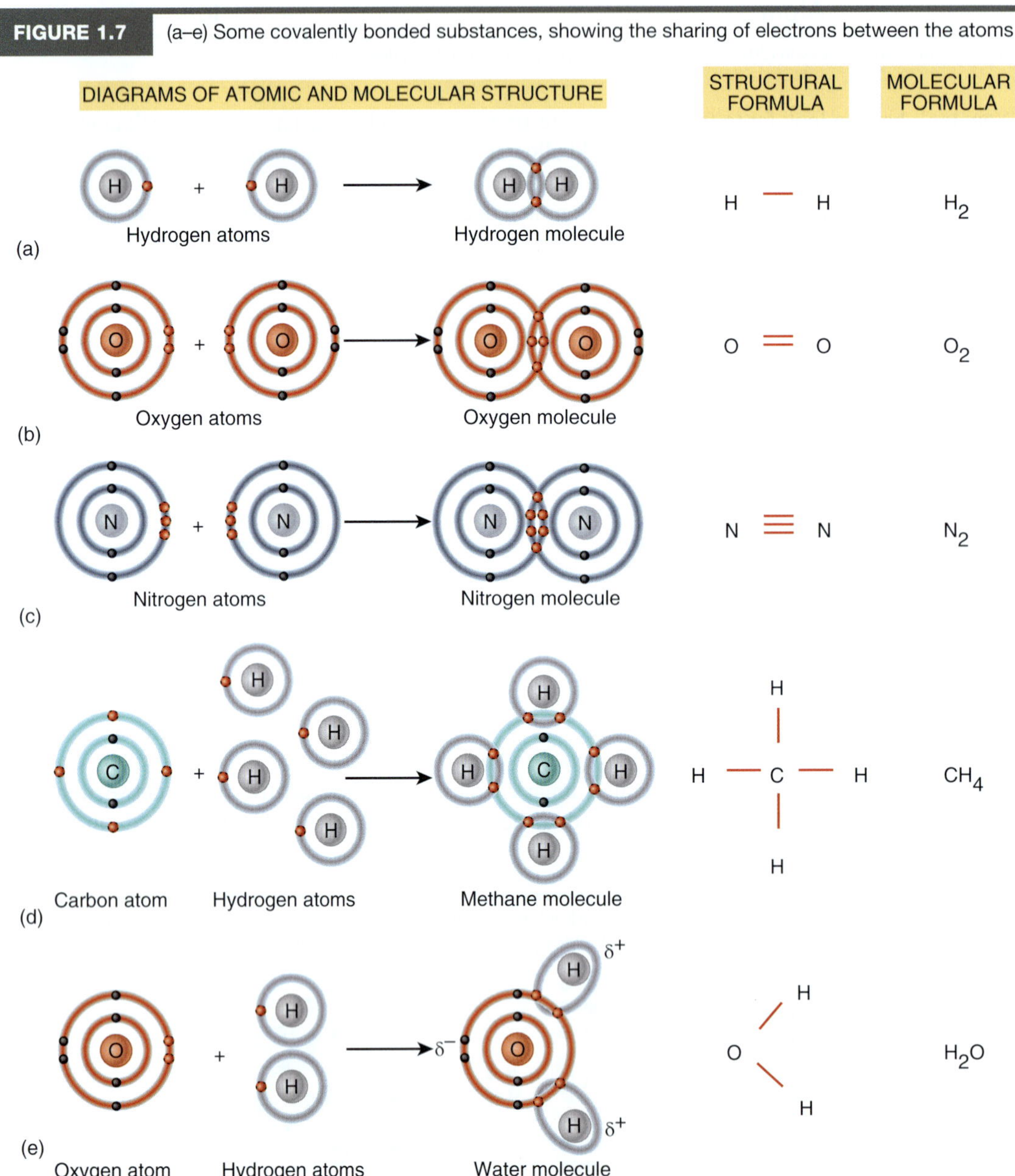

Source: Tortora and Derrickson (2014). Reproduced with permission of John Wiley & Sons.

Notice that some of the common covalent compounds shown in figure 1.7 contain double and triple covalent bonds, in which four or six electrons are shared to create the bonds.

Polar molecules

Sometimes, covalently bonded molecules do not share their electrons equally and the shared electron may spend more time orbiting one end of the covalent bond than the other, giving a more negative charge to that part of the molecule. This difference in charge between one end of a molecule and the other is called polarity, and a molecule that has a charge disparity between its two ends is known as a polar molecule. Water is a polar molecule because the two shared electrons that form each of the bonds between the oxygen atom and the hydrogen atoms spend more time orbiting the oxygen nucleus, thereby making the oxygen end of the molecule more negative than the hydrogen end. When we illustrate the molecule (figure 1.8), the polarity is indicated by the Greek letter delta (δ) followed by a plus or minus sign to indicate the relative charge at each end of the molecule.

FIGURE 1.8 Water, a polar molecule, with its positive and negative poles shown

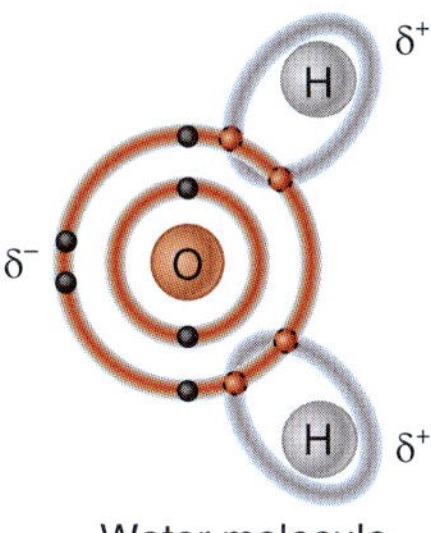

Source: Tortora and Derrickson (2014). Reproduced with permission of John Wiley & Sons.

Because of this charge difference within the molecule, polar molecules can attract ions or other polar molecules of the opposite charge, just like ions, and this attraction forms weak bonds. Polar molecules will often swing round and line up with their more negative ends towards a positive charge, or away from a negative charge. The most important weak bond of this type occurs between water and other polar molecules or ions. Because the weak attraction is between the more positive hydrogen end of one water molecule and the more negative end of another water molecule, this type of bond is known as a hydrogen bond (figure 1.9).

FIGURE 1.9 Hydrogen bonds and water. The weak bonds between the hydrogen of one water molecule and the oxygen of a neighbouring water molecule are known as hydrogen bonds, and account for the cohesion, or 'stickiness' of water, for surface tension effects and for its tendency to mix well with other polar molecules and ions.

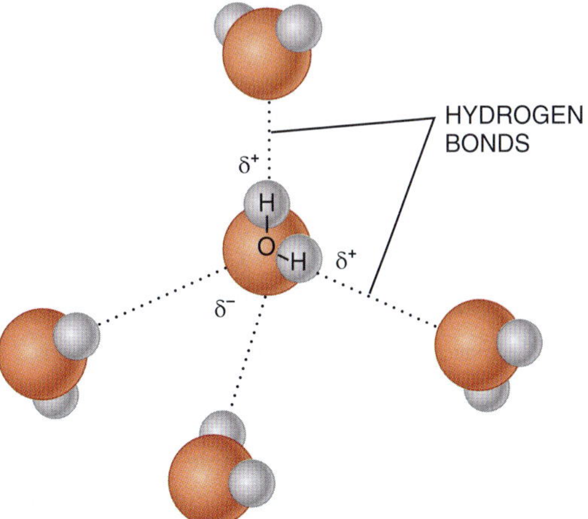

Source: Tortora and Derrickson (2014). Reproduced with permission of John Wiley & Sons.

Electrolytes

When ionically bonded substances are placed in water, the ionic bonds break, and the ionically bonded substances 'dissociate' or fall apart, and the ions are released into the water as separate entities, no longer bound to each other. If you were to apply an electrical potential to a solution like this, by placing electrodes attached to a battery into the water, the ions in solution would respond by moving through the solution — the positively charged ions would move in one direction (towards the negatively battery pole) and the negatively charged ions in the other (towards the positively charged battery pole). By this movement, the ions would effectively carry their charge through the solution, thereby allowing electrical current to pass through the solution. Because of this, ions in solution are known as **electrolytes**, and an electrolyte solution will allow current to pass through it. As you'll come to see, electrolytes are a key component of many processes in the body, therefore having the correct amount of these in the right places is vital.

1.4 Acids and bases

LEARNING OBJECTIVE 1.4 Describe the pH scale and its importance to life.

The concept of acidity is an extremely important one to understand, as maintaining **acid–base** balance in the body is essential for life. The acidity of a solution is a measure of the number of hydrogen ions in that solution; the more hydrogen ions in a solution, the more acidic it is. **Acids** are compounds, which when placed in water dissociate into hydrogen ions and a second ion (which will vary depending on the acid). Any substance, therefore, which releases free hydrogen ions when it is put into a solution is an acid. The more hydrogen ions it releases, the stronger the acid it is. Conversely, an **alkali** (or **base**) is a substance which removes hydrogen ions from a solution, usually by releasing hydroxyl ions (OH^-) into a solution. Hydroxyl ions are attracted to and readily bind with H^+ ions, resulting in water.

A substance, therefore, which removes free hydrogen ions from a solution by providing another ion to bind them up is an alkaline substance. Because of this ability to bind with H^+ ions, the acid and base can balance out, or 'buffer', each other.

Acidity and alkalinity are measured on the **pH** scale, which extends between 0 and 14, the most acidic being 0 (many more hydrogen ions than hydroxyl ions in solution) and the most alkaline being 14 (many more hydroxyl ions than hydrogen ions in solution). This means that as the pH value goes down (towards 0), the acidity increases — this is an important distinction to remember! Halfway between these two extremes, 7 on the pH scale, is the neutral point (an equal number of hydrogen ions and hydroxyl ions), as indicated on the pH scale accompanied by hydrogen and hydroxyl ion concentrations in figure 1.10.

FIGURE 1.10 The pH scale

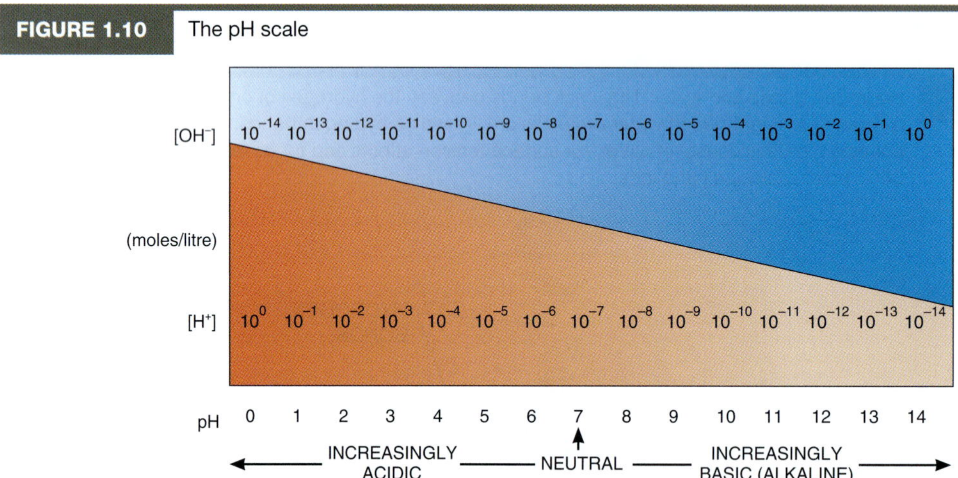

Source: Tortora and Derrickson (2014). Reproduced with permission of John Wiley & Sons.

The pH scale is a logarithmic scale, which means that each unit on the scale corresponds to a tenfold change in the concentration of hydrogen ions. For example, a solution with a pH 3 is 10 times more acidic than a solution of pH 4, 100 times (10 × 10) more acidic than a solution of pH 5, and 1000 times (10 × 10 × 10) more acidic than a solution of pH 7. The same applies to pH values that are above 7 (i.e. alkaline solutions).

Blood and pH values

The normal pH range in blood is slightly above 7 on the pH scale — it is therefore slightly alkaline. However, for the purposes of physiology, a blood pH lower (more acidic) than 7.35 is considered to be too acidic, and one greater than 7.45 is too alkaline, and when either of these events occurs it can have a serious effect on physiological function — as is discussed in other chapters within this book. The pH range for blood may seem very narrow, but because the scale is a logarithmic one, just a small change in pH indicates a very significant alteration in H^+ concentration. An alteration of pH from pH 7.4 to pH 7.3 actually represents a doubling of the H^+ ion concentration (figure 1.11). Notice the large range of pH for urine — as a means of removing or retaining acid in the body, this can vary quite significantly.

FIGURE 1.11 The pH of some common household substances and some body fluids

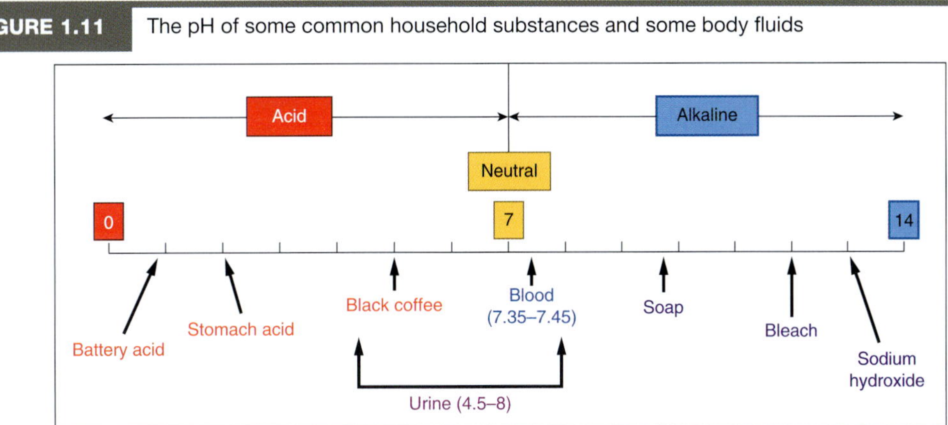

Representing chemical reactions in written form: chemical equations

As already mentioned, to make writing chemistry quicker and easier, we use symbols to represent each element in the periodic table. When one element reacts with another to form a new compound, we can represent that reaction using the same symbols, showing the compounds reacting (the **reactants**) and the new compounds resulting from the reaction (the **products**).

As an example, let us look at a reaction which produces water, one of the most important and ubiquitous compounds on Earth. We all know water as a liquid at room temperature, yet it is formed by the reaction between the gases hydrogen and oxygen. Two atoms of hydrogen bond with one atom of oxygen to create the new molecule we know as water. However, because in nature hydrogen gas exists as a hydrogen molecule (two hydrogen atoms bound together) as does oxygen gas (two oxygen atoms bound together), this means that two hydrogen molecules will actually react with one oxygen molecule, producing two water molecules. That equation is represented as:

$$2H_2 + O_2 = 2H_2O$$

Since each water molecule contains two hydrogen atoms and only one oxygen atom, the chemical formula indicates this by placing a subscript 2 after the symbol for hydrogen, and since two hydrogen molecules are required for the reaction, a large 2 before hydrogen indicates this. As the reaction produces two water molecules, you can also see a large 2 before them on the right-hand side of the equation.

Chemical reactions can also be shown in a more graphical way, using not only the chemical symbols, but also diagrams of the atoms and molecules themselves, to give a better idea of their structure, as shown in figure 1.12.

So, a chemical equation is just a shorthand way of showing a chemical reaction.

It is important to understand that chemical reactions involve a rearrangement of atoms and molecules to form different molecules and compounds — nothing can be created and nothing destroyed in these reactions, so the total number of atoms and molecules must be the same on each side of a chemical equation. Remember that chemical bonds form in the first place to allow atoms and molecules to achieve a lower energy, more stable state, so it follows that if a chemical rearrangement is to take place, then the rearranged form of the chemicals must be a still lower energy state. Therefore, when these reactions occur, energy is released as heat when chemical bonds are broken and different ones formed. This means that heat is one of the products of the reaction, along with the chemical products. Chemical reactions which produce heat as a by-product of the reaction are known as exothermic reactions. Humans often put exothermic reactions to good use — the best example in the body is how we shiver when we are cold. The muscle contractions required to shiver need energy, and as the body increases production of energy for these contractions, heat is produced by the exothermic chemical reactions involved. This is also why your body temperature increases when you exercise!

FIGURE 1.12 Pictorial depiction of the reaction between two hydrogen molecules and one oxygen molecule to produce two water molecules

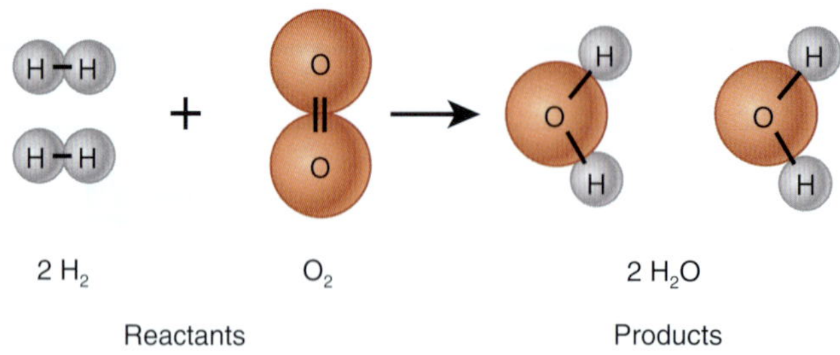

Source: Tortora and Derrickson (2014). Reproduced with permission of John Wiley & Sons.

The arrow in the middle of a chemical equation indicates the direction of the reaction; in other words, it points towards the products of the reaction. This is not to say that the reaction cannot also reverse and proceed from right to left as written, but it does mean that if the reaction from left to right is exothermic (produces heat), then energy will need to be supplied in order to get it to go back the other way. Take the example shown earlier of the gases hydrogen and oxygen combining to form water; that reaction is exothermic. It is also possible for the reaction to proceed in the opposite direction, and water to break apart to yield hydrogen and oxygen, but energy would have to be supplied to drive this reaction, so it would not happen spontaneously.

In a chemical equation, the reactants and the product may be separated by a single arrow (→) as in the earlier example of H_2O. This indicates that the reaction occurs only in the direction that the arrow is pointing. If a reaction can proceed in either direction, it is known as a reversible reaction, and is written with arrows pointing in both directions.

An example of a reversible reaction, and one which is a very important reaction in the control of acid–base balance in the body, is the reaction between carbon dioxide and water to form carbonic acid.

$$CO_2 + H_2O \rightleftharpoons \underset{\text{Carbonic acid}}{H_2CO_3} \rightleftharpoons \underset{\text{Bicarbonate ion}}{HCO_3^-} + \underset{\text{Hydrogen ion}}{H^+}$$

Not only does the reaction take place in two stages, but, as the arrows indicate, the reactions can also proceed in both directions, with bicarbonate and hydrogen ions combining to form carbonic acid, which then rearranges to produce carbon dioxide and water. Reactions like this, which can proceed in either direction, will create an equilibrium, a point at which there is a mix of products and reactants. This means that changes in the balance between the reactants and the products would therefore be expected to 'tip' the reaction in one direction or the other. This behaviour is very important in the rapid buffering of acids and alkalis in the blood, to help maintain normal blood pH.

1.5 Organic molecules

LEARNING OBJECTIVE 1.5 List the differences between organic and inorganic substances.

Chemicals can be classified as being either organic or inorganic. These terms derive from the observation that the molecules that make up living things are large, carbon-containing compounds, and these became known as organic compounds, because they formed living (organic) material. Organic molecules (or **organic substances**) contain carbon, often in long chains, with hydrogen, and are usually very large molecules. Inorganic molecules (or **inorganic substances**), on the other hand, do not contain carbon and hydrogen atoms arranged in long chains, although some do contain carbon (carbon dioxide, for example, is an inorganic compound) and some contain hydrogen (water, for example). Inorganic molecules tend to be much smaller.

There are other characteristics which set organic and inorganic compounds apart.

- *Organic* molecules:
  - contain carbon (C) and hydrogen (H)
  - are usually larger than inorganic molecules
  - dissolve in water and organic liquids (but not all)
  - include carbohydrates (sugars), proteins, lipids (fats) and nucleic acids (part of DNA) — see the chapter on genetics. Organic molecules are sometimes known as the 'molecules of life' for this reason.
- *Inorganic* molecules:
  - include water (H_2O), carbon dioxide (CO_2) and inorganic salts such as sodium chloride
  - are usually smaller than organic molecules
  - usually dissolve easily in water or react with water to produce ions.

Examples of organic substances

Carbohydrates

This group of organic molecules, also known as saccharides, makes up one of our major food groups, and includes sugars, starch and cellulose. The smallest and simplest members of the group, the monosaccharides, provide energy to cells as well as forming part of some of the structures in cells (see the chapter on cells, cellular compartments, transport systems, fluid movement between compartments). They contain carbon (C), hydrogen (H) and oxygen (O), usually in the proportion CH_2O; that is, with two hydrogen atoms to every one oxygen and carbon atom.

Carbohydrates are classified into three groups based on their molecular size.

Monosaccharides	Glucose (dextrose), formula $C_6H_{12}O_6$ Fructose (fruit sugar), formula also $C_6H_{12}O_6$
Disaccharides	Sucrose (table sugar), formula $C_{12}H_{22}O_6$ Lactose (milk sugar), formula $C_{12}H_{22}O_{11}$
Polysaccharides	Starch (amylose), formula $(C_6H_{10}O_5)n$ Glycogen, formula $(C_6H_{10}O_5)n$ Cellulose, formula $(C_6H_{10}O_5)n$

Monosaccharides and disaccharides can be referred to collectively as simple sugars or simple carbohydrates. Disaccharides, as the name suggests, consist of two monosaccharides bonded together — a sucrose molecule is one molecule of glucose bound to one molecule of fructose. The much larger polysaccharides are referred to as complex sugars or complex carbohydrates. It is the foods containing complex carbohydrates that are often listed as having a low glycaemic index, since larger sugars require digestion before they can be absorbed and thus arrive in the bloodstream more gradually.

Fats

Fats are one part of a larger group of chemicals known as lipids. They form another major food group, and are used in the diet to provide energy, but cell membranes are made of lipids and the group of hormones known as the steroids are also lipids, so this group plays a range of important roles in human function. Like carbohydrates, they consist of carbon (C), hydrogen (H) and oxygen (O), but because the relative proportions of these atoms are different from the carbohydrates, the lipids have different properties. They are only soluble in non-polar solvents like alcohol, for example, and not in water.

There are several types of lipids, but some of the most common are the following.

Fatty acids

These molecules are the 'building blocks' of larger, more complex lipids, and do not often exist on their own. They consist of long chains of carbon and hydrogen, with an organic acid group at the end (figure 1.13). There are many different types of fatty acids, three common examples being oleic acid (found in olive, sunflower, peanut and palm oil), palmitic acid (found in palm oil, meat and dairy) and stearic acid (found most commonly in animal fats).

FIGURE 1.13 The fatty acids — palmitic acid and oleic acid — indicating the general structure of fatty acids (note the organic acid group (–COOH) found at the left end of each fatty acid)

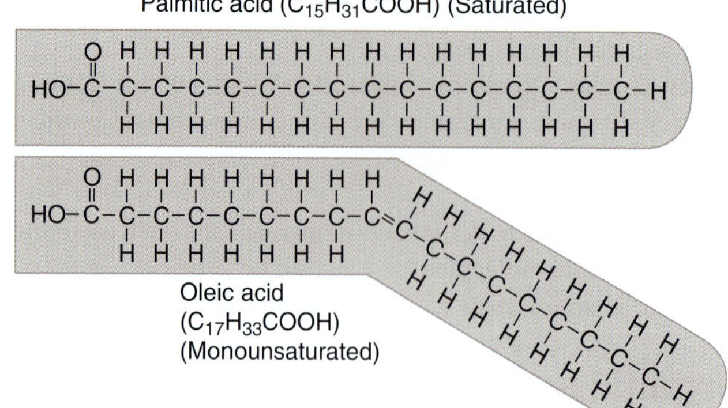

Source: Tortora and Derrickson (2014). Reproduced with permission of John Wiley & Sons.

Triglycerides (triacylglycerols)

These molecules consist of three fatty acid molecules attached to a glycerol molecule (figure 1.14). The long chains of the fatty acid molecules anchored to the glycerol molecule make the triglycerides look a little like three ties on a hanger, or a capital letter 'E'.

FIGURE 1.14 Triglyceride molecule

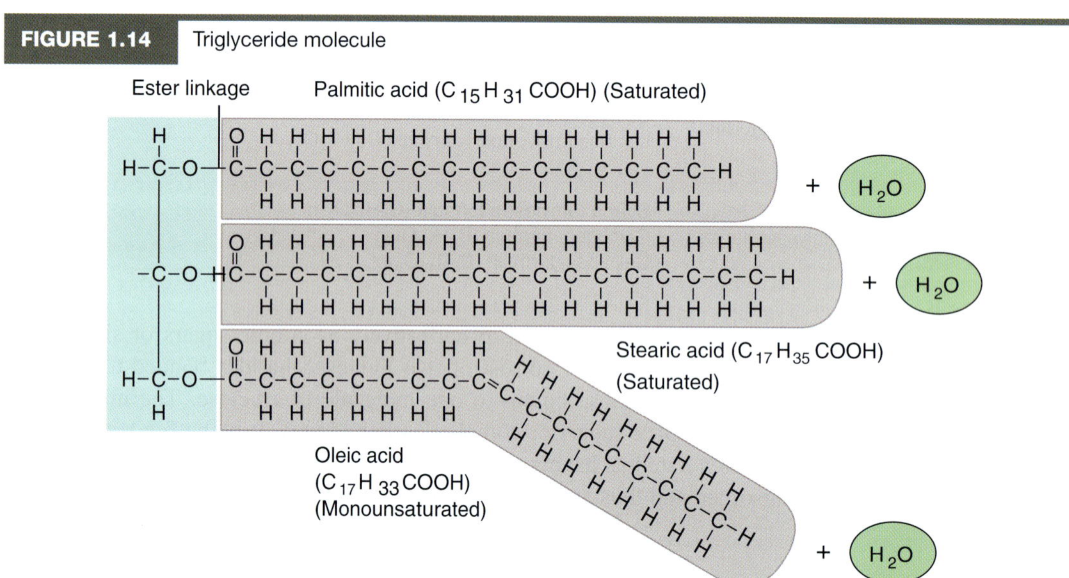

Source: Tortora and Derrickson (2014). Reproduced with permission of John Wiley & Sons.

These are the lipids that our cells can use for energy, and we often measure triglycerides circulating in the blood when checking a person's blood lipid profile.

CLINICAL CONSIDERATIONS

Cholesterol, blood lipids and health

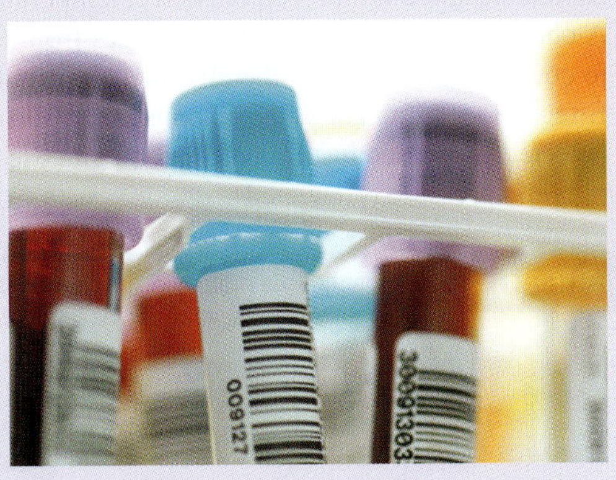

Routine measurement of blood lipids includes measurement of a number of lipids carried in the bloodstream, and usually includes triglycerides, low-density lipoprotein (LDL), high-density lipoprotein (HDL) and total cholesterol. While fats are an excellent source of energy, excessively high levels of triglycerides, LDL and total cholesterol are linked with an increased risk of cardiovascular disease. High levels of HDL, on the other hand, are associated with reduced risk of cardiovascular disease — it helps to regulate cholesterol levels, among a wealth of other protective effects. Improving blood lipid profiles to improve health can be achieved through lifestyle modification such as dietary changes and increasing physical activity — this is the first-line treatment in Australia. Should a patient's blood lipids continue to suggest a high risk of a cardiovascular event, the use of drugs known as statins also has a powerful effect on cholesterol levels, and these drugs are widely prescribed for this purpose in Australia. As with any drug, the benefits of taking it have to be carefully weighed against the risks. The data suggests that raising HDL to provide a protective effect is just as, or perhaps more, important than reducing LDL, and researchers are continually looking to refine the way in which the problem of high blood lipids is managed.

Phospholipids

As the name suggests, these lipids have a phosphate group as a component of their molecules. A double layer of these molecules makes up the basis of our cell membranes (called the lipid bilayer), as will be discussed in the chapter on cells, cellular compartments, transport systems, fluid movement between compartments (figure 1.15).

Steroids

Steroids are substances that are quite different chemically from lipids, but are considered lipids because they are insoluble in water. A number of very important hormones are steroids, as is cholesterol, which is a vital component of cell membranes. The names of these substances usually indicate the chemical group they belong to, by including -sterol or -sterone in the name (e.g. cholesterol, corticosterone, aldosterone, progesterone, testosterone).

Proteins

Proteins are large molecules built from amino acids strung together to form long chains. The body makes many different proteins, each one with a different sequence and number of amino acids joined together. The structural material that makes up the body is protein, and many vital molecules such as hormones receptors, **enzymes** and **antibodies** are proteins. It is useful to think of protein function in two major categories: structural proteins (make up our structures) and functional proteins (part of our biochemical machinery, including receptors, enzymes and antibodies). Proteins will be discussed in much greater depth in the chapter on genetics.

1.6 Homeostasis

LEARNING OBJECTIVE 1.6 Outline the regulation of homeostasis in the body.

Homeostasis is the maintenance of a relatively stable internal environment in the face of a constantly changing external environment — from cold to hot, from dry to wet, from acid to alkaline and so on. Homeostatic mechanisms are continuously monitoring and controlling variables in the body such as blood pH, core temperature, blood pressure, blood glucose levels and many others — we have specific receptors to monitor such variables (see the chapter on the nervous system). Regardless of the variable being controlled, homeostatic systems all follow a general scheme.

1. A detector system to monitor changes in the variable. These detectors are collectively known as receptors, and we have many types — each one specialised to detect a particular variable (e.g. baroreceptors detect pressure changes in blood vessels, chemoreceptors detect changes in the concentration of some chemicals and thermoreceptors detect temperature changes).
2. A control centre to receive the messages from the detectors about changes, and to organise a response to counteract the change, thereby maintaining stability.
3. Effectors, to bring about the response (e.g. shivering and 'goosebumps' when a drop in temperature is detected, increased insulin when blood glucose level increases or an increase in heart rate when a drop in blood pressure is detected).

FIGURE 1.15 Phospholipid molecule. This molecule has a 'head', where the phosphate group is located, and two 'tails', consisting of two fatty acid molecules.

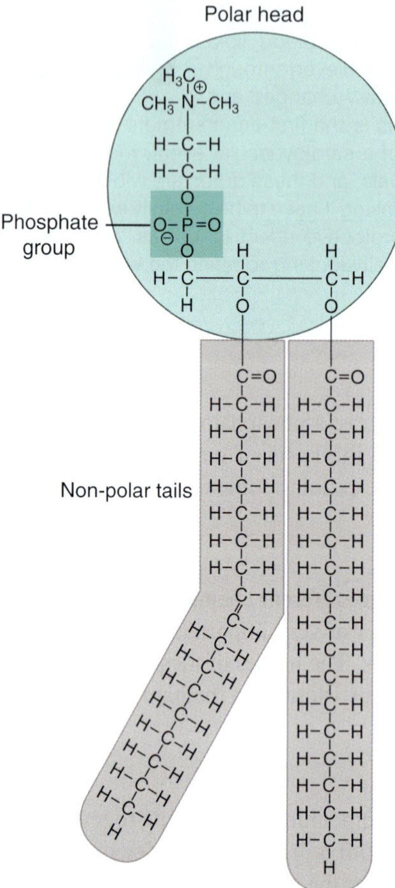

Source: Tortora and Derrickson (2014). Reproduced with permission of John Wiley & Sons.

Since the tendency of homeostatic control is therefore to resist, or at least limit, the size of changes occurring within the internal environment, the mechanism which achieves this is often referred to as a negative feedback loop, since the response of the system is opposite to (a negative of) the change that triggered it (i.e. it reverses the initial stimulus). For example, if the blood pressure drops slightly, the homeostatic mechanism that controls blood pressure will respond by producing an increase in blood pressure — the response is therefore opposite to the change, hence the feedback to the change is negative to it. Once blood pressure returns to normal, this response will stop. Systems that work like this are inherently stable, as they tend to resist change within the system.

Much of the study of human function is the study of these complex homeostatic control mechanisms, and the maintenance of good health depends on their effectiveness. It is important to remember that homeostasis does not 'lock' a variable at one setting, but limits the degree to which a variable can change, so that our systems are flexible enough to adapt to changing demands and conditions, but stable enough to maintain an internal environment that is consistent with healthy function of our body systems. Maintaining our internal environment in this way is essential to our optimal function and survival — many diseases impact our ability to do this, hence their negative effects to our health.

Units of measurement

To conclude this chapter, which introduces certain scientific concepts and prepares the reader for the remaining chapters, there are some brief notes about units of measurement. This is an important section because the ability to identify and understand units of measurement will enhance the understanding of the complex human organism.

A unit is a standardised, descriptive word that specifies the dimension of a measured property. Traditionally there have been seven properties of matter that have been measured independently of each other, namely:

- *time* — measures the duration that something occurs
- *length* — measures the length of an object
- *mass* — measures the mass (commonly taken to be the weight) of an object
- *current* — measures the amount of electric current that passes through an object
- *temperature* — measures how hot or cold an object is
- *amount* — measures the amount of a substance that is present
- *luminous intensity* — measures the brightness of an object.

Originally, each country had its own units of measurement. In the UK, for example, there were such units as furlongs, miles, poles, gallons, quarts, bushels and pecks. This made it difficult for people, particularly scientists, from other countries to work with each other, so several years ago an international system of units was agreed upon by most major countries including Australia (a notable exception to this agreement is the USA). This new agreed system became known as the Système International d'Unités (or SI units for short). It is a system of units that relates present scientific knowledge to a unified system of units. There are still some instances in healthcare when other units are referred to, such as new parents reporting their baby's birth weight in pounds and ounces or a person stating their height in feet and inches, which may need conversion to SI units for comparison. Tables 1.1, 1.2, 1.3, 1.4, 1.5, 1.6 and 1.7 give the SI units, unit prefixes and some Imperial unit equivalents that will be useful as reference while working through this book.

TABLE 1.1 **The fundamental SI units**

Quantity	Name	Symbol
Length	metre	m
Mass	kilogram	kg
Time	second	s
Current	ampere	A
Temperature	Kelvin	K
Amount of substance	mole	mol
Luminous intensity	candela	cd

TABLE 1.2 **Other common SI units**

Physical quantity	Name	Symbol
Force	Newton	N
Energy	Joule	J
Pressure	Pascal	Pa
Potential difference	Volt	V
Frequency	Hertz	Hz
Volume	litre	L

TABLE 1.3 Multiples of SI units

Prefix	Symbol	Meaning	Scientific notation
tera	T	one million million	10^{12}
giga	G	one thousand million	10^{9}
mega	M	one million	10^{6}
kilo	k	one thousand	10^{3}
hecto	h	one hundred	10^{2}
deca	da	ten	10^{1}
deci	d	one tenth	10^{-1}
centi	c	one hundredth	10^{-2}
milli	m	one thousandth	10^{-3}
micro	μ	one millionth	10^{-6}
nano	n	one thousandth of a millionth	10^{-9}
pico	p	one millionth of a millionth	10^{-12}
femto	f	one thousandth of a pico	10^{-15}
atto	a	one millionth of a pico	10^{-18}

TABLE 1.4 Measures of weight

1 kg = 1000 g
1 g = 1000 mg
1 mg = 10^{-3} g
1 μg = 10^{-6} g
1 pound = 0.454 kg/454 g
1 ounce = 28.35 g
25 g = 0.9 ounce
1 ounce = 8 dram

TABLE 1.5 Measures of volume

1 L = 1000 mL
100 mL = 1 dL
1 mL = 1000 μL
1 UK gallon = 4.5 L
1 pint = 568 mL
1 fluid ounce = 28.42 mL
1 teaspoon = 5 mL
1 tablespoon = 15 mL

TABLE 1.6	Measures of length
1 m = 10^{-3} km	
1 cm = 10^{-2} m	
1 mm = 10^{-3} m	
1 m = 39.37 inches	
1 mile = 1.6 km	
1 yard = 0.9 m	
1 foot = 0.3 m	
1 inch = 25.4 mm	

TABLE 1.7	Measures of energy
1 calorie = 4.184 J	
100 calories = 1 dietary Calorie or kilocalorie	
1 dietary Calorie = 4184 J or 4.184 kJ	
1000 Calorie = 4184 kJ	
1 kJ = 0.238 Calories	

SUMMARY

This concludes our brief introduction to some of the basics of chemistry and biology. As you will appreciate, the study of body function at any level, whether it be at the level of molecules reacting or at the level of the whole person, is extremely complicated, but also fascinating.

Learning something about how bodies function and how they respond to the challenges placed upon them in both health and disease can equip you with the knowledge and power to save lives in your future practice. It is only through gaining an understanding of the wonderful machines we inhabit that we can learn how to best care for them. Enjoy the discoveries that await you.

KEY TERMS

acids A chemical substance with a pH below 7.

acid–base balance The maintenance of pH within controlled limits. This is essential for good health. See pH.

alkali A chemical substance with a pH above 7.

anatomy The study of the structures of the body.

anion An ion with a negative charge.

antibodies Proteins that recognise and attach to specific infectious agents in the body.

atomic number The number of protons in the nucleus of an atom.

atom The smallest unit of matter.

base An alkaline substance.

bonds The joining together of various substances, particularly atoms and molecules. See chemical bond, covalent bonding, ionic bonds, and polar bonds.

cation An ion with a positive charge.

chemical bond The 'attractive' force that holds atoms together.

chemical reactions A process in which chemical substances react together to produce a different chemical form. This is usually expressed by a chemical equation.

compounds A substance that is made up of two or more elements chemically bonded together.

covalent bonding Bonds between atoms formed by the sharing of electrons between the atoms.

electrolytes Substance that produces a solution that conducts electricity when placed in water. Physiologically important electrolytes include sodium and potassium ions.

electrons The parts of an atom that orbit the atomic nucleus and carry a negative electrical charge. See also neutrons and protons.

elements A chemical substance that cannot be broken down into anything simpler by chemical means.

enzymes Proteins produced by cells that increase the rate of biochemical reactions in the body.

homeostasis The maintenance of a stable internal environment by the use of systems of detectors, control centres and effectors.

inorganic substances Substances that do not contain long chains of carbon and hydrogen molecules (although they may contain carbon and hydrogen).

ionic bonding Bonds that form between ions with opposite charges.

ions The entities formed when atoms lose or gain electrons, thereby becoming positively or negatively charged.

mole The unit of measurement of the amount of a substance.

molecules Electrically neutral group of two or more atoms bonded together.

neutral A chemical substance that is neither acidic nor alkaline.

neutrons The parts of an atom that carry a neutral electrical charge (i.e. they have no electrical charge). See also electrons and protons.

organic substances Substances that contain carbon molecules (e.g. carbohydrates, lipids, proteins).

pH A measure of the acidity or alkalinity of a solution. See acid–base balance.

physiology The study of the way in which the body structures function.

polar bonds Bonds that form between polar molecules, in which the increased negativity of one pole of a polar molecule is attracted to the increased positivity of the opposite pole of another molecule. Hydrogen bonds are polar bonds.

products (chemical reactions) The new substance/s formed following a chemical reaction.

protons Subatomic particles found in the atomic nucleus which carry a positive electrical charge. See also electrons and neutrons.
reactants (chemical reactions) The individual substances involved in a chemical reaction.
shells (of an atom) The name given to the orbits of electrons moving around the nucleus of an atom.
valency The number of hydrogen atoms an element is able to combine with. This is the bond-forming power of an element, and depends on the number of electrons in its outermost shell.

ACTIVITIES

TRUE OR FALSE

1 An ion is an atom that is in an electrically neutral state.
2 Molecules are combinations of atoms.
3 Many electrolytes are essential minerals.
4 Organic substances contain carbon and hydrogen.
5 Lipids are examples of inorganic substances.
6 Proteins are built up from amino acids and provide the structural material for the body.

TEST YOUR LEARNING

1 What is the importance of respiration for the body?
2 Why is water essential for all organisms, including humans?
3 How is the atomic number of an atom calculated?
4 What is an ion, and what is its importance for us?
5 Make a list of some of the common elements found in the body.
6 Explain what is happening in the chemical reaction as depicted by this chemical equation:

$$C_6H_{12}O_6 + 6O_2 + 6H_2O + ATP\,(\text{cellular energy})$$

7 Discuss the importance of the pH of blood.
8 Discuss the importance of carbohydrates to the body.

FIND OUT MORE

1 Look at a copy of the periodic table of elements and mark off the ones you have come across in this chapter and that are important for humans.
2 Many electrolytes are essential minerals for the body. Find out which these are.
3 Find out about, and make notes on, the process of osmosis and its importance for human functioning and health.
4 Discuss the acid–base balance and its importance for maintaining good health — and, indeed, for life itself.
5 Discuss what is happening in these two equations — you will need to have access to chemical abbreviations to help you understand the symbols.

$$N_2 + 3H_2 \rightarrow 2NH_3$$

$$H_2CO_3 \rightarrow H^+ + HCO_3^-$$

6 Find out the normal range of human pH and then discuss why it is important for the nurse to alert medical staff if a patient's pH is found to be outside the normal range.
7 Find out more about the importance of homeostasis to health.
8 Lipids/fats can be either saturated on unsaturated — find out from the foodstuffs that you normally eat which of them contain either or both of these types of lipids and their role(s) in healthy nutrition.
9 Take one day, and on that day look at your breakfast, lunch and tea/dinner (as well as snacks, etc.) and try to find out the contents of them all in terms of carbohydrates, lipids and proteins.
10 How can a nurse help to provide a healthy diet for their patients while they are in hospital and/or the community?

REFERENCE

Tortora, G.J. and Derrickson, B.H. (2014) *Principles of Anatomy and Physiology*, 14th edn. Hoboken, NJ: John Wiley & Sons.

ACKNOWLEDGEMENTS

Photo: © Tyler Olson / Shutterstock.com
Photo: © Cultura RF / Getty Images

CHAPTER 2

Cells, cellular compartments, transport systems, fluid movement between compartments

TEST YOUR PRIOR KNOWLEDGE

- Where do cells come from?
- What, approximately, is the average size of a human cell?
- What are the various forms human cells can take?
- How are human cells taken and examined for diagnostic purposes?
- An understanding of cell biology is particularly vital for finding a cure for which group of diseases?

LEARNING OUTCOMES

After reading this chapter you will be able to:

2.1 describe the functions of the major cell organelles

2.2 describe how the structure of the plasma membrane determines its permeability

2.3 list the various ways in which substances move into and out of cells

2.4 list the major differences in ionic composition between intracellular and extracellular compartments

2.5 predict the movements of water by osmosis, based on the circumstances, and explain the reason for its importance to living organisms.

Introduction

Cells are the basic structural and functional units that make up all living organisms. Some organisms, such as bacteria and protozoans, are unicellular, consisting of a single cell, but many are multicellular, made up of billions of cells sometimes, as in the case of humans. Multicellular animals possess a range of cells that are specialised to perform various special functions (figure 2.1) — these are some great examples of the relationship between anatomy and physiology (i.e. structure and function) that was introduced in the chapter on basic scientific principles of physiology.

FIGURE 2.1 Examples of some cells of the human body

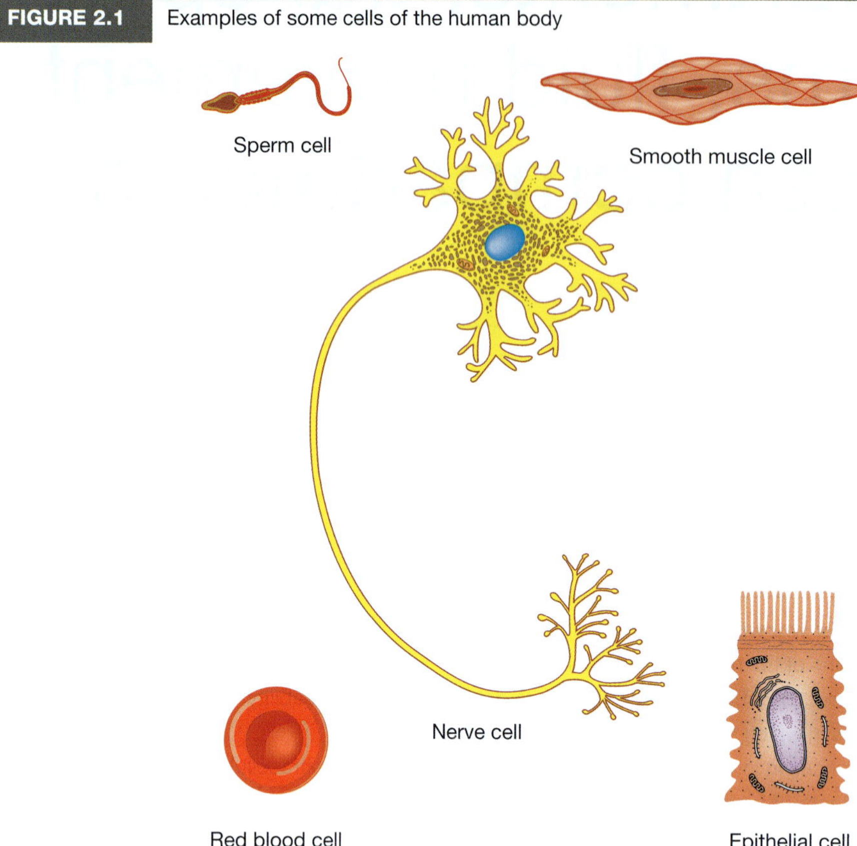

Source: Tortora and Derrickson (2009). Reproduced with permission of John Wiley & Sons.

2.1 Inside the cell

LEARNING OBJECTIVE 2.1 Describe the functions of the major cell organelles.

Regardless of their specialisation, almost all cells contain the same structures and **organelles** needed to perform the basic functions of the cell, such as growth, metabolism and reproduction (briefly outlined in table 2.1). Each cell (with the exception of mature red blood cells) also contains its own complete set of instructions for carrying out these activities in the form of genetic material or DNA (see table 2.1 and figure 2.2).

Cells are filled with a jelly-like fluid known as cytosol, in which the cell's organelles are suspended. The cytosol is 90 per cent water, with various dissolved ions, amino acids, sugars and lipids. The entire cell is bounded by a protective cell membrane, which maintains the integrity of the cell. In order to carry out their activities, however, cells need to obtain a supply of nutrients and water from their surroundings, and they need to be able to expel waste products from the cell into their surroundings, so there is a requirement for transport of selected substances across the membrane.

TABLE 2.1 Important typical components of a cell

Organelle	Function
Cell membrane	Protective outer layer; controls entry and release of substances (semi-permeable)
Nucleus	Houses the genetic material (DNA) of the cell; directs development, function and replication
Ribosomes	Carries out protein synthesis
Rough endoplasmic reticulum	Site of protein synthesis within the cell (covered in ribosomes)
Smooth endoplasmic reticulum	Site of lipid synthesis within the cell
Golgi apparatus	Packages up substances for transport within/release from the cell (e.g. hormones to be released into the blood)
Lysosomes	Contain enzymes to help break down wastes and invading substances (e.g. bacteria)
Mitochondria	Site of energy (ATP) production within the cell (see the section on active transport)
Cytoplasm	Total content of fluids within the cell (cytosol plus that within all organelles)

FIGURE 2.2 Structure of a cell

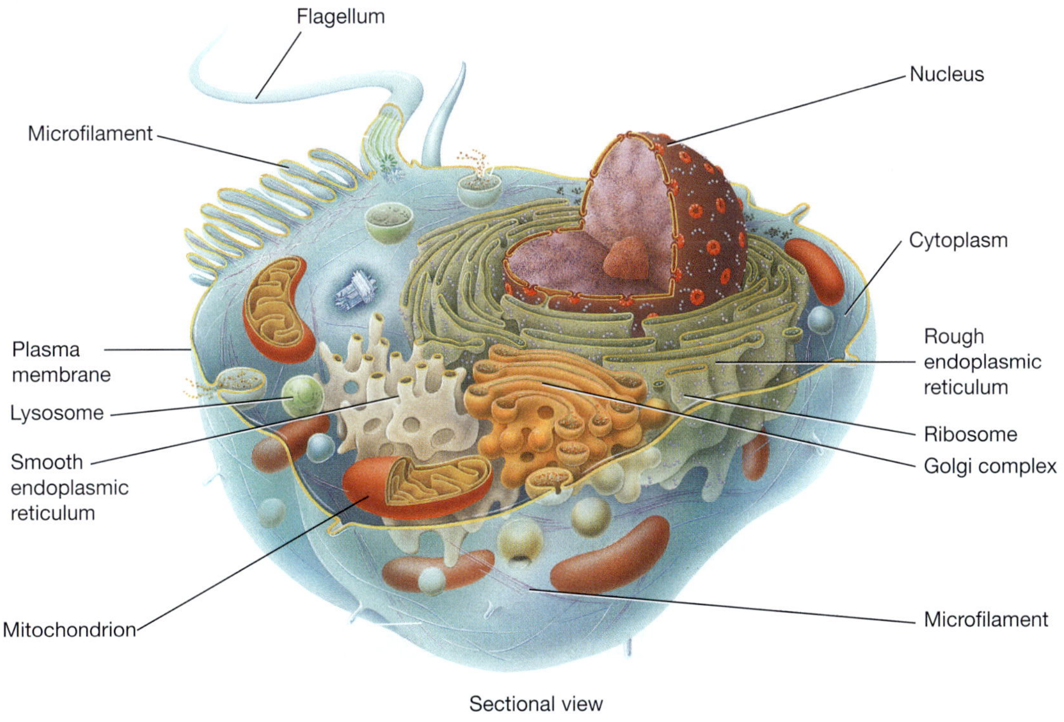

Source: Nair and Peate (2009). Reproduced with permission of John Wiley & Sons.

2.2 Structure of the cell membrane

LEARNING OBJECTIVE 2.2 Describe how the structure of the plasma membrane determines its permeability.

The cell membrane (also known as the **plasma membrane**) consists of a double layer (a 'bilayer') of phospholipid molecules, which forms a stable barrier between the two aqueous **compartments** (i.e. the inside and the outside of the cell). As discussed in the chapter on basic scientific principles of physiology, the phospholipid molecule has a globular head and two thin tails, which are the fatty acids (see also O'Connor & Adams 2010). While the charge on the fatty acid tails is evenly distributed, the charge on the head of the molecule is unevenly distributed, giving the head of the molecule areas that are somewhat positive and others that are somewhat negative (making the head 'polar'). Polar molecules tend to mix with other polar molecules and ions (including water), whereas non-polar molecules do not. The polar heads of the phospholipid molecules therefore mix with water, meaning they are '**hydrophilic**' (water-loving). The fatty acid 'tails' of the molecules, on the other hand, do not mix with water, so they are '**hydrophobic**' (water-hating). When placed in water, this means that phospholipid molecules line up so that their heads are in contact with the water, and their tails are not. The only way this can be achieved, of course, is for the molecules to form a double layer, with the molecules effectively 'back to back', with their heads orientated outwards, in contact with the water, and the tails orientated inwards, away from the water (see figure 2.3). As such, the bilayer is self-sealing, and is able to control what can pass through; for example, water and water-soluble substances would be repelled by the water-hating tails in the middle of the bilayer, making the bilayer waterproof. However, since the cell needs to receive nutrients and other vital substances from its surroundings, there must be ways to transport certain substances across the membrane. This special transport is carried out by protein molecules embedded in the membrane (figure 2.3). These **transport proteins** form channels through which water and selected ions can cross the lipid bilayer, they form transporters that carry certain substances across the membrane, and they form receptors, responsible for cell–cell recognition and cell–cell signalling.

FIGURE 2.3 Cell membrane

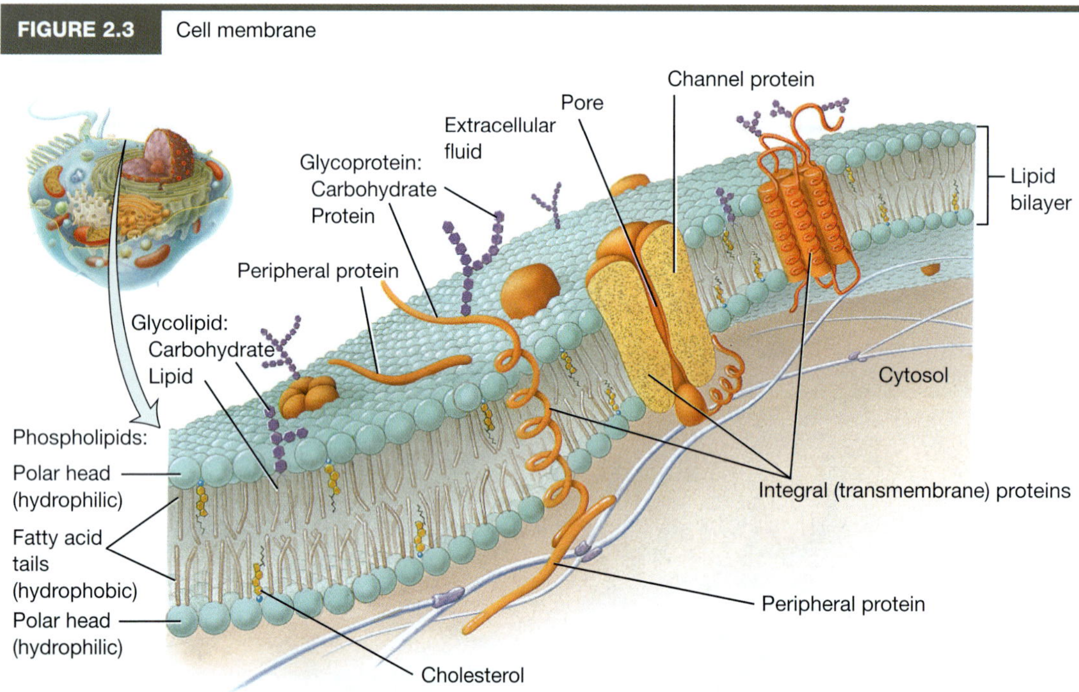

Source: Tortora and Derrickson (2009). Reproduced with permission of John Wiley & Sons.

2.3 Transport of substances across the cell membrane

LEARNING OBJECTIVE 2.3 List the various ways in which substances move into and out of cells.

All organisms, whether single-celled or multicellular, need to be able to obtain essential nutrients and oxygen from their surroundings, and the bigger and more complex the organism, the greater the need for transport mechanisms to quickly and efficiently get substances to where they are needed in the body. Because all cells are surrounded by the cell membrane, transport into a cell requires that substances can get across the cell membrane somehow.

Transport can occur via passive or active mechanisms. **Passive transport** does not require the input of energy in order to drive the process (e.g. rolling a car down a hill), but **active transport** does (e.g. driving a car up a hill).

Passive transport

The simplest form of passive transport is a process known as **diffusion**. Diffusion comes about because all atoms and molecules are in constant motion — the molecules in a gas can move more freely than those of a liquid, which in turn move more freely than molecules in a solid, but all are constantly vibrating. The speed of this movement is related to the temperature; as the temperature of a substance increases, the molecules will vibrate more rapidly, and as temperature drops, the molecular movement slows down (hence why solid ice melts into liquid water when it heats). Because of this constant motion, molecules do not stay exactly where they have been placed and will move and spread out evenly by the process of diffusion. For example, if you carefully place some crystals of solid dye at the bottom of a flask of water and do not stir it, you will find that over time the dye will gradually spread throughout the water in the flask, until the water is evenly coloured (figure 2.4).

FIGURE 2.4 Diffusion in a fluid. At the beginning of our experiment, a crystal of dye placed in a cylinder of water dissolves (a) and then diffuses from the region of higher dye concentration to regions of lower dye concentration (b). At equilibrium (c), the dye concentration is uniform throughout, although random movement continues.

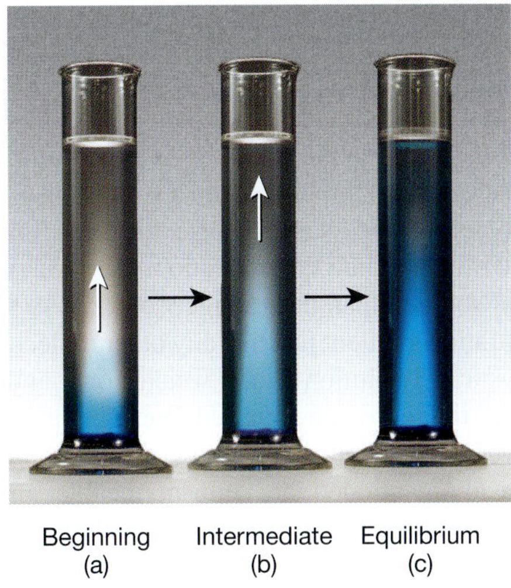

Beginning (a) Intermediate (b) Equilibrium (c)

Source: Tortora and Derrickson (2009). Reproduced with permission of John Wiley & Sons.

Diffusion therefore results in the distribution of a substance being 'evened out'. Another way of expressing this would be to say that diffusion is the passive movement of a substance from where it is in high concentration to where it is in lower concentration, or the passive movement of a substance down its concentration gradient. The rate at which diffusion occurs depends on a number of factors.

1. *Whether the substance is a gas, a liquid or a solid.* Because the random movement of the molecules is much greater in a gas then a liquid or a solid, diffusion will occur more rapidly in gases, than in liquids, and diffusion in liquids will be much faster than in solids.
2. *The temperature.* Diffusion becomes more rapid as temperature increases.
3. *Molecular size.* Small molecules will move faster than large ones.
4. *Concentration.* The bigger the difference in concentration, the faster the diffusion will occur to even out that difference.
5. *Distance over which diffusion is occurring.* Molecules will even out their concentration over a small area more rapidly than over a large area.

Diffusion does not only occur in a single compartment though; molecules will also diffuse across a cell membrane if their concentration on the other side of the membrane is different (and provided, of course, that they can get through the membrane). Small, hydrophobic molecules and gases such as oxygen and carbon dioxide readily cross cell membranes by diffusion (figure 2.5). The exchange of respiratory gases in the lungs occurs by simple diffusion and occurs rapidly enough to provide enough oxygen for our needs and remove the carbon dioxide we produce, even when we are working hard. In another example of the link between anatomy and physiology, structures such as alveoli (air sacs) and capillaries have very thin walls, to help this diffusion occur.

FIGURE 2.5 Simple diffusion

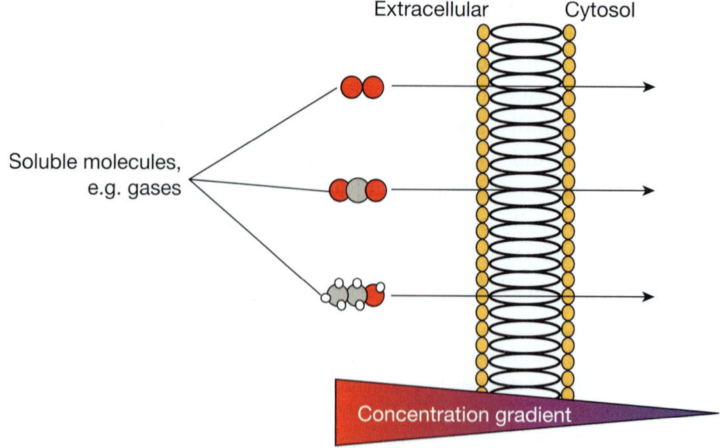

Source: Nair and Peate (2009). Reproduced with permission of John Wiley & Sons.

Osmosis: a special case of simple diffusion

Figure 2.6 shows a container that is divided in the middle by a structure that is similar to a cell membrane. A weak sugar solution is on one side of this membrane, and a strong sugar solution on the other. According to the principle of diffusion, therefore, we would expect the sugar molecules to diffuse down their concentration gradient in order to even out their concentration. However, water will be present at a greater concentration in the weaker sugar solution than the stronger solution, so we should also expect that water will diffuse down its own concentration gradient just like any other molecule. In this scenario, sugar should be moving from the more concentrated solution to the weaker one, and water should be moving from the less concentrated solution into the more concentrated one. This is indeed what would happen if the membrane dividing the two halves of the container were permeable to both sugar and water, but in fact, it is not. Cell membranes, as already mentioned, are semi-permeable, and only allow certain substances to cross them. Water is able to cross the membrane relatively freely by means of pores or water channels created by proteins in the membrane, but ions and larger molecules cannot cross freely.

FIGURE 2.6 Osmosis — water passing through a semi-permeable membrane into a region of higher sugar concentration

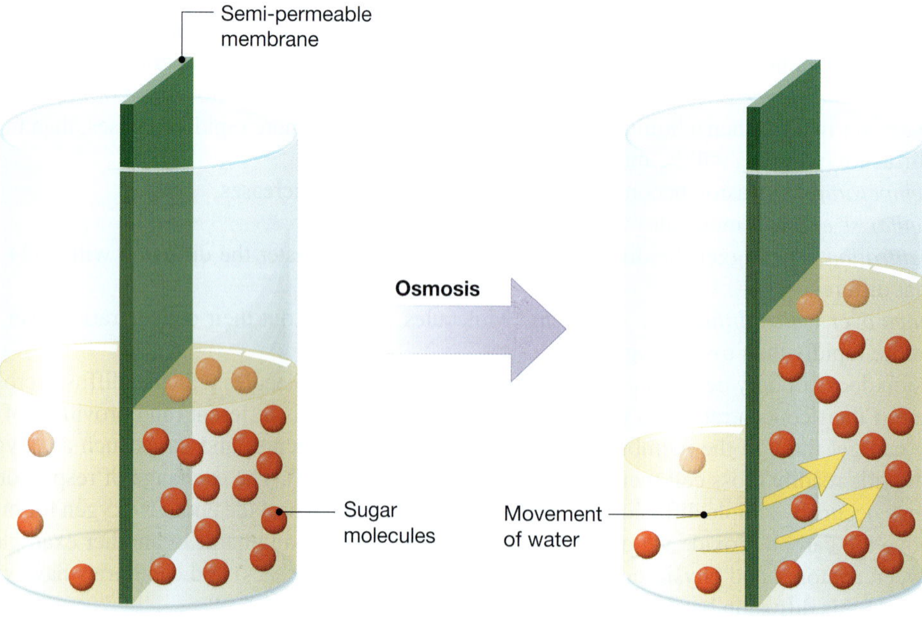

Going back to our scenario in figure 2.6, since the sugar would not be able to cross the membrane, only water would be moving, and it would be moving from the weaker to the more concentrated solution (to balance it out). Over time, we would see water accumulating on the side of the container with the stronger sugar solution in it. The water level on this side would increase above the water level on the other side, and the solution would be diluted so that its concentration was closer to that of the weaker solution on the other side. Whether the two solutions could ever reach a situation where their concentrations were exactly the same would depend on a number of things: how different the concentrations were to start with, how much room there was for water to accumulate on the side with the stronger solution, and whether the movement of water was being opposed by any other force (e.g. an increasing pressure due to more and more water arriving on one side of the membrane, known as **'osmotic pressure'**).

The presence of a semi-permeable membrane, such as a cell membrane, therefore prevents the simple diffusion of many substances down their concentration gradients, by virtue of the simple fact that they cannot get across, but it does not prevent water from diffusing. This means that where cell membranes are involved, it is the diffusion of water across these membranes that will dominate above all else. It is this movement of water down its concentration gradient across a semi-permeable membrane that is termed **osmosis**.

Osmosis is an incredibly important process for living things, since the inside and outside of their cells, and their various body compartments, are separated by semi-permeable membranes. This means that whenever there is a difference in the concentration of solutions between the inside and the outside of cells, or between one body compartment and another, the movement of water by osmosis will inevitably occur.

Understanding and being able to predict the process of osmosis is a vital skill for nurses, and yet it is one that students of nursing often struggle to grasp. Remember that osmosis is quite simply the diffusion of water across a membrane from where it is present in higher concentration to where it is present at a lower concentration. Because water is one of the few molecules that is able to cross the membrane freely, and because our body fluids are watery, osmosis plays a central role in our normal function. Osmosis dictates that any change in total **solute** (dissolved substances) concentration in any of our fluid compartments will trigger a flow of water between compartments to even out this change.

An often-used example of the importance of osmosis that is highly relevant for nursing is what happens when the concentration of the solution outside red blood cells does not match the concentration inside the cells. Red blood cells spend their lives circulating in the blood, suspended in plasma. The plasma is, like all body fluids, a watery solution. The composition of the blood plasma may be very different to the composition of the **intracellular** fluid (ICF) of the red blood cell in terms of the actual solutes, but because most solutes cannot freely cross the membrane, they will not be able to diffuse down their concentration gradients, and so those differences in composition will be maintained. However, if the concentration of water in the plasma is different from that inside the red blood cell, then water will move to even the concentration out. The experiment illustrated in figure 2.7 shows us how an imbalance in the water concentration between the intracellular and **extracellular** compartments can result in damage to, or destruction of, cells. If this were allowed to happen in a person's bloodstream to any great extent, the person could die as a result — there wouldn't be enough 'healthy' red blood cells to carry out their function.

FIGURE 2.7 (a–c) Osmotic effects of the concentration of a solution on a red blood cell. In (a) a cell is placed in a solution that has the same total solute and therefore water concentration as the intracellular fluid (an isotonic solution); in (b) a cell is placed in a solution that has a lower total solute and therefore higher water concentration than the inside of the cell (a **hypotonic** solution); and in (c) a cell is placed in a solution that has a higher total solute concentration and therefore lower water concentration than the inside of the cell (a **hypertonic** solution).

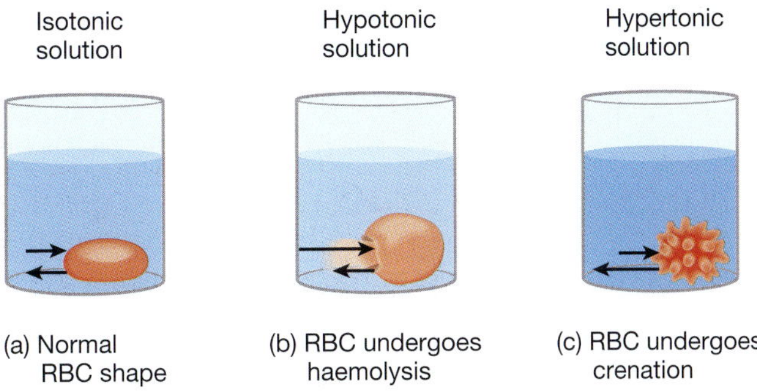

Source: Tortora and Derrickson (2009). Reproduced with permission of John Wiley & Sons.

Facilitated diffusion

Highly charged molecules, such as ions, and large molecules, such as sugars and amino acids, cannot cross cell membranes by simple diffusion, so special transport arrangements are needed for these substances if they are to gain access to cells down their concentration gradient. In these cases, transport is 'facilitated' by proteins that span the cell membrane and provide a passageway for these substances.

Ions pass through specific proteins that create channels for them to pass through (known as ion channels). The ions still diffuse passively (i.e. they use no energy), but they do so through the channel rather than passing through the lipid bilayer directly. These channels are usually specific to one ion, and they are usually gated, so that ions can only pass through the channels under conditions which cause the channels to open. Larger molecules, including organic molecules such as glucose, bind to specific protein 'carrier' molecules, located in the membrane. These more complex passive processes are known as **facilitated diffusion** (figure 2.8). Note, though, that these are still passive transport processes, because the substances are moving down their concentration gradients (i.e. from an area of where they are at higher concentration to one where they are at a lower concentration).

FIGURE 2.8 Passive transport mechanisms

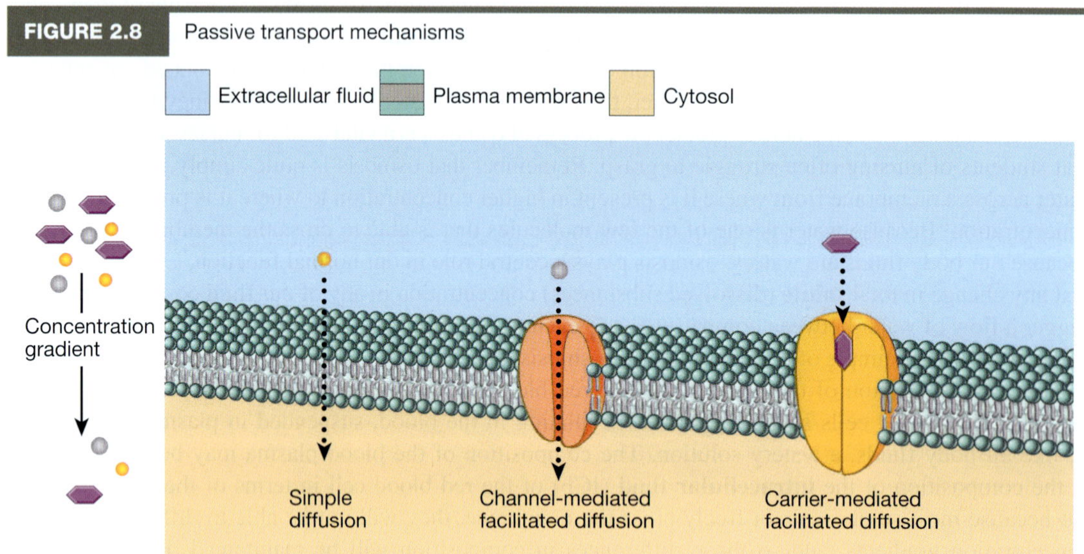

Source: Nair and Peate (2009). Reproduced with permission of John Wiley & Sons.

Active transport

In some situations, for example when taking up glucose or other nutrients, cells need to concentrate large amounts of substances, meaning that they will need to be moved from an area of lower concentration to an area of higher concentration (i.e. they travel up their concentration gradient). In these situations, active transport is required, and this transport requires energy to drive it. Examples of active transport include the glucose transporter which moves glucose into cells for use or storage, and the sodium-potassium (Na^+/K^+) pump — a transport system present in all cell membranes, which actively transports sodium ions out of the cell and potassium ions into the cell (figure 2.9). These ions are both being moved up their concentration gradients, as sodium ions are at a greater concentration outside the cell and potassium ions are present at greater concentration inside the cell — correct distribution like this is vital for maintaining normal cell function.

FIGURE 2.9 The Na^+/K^+ pump

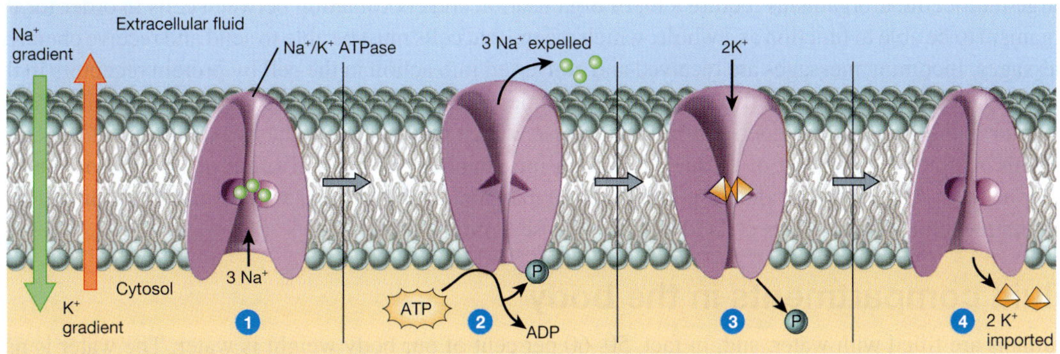

Source: Tortora and Derrickson (2009). Reproduced with permission of John Wiley & Sons.

MEDICINES MANAGEMENT

Tiny pumps, big consequences ...

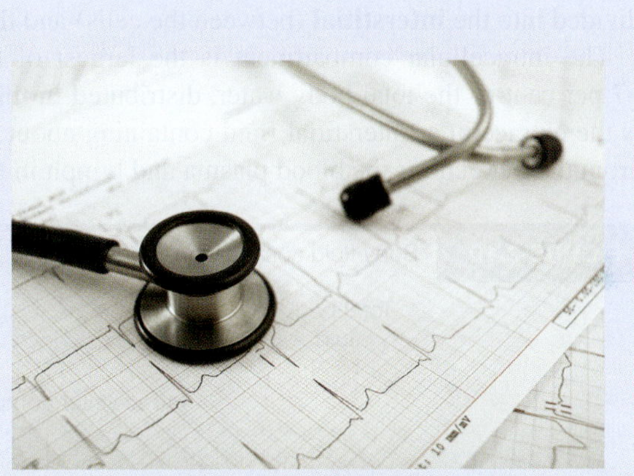

Digoxin has been used to manage heart failure for centuries, and is still an important part of the management of congestive heart failure and some irregular heart rates (cardiac arrhythmias) in Australia today. The drug makes the heart beat more strongly, by increasing the strength of contraction of the heart muscle — a very beneficial effect for a patient with a failing heart. The drug must be used carefully though, as at high doses it has the potential to cause cardiac arrhythmia and palpitations, among other adverse effects. Digoxin has its action by inhibiting (i.e. blocking) the sodium-potassium pump on the cell membranes of heart muscle cells. This transporter pumps sodium ions out of the cell in exchange for potassium ions, thus maintaining the sodium ion concentration gradient across the membrane. This gradient, in turn, drives an exchange transporter which removes calcium ions from the cell in exchange for sodium ions. When digoxin is used, the inhibition of the sodium-potassium pump reduces the concentration gradient for sodium across the cell membrane (i.e. more sodium ions are 'trapped' inside), thus reducing the transport of calcium out of the cells and resulting in an increased intracellular concentration of calcium in the heart muscle cells. Because calcium has a central role in muscle contraction, more calcium equals stronger contractions, and so the heart beats harder.

The energy to power active transport comes from the cell's mitochondria

In the same sense that you need to convert Australian dollars (AUD) into American dollars (USD) to spend in America, the energy contained in the food you eat needs to be converted into a form usable by your body. To do this, mitochondria in your cells take in oxygen and nutrients such as glucose and fatty acids, and from these raw materials produce a supply of a high-energy molecule, **adenosine triphosphate (ATP)**. This molecule contains high-energy bonds with the phosphate groups which, when broken, release energy that can power cellular functions. Once the ATP has been split and the resulting energy released for use, **adenosine diphosphate (ADP)** and phosphate remain, and the ATP molecule can be regenerated by the mitochondria to supply more energy.

How do cells communicate?

Large multicellular organisms require a lot of organisation and coordination between cells in order for the organism to be able to function as a whole, which means that cells must be able to send and receive chemical messages. Incoming messages are received and converted into action in the cell by protein receptors in the membrane that recognise specific signalling molecules. The 'docking' of the molecule with its protein receptor in the membrane triggers a cellular response, which may be the synthesis and release of a specific protein or lipid, the opening or closing of certain ion channels, or the activation of an enzyme, among other actions. An example of this response that you may already be familiar with is insulin binding with a protein receptor, which causes cells to take in glucose from the blood.

Fluid compartments in the body

Humans are filled with water, and, in fact, 50–60 per cent of our body weight is water. The water is not, of course, pure — it contains many dissolved substances (solutes) and larger suspended particles (which are not fully dissolved). In addition, the watery solutions in our bodies are separated into a number of compartments, and the composition of the solutions in each compartment can differ significantly. We can divide these body compartments firstly into the intracellular compartment (the fluid contained inside cells) and the extracellular compartment (the fluid outside cells). The extracellular compartment is then further divided into the **interstitial** (between the cells) and the intravascular (blood and lymph) compartments.

The intracellular compartment is the largest of the body's fluid compartments, containing around 67 per cent of the total body water, distributed in millions of tiny volumes in the cells. The next largest is the extracellular interstitial fluid containing about 25 per cent of total body water, and the smallest, at around 8 per cent, is the blood plasma and lymph in the intravascular compartment (figure 2.10).

FIGURE 2.10 Body fluid compartments

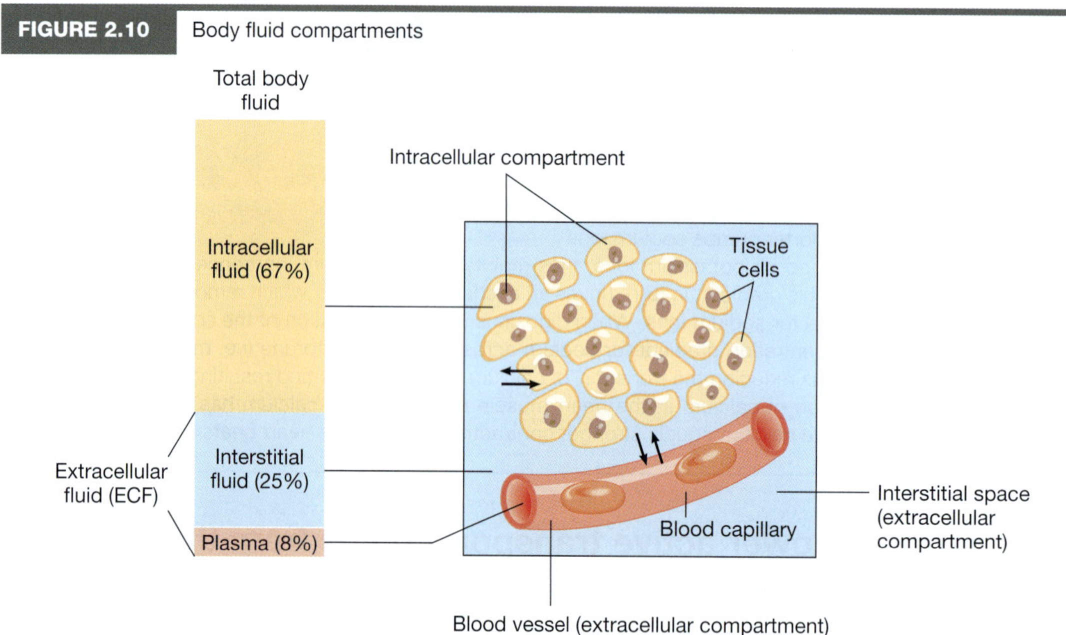

Source: Nair and Peate (2009). Reproduced with permission of John Wiley & Sons.

The major fluid compartments in the body have been discussed but it should also be noted that a very small portion of extracellular fluid (ECF) is represented by specific body fluids such as cerebrospinal fluid, gastrointestinal tract fluids, aqueous humour in the eye and joint fluid. These fluids, which are produced by epithelial tissue lining the spaces in which they are found, are collectively known as transcellular fluid. While small in volume, these fluids are vitally important to the normal function of the tissues and organs in which they are found, as you will discover.

Bulk transport across the cell membrane

So far, this chapter has covered the ways in which individual molecules of a substance can cross cell membranes, either by active or passive processes. However, there are many situations in which larger amounts of a substance need to be moved into or out of a cell quickly. For this to occur, the items to be transported are bundled up in a membrane of their own, forming a small, membrane-bound package called a vesicle. On contact with the cell membrane, the membrane of the vesicle melts into (fuses with) the cell membrane, and the contents are released into or outside the cell, depending on the direction of transport. This kind of bulk transport is used to remove unwanted substances from cells and to secrete substances such as hormones, enzymes or neurotransmitters from cells, and to bring large items into cells.

Endocytosis: bulk transport into cells

Endocytosis is the process by which cells take in molecules such as proteins from outside the cell by engulfing them with their cell membranes (figure 2.11). It is used by all cells of the body to bring polar and large molecules into the cell in bulk. The cell membrane folds around the substances to be transported and a vesicle is formed, containing the substance. Endocytosis may involve small droplets of a substance, in which case it is known as pinocytosis (from the Greek meaning 'cell drinking'). All cells use pinocytosis to supply their needs. Certain cells of the immune system are also able to carry out another form of endocytosis called phagocytosis (from the Greek meaning 'cell eating'). In phagocytosis, whole cells, such as bacteria, or large pieces of cells can be ingested by a cell. The object in this case, though, is to engulf and destroy something harmful as a protective measure, rather than to obtain nutrients or useful substances. Our immune systems are equipped with a number of phagocytic white blood cells which perform a vital role in defending us against bacteria and other disease-causing organisms by engulfing and destroying those organisms.

FIGURE 2.11 Phagocytosis and pinocytosis

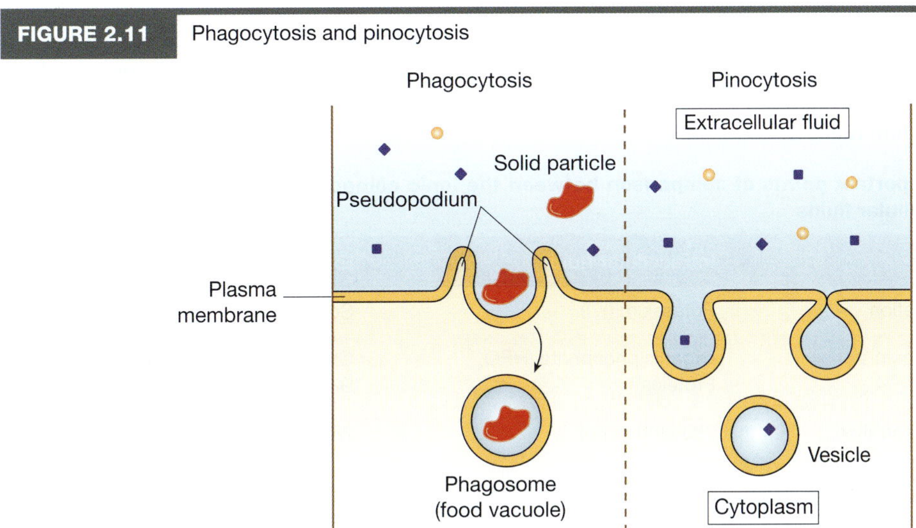

Source: Peate and Nair (2011). Reproduced with permission of John Wiley & Sons.

Exocytosis: bulk transport out of cells

Exocytosis is the process by which the cell moves packages of substances from the inside of the cell to the outside (use the similarity between 'exo-' and 'exit' to remember this!). Newly synthesised products, such as hormones or enzymes to be secreted, are packaged into vesicles by the Golgi apparatus, and transported to the cell membrane. At the cell membrane, the vesicle membrane fuses with the cell membrane and the contents of the vesicle are deposited outside the cell (figure 2.12).

FIGURE 2.12 Exocytosis. Proteins, lipids and other products produced in the cell are packaged into vesicles by the Golgi apparatus to be moved out of the cell. Exocytosis can be stimulated by an incoming signal.

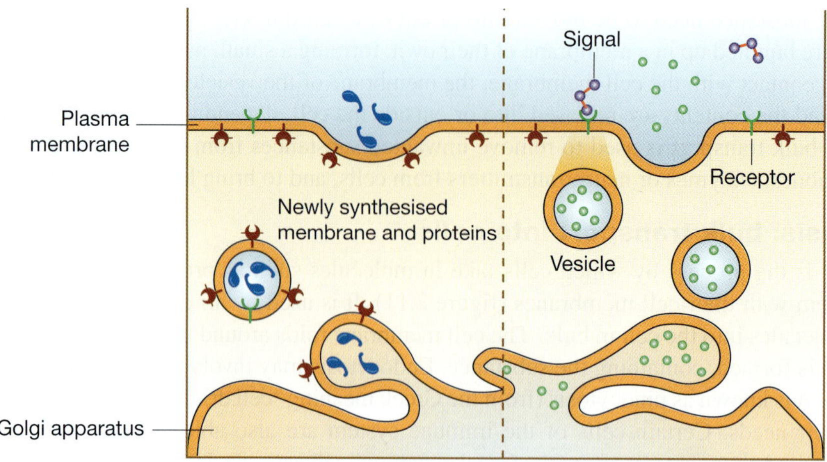

Source: Nair and Peate (2009). Reproduced with permission of John Wiley & Sons.

2.4 The composition of body fluids

LEARNING OBJECTIVE 2.4 List the major differences in ionic composition between intracellular and extracellular compartments.

The composition of the intracellular fluid differs from that of extracellular fluid in a number of ways, but the most important differences are in the ions. Extracellular fluid contains a high concentration of sodium and chloride ions, and a relatively low concentration of potassium and organic ions, and the reverse is true for intracellular fluid (table 2.2).

TABLE 2.2 **Important points of comparison between the ionic composition of intracellular vs extracellular fluids**

	Intracellular fluid	Extracellular fluid
Most abundant cation	Potassium (K^+)	Sodium (Na^+)
Most abundant anion	Organic phosphate (HPO_4^{3-}) Proteins	Chloride (Cl^-) Bicarbonate (HCO_3^-)
Total solute concentration	280–300 mmoL L^{-1}	280–300 mmoL L^{-1}
Cations vs anions	Equal numbers	Equal numbers

The differences between intracellular and extracellular fluid composition will mean that for the various solutes, concentration gradients exist between the intracellular and extracellular compartments. However, as already mentioned, ions and large molecules such as proteins do not have free passage across cell membranes, so they are not free to diffuse down their concentration gradients and equalise the fluid compositions. In order to ensure that there is no net movement of water between these compartments, though, the intracellular and extracellular compartments must contain the same concentration of water, or put another way, they must have the same total concentration of solutes. It does not matter that the solutes are not of the same type — it just matters that they are present in the same total concentration in both compartments. Notice also that both extracellular and intracellular compartments contain an equal number of positive and negative ions, making each compartment electrically neutral.

Electrolyte and water balance

Both intracellular and extracellular fluids contain several **electrolytes**, such as sodium chloride and sodium bicarbonate, which split up (dissociate) to yield ions in solution (shown in table 2.2). These ions, since they carry charge and can move through the solution, carry current when they move (this is where the term electrolyte originated). In fact, they perform this function in our nerve and muscle cells, which are electrically powered, as you will see in the chapters on the muscular system and the nervous system.

Table 2.3 provides a summary of the most important electrolytes and their main functions.

TABLE 2.3 Principal electrolytes and their functions

Electrolytes	Function	Distribution
Sodium (Na^+)	Important extracellular cation, which is key to the generation of action potentials in nerve cells; as the most abundant extracellular cation, it plays an important role in maintaining extracellular fluid volume	Mainly in ECF
Potassium (K^+)	Important intracellular cation, which is key to establishing the resting membrane potential of a cell, and in the activity of nerve and muscle cells	Mainly in ICF
Calcium (Ca^{2+})	Physiologically, a very important ion; it is a vital factor in many functions, such as the release of neurotransmitter from activated nerve cells, activation of clotting factors, muscle contraction after activation of muscle cells and many more	Mainly in ECF
Magnesium (Mg^{2+})	Helps to maintain normal nerve and muscle function	Mainly in ICF
Chloride (Cl^-)	Abundant anion in ECF, therefore important for fluid balance; used to produce hydrochloric acid in the stomach	Mainly in ECF
Bicarbonate (HCO_3^-)	Important in acid–base balance, as buffer of hydrogen ions in plasma	Mainly in ECF
Phosphate (HPO_4^{2-})	Essential for bone formation and maintenance	Mainly in ICF

Because of the central roles of many of these ions in physiological functions, it is important that their levels are maintained within narrow limits, as too much or too little of any of them could cause a number of failures, in nerve and muscle function, body fluid maintenance, blood clotting, bone health and so forth. In addition, water in the body is inextricably linked to electrolyte balance, thanks to osmosis: if the concentration of electrolytes in any fluid compartment increases, then by definition the concentration of water in that same fluid compartment will be decreased, and water will move by osmosis from another fluid compartment (as shown earlier with the red blood cells in figure 2.7). In this way, water can be said to 'follow' electrolytes in the body. This means that electrolyte and fluid levels are locked together by osmosis. The levels of the most important electrolytes and water are separately controlled to keep them all within physiological limits. The major hormones (chemical messengers) involved in their homeostatic control are shown in table 2.4.

TABLE 2.4 Homeostatic control mechanisms for the major body fluid ions and water

	Monitored by	Controlled by	Action of hormone
Plasma Na^+	Specialised cells in the kidney detect Na^+ concentration and blood volume	Aldosterone	Works at the kidneys to increase the retention of Na^+ and the excretion of K^+, therefore increases Na^+ and decreases K^+ in body fluids
Plasma K^+	No specialised cells known	Aldosterone	
Plasma Ca^{2+}	Specialised cells in the parathyroid gland detect plasma Ca^{2+} concentration	Parathyroid hormone	Works at the gut to increase the absorption of Ca^{2+}; directs the kidneys to reduce the excretion of Ca^{2+}, and the bones to release calcium to replace deficits in the plasma
Water	Specialised cells in the brain (osmoreceptors) detect shrinkage due to dehydration and kidney cells detect blood volume changes	Antidiuretic hormone (ADH)	Works at the kidneys to increase the retention of water; increases water in body fluids, thereby also increasing volume of body fluids

CLINICALLY REASONED EPISODE OF CARE

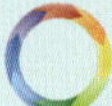

Hyponatraemia

Consider the patient situation

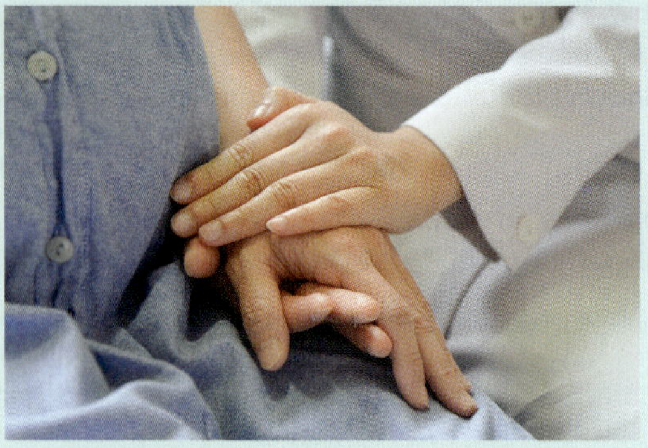

Meria is 65 years old. She has presented to the emergency department. According to her daughter, Meria was falling frequently and finding it difficult to walk, and her speech had become difficult to understand. Despite these reported symptoms, Meria was observed conversing with her daughter in the waiting room.

Collect cues and information

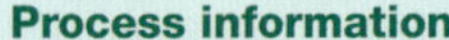

- Health history: approximately 2 weeks of flu-like symptoms, 4 days of vomiting; Meria reported she had been drinking large amounts of water to 'flush toxins from her system'.
- Abdominal assessment: reporting 6/10 occasional cramping pain.
- Neurological assessment: reduced attention span, slowed speech, altered gross motor function.
- Blood results: electrolytes — serum sodium 100 mmol/L (ref range 135–145 mmol/L).

Process information

Meria is experiencing severe hyponatraemia (serum sodium < 110 mmol/L). This is a common electrolyte imbalance presentation, especially for elderly people. Milder presentations do not often result in significant symptoms.

For Meria, this imbalance has occurred due to 4 days of vomiting, probable sweating with the 'flu-like symptoms', and drinking large amounts of water. Other causes can include excessive secretion of antidiuretic hormone from the posterior pituitary, resulting in reduced urine production and fluid retention, diuretic medications and excessive diarrhoea. People living with heart failure and renal failure can also develop hyponatraemia.

Loss of sodium from the blood lowers the tonicity of the ECF (extracellular fluid) compared with the fluid in the tissues, and water leaves the blood, moving through the tissues and into the cells (ICF, or intracellular fluid), causing cellular oedema. This is the basis of Meria's neurological symptoms.

Nursing actions

1. Administer fluids as charted by medical officer: 100 ml bolus 3% (hypertonic) saline solution.
   Rationale:
   - A bolus can correct the deficit quickly, providing additional sodium but not too much additional water, which would create the risk of worsening a likely fluid volume excess due to Meria's large fluid intake.
   - Restricting fluid intake and waiting for the sodium and water balance to normalise may take too long, and there is a risk Meria will suffer permanent neurological damage.
   - Increasing the serum sodium by 0.5 mmol/L/hour reduces the risk of central nervous system damage.
2. Restrict fluid intake.
   Rationale:
   - Meria has been drinking excessive amounts of water, which has contributed to dilutional hypona traemia; restricting fluid intake will help to correct this.
   - Meria is likely experiencing fluid volume excess and restricting fluids will assist in restoring a normovolaemic status.
3. Monitor sodium levels as requested by the medical officer; blood tests at 3 hours, 5 hours and 12 hours.
   Rationale:
   - Monitoring sodium levels will help to determine the efficacy of the management.
4. Monitor hourly vital signs and neurological assessment.
   Rationale:
   - This will monitor Meria's improvement and detect deterioration.
5. Refer to dietician for assessment and advice.
   Rationale:
   - Education around sodium and water intake will help to prevent a recurrence of this event.

Evaluate outcomes

Meria's serum sodium rose: 107 mmol/L, 114 mmol/L and then > 135 mmol/L. Neurological symptoms resolved. Abdominal discomfort resolved.

Source: Based on the Clinical Reasoning Cycle, Levett-Jones (2013); Therapeutic Guidelines (2020).

2.5 Fluid movement between compartments

LEARNING OBJECTIVE 2.5 Predict the movements of water by osmosis, based on the circumstances, and explain the reason for its importance to living organisms.

Movement of fluid between the intracellular and the extracellular compartments (i.e. in and out of the cell) will be by osmosis, and so will occur if there is a concentration gradient for water (a difference in solute concentration) across the cell membrane. Normally this gradient does not exist, as there is an equal total solute concentration between inside the outside the cell, as shown in table 2.2, but if such a gradient were introduced by changes in the water or solute concentration in one of the compartments, then osmotic movement of water would occur. How much water would move would depend on the size of the gradient. We use the term osmotic pressure to give us an idea of the size of any concentration gradient for water across a cell membrane, since this gives us a sense of how much water would move. The osmotic pressure is in fact the pressure that would have to be exerted on a solution to resist the movement of water due to osmosis (essentially to push back against the water). This is useful because it allows us to measure and therefore put a number to the water-driving power of osmosis.

The movement of extracellular fluid between the intravascular and the interstitial compartments is determined by two forces: the osmotic pressure and the hydrostatic pressure that the blood exerts against the walls of the vessel (we usually just call this blood pressure). The hydrostatic pressure in blood vessels is at its highest in the arteries (taking blood away from the heart), and gradually decreases as the blood travels through the network of blood vessels; from arteries to arterioles to capillaries, then to venules and finally to veins. As blood enters a capillary from an arteriole, it is therefore at a higher pressure at that point than when it reaches the end of the capillary just before it enters a venule. Capillaries, of all the blood vessels in the circulatory system, are the ones that are adapted to allow exchange of substances between the blood and the interstitial fluid, and their walls are perforated to allow this to happen. Changes in pressure inside and outside the capillary will therefore determine whether substances will move out of or into the capillary.

There is a greater tendency for fluid to move out of the blood vessel and into the interstitial fluid at the start of the capillary (the arterial end), because the hydrostatic pressure is greater there, and a tendency for fluid to move into the capillary at the venous end of the capillary where the hydrostatic pressure is lower. Fluid and solutes therefore leave the arterial end of the capillaries and move into the interstitial fluid, whereas they return to the capillaries at the venous end. It is important to note that although a bulk flow of fluid and its solutes occurs at the capillary level, the process of diffusion is also continuing, so that as oxygen-rich blood flows into the capillary at the arterial end, the oxygen in the plasma will diffuse rapidly down its concentration gradient out of the capillary and into the surrounding interstitial fluid, and from there into the cells in the area, and carbon dioxide will move into the blood in the same way. Glucose will also be able to diffuse from the capillaries into interstitial fluid because, unlike the cell membrane, the capillary wall is readily permeable to solutes, which means that the osmotic pressure within the capillary is principally determined by only the largest molecules, the plasma proteins such as albumin, that cannot leave the capillaries. The osmotic pressure exerted by the proteins inside the capillaries is referred to as 'oncotic' or 'colloid osmotic' pressure and is typically 25–30 mmHg. It increases as the blood flows along the capillary from the arterial to the venous end, because the fluid and smaller solutes leaving the capillary as a result of the hydrostatic pressure leave behind proteins in the blood and less water, which results in an increased protein concentration (and therefore a lower water concentration). Water will thus move into the capillary at the venous end as a result of osmosis (figure 2.13).

In normal conditions, therefore, the flow of fluid out of the capillary at the arterial end would be balanced by the subsequent flow back into the capillary at the venous end, and there would be no net gain or loss of fluid by the intravascular or interstitial compartments. However, if anything occurs to alter the hydrostatic or osmotic pressures in either compartment, the situation may rapidly change. For example, higher than normal hydrostatic pressure in the blood vessels (i.e. a high blood pressure) can increase the tendency of fluid to move out of the capillaries into the interstitial fluid and remain there, leading to oedema (excess fluid in tissues).

FIGURE 2.13 Capillary hydrostatic and osmotic pressures

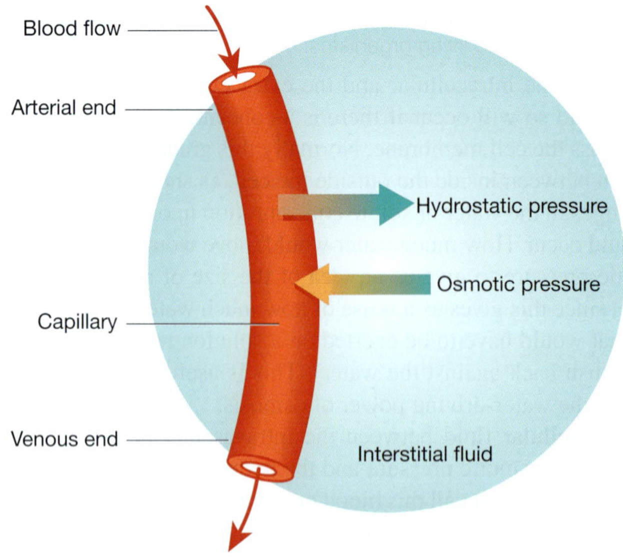

Source: Peate and Nair (2011). Reproduced with permission of John Wiley & Sons.

CLINICAL CONSIDERATIONS

Dehydration

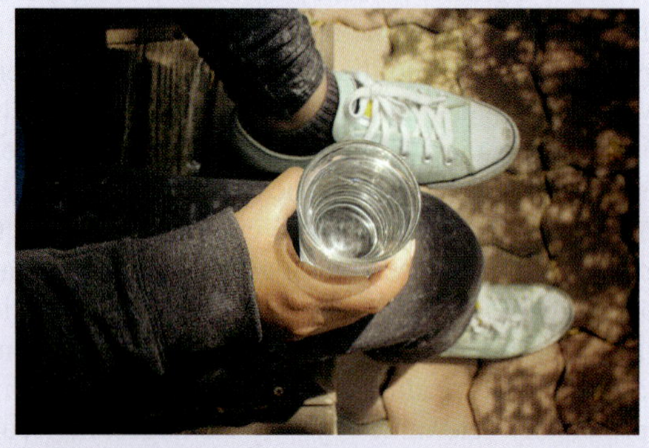

Dehydration may be caused by insufficient water intake, excessive water loss or a combination of both. The most common cause of dehydration is failure to drink enough liquid. The average person loses water from the body on a daily basis in urine, in expired air, through perspiration and from the gastrointestinal tract. This water needs to be replaced to prevent dehydration. If water loss is greatly increased, for example due to intense perspiration, and the water lost is not replaced by drinking, dehydration will occur, which could result in shock and death within only a few hours. The risk of this is greatly increased when patients have difficulty swallowing, or a reduced sense of thirst or capacity to respond to thirst — something particularly true in both paediatric and elderly patients. Severe vomiting or diarrhoea can result in loss of a large volume of body water and electrolytes which need to be consistently replaced as long as the illness persists if dehydration is to be avoided; if the patient is unable to replace the loss of body water and electrolytes themselves, the administration of intravenous fluids may be required.

Signs and symptoms of dehydration include headache, thirst, dry mouth, low volume of very concentrated urine (darker in colour), dizziness and lethargy. The skin may also appear shrunken, blood pressure may drop and the heart rate may increase (to try and compensate/maintain adequate blood flow). If the dehydration is due to excessive perspiration in high temperatures, the loss of fluid can result in a shutting down of sweating (often observed in heat stroke), which can then allow core temperature to rise dangerously.

CLINICALLY REASONED EPISODE OF CARE

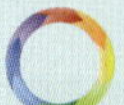

Burns

Consider the patient situation

Boon Sew, a 48-year-old male, is rushed to the emergency department after being rescued from his burning house. He was asleep when a spark from the fireplace started a fire, leaving him trapped in his bedroom. By the time the fire rescue team arrived, he had suffered severe burns and smoke inhalation.

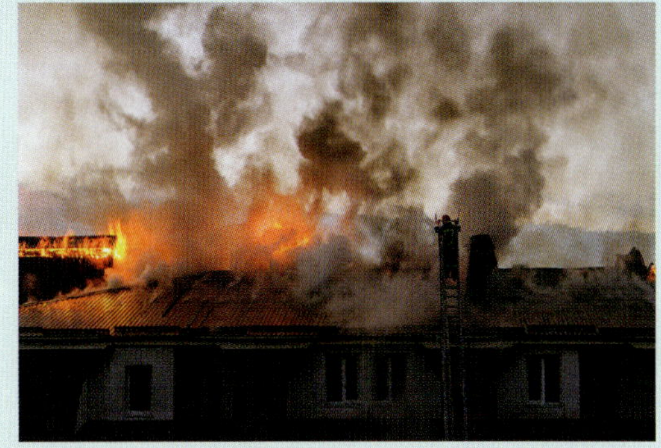

Collect cues and information

- Neurological assessment: unconscious.
- Skin assessment: third-degree burns to > 20% of body, second-degree burns to > 5% of body — thoracic, abdominal regions and right elbow.
- Vital signs: respiratory rate 38 breaths/min, heart rate 200 beats/min, blood pressure 53/35 mmHg.

Process information

Burnt skin no longer functions as an adequate body covering, and fluid and solutes escape at a rapid rate from the extracellular fluid compartment through the burnt areas (heat also escapes from the blood at the burn site and the person with burns can get cold very quickly as a result). The loss of fluid from the burns results in a large drop in blood volume and therefore blood pressure, which would explain Boon's low arterial pressure, despite the heart beating rapidly in an attempt to maintain it.

Boon is experiencing circulatory shock and the resulting poor circulation means that the supply of oxygen and nutrients to the cells and the removal of waste products is being compromised at the same time that the airways themselves are damaged by heat and smoke. This would explain the elevated respiratory rate.

The administration of intravenous fluids helps to restore the lost volume in the blood, thereby improving blood pressure and circulation; however, intravenous fluids with electrolytes need to be maintained for some time, as extracellular fluid will continue to seep from the burns. While fluids will help to stabilise vital signs, consideration will need to be given as to how much damage the blood tissue has sustained — burns over a large area can result in the destruction of a large number of blood cells as they are carried to the burnt area and destroyed by heat or lost from the body through the open burn. Third-degree burn damage to the cutaneous membrane will readily allow the entry of bacteria and other disease-causing organisms.

Nursing actions

1. Administer intravenous fluids and electrolytes as charted by the medical officer.
   Rationale:
   - Infusing fluid directly into the veins will increase blood volume and maintain cardiac output, reversing circulatory shock.
   - Infusing fluid directly into the veins will replace the fluid being lost through the damaged cutaneous membrane.
   - Replacement of electrolytes will prevent neurological, cardiac and muscular impairment.
2. Administer blood transfusion as prescribed by the medical officer.
   Rationale:
   - Blood or blood product transfusion will replace the damaged red blood cells and ensure adequate oxygen-carrying capacity.
3. Prevent infection by ensuring burns are clean and that all contact with the open wounds uses sterile techniques.
   Rationale:
   - Infection results in further tissue damage and creates a risk of systemic sepsis (septicaemia).
4. Refer to a dietician for nutritional support.
   Rationale:
   - Tissue healing requires a diet high in protein and kilojoules.

Evaluate outcomes

Boon regains consciousness and his vital signs stabilise into normal range. Boon has no signs of clinical infection. His wounds heal rapidly.

Source: Based on the Clinical Reasoning Cycle, Levett-Jones (2013); Agency for Clinical Innovation (2019).

CLINICAL CONSIDERATIONS

Administration of intravenous fluids

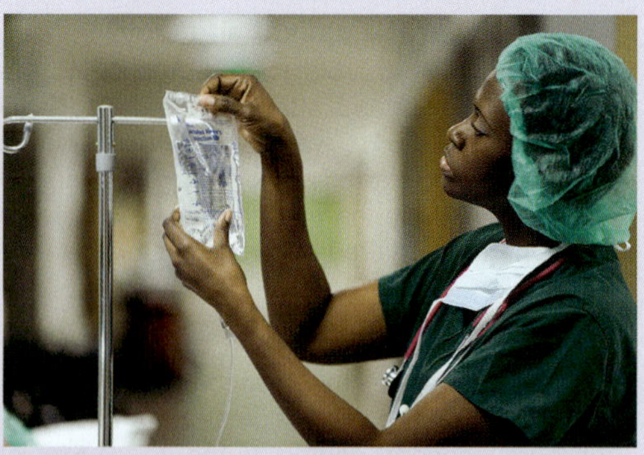

Administration of fluids and electrolytes in situations where body fluids have been lost and blood volume is low can save lives. The aim is to expand the circulating plasma volume, thereby increasing blood pressure. The fluid solution used must be isotonic and non-toxic. A crystalline solution such as sodium chloride is often used at a concentration of 0.9% (this is known as normal saline), but other solutes such as sodium lactate (Ringer's lactate and Hartmann's solutions) can also be used. Crystalline fluids given intravenously will not remain in the bloodstream, however, since the solutes will leave the capillaries and move into the interstitial space along with water. This will mean that a much greater volume of fluids will need to be given, to compensate for the volume of fluid that moves out of the intravascular compartment (third spacing). Colloid solutions provide an alternative, as they contain large molecules such as the protein albumin (5% solution), or the polysaccharide dextran that are too large to escape from the capillaries. Since the molecules cannot leave the blood, the water will not either, as a result of the osmotic pull of the colloids trapped in the blood vessel. This means that less fluid is needed to expand the plasma volume. Colloidal solutions are much more expensive, however, and can produce an allergic response in some patients.

Although fluid replacement is necessary for a patient who has low blood volume (hypovolaemia), overzealous administration of fluids, or administration when fluids are not needed can be detrimental to a patient's health. If fluids are administered to a patient with normal blood volume, fluid overload may occur, causing fluid to enter lung spaces, increased excretory demands to be placed on the kidneys, and increased workload on the heart. Nurses need to be aware of this and monitor patients carefully for signs of fluid overload, such as respiratory difficulty, abnormal lung sounds, high blood pressure and oedema (see Hilton et al. 2008).

SUMMARY

The cell, as the smallest living unit in the body, represents the smallest scale on which we are able to study physiological function; at higher levels — tissue, organ, organ system and organism levels — we are observing the concerted and coordinated functions of cells working together. Everything the organism is able to do is due to the correct functioning of billions of cells. How the cell does what it does is therefore a fundamental part of the study of physiology. The health and life cycle of individual cells also comes to the fore in cancer research, as the search for ways to cure cancer focuses around the study of the mysteries of individual cells, and what makes them start to divide in an uncontrolled manner. The fluids which our cells are filled with and bathed in are also vital to normal function. Our bodies are filled with salty solutions, and the semi-permeable nature of our plasma cell membranes ensures that those salty solutions cannot mix freely. This control of what can and cannot cross cell membranes explains the various specific transport mechanisms that cells have developed in order to be able to supply their needs, and it explains the electrical potentials that are created between one side of the membrane and the other, due to the distribution of electrolytes between the intracellular and extracellular fluids. This electrical potential can be converted to electrical current by the membrane opening ion channels and allowing ions to flow, carrying their charge, and this is the basis of our electrically operated nerve and muscle cells.

For the nurse, a sound understanding of osmosis and electrolyte and fluid balance is absolutely essential. All patients, regardless of their age or health status, can become vulnerable to dehydration, overhydration or electrolyte imbalance as a result of drugs, stress, infection, renal problems or inappropriate fluid intake. Being aware of what water and electrolytes do and where they go in the body is the first step to understanding how watery creatures like humans function, and to ensuring that they are safe when in your care.

KEY TERMS

active transport The energy-requiring process by which substances are moved up their concentration gradient (i.e. from an area with lower concentration to one with a higher concentration).

adenosine diphosphate (ADP) The product produced when adenosine triphosphate (ATP) is metabolised with the breaking of its high-energy phosphate bond to release energy.

adenosine triphosphate (ATP) High-energy compound which provides energy for the cell when its high-energy bonds with phosphate groups are broken.

compartments Spaces within the body that are separated by living membranes.

cytoplasm The fluid and contents of a cell.

diffusion The movement of substances down their concentration gradients from a higher to a lower concentration.

electrolytes Substances that dissociate in water to form ions.

endocytosis Bulk movement into a cell.

extracellular Outside cells.

exocytosis Bulk movement out of a cell.

facilitated diffusion Diffusion with the aid of a transport protein.

hydrophilic Water-loving, soluble in water.

hydrophobic Water-hating, insoluble in water and soluble in lipids.

hypertonic A solute concentration higher than that of intracellular fluid. Cells placed in a hypertonic solution would shrink, as water would flow out into the hypertonic solution by osmosis.

hypotonic Solute concentration lower than that of intracellular fluid. Cells placed in a hypotonic solution would swell, as water would flow from the hypotonic solution into the cells by osmosis.

interstitial Between cells.

intracellular Inside the cell.

organelles 'Mini organs' that perform the vital functions of the cell.

osmosis Movement of water through a selectively permeable membrane to even out the solute concentration on either side of the membrane.

osmotic pressure The pressure that must be exerted on a solution into which water is flowing by osmosis in order to completely oppose that osmotic movement.

passive transport The process by which substances move down a concentration gradient without requiring energy.

plasma membrane Outer layer of the cell.

solute Dissolved substance.

transport proteins Large protein molecules that move specific substances across a cell membrane.

ACTIVITIES

TRUE OR FALSE

1. A molecule will move from where it is at a lower concentration to where it is at greater concentration (i.e. up its concentration gradient).
2. Facilitated diffusion does not require energy.
3. The interstitial compartment is part of the extracellular compartment.
4. The cell membrane contains cholesterol.
5. Potassium is the principal extracellular ion.
6. Chloride ions are negatively charged.
7. Hyponatraemia means high sodium levels.
8. 0.9% normal saline is a hypertonic solution.
9. ADH reduces the loss of water in the urine.

FIND OUT MORE

1. What are organelles and their functions?
2. What are the factors affecting diffusion?
3. Discuss the effects of low potassium level on the cardiovascular system.
4. What do you understand by the term 'third fluid space'? What role does it play in fluid balance?
5. Explain what happens to fluid in the fluid compartments when a person is:
   (a) dehydrated
   (b) overhydrated.
6. What do you understand by the term secondary active transport?
7. Do mitochondria contain DNA?
8. In an active transport system, from where do the cells get their energy?

CHEMICAL SYMBOLS

Write the correct chemical symbols for the following electrolytes:

Potassium ____________________

Sodium ____________________

Bicarbonate____________________

Chloride ____________________

Organic phosphate ____________________

Sulphate ____________________

Calcium____________________

CONDITIONS

The following is a list of conditions that are associated with the subjects discussed in this chapter. Take some time and write notes about each of the conditions. You may make the notes taken from textbooks or other resources (e.g. people you work with in a clinical area) or you may make the notes about people you have cared for. If you are doing this, you must ensure that you adhere to the rules of confidentiality.

Water intoxication
Pulmonary oedema
Nausea and vomiting
Acidosis
Alkalosis

REFERENCES

Agency for Clinical Innovation (2019) Clinical guidelines. Burn patient management, 4th edn. https://aci.health.nsw.gov.au/__data/assets/pdf_file/0009/250020/Burn-patient-management-guidelines.pdf (accessed December 2020).

Hilton, A.K, Pellegrino, V.A. and Scheinkestel, C.D. (2008) Avoiding common problems associated with intravenous fluid therapy. *Medical Journal of Australia* 189(9): 509– 513.

Levett-Jones, T. (2013). *Clinical Reasoning: Learning to Think Like a Nurse.* Pearson Australia.

Nair, M. and Peate, I. (2009) *Fundamentals of Applied Pathophysiology: An Essential Guide for Nursing Students*. Oxford: John Wiley & Sons, Ltd.

O'Connor, C.M. and Adams, J.U. (2010) *Essentials of Cell Biology*. Cambridge, MA: NPG Education, 2010. www.nature.com/scitable/ebooks/essentials-of-cell-biology-14749010/122997196 (accessed June 2019).

Peate, I. and Nair, M. (2011) *Fundamentals of Anatomy and Physiology for Student Nurses*. Chichester: John Wiley & Sons, Ltd.

Therapeutic Guidelines (2020) Electrolyte abnormalities: hyponatraemia. eTG complete. www.tg.org.au (accessed December 2020).

Tortora, G.J. and Derrickson, B.H. (2009) *Principles of Anatomy and Physiology*, 12th edn. Hoboken, NJ: John Wiley & Sons, Inc.

FURTHER READING

DIABETES INSIPIDUS

Better Health (2020) Introduction. www.betterhealth.vic.gov.au/health/ConditionsAndTreatments/diabetes-insipidus (accessed 4 December 2020).

Useful Australian government website for up-to-date information on diseases you may come across in practice.

ELECTROLYTES AND ELECTROLYTE BALANCE

Best Practice Advocacy Centre New Zealand (2011) A primary care approach to sodium and potassium imbalance. https://bpac.org.nz/BT/2011/September/docs/best_tests_sep2011_imbalance_pages_2-14.pdf (accessed 20 June 2019).

Felman, A. (2017) Everything you need to know about electrolytes. www.medicalnewstoday.com/articles/153188.php (accessed 25 February 2020).

Lederer, E., Nayak, V., Alsauskas, Z.C. and Mackelaite, L. (2018) Hyperkalemia treatment and management. http://emedicine.medscape.com/article/240903-treatment (accessed 20 June 2019).

ACKNOWLEDGEMENTS

Photo: © shansekala / iStockphoto / Getty Images

Photo: © Nonlani / Shutterstock.com

Photo: © successo images / Shutterstock.com

Photo: © Farion_O / Shutterstock.com

Photo: © Odilon Dimier / PhotoAlto / Getty Images

Figure 2.6: © Designua / Shutterstock.com

CHAPTER 3

Genetics

TEST YOUR PRIOR KNOWLEDGE

- What are the four bases that are found in DNA and what is their role in the double helix?
- If we have a DNA base sequence of ACATGGCTA, what would the corresponding RNA bases be?
- What is happening during the interphase stage of the cell cycle?
- What do we mean by Mendelian inheritance?
- What is the difference between autosomal recessive inheritance and autosomal dominant inheritance?

LEARNING OUTCOMES

After reading this chapter you will be able to:

3.1 explain what genes and alleles are and their importance to our health
3.2 describe the basics of the DNA double helix and chromosomes
3.3 understand and describe protein synthesis, including transcription and translation
3.4 explain the cell cycle and cell division
3.5 understand Mendelian inheritance patterns: autosomal dominant, recessive and X-linked
3.6 describe the basics of non-Mendelian inheritance patterns.

Cellular anatomical map

FIGURE 3.1 (a–c) The cell nucleus

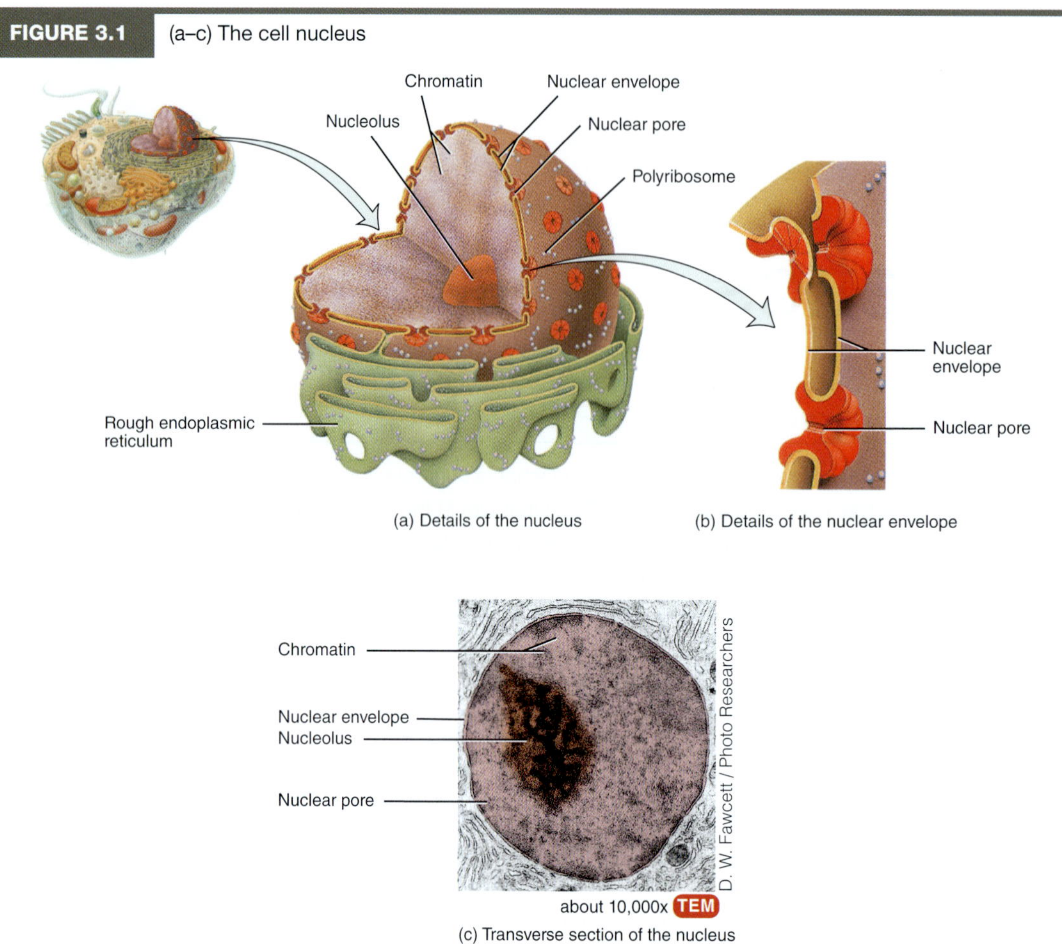

(a) Details of the nucleus

(b) Details of the nuclear envelope

(c) Transverse section of the nucleus

Source: Tortora and Derrickson (2014). Reproduced with permission of John Wiley & Sons.

Introduction

Genetics is an area of rapid knowledge expansion, which makes it fascinating and increasingly complex. Genetics is also incredibly important as it includes the understanding of what makes us human: our **DNA** and the **genes** it carries. In addition, many health problems are directly caused by errors to genes and other health problems are influenced by our genetics.

So, what are genes? Genes are sections of deoxyribonucleic acid (DNA) that are carried within our **chromosomes**. Genes contain sets of instructions to make particular proteins, which allow us to function. Your genes direct all your activities including growth, development and ageing, reproduction, general health and functioning, in conjunction with the environmental influences you experience. Our genetic material, which is inherited from our parents, gets expressed as characteristics or traits, known as **phenotypes**. So, although we share many similar features with our biological relations, each of us is genetically unique. In this chapter we will understand the role our genes play in these similarities and differences and how this is important to health and disease.

3.1 Deoxyribonucleic acid (DNA) and ribonucleic acid (RNA)

LEARNING OBJECTIVE 3.1 Explain what genes and alleles are and their importance to our health.

Genes are sections of DNA that contain the information for making the proteins that are vital to normal function. To assist in understanding how DNA determines our individuality and function, let's start by defining a few terms.

DNA	Deoxyribonucleic acid — part of the two polynucleotide chains wrapped around each other to form the three-dimensional **double helix** structure
RNA	Ribonucleic acid, normally single-stranded, transcribed from DNA
mRNA	Messenger RNA — RNA that carries information from DNA to the **ribosomes**, working together with ribosomes to assemble proteins from **amino acids**
tRNA	Transfer RNA — plays a key role in the **translation** process by delivering specific amino acids to the ribosome according to the mRNA sequence

The capacity of our cells to replicate their own DNA constitutes the basis of all **hereditary** transmission. This is because it allows us to produce new cells that have the identical information to existing cells, and to make the reproductive cells, the **gametes** (eggs and sperm), that create new life. We will examine these processes in more detail later. The other major function of DNA is as a template for the synthesis of RNA. There are many types of RNA, with mRNA holding the message from DNA that provides the instructions to synthesise proteins with the assistance of tRNA, rRNA and some enzymes. Proteins perform many of the functions of cells and hence are important in determining our own unique features.

DNA is contained within the nucleus of our cells as a molecular structure known as chromatin — a complex of DNA wound around a particular type of protein (**histone protein**). Each length of chromatin, known as a chromosome, houses a proportion of the roughly 30 000 genes that are needed to make a human. Each nucleated cell has 23 pairs of chromosomes within its nucleus. Chromosomes are considered a pair if they have the same genes on them. As each pair has a different number and set of genes, each pair is unique and so we can identify each of the 23 pairs of human chromosomes by their **nucleic acid** structure. The human chromosomes are designated as chromosomes 1 through 22, known as autosomal chromosomes, and the 23rd pair are the sex chromosomes, X and Y: either two X chromosomes in females or one X chromosome and one Y chromosome in males. The only exception to this is the cells involved in reproduction. These cells, called gametes — **ova** (eggs) from the mother and **spermatozoa** (sperm) from the father, have just one copy of each chromosome (i.e. 23 chromosomes in total).

Some people do not have 46 chromosomes. These individuals have an aneuploidy, which is an abnormal number of chromosomes in cells. People with Down syndrome, for example, have 47 chromosomes, with three copies of chromosome 21 (a condition known as trisomy 21), while people with Turner syndrome (also known as 45,X), have only 45 chromosomes, as they have only one sex chromosome, an X chromosome (Crespi 2008). There are also instances where people have extra or missing parts of chromosomes. We will consider this and other gross chromosomal abnormalities later in this chapter.

CLINICALLY REASONED EPISODE OF CARE

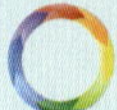

Turner syndrome

Consider the patient situation

Carly is a school-aged girl who has presented to the school nurse with recurrent ear infections. She communicates with the nurse that she has Turner syndrome. Carly has not previously disclosed this information as it is important to her to live a 'normal' life.

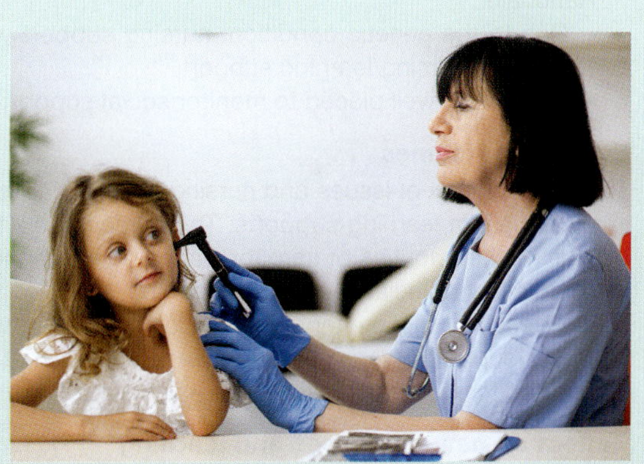

Collect cues and information

The nurse observes that Carly does not have some of the typical markers of Turner syndrome; for example, stature, thickened neck or swollen hands. Carly states that she is currently on growth hormone treatment.

Carly expresses concern about the social implications of her condition and her desire to remain independent.

Process information

Turner syndrome is a genetic condition that affects 1 in 2000 girls born in Australia each year (NSW Government, Centre for Genetics Education 2018). Females with this condition experience a variety of symptoms that vary in severity with the degree of chromosomal abnormality. Girls with Turner syndrome may be missing a complete X chromosome, or just part of one, and it may be missing from all their cells, or only some cells (a phenomenon known as mosaicism). A diagnosis of Turner syndrome is made by counting the chromosomes in the nuclei of white blood cells from a sample of the child's blood — a procedure known as a karyotype analysis.

Turner syndrome is characterised by several physical abnormalities and learning disabilities, particularly around mathematics and spatial awareness. It can affect the onset of puberty and lead to social isolation.

Narrowed eustachian tubes within the ear are characteristic of Turner syndrome, hence recurrent ear infections are common. Frequent ear infections and build-up of fluid in the middle ear can lead to permanent damage to the eardrum and other structures and may result in permanent hearing loss. Hearing loss can delay learning and may result in poor school performance.

Additionally, those with Turner syndrome have difficulties with mathematics and map reading due to impaired spatial awareness, which contributes to impaired learning and development. Approximately 8 in 10 girls will experience difficulties in this area, along with challenges in understanding social relationships.

This is a lifelong issue for Carly, who is at a vulnerable age. Adolescence, and the associated hormonal, physical and social changes associated with puberty, can be a difficult time for young people, and particularly so for those with genetic conditions and learning disabilities.

Identify problems/issues

1. Recurrent ear infections
2. Hearing loss and learning
3. Genetic disposition to learning difficulties
4. Social implications

Nursing actions

1. Assess the need for medical input/treatment for ear infection.
   Rationale:
   - Ear infections are often painful and distressing for individuals.
   - A current ear infection represents an acute issue and may require treatment to avoid ongoing damage such as tympanic membrane scarring, mastoiditis, and in severe cases meningitis. It is important that recurrent ear infections are treated in a timely manner to avoid damage to the ear structures and subsequent hearing loss.
2. In consultation with Carly and her parents, refer to audiology.
   Rationale:
   - A hearing specialist can assess Carly's current hearing status.
   - Appropriate interventions and monitoring of hearing can ensure that Carly's hearing loss is minimised.
   - This information may inform learning plans and school support.
3. In consultation with Carly and her parents, liaise with school departments.
   Rationale:
   - This provides an avenue to educate other education professionals on the effects of genetic issues and hearing loss on learning. It ensures ongoing support to facilitate learning.
   - It provides an avenue for ongoing social support.
4. Monitor progress and provide ongoing support to Carly and her family.
   Rationale:
   - Due to the genetic condition, nursing support will likely be ongoing. This provides an avenue for ongoing nursing/learning support.
   - Nurses are well placed to monitor social support needs.

Evaluate outcomes

The identification of issues and nursing actions has led to investigation of Carly's hearing status and an improvement in learning supports. The nurse is able to use a variety of clinical and non-clinical cues to determine the priorities of care for Carly and relate these back to the context of learning. These include the medical and social needs of the person.

As a result of these interventions, Carly's hearing was assessed and a hearing deficit was identified. Learning supports were put in place to ensure that her identified deficits in spatial awareness were accounted for in learning situations. As a result, Carly reports feeling more confident at school.

Reflect on new processes and learning

Reflect on the scenario above and the clinical reasoning cycle. How has the disclosure of the genetic anomaly Turner syndrome impacted nursing actions for Carly?

Source: Based on the Clinical Reasoning Cycle, Levett-Jones (2013).

3.2 The DNA double helix

LEARNING OBJECTIVE 3.2 Describe the basics of the DNA double helix and chromosomes.

The structure of the DNA double helix was determined in the 1950s by James Watson and Francis Crick, following the work in X-ray diffraction by Rosalind Franklin. The structure is vital to our cellular functioning, as it allows cells to make exact copies of their DNA and assists in repairing small errors. The double helix is made up of two **strands** of DNA, which consist of chemical complexes known as **nucleotides** strung together. A nucleotide consists of three chemical groups:

- **deoxyribose** — a five-carbon cyclic sugar
- *phosphate* — an inorganic, negatively charged phosphorous-containing molecule
- **base** — a nitrogen-carbon ring structure, of which there are four types found in DNA:
  - **adenine (A)**
  - **thymine (T)**
  - **guanine (G)**
  - **cytosine (C)**.

> Adenine (A) and guanine (G) are **purines** with two-carbon nitrogen rings.
> Thymine (T) and cytosine (C) are **pyrimidines** with one single ring.

These strings of nucleotides twist around forming a spiral molecule resembling a ladder. The sides of the ladder are formed by the deoxyribose-phosphate groups of the nucleotides. The rungs are formed by the bases of one strand interacting with the bases of the other strand and therefore hold the sides of the ladder together. The double helix is said to be antiparallel. The two strands that interact to form the double helix run in opposite ends to form a stable helix — one strand runs from 5' to the 3' end, while the other runs from 3' to 5', permitting complementary base pairing between the bases to form a stable double helix. It is the sequence of these nucleotides and their specific bases (the rungs) along the length of the ladder-like DNA molecule that holds the genetic code. There is a strict rule governing which bases will interact with each other to form the rungs of the DNA ladder, and it is that adenine (A) will only bind to thymine (T), and guanine (G) will only bind to cytosine (C). So if, for example, one strand of DNA has a base sequence AGGCAGTGC, then the opposite strand will have the complementary base sequence, which will be TCCGTCACG; you can see this in figure 3.2.

FIGURE 3.2 A pictorial representation of a portion of the double helix

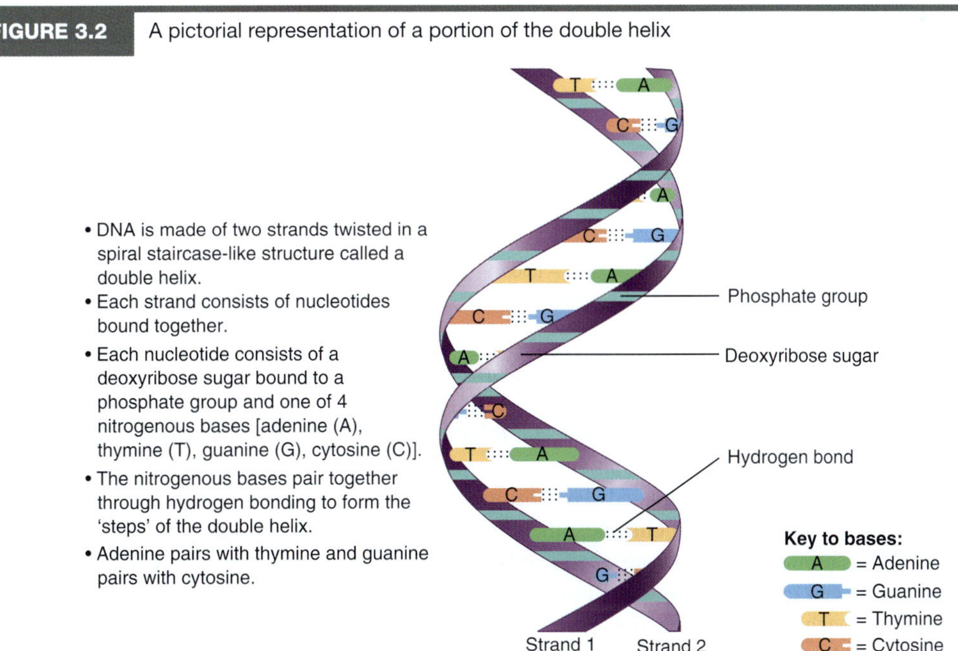

Source: Tortora and Derrickson (2014). Reproduced with permission of John Wiley & Sons.

The complementary bases are held together by hydrogen bonds, whereas each nucleotide is held to the next with covalent bonds (these bonds were discussed in the chapter on basic scientific principles of physiology). Of the two types of chemical bonds, hydrogen bonds are weaker, which has implications for the processes of DNA replication and **transcription**, as you will see.

Chromosomes

Within the nucleus, the DNA of eukaryotes (organisms, including humans, whose cells contain a nucleus and other organelles enclosed within membranes) is contained as lengths of chromatin known as chromosomes. The histones are packaging proteins that bind to the DNA, providing structural integrity. As shown in figure 3.3, the DNA winds around the histones forming a **nucleosome**. Many nucleosomes are required to package one strand of DNA. If the DNA inside the nucleus of a human cell were stretched out, it would be approximately 2 metres long, but because it is so tightly coiled it fits into the nucleus, which is about six micrometres in diameter. Chromatin can either be loosely structured to allow the cell to expose the sequence of bases and use these instructions for making proteins, or at other times, tightly packaged into the 'X' structure, of the chromosome, which is the form it takes during cell division, which will be explained later.

FIGURE 3.3 DNA from double helix to chromosome

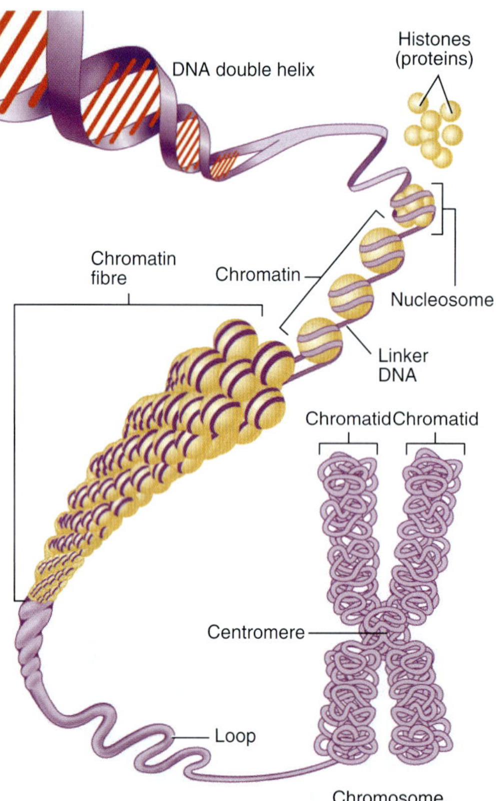

Source: Tortora and Derrickson (2009). Reproduced with permission of John Wiley & Sons.

The term chromosome can be confusing because it refers to each length of double-stranded DNA found in the nucleus (remember we have 46 in total), and also to a couplet of two strands of DNA, one a copy of the other, after the DNA has been replicated. The chromosome structure shown in figure 3.3 depicts DNA that has already been copied, so each chromosome is made up of two **chromatids** joined together at the **centromere**. DNA is replicated just before a cell needs to divide itself to make two new cells. This process occurs as part of the **cell cycle**, which we will look at later in this chapter.

In most humans, each nucleated cell (i.e. each cell with a nucleus) has 46 chromosomes, which occur as 23 pairs (figure 3.4). Of those 23 pairs, one pair determines the gender of the person.

- Females have a matched **homologous** (the same) pair of X chromosomes.
- Males have an unmatched **heterologous** (different) pair — one X and one Y chromosome.

- The remaining 22 pairs of chromosomes are known as **autosomes** (each pair is homologous as they have the same genes on them). In biology, the suffix 'some' means body, so autosome means 'self body'. Thus, 'autosomes' can be defined as the chromosomes that determine physical characteristics — in other words, all the characteristics of a person that are not connected with gender. This is not to say that the X and Y chromosomes only have genes for gender determination. The X chromosome contains hundreds of genes, including those for red-green colour vision, blood clotting and tooth enamel, to name a few. In contrast, the Y chromosome has only 70 genes or so, most of which are involved in determining male gender. So the majority of the genes of the X chromosome are not matched by a corresponding gene on the Y chromosome. This means that although the Y chromosome contains some of the same genes as the X chromosome, such as that for tooth enamel, most do not match the X chromosome genes, which has important implications for the inheritance of some genetic conditions, as discussed later in this chapter.

FIGURE 3.4 The chromosomes of a human male — a karyotype. Chromosomes only take on this particular shape during cell division. The assessment of karyotype can be performed to identify the presence of some genetic disorders. Each chromosome is identified by its size and 'banding' pattern following staining with particular dyes.

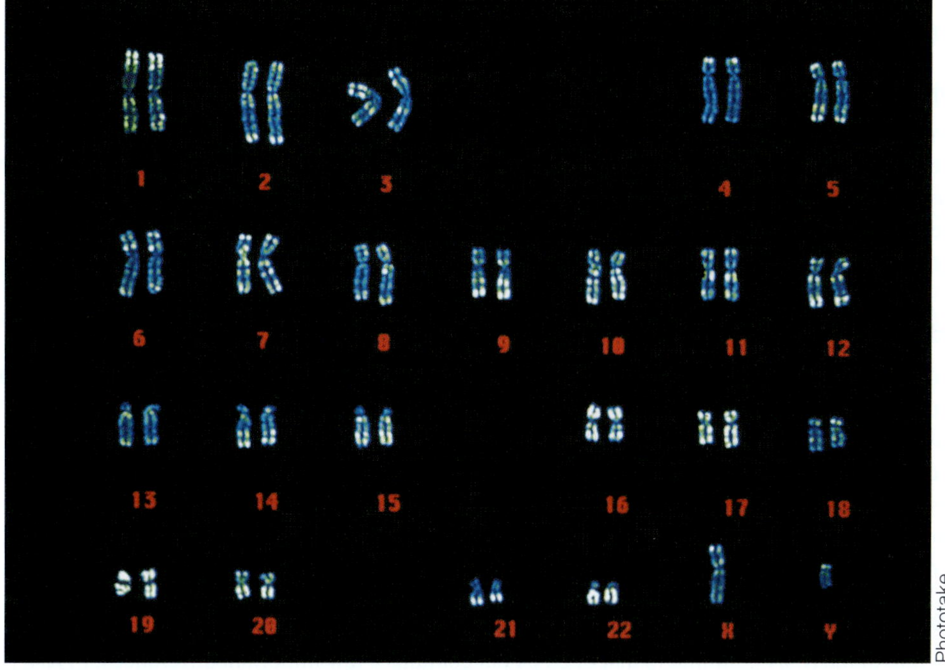

Source: Snustad and Simmons (2012). Reproduced with permission of John Wiley & Sons.

The position a gene occupies on a chromosome is called a **locus**, and there are different loci for eye colour, height, hair type, and so on ('loci' is the plural of 'locus'). Think of the locus as the address of that particular gene on Chromosome Street in the same way that a house number signifies where you live on your street.

Our autosomes occur in pairs, which means we have two pieces of DNA for each autosomal gene. Each version of a gene is known as an **allele**. So, we can say that alleles for each gene occur at the same loci on homologous chromosomes. As you inherited one of the chromosomes in the homologous pair from your mother and the other from your father, you therefore received one allele for each gene from your mother and one from your father. Alleles do not have to have exactly the same sequence of bases, although they will be very similar, but they do provide information for alternative forms of proteins that perform a particular function. Eye colour is a good example — if we consider that eyes are either brown or blue (there are other alternatives but these are governed by more complex factors that we will not consider here), then we know that there is one gene that determines eye colour located at the same place on each of the two chromosomes of a homologous pair. One allele of this gene will come from the father and the other from the mother. If a child's mother has blue eyes and the father has brown eyes, the child may have blue or brown eyes, depending upon factors that will be discussed later.

In the human population, a gene may have more than two possible alleles, but each individual person will only have two. A person with a pair of identical alleles for a particular gene locus is said to be **homozygous** for that gene, whereas someone with two different alleles is **heterozygous** for that gene. Whether you are homozygous or heterozygous for one gene will not influence whether you are homozygous or heterozygous for another gene. The alleles you have for a gene determine your **genotype** for that gene, so each individual has thousands of genotypes (one for each gene).

The allele combinations for a particular gene can interact in different ways to produce variations on the characteristic the gene is coding for. This is because some alleles are recessive and some are dominant.

- A **dominant allele** exerts its effect and is physically manifested (the phenotype) when present on at least one of the chromosomes of the pair, so you could have two dominant alleles (homozygous genotype) or have one dominant and one **recessive allele** (heterozygous genotype) and still show the same physical characteristic (phenotype).
- A recessive allele has to be present on both chromosomes to manifest itself physically (phenotype). So, to see the effect of a recessive allele, you have to have a homozygous genotype for that gene (or lack the dominant allele).

This will be explained more fully later in this chapter, but it is very important because of the significance that it has in hereditary disorders.

3.3 Gene expression: from DNA to proteins

LEARNING OBJECTIVE 3.3 Understand and describe protein synthesis, including transcription and translation.

Gene expression is the process by which the information contained in DNA (within the nucleus) is made available to the cell. DNA molecules within nucleic acid strands have two major functions: to direct protein synthesis, and to faithfully carry genetic information from one generation of cells to the next, and from one generation of individuals to the next. This occurs in two processes called transcription and translation, whereby the DNA information is transferred from DNA to RNA to proteins.

Protein synthesis

Synthesis simply means 'production'; hence the production of protein from raw materials. The instructions for making proteins are found in DNA, so to synthesise proteins the genetic information encoded in the DNA has to be turned into a corresponding sequence of protein building blocks (amino acids).

This occurs in two processes: transcription and translation. The process of transcription creates a messenger RNA (mRNA) copy of the DNA. Transcription of a gene is similar to transcribing information from a textbook onto a piece of paper that we can take with us, leaving the book in the library. During translation, the mRNA code is 'read' and turned into a protein molecule.

Structural differences between DNA and RNA

The structure of the RNA is similar to that of DNA but contains a few important differences. In RNA, ribose replaces 2' deoxyribose, and the base thymine is replaced by another base, **uracil**, which in turn forms a base pair with adenine (further details are discussed later in this chapter). Moreover, RNA molecules usually exist as a single polynucleotide strand that does not form a double helix like the DNA.

Transcription

DNA has to be transcribed into RNA, because DNA is 'stuck' in the nucleus due to its size, whereas proteins need to be synthesised in the ribosomes, within the cell's cytoplasm (see the chapter on cells, cellular compartments, transport systems, fluid movement between compartments). Using a specific portion of DNA (a gene) as a template, the genetic information stored in the sequence of bases of DNA is rewritten so that the same information appears in the bases of RNA. To do this, the two strands of the DNA have to separate (figure 3.5). This is achieved by momentarily breaking the hydrogen bonds that pair each of the bases in the double helix strands together. The exposed bases are now available to pair with their complementary bases by hydrogen bonding (remember the base-pairing rule) with the aid of an enzyme called **RNA polymerase**. However, this time the bases are on RNA nucleotides, so the new molecule is RNA, specifically messenger RNA (mRNA).

As with DNA, guanine can only pair with cytosine in RNA. But while the thymine in DNA only binds to adenine in the RNA, there is no thymine in RNA, so adenine binds to the RNA base uracil (U), which does not occur in the DNA molecule.

DNA	mRNA
guanine (G)	cytosine (C)
cytosine (C)	guanine (G)
thymine (T)	adenine (A)
adenine (A)	uracil (U)

FIGURE 3.5 The separation of DNA for transcription. A small segment of DNA containing the gene to be transcribed opens up as the hydrogen bonds between complementary bases are temporarily broken. A strand of RNA with the help of an enzyme called RNA polymerase is then formed. Once finished, the DNA bonds itself back to the original helical structure and is released.

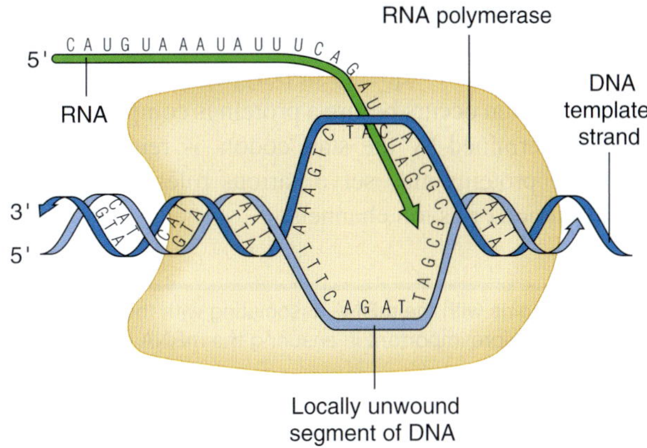

Source: Snustad and Simmons (2012). Reproduced with permission of John Wiley & Sons.

For example, if DNA has a base sequence AGGCAGTGC, then the complementary base sequence on mRNA will be UCCGUCACG. Figure 3.5 demonstrates the way in which the DNA separates to allow the RNA to be formed with the same information as one of the DNA strands in that region.

In addition to the sequence of bases in DNA that provide the code for the body's proteins, some regions of DNA provide important regulatory information. DNA can therefore be loosely classified as being part of an exon or an intron (also referred to as coding or non-coding regions respectively). Bases within exons provide the amino acid order for the protein and bases in introns direct regulation of protein synthesis activities, such as when and how much of each protein should be made. Other non-exon parts of DNA determine where each individual gene starts and finishes. The interspersing of introns among the exons of a gene also allows alternate forms of mRNA to be generated from the same gene, and this partly explains why we have over 100 000 proteins but only around 30 000 genes.

The removal of introns following transcription is known as splicing and results in the formation of the mature mRNA molecule. The mRNA is therefore a copy of a section of a chromosome small enough to be transported out of the nucleus ready for the next step: translation. However, in addition to serving as the template for the synthesis of mRNA, DNA also provides the information for the synthesis of other kinds of RNA (more research continues to find new types of RNA), two of which, ribosomal RNA (rRNA) and transfer RNA (tRNA), are also essential for the translation step of protein synthesis. rRNA, together with the ribosomal proteins, makes up the ribosomes, and tRNA matches the code on the mRNA with the correct amino acids.

Translation

In genetics, translation is the process by which the specific sequence of bases in mRNA is used to specify the amino acid sequence of a protein. There are 20 different amino acids from which our proteins are assembled.

Translation occurs in the cell's cytoplasm and involves the three types of RNA, mentioned above, as well as ribosomal proteins. The following depicts the sequence of the major steps of protein synthesis, also shown in figures 3.6 and 3.7.

- In the cytoplasm, a small and a large ribosomal subunit assemble around the start of the mRNA molecule to provide the platform where the mRNA is decoded into amino acids.

- Each mRNA has a group of three bases (**codon**) which the tRNA matches by complementary base pairing. Each amino acid is also attached to a specific tRNA molecule. Each tRNA has a unique sequence of three bases, known as an **anticodon**, which determines the particular amino acid it is attached to. The translation process is initiated when the first tRNA (with the corresponding amino acid, methionine) is attached to the start codon on the mRNA.
- Subsequently, the next tRNA with complementary anticodon matching the mRNA codon attaches itself to the adjacent site. An enzyme called **peptidyl transferase** forms a peptide bond between the amino acids, allowing the nascent protein molecule to grow. In this way the mRNA is decoded by tRNAs and the correct amino acids are added to the growing protein molecule, as determined by the sequence of codons in the mRNA. This step is called **elongation**. Sequences of three bases in DNA (known as **triplets**) therefore relate to the sequence of codons in mRNA. Correspondingly, the four bases present in DNA can combine in various ways to form 64 different mRNA codons, of which three codons act as stop signals for the translation process to terminate, and the remaining 61 (including the start codon) encode the 20 amino acids that present as building blocks for proteins.
- The translation process is terminated when a stop codon is reached. The ribosome then detaches itself from the mRNA and releases the protein sequence or polypeptide. Subsequently, moderate to extensive post-translational modification often occurs before a protein is complete. For example, the initial amino acid called methionine, as determined by the start codon, is removed from the polypeptide chain. Depending on the type, these proteins may serve various roles in the organism such as enzymatic reactions, cellular support function or as ion channels.

FIGURE 3.6 (a, b) Translation begins with the mRNA associating with the small and large ribosomal subunits. The ribosome is therefore important in ensuring the mRNA is decoded as the correct groups of three bases (codons).

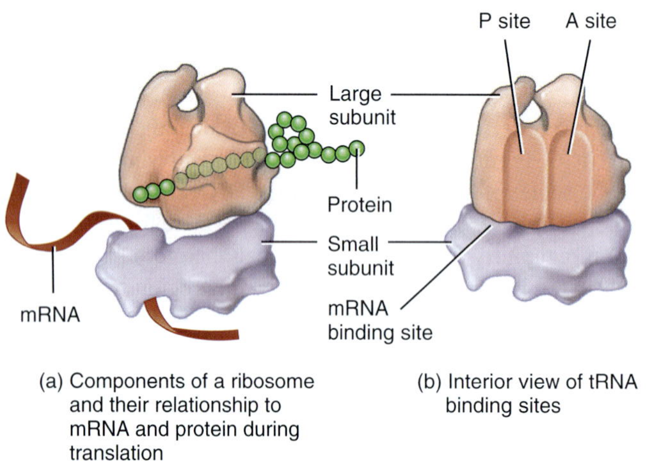

Source: Tortora and Derrickson (2009). Reproduced with permission of John Wiley & Sons.

Let's look at this process in a little more detail, as shown in figure 3.7.

- The tRNAs attach to their associated amino acids.
- The ribosome attaches to the mRNA at the site that designates the start of the protein.
- The ribosome has 'sites' within it that line up with the codons of the mRNA.
- The tRNAs attempt to bond their anticodons with the mRNA codon that is lined up with the ribosome. Only the tRNA with the complementary anticodon to the codon will be able to bind (because of complementary base pairing). For example, only the tRNA with the anticodon UAC can bind if the mRNA codon is AUG (start codon) to begin the protein translation **initiation** step. As a result, the 'correct' amino acid is put into the right place in the amino acid chain. Note this base pairing of codon and anticodon only occurs when the mRNA is attached to a ribosome.
- The ribosome now moves along the mRNA strand to initiate the elongation step in the translation process so that the next codon is lined up in the ribosome; now the second tRNA anticodon moves into position.
- The adjacent amino acids on the two tRNAs are joined to each other by a peptide bond (through the action of the ribosome). The first tRNA detaches itself from the mRNA strand and binds a new molecule of its specific amino acid. This continues the elongation process.

- Meanwhile, the ribosome continues moving along the strand of mRNA, and the process repeats, creating a progressively larger protein chain during the elongation step until the protein specified by the mRNA strand (which was initially specified by the genes on the DNA strand) is complete — in other words, the correct number of amino acids have been joined together in the correct order.
- The addition of amino acids is stopped when the stop or **termination codon** (a combination of three bases that signals the protein is complete) on the mRNA is reached. This process is called **termination**. The newly assembled protein and the mRNA are released from the ribosome.

FIGURE 3.7 Summary of the movement of the ribosome along mRNA

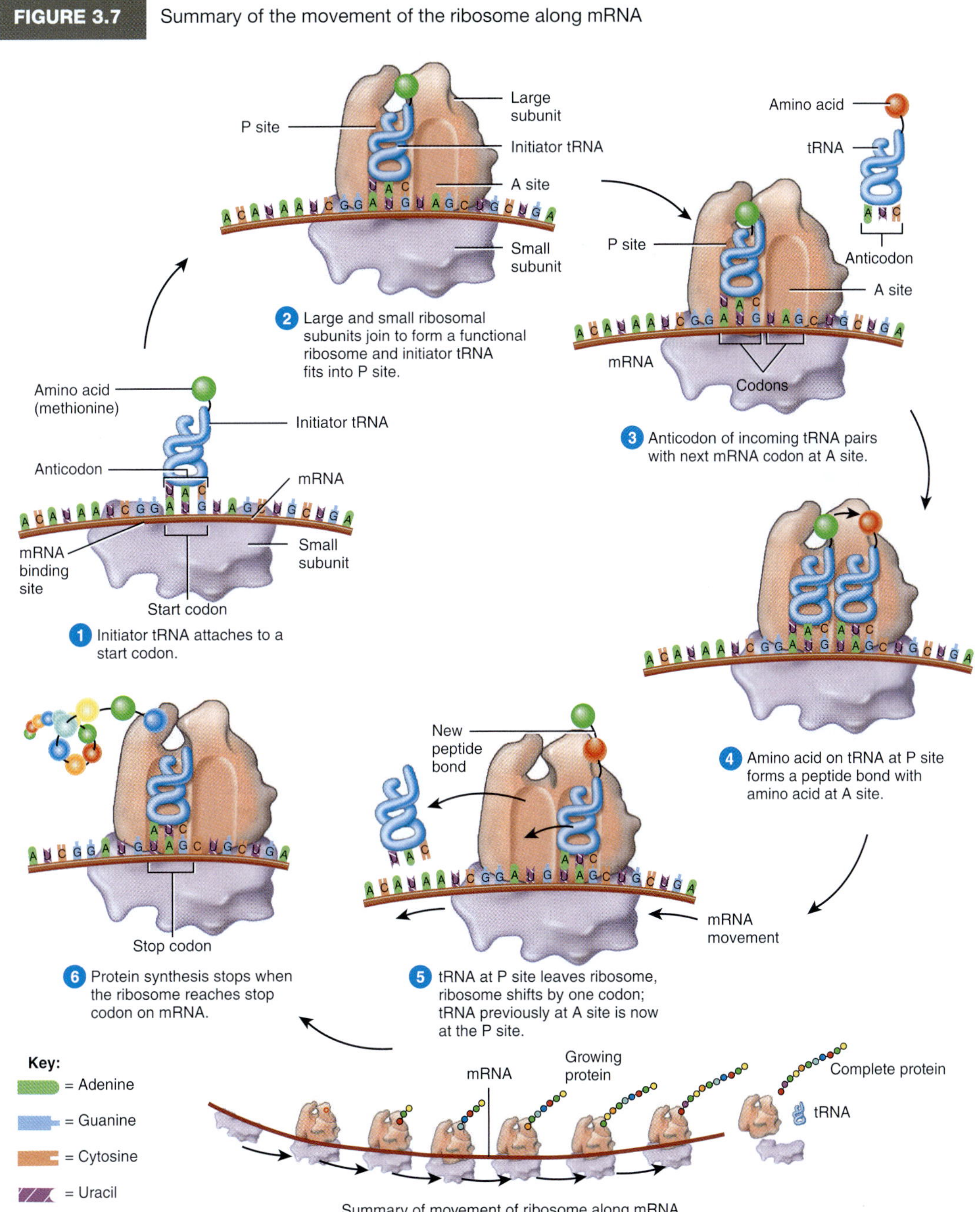

Source: Tortora and Derrickson (2009). Reproduced with permission of John Wiley & Sons.

Although understanding the process of protein synthesis may take a while, the process itself is very quick. In fact, protein synthesis progresses at the rate of about 15 amino acids per second. In addition, as the ribosome moves along the mRNA strand it vacates the starting point of the mRNA allowing another ribosome to assemble at that place (figure 3.7). In this way, many molecules of the same protein are made from a single strand of mRNA at one time. Hence, more protein will be made than the amount of mRNA that was made.

In genetics, the concept of mutation is an important one, with many implications for health. Mutation is a permanent change to the sequence of bases in the DNA double helix. Mutations can be brought about by external agents (like UV radiation from the sun) or internal agents (like highly reactive free radicals) that damage the DNA. They can also result from a copying error when DNA is replicating (making a copy of itself) prior to a cell dividing. Fortunately, cells are equipped to repair much of the damage that occurs, but major errors may be irreparable. A mutation that causes a change to the sequence of DNA bases will flow on and result in an incorrect mRNA and amino acid sequence, resulting in an incorrect protein structure. This can lead to dysfunctional proteins and genetic disease. Further, if a mutation is present in one or both of our gametes (i.e. ovum or sperm), then it can be passed on to our children, leading to familial genetic disorders such as Huntington's disease (autosomal dominant), cystic fibrosis (autosomal recessive) and haemophilia (X-linked).

Summary of relationship between DNA, RNA and protein

We can now define a gene as a sequence of nucleotides on a DNA molecule that serves as the master recipe for manufacturing a specific protein.

- Genes are on average about 1000 pairs of nucleotides long.
- The base sequence of the gene determines the base sequence of the mRNA.
- The base sequence of the mRNA determines the amino acid sequence of the protein coded by that gene.
- No two genes have exactly the same sequence of nucleotides. Each gene has a number of possible alleles (slight variations in nucleotide sequence) that will produce variation in the mRNA and therefore in the protein sequence and this is the fundamental reason for variation between individuals in our population.

MEDICINES MANAGEMENT

Three-parent babies

This is a very new procedure aimed at preventing mitochondrial disorders being passed on to new generations. Mitochondria, the ATP-producing organelles, also contain their own piece of DNA that houses the genes required for the cell's energy production. Mutations in mitochondrial DNA can result in serious, often fatal, diseases resulting in muscle wastage, nerve damage, loss of sight or heart failure. These diseases are passed on to offspring from the mother, as the mitochondria in the cells of any offspring come from the mother. Approximately 1 in 4000 women are clinically affected or are at risk for developing a mitochondrial mutation in their eggs.

In January 2015, the UK became the first country to allow what have become known as 'three-parent babies'. The DNA from the mother's egg is placed into a donor egg that has had its nuclear DNA removed. This egg is then fertilised in vitro by the father's sperm (so the nuclear DNA is the usual combination of maternal and paternal DNA). The mitochondria of the donor egg remain and will be the source of new mitochondria in the cells of the child. The resulting child will have three biological parents — the mother and father (who supplied the nuclear DNA), and the woman who supplied the mitochondria and other organelles. The child will be the genetic offspring of the mother and father as the nuclear DNA is the major determinant of a person's phenotype. But, as a result of the donor mitochondria, which are free of mutations, the child, and, if a girl, her descendants, will not suffer the effects of mutations carried in the DNA of her mother's mitochondria.

Since this procedure introduces genetic changes that will be passed on from female three-parent babies, there are ethical concerns about the use of this process. There are also health concerns, as this technology is still in its infancy and the long-term effects of manipulating an egg in this way have not yet been established. Therefore, more research and tight regulatory controls around procedures such as these need to be in place, to ensure that the risks of the procedure do not outweigh the benefits.

See Poulton (2016).

3.4 The transference of genes — the cell cycle

LEARNING OBJECTIVE 3.4 Explain the cell cycle and cell division.

This section explains how genetic information is transferred from existing cells to new cells, and also from parents to children. First, we will look at how cells pass on genetic information to new cells.

Cells must be able to divide and create new cells for growth and to replace dead and damaged cells. The new cells must all contain a complete set of the genetic information (the DNA) that was in the original cell, which means cells must replicate their DNA accurately prior to dividing into two cells. The process by which cells divide their DNA to produce two new cells is known as **mitosis**. All human cells undergo a cell cycle, during which they are either actively undergoing mitosis, or undertaking their normal functions and preparing for mitosis.

While cells reproduce themselves by simple mitotic division, individuals reproduce by sexual reproduction, a process which involves the joining and mixing of genetic material from two different individuals (the father and the mother). In order to mix the chromosomes from two individuals and not end up with twice the normal amount of chromosomes, gametes (sperm and egg) which contain only half the normal number of chromosomes are used. The process by which gametes are produced is known as **meiosis**.

Whether mitosis or meiosis is occurring, an exact copy of the cell's DNA must first be made (replication). During this process the two strands of the DNA separate, exposing the bases, which can now pair with their complementary bases on free nucleotides, and a new copy of each strand of the DNA is made (see figure 3.8).

FIGURE 3.8 DNA replication. To make additional chromosomes to distribute to new cells, DNA has to be replicated by first separating the two strands, and then creating a new complementary strand for each of the original strands. At the end of this process the cell will have two identical chromatids, each consisting of an 'old' and a 'new' strand.

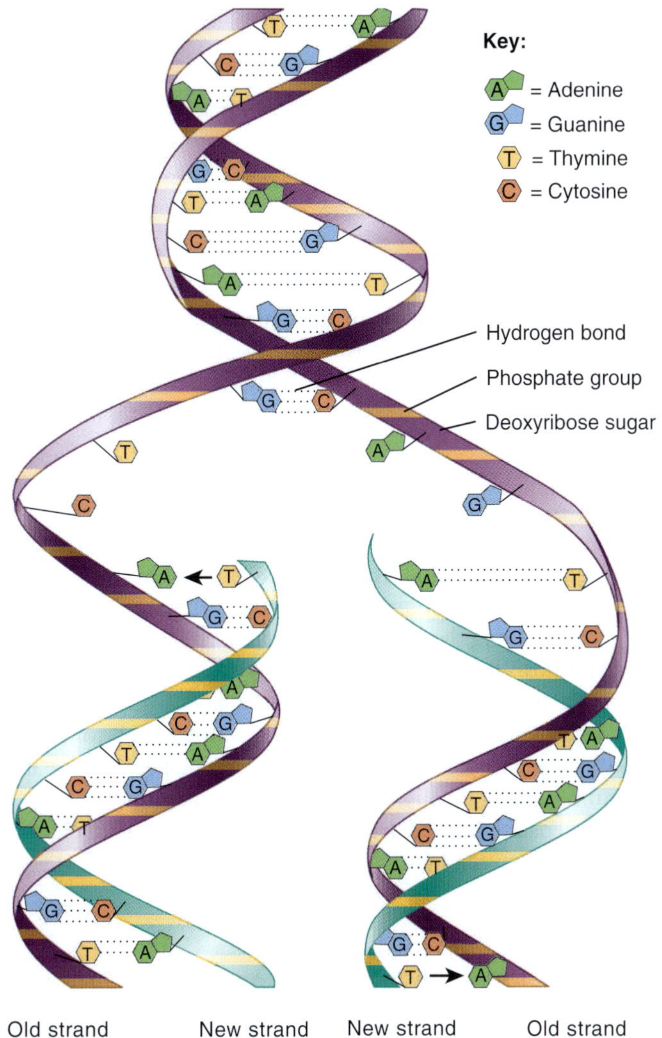

Source: Tortora and Derrickson (2009). Reproduced with permission of John Wiley & Sons.

At the end of DNA replication, each of the 46 chromosomes will have an exact duplicate of itself. Each chromosome will exist as two identical chromatids joined by a centromere. This process occurs in the stage of the cell cycle known as **interphase**. Interphase is also the stage during which the cell will undertake its normal everyday functions. At the end of interphase, the cell will commence mitosis if it is one of the body's somatic cells or meiosis if it is one of the body's gamete-producing cells. Note that once mitosis/meiosis is complete, the cell will again be in interphase. Indeed, if we look at the cell cycle (figure 3.9), we see that the cell spends the majority of time in interphase. During this period, in addition to producing the extra DNA, the cell must also increase the number of organelles such as mitochondria.

FIGURE 3.9 The cell cycle

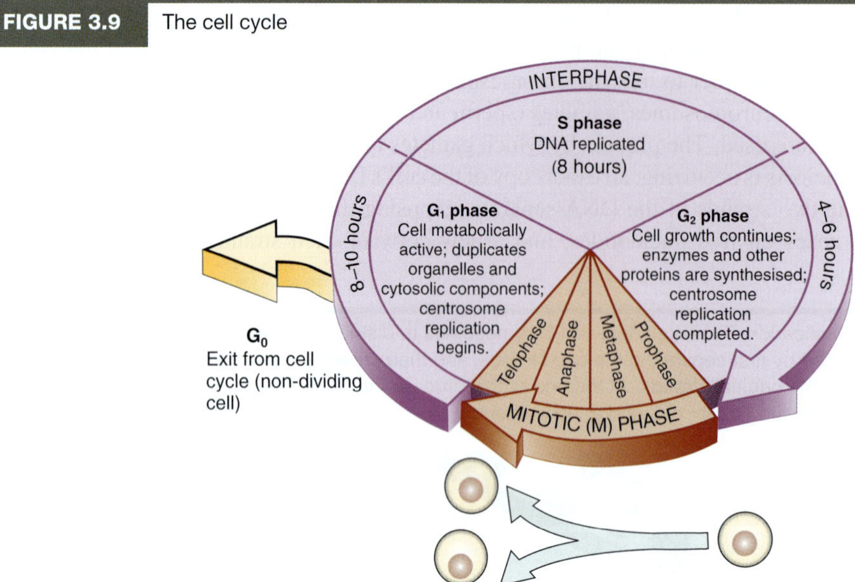

Source: Tortora and Derrickson (2009). Reproduced with permission of John Wiley & Sons.

Mitosis

The process of mitosis produces two identical diploid daughter cells, each with 46 chromosomes, from one cell. This process occurs in four stages (after interphase): prophase, metaphase, anaphase and telophase, with specific events occurring in each stage (shown in figure 3.10). Note that for simplicity, only a few chromosomes are shown. In adults, mitosis plays a role in cell replacement, wound healing and tumour formation.

During interphase, the individual chromosomes in the nucleus are difficult to see because they are in the form of uncoiled threads so that they can be replicated and used for transcription. However, during mitosis the chromosomes are tightly packaged into discrete units (chromosomes, depicted in figure 3.3) so they can be accurately and equally divided to form daughter cells, and not be damaged during this process. During this first step in mitosis the cell also produces spindle fibres, specialised structures that attach to the chromosomes and assist in aligning them along the centre of the cell.

During the early stages of mitosis the nuclear envelope dissolves, leaving the chromosomes temporarily in the cytoplasm. The spindle fibres extend from opposite sides of the cell (**poles**) and attach to each chromosome, one from each pole. The spindle fibres then contract back towards the poles, pulling the chromatids apart and towards each pole. The spindle fibres disappear, and a nuclear envelope forms around each set of 46 chromosomes. Finally, the cytoplasm is also divided via cytoplasm constriction (cytokinesis) to produce two separate and identical cells, each containing 46 chromosomes. The cell then enters interphase — the interval between mitotic divisions.

Meiosis

Meiosis is the form of cell division used only to produce the gametes (i.e. male sperm and female ova).

The cells of the human body that contain 23 pairs of chromosomes (46 in total) are referred to as **diploid cells**. Gametes, on the other hand, possess only 23 chromosomes, and are referred to as **haploid cells**. Therefore, when gametes fuse during reproduction, the combined DNA from both gametes equals 46 chromosomes. Gametes develop from cells with 46 chromosomes, and through the process of meiosis end up with 23 chromosomes.

Meiosis is divided into eight stages, in contrast to the four of mitosis, occurring as two meiotic divisions: meiosis I and meiosis II. The stages have the same names as those occurring during mitosis, since they describe similar events. There are, however, some important differences between the two meiotic divisions, so to distinguish these we identify the four stages of meiosis I as prophase I, metaphase I, anaphase I, telophase I, and the four stages of meiosis II as prophase II, metaphase II, anaphase II and telophase II. As with mitosis, these stages occur in a sequential fashion with the progression from one stage to the next tightly controlled.

FIGURE 3.10 The stages of the somatic cell cycle. Somatic cells are all the cells of the body except the gametes. When we need a new somatic cell, (a) the DNA is replicated during interphase, (b–e) the nucleus is divided by mitosis, (f) resulting in the formation of two identical daughter cells.

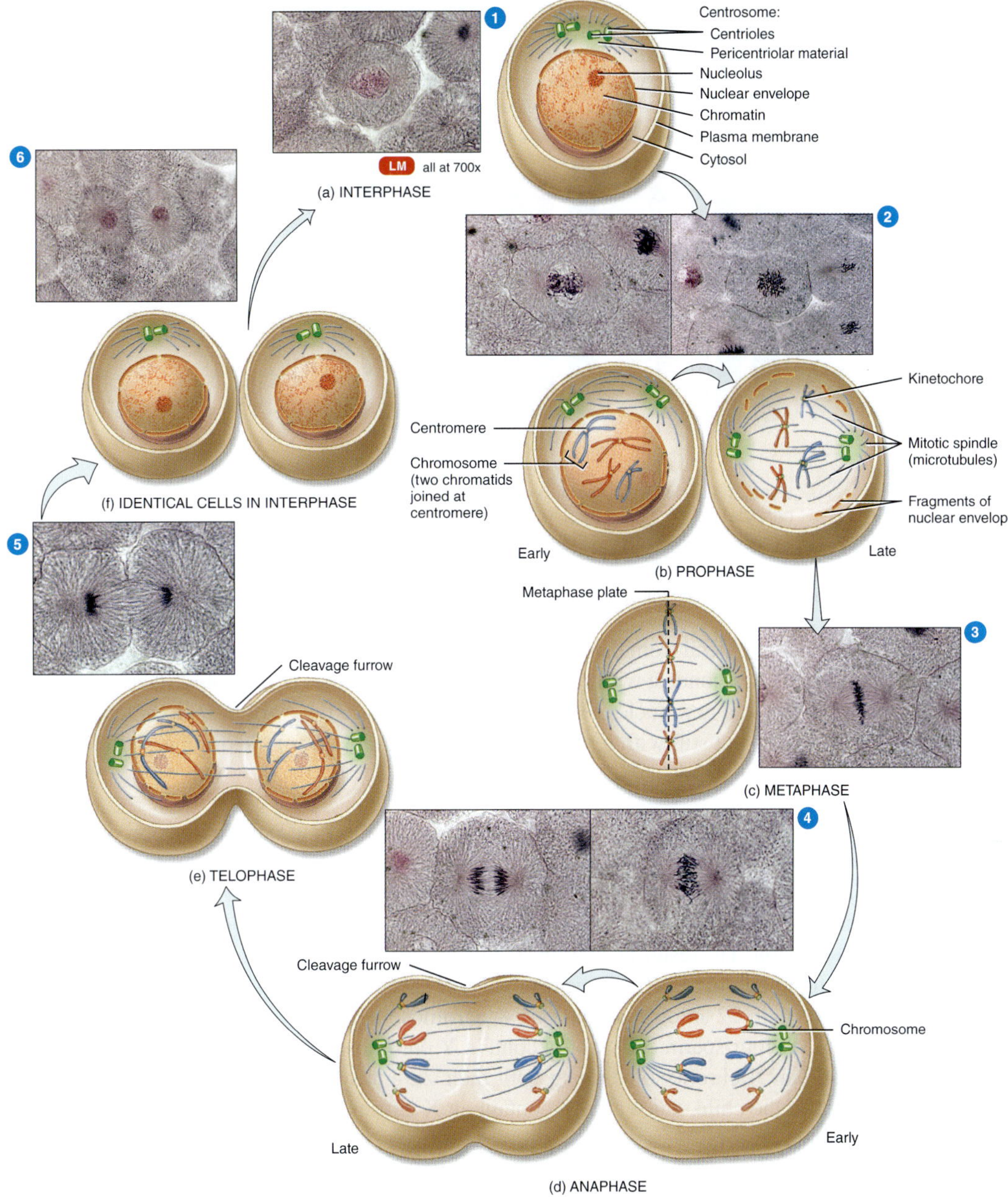

Source: Tortora and Derrickson (2009). Reproduced with permission of John Wiley & Sons.

Meiosis I

Prior to the first meiotic division, the cell is in interphase, just as it is prior to mitosis, and would have replicated all its chromosomes. The early events of the first meiotic division are similar to mitosis with the tight coiling of the chromosomes, dissolution of the nuclear envelope and generation of the spindle fibres. However, instead of lining up along the middle of the cell as 46 individual chromosomes (as in mitosis), the chromosomes line up in their pairs so that there are 23 pairs of chromosomes lying side by side across the **equator of the cell**. While next to each other this way, the paired chromosomes are able to swap some of their DNA. Each chromosome pair includes one maternal and one paternal chromosome, containing the same genes (but not necessarily the same alleles). Some of the DNA can be swapped between the maternal and paternal versions of the genes at this point, in a process called 'crossing over' or recombination (see figure 3.11). The genes still remain in the correct loci, but some alleles that were originally on the paternal chromosome may swap to the maternal one, and vice versa. This creates entirely new versions of the chromosomes with a mix of alleles that did not exist in the parent — a process which adds genetic variation to the offspring.

FIGURE 3.11 **Gene crossover** (recombination). During meiosis I homologous chromosomes pair together. The chromatids can then exchange information between non-sister chromatids in the homologous pair (sister chromatids are the exact copies made by DNA replication). This creates chromosomes that have a mix of alleles of the genes of the original chromosomes.

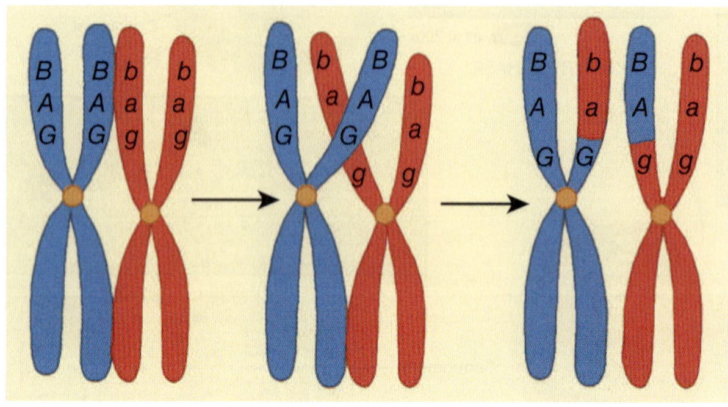

Source: Tortora and Derrickson (2009). Reproduced with permission of John Wiley & Sons.

As in mitosis, the spindles extend from the poles of the cell, but instead of connecting and pulling single chromatids (as in mitosis), they connect with and pull whole chromosomes to the poles. Each pole now has 23 chromosomes contained in a new nuclear envelope. The division of the cytoplasm completes meiosis I producing two haploid cells (but still with replicated sister chromatids) from the original diploid cell.

Meiosis II

During the second meiotic division, both of the cells produced by the first meiotic division divide again. However, as there is no interphase between meiosis I and meiosis II, the DNA is not replicated prior to this division. Meiosis II is similar to mitosis, with the main difference being that there are only 23 chromosomes to line up at the equator. The individual chromatids of these 23 chromosomes are pulled apart and moved to the poles during this division. The resulting cells each contain 23 single chromatids. Note that at the end of this process there are four haploid cells from one original parent cell. If an egg (ovum) was being produced, then each cell would contain 22 autosomes and one X chromosome. If sperm (spermatozoa) were being produced, then two of the four sperm cells would contain Y chromosomes along with the 22 autosomes, and two would contain an X chromosome along with their 22 autosomes. It is therefore the sperm that determines the gender of the child, since all ova contain an X chromosome, but a sperm cell can contain an X or a Y chromosome.

3.5 Inheritance

LEARNING OBJECTIVE 3.5 Understand Mendelian inheritance patterns: autosomal dominant, recessive and X-linked.

We are a product of our genes, or perhaps more precisely a product of our genes acted on and influenced or changed by our environment. Our environment in this context includes factors such as time, space, relationships, education, nutrition, physical activity, sleep quality, sun exposure, air quality, and so on. Epigenetics is a term used to describe inheritance by mechanisms (e.g. the environmental factors mentioned above) other than through the direct DNA sequence of genes, which may influence the development of phenotypic traits. In the past two decades, this field has taken great importance in human health and disease (see the medicines management box on monozygotic twins and epigenetic influence).

We inherit our genes from our parents through the direct transfer of their chromosomes into the gametes that fused to produce us. But why are we still unique? The answer lies in the behaviour of the alleles of each gene. This concept was first investigated in the 1860s by the monk Gregor Mendel. Mendel was assigned to care for the monastery garden. Mendel was very curious and began to wonder why the offspring of plants differed from their parents. He carried out controlled experiments in cross-breeding of plants and used statistics to interpret his results (the use of statistics was not common in biology at that time).

In 1866, Mendel published a paper of his work and the response from the scientific community was a deafening silence — his observations and theories were completely ignored until their 'rediscovery' in the early 1900s. It is this work that forms the basis of the science of inheritance that we now understand. Any human characteristic or genetic disorder that fits with his theories is said to follow a Mendelian (or classical/simple) inheritance pattern (**Mendelian genetics**), with characteristics/disorders that fit the more recently identified inheritance patterns referred to as being non-Mendelian (or complex).

Without any knowledge of DNA or genes, Mendel was able to postulate that there were factors that controlled an organism's characteristics. He determined that these occur in pairs and he discovered that within the pair, the information could be identical (what we now call homozygous) or the pieces of information could be slightly different (heterozygous). This allowed him to explain the concepts of dominance and recessivity that were explained earlier in this chapter. Mendel derived two laws of inheritance from his experimental work: **Mendel's law of independent assortment** and **Mendel's law of segregation**.

The law of segregation states that the members of a gene pair separate equally into the gametes. This law means that during meiosis I, when the homologous chromosomes pair up together and separate into the daughter cells, the paired alleles for each gene (i.e. the paternal and maternal chromosomes) will separate into two separate cells — both chromosomes of a pair will not end up in the same cell. Therefore, the offspring will have new 'pairings' created from the single sets of chromosomes contained in the egg and sperm when they fused together.

The law of independent assortment states that the chromosomes contained in each gamete will contain a random mix of maternally and paternally derived chromosomes — the pairs of chromosomes that line up on the cell equator prior to separation do not have paternal chromosomes on one side and maternal on the other; they are randomly assorted, and so each new cell/gamete will receive an unpredictable number of maternal and paternal chromosomes as each chromatid is pulled into its new cell. The diagrams in figure 3.12 illustrate these concepts with cells that have two pairs of chromosomes instead of 23.

Mendelian inheritance

We inherit our DNA from our parents, who inherited theirs from their parents. So we share some of our DNA with our grandparents and great-grandparents, and so on. The phenotypes which result from our inherited DNA will depend on the inheritance patterns of the genes. For characteristics that follow a Mendelian inheritance pattern, genes can be autosomal dominant, autosomal recessive or X-linked recessive.

Remember, that at each locus (gene), the alleles can be either dominant or recessive. If a dominant allele is present, then it will always be reflected in the phenotype, regardless of the other allele, but a recessive allele will only appear in the phenotype if there is no dominant allele. Note that when we represent these alleles in written form, dominant alleles are usually given capital letters, while recessive alleles are usually given lower-case letters.

In genetics we are often interested in calculating the probability of inheriting certain dominant or recessive alleles. We do this by considering the possible alleles that any gamete produced by the parents could have for a particular gene, and then work out the possible combinations that could come together in the offspring. When calculating the probability of inheriting any particular genotype, it is important to remember that the probability applies independently to each child born. For example, if the risk of inheriting a particular pair of alleles of a gene is 25 per cent or 1 in 4, it does not mean that the couple has to have 4 children before they are likely to have a child with those alleles; it means that each child will have a 25 per cent chance of having the alleles in question. So, while we report a risk as a percentage, all of the children of a couple may inherit the same pair of alleles for a locus or they may have different combinations.

Using our knowledge of dominant and recessive alleles and probability we can also identify which traits are dominant and which recessive. If a man with red hair and a woman with brown hair have many children, and all of them have brown hair, then this would suggest that the brown allele is dominant and the red allele recessive. If this is true, the father must be homozygous for the red allele in order to have red hair. Therefore, he only has a red allele to pass to his children. So, what can we say about his children's genotype? Since they all have brown hair, they must all have at least one dominant (brown) allele, and we also know they must all have a recessive (red) allele, as they had to get one allele from their father. Therefore, they must be heterozygous for this particular gene.

FIGURE 3.12 Mendel's laws of genetic inheritance. The two diagrams show the effects during meiosis of random assorting of chromosomes on the combinations of chromosomes in the gametes. The law of segregation is also shown for each chromosome pair of the original cell; only one is found in each gamete.

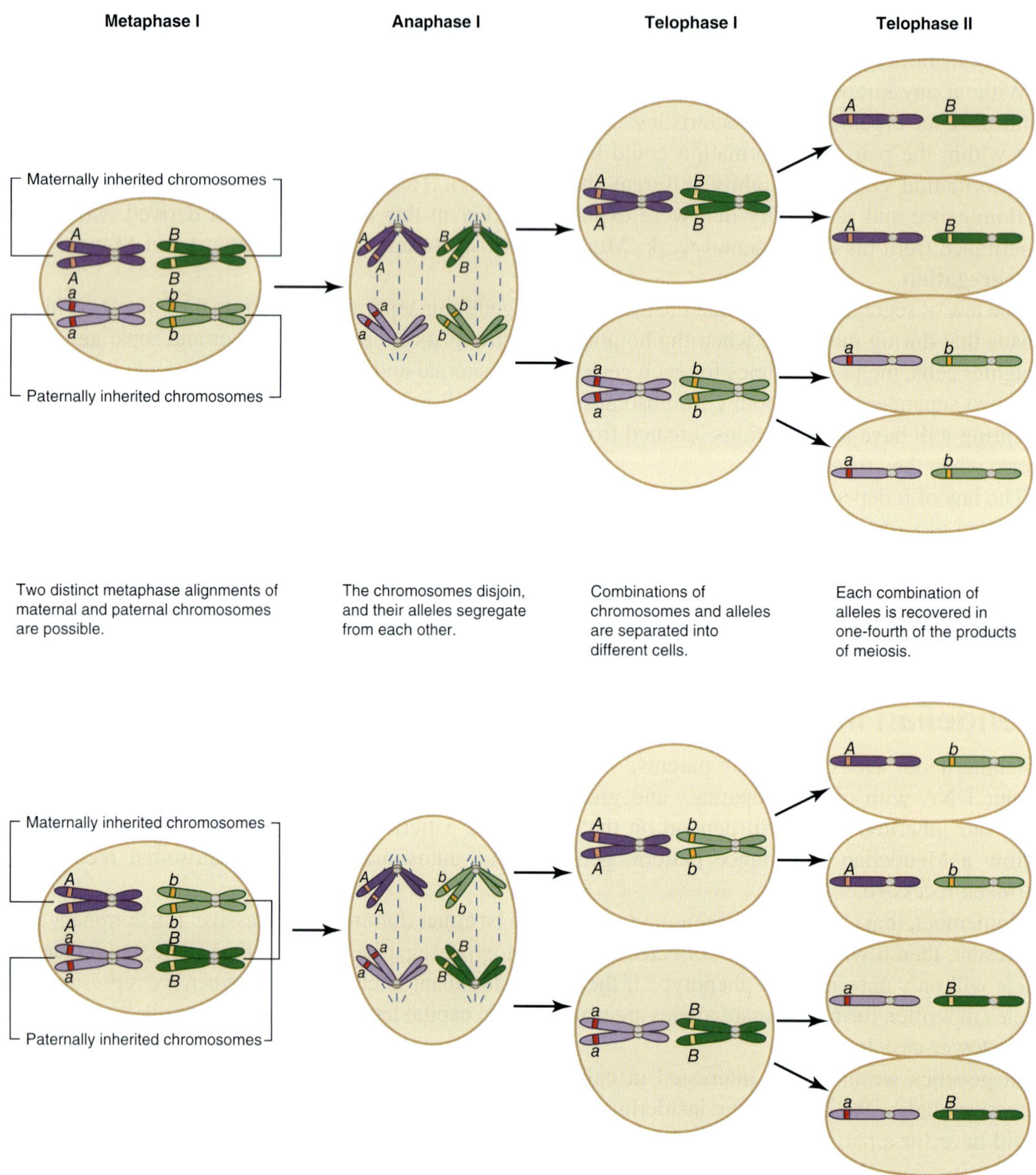

Source: Snustad and Simmons (2012). Reproduced with permission of John Wiley & Sons.

If one of these children goes on to have a child with red hair, like their grandfather, then we know that the child must have inherited a red allele from their mother to complement the red allele from their brown-haired father, since the child would have to possess two red alleles to have red hair. Both parents must therefore have been heterozygous for hair colour. This is often referred to as a trait 'skipping a generation' and is something that we can only see with recessive traits.

Autosomal dominant inheritance

If a person has one dominant allele that causes disease, such as Huntington's disease or neurofibromatosis, the person will have the disease, since the allele is dominant and will therefore determine the phenotype, but what is the risk of any of the person's children having the disease?

To determine the probability, we need to know the genotypes of both parents. If we assume the other parent does not have the disease, they are homozygous for the recessive allele, and therefore cannot possess the dominant disease-causing allele. This parent can therefore only pass on a recessive allele to his or her children. However, the parent with the disease has a 50 per cent chance of passing the dominant allele to their children, as this person has one dominant and one recessive allele. There is therefore a 50 per cent probability that a child will have the **autosomal dominant disorder**. If the affected parent was homozygous for the dominant allele, the risk of it being passed to any offspring would be 100 per cent (as all offspring would get one of the dominant alleles). Alternatively, if both parents were heterozygous for the dominant condition the risk of a child inheriting the condition would be 75 per cent. We can use a device known as a punnet square to show us why. Figure 3.13 shows an example for parents who are heterozygous for the gene involved in the disorder phenylketonuria (PKU). The dominant allele for this gene is the normal allele that protects the individual from having PKU.

FIGURE 3.13 Punnet squares are used to assess risk of offspring having a particular condition. The interpretation relies upon knowing whether the condition is dominant or recessive. The punnet square is created by putting together the alleles carried by both parents from the column and row that form the boxes of the square. This then offers four possible genotype combinations, which, depending on the original parental alleles, may include the same genotype repeated. The number of combinations resulting in disease can then be determined.

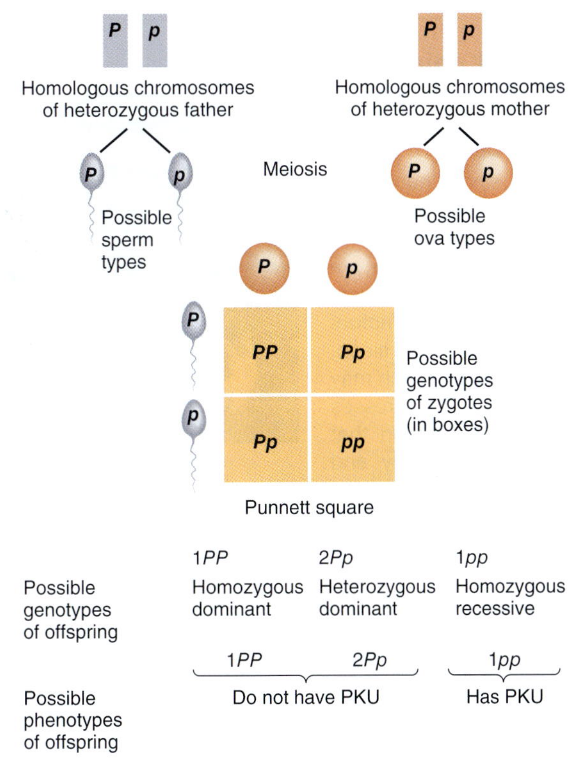

Source: Tortora and Derrickson (2009). Reproduced with permission of John Wiley & Sons.

Autosomal recessive inheritance

Autosomal recessive diseases occur when a disease-causing allele is recessive, which means an individual must have two of these alleles to have the disease. The parents of that individual must each have passed on one recessive allele to their child, and they would each have been heterozygous (or homozygous) for the condition. When a person is heterozygous for a recessive disease, they are said to be a carrier, as the disease allele is present in their genotype (and could possibly be passed to their offspring) but they do not have the disease themselves. A genetic disease can be carried through many generations and not seen until a carrier has children with someone who is also a carrier for the same condition (or is affected from the condition). The approach to calculating the probability of inheriting an autosomal recessive disease is the same as that used for dominant disease-causing traits.

Let's consider an example of a couple who are both carriers of the mutant allele that causes cystic fibrosis. As both parents are carriers then they have the same genotype, Cc (remember upper case is used for dominant alleles), which means that half of each parent's gametes will have the C allele and the other half the c allele. To determine the likelihood that these parents have a child with cystic fibrosis or who is a carrier we can use a punnet square (see figure 3.13). From this we see that there is a 25 per cent chance of the child inheriting the C allele from both of their parents. Any child with this genotype (CC) would be phenotypically normal (since the dominant allele in this case is not the disease-causing one) and, in the future, cannot pass on the disease-causing allele to their children, since they do not possess it. There is also a 25 per cent (or 1 in 4) chance that the child would inherit the c allele from both their parents. This child would have cystic fibrosis. The other two possible combinations result in the same Cc genotype (but with the C allele coming from a different parent in each case); therefore there is a 50 per cent (or 1 in 2) chance that they will have a child who is a carrier of the cystic fibrosis allele. Any child with the cc (affected) or Cc (carrier) genotype has a possibility of having affected children in the future, depending on their partner's genotype. It is important to remember that the calculated probabilities apply to each pregnancy separately (LeMone et al. 2015). So, if these parents have four children it does not mean that they will have one child with each of the possible genotypes in the punnet square. Each pregnancy has the same chances of inheriting one of the genotypes as the other pregnancies.

CLINICAL CONSIDERATIONS

Monozygotic twins and epigenetic influence

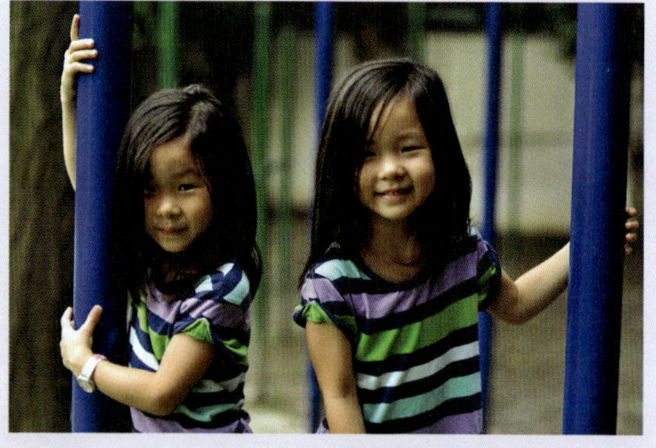

Monozygotic identical twins share identical genetic makeup but have different epigenomes. In the past two decades, over 100 genetic variants, also referred to as single nucleotide polymorphisms, have been identified as playing a key role in health and the development of certain diseases. As explained earlier, we are a product of our genes, and our genes are influenced or changed by environmental factors such as poor diet, lack of exercise or sleep, stress and increased smoking habits, which may cause cellular or DNA stresses. The stresses can lead to changes in DNA methylation that cause increased immune cellular activity and subsequent progression of autoimmune diseases such as rheumatoid arthritis or type 1 diabetes. The study of inherited traits caused by mechanisms other than changes to the underlying DNA sequence is called epigenetics.

Monozygotic twins share the same genetic variants and undergo similar early-life environments until early adulthood. Epigenetic studies using these twins allow the control of most genetic, maternal, environmental and cohort effects. Past studies have revealed that monozygotic twins often show divergent patterns for developing the most common diseases such as type 1 diabetes, type 2 diabetes, multiple sclerosis, autism, schizophrenia and various cancers. Thus, the older the twin pairs were, the greater the dissimilarity in their health and medical histories as they spent more years apart. This shows that for many complex traits, genotype alone may not fully reveal phenotypic variation, with genetic and environmental interactions needing to be taken into consideration. The use of twins in studies is useful for scientists to control for confounding differences in the DNA sequence and to see DNA methylation changes very clearly.

MEDICINES MANAGEMENT

Gene replacement therapy

Gene therapy, under the umbrella of regenerative medicine, is the technique of using a vector, usually viral, to apply a piece of DNA with the correct sequence to the faulty gene. This allows the identified faulty or missing gene to be replaced with the correct copy onto the corresponding cells. One of the pioneers in this field is Professor Ian Alexander, who heads the Gene Therapy Research Unit at Sydney University.

Gene therapy is one way in which genetic disorders can be treated, or at least ameliorated, by:

- replacing the mutated or malfunctioning gene
- manipulating or turning off the gene that is causing the disease
- stimulating other bodily functions to fight the disease.

The most common form of gene therapy is replacement of a malfunctioning or missing gene with a healthy one, and there have been attempts to cure diseases using this form of therapy. Since 1990, there have been many clinical trials for gene therapy, and the first trial was performed on a child with severe combined immunodeficiency (SCID), but with insignificant therapeutic benefits. In the late 1990s, unsuccessful attempts were made to treat cystic fibrosis; and in the early 2000s, gene replacement therapy for the adenosine deaminase deficiency that causes SCID was successfully carried out in several children. However, complications and mortality in children who had received gene therapy prompted subsequent suspension of this program.

Despite many refinements, gene therapy still poses a risk of serious complications, partly due to the method of using modified viruses to 'carry' and insert the 'new' corrective genes into the DNA of the body cells. Insertion of a healthy gene, essentially a length of DNA, into an existing genome at exactly the correct point to override the abnormal gene is a difficult and complex manoeuvre. In the earliest gene therapy trials, despite the therapy being initially successful, two children went on to develop leukaemia as a result of the 'new' gene inserting into the wrong place in the genome. Fortunately, this problem has now been largely eliminated, and gene replacement for this and other primary immunodeficiencies is regularly carried out in specialist centres.

The latest revolutionary technique which allows an easier, cheaper and efficient strategy for gene editing is called CRISPR. In Australia and New Zealand, this whole field is tightly regulated by the TGA and Medsafe respectively, to ensure that the practice adheres to stringent local and international legislation (O'Sullivan et al. 2019). In addition to the risk of cancer developing, other problems can arise with this therapy. For instance, the inserted virus could be perceived as a foreign invader by the immune system, which could lead to the body attacking the virus and its own organs. So far, in the case of children with specific severe primary immunodeficiencies, this has not been a problem, but it is an ever-present risk. These risks must be weighed against the fact that there are no completely effective alternative treatments. Like every advancement in medical science, both failures and small successes spur on researchers and doctors to refine, correct and improve the treatments for these and other genetic conditions.

CLINICAL CONSIDERATIONS

Genetic counselling

Generally, the clinical application of genetics in health is the responsibility of doctors and scientists. However, genetic counselling is an extremely important aspect of genetics that is within the nurse's scope of practice. While there are professionals (i.e. genetic counsellors) who are specially trained in genetics and genetic counselling, on a day-to-day basis the nurse is the health practitioner that spends the greatest time with a patient and builds rapport.

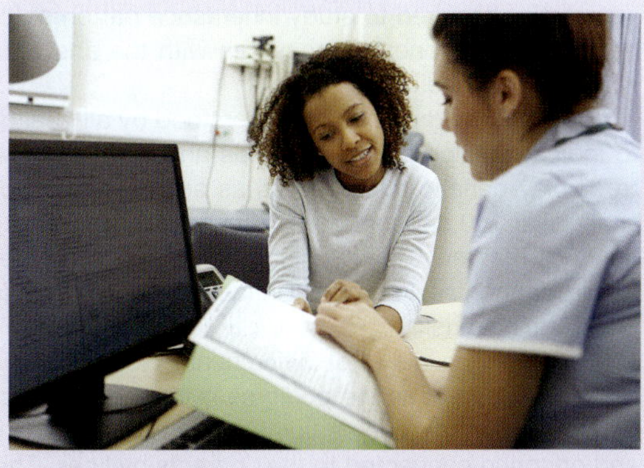

Genetic counselling involves providing information and support to patients and their family, and answering their specific questions about their genetic conditions and potential risks from certain genetic inheritance patterns. Genetic counsellors have trained knowledge and experience in human genetics, counselling and health communication. In Australia, they are part of the Allied Health Professions Australia network, after completing appropriate qualifications and a period of in-job training. Almost all medical specialties may require genetic counselling since abnormal genetic conditions can affect individuals in a variety of ways. Genetic counsellors may be employed in a variety of clinical settings, such as hospitals, medical specialist clinics, obstetric practices, community health centres, research clinics within institutes or genetics laboratories, and in government departments for strategic policy planning.

The inclusion of the family is very important when dealing with inherited disease as there are ramifications for the whole family. If requested, counselling may occur privately with individual family members who have questions that are particularly relevant to them.

For a consultation, a genetic counsellor will need:

- knowledge of genetics, genetic diseases and current treatment options
- respect for the patient and family
- time, patience and empathy.

During a consultation, the genetics counsellor will:

- begin building rapport and trust
- provide information in appropriate language so that the patient and family can make informed and independent decisions; this may include explaining familial inheritance patterns and showing associated risks of genetic diseases with a pedigree tree (after gathering information from close family members)
- allow the patient/family time to process the information, and be patient and innovative in repeat explanations so that they can absorb and understand the situation
- allow the patient and family time to think things over, arrange for them to be seen again in the near future, and be available to answer questions as they arise
- maintain privacy and confidentiality
- be truthful about potential consequences, discuss the positives and negatives, and clearly explain the risks of passing on a genetic disease
- provide emotional and practical support to patients and their families, helping them to adjust to (or being at risk for) a known genetic condition
- respect the patient's/family members' beliefs and feelings rather than imposing their own
- not make decisions for the individuals involved; for example, do not tell a couple to end a pregnancy, or have a specific treatment.

While most hospitals now have specialist genetics counsellors, they are not always immediately available to patients or their families, which is where the nurse on the ward or in the clinic comes into their own. The nurse will be trusted and available to discuss these matters without the formality of an appointment and official consultation. Consequently, the nurse needs to have knowledge of the conditions and their treatments and outcomes, especially when it comes to genetic inheritance medical problems. The nurse plays a vital role in providing patients with the support and information they require, as they become ready to receive it. Much of what the genetics counsellor has discussed with the patient/family may need to be repeated and reinforced during the patient's stay in hospital. This, of course, places additional responsibility on the nurse to be well informed about genetic inheritance patterns.

SKILLS IN PRACTICE

Constructing a family pedigree to assess risk

When guiding a couple on the risk of having a child with a genetic condition present in their family, it can be useful to construct a family pedigree chart. This is a family tree which includes the pertinent genetic information required to study inheritance patterns. It is important to advise the family involved that they need to be as honest as they can with the answers to the questions you will need to ask in order to construct the pedigree.

So that a pedigree can be understood by all health care professionals, conventional symbols are used to indicate biological relationships and the presence of the condition in question. It is very important to display genetic relationships as accurately as possible. For instance, identical (monozygotic) twins share near 100 per cent genetics, whereas non-identical (dizygotic) twins have no more similarity in their genetics than any other siblings from the same parents. However, non-identical twins may share many more common environmental influences than non-twin siblings. These considerations are often important in determining risk.

Many families may not differentiate biological relatives from non-biological relatives, and this may become apparent as the pedigree is constructed, as the biological inheritance lines are shown for their family. An example of a pedigree is shown in figure 3.14. Men are identified by squares, women by circles, and offspring connected to their parents by lines. The circles or squares of individuals with the condition in question are filled in to allow the inheritance pattern to be seen.

FIGURE 3.14 Mendelian inheritance in human pedigrees: (a) Pedigree conventions; (b) inheritance of a dominant trait — the trait appears in each generation; and (c) inheritance of a recessive trait — in this instance, the two affected individuals are the offspring of relatives, although this is not required to inherit a recessive trait

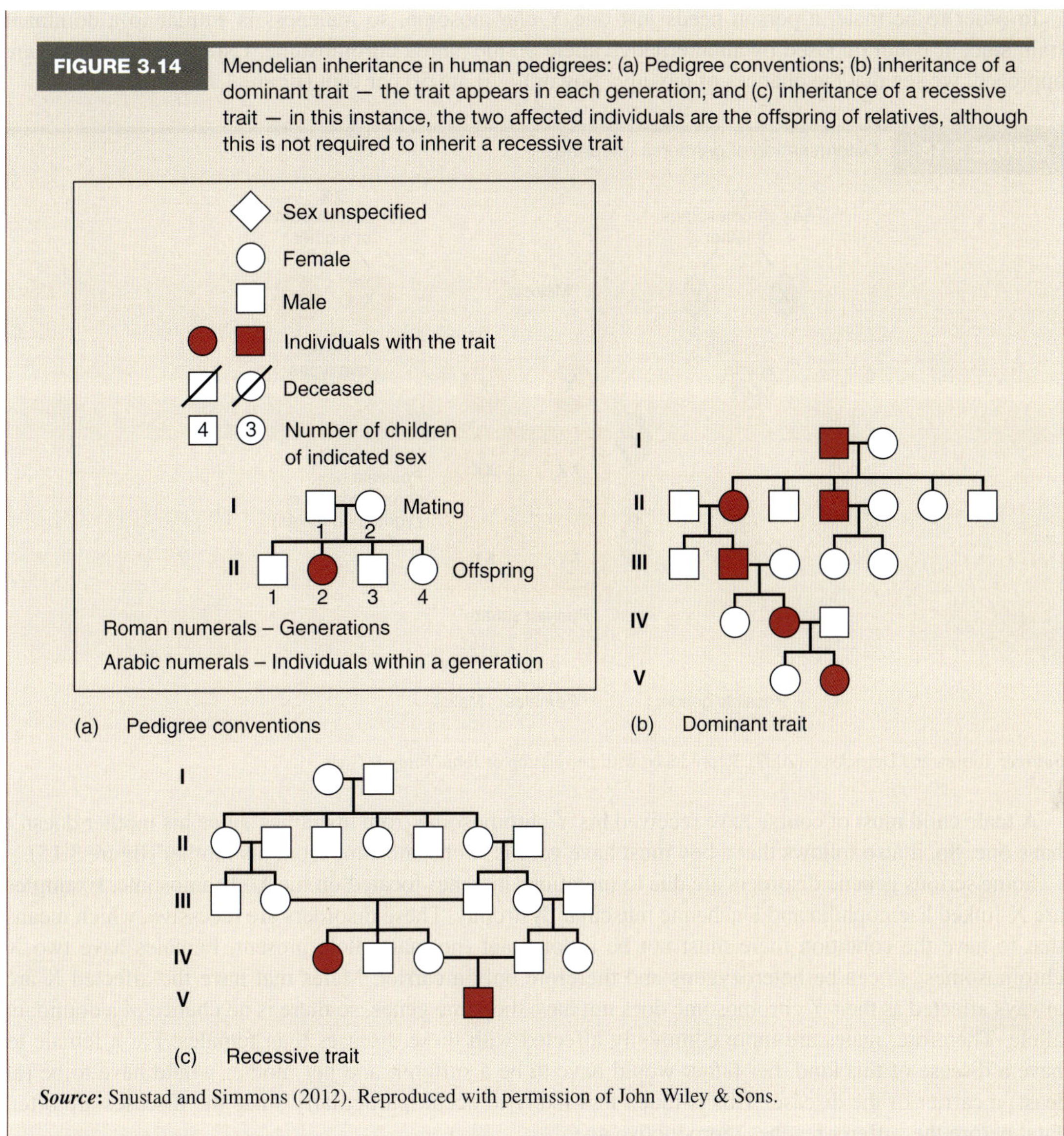

Source: Snustad and Simmons (2012). Reproduced with permission of John Wiley & Sons.

Morbidity and mortality of dominant versus recessive disorders

Autosomal dominant disorders are generally less severe than recessive disorders, because everyone with the disease allele also has the disease. If an autosomal dominant disorder produced severe or fatal effects, then people with the allele would be more likely to die before reaching an age to reproduce. In this way, the alleles for severe autosomal dominant disorders cease to exist in the population. The only ones that remain are those that do not cause the death of the sufferer before they reach sexual maturity. Huntington's disease is a fatal autosomal dominant disorder that survives in the population because the disease does not tend to show itself until adulthood, giving time for the sufferer to have unknowingly passed the affected gene on to the next generation. **Autosomal recessive disorders**, on the other hand, are often severe as a person can be a carrier of the allele and pass it on to their offspring without having any disease at all.

X-linked recessive disorders

Disorders can be inherited on the sex chromosomes in addition to the autosomes. The sex chromosomes determine gender, as possession of two X chromosomes results in a female, while one X and one Y results in a male. Since most of the genes on the X chromosome do not have an equivalent on the Y chromosome, and males and females have different X and Y combinations, inheritance patterns of genes located on the sex chromosomes require different interpretation to autosomal gene inheritance.

In order to be male, a person needs just one Y chromosome, so maleness is similar to a dominant trait, since it is not opposed by an alternative allele on the paired chromosome. Using the punnet square approach, we see that the chances of having a boy or a girl are 50 per cent (figure 3.15).

FIGURE 3.15 Determination of gender in offspring

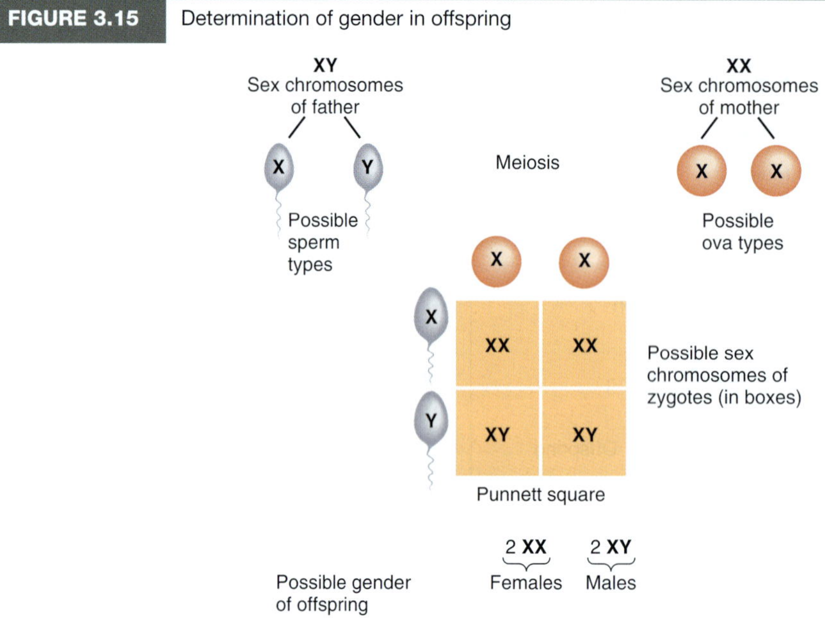

Source: Tortora and Derrickson (2009). Reproduced with permission of John Wiley & Sons.

A male child must of course have received his Y chromosome from his father, since his mother doesn't have one. So, it also follows that a boy must have got his X chromosome from his mother (figure 3.15).

Some serious genetic disorders are due to mutations in genes located on the X chromosome. Examples are X-linked haemophilia and Duchenne muscular dystrophy. These disorders are recessive, which means that to have the condition there must not be a dominant (normal) allele present. Females have two X chromosomes, so can be heterozygous and therefore only a carrier. Males that have the affected X are always affected as their Y chromosome does not have the same genes, so there is no chance of a dominant allele. Therefore, males are more commonly affected with these diseases than females. For a female to have a disease of this kind, her father would have to be a sufferer, and her mother would have to be (at least) a carrier of the disease. This is much less likely to occur, particularly since the diseases are often fatal before the sufferer reaches reproductive age.

Therefore, with **X-linked recessive diseases**, the risk is completely dependent on gender. To indicate this in pedigrees, X chromosomes bearing mutated (recessive) alleles are marked with a superscript lower-case letter (e.g. X^h, figure 3.16). Using this example of red-green colour blindness, the possible genotypes of offspring from these parents are:

- a girl who does not carry the affected allele, so is neither a carrier nor affected
- a boy who does not carry the abnormal allele, so has a normal X and a Y and is neither a carrier nor affected
- a girl who carries the abnormal allele (X^c), but the action of that gene is blocked by her other X allele, so she is not affected, but is a carrier
- a boy who carries the abnormal X allele (X^c). As the Y chromosome does not have this gene it is unable to block the action of the abnormal gene, so he is affected (and can of course pass the allele on to any female offspring he produces).

Consequently, we can say that:

- 50 per cent (or 1 in 2) of female children will be carriers
- 50 per cent (or 1 in 2) of male children will have the disease.

FIGURE 3.16 X-linked inheritance

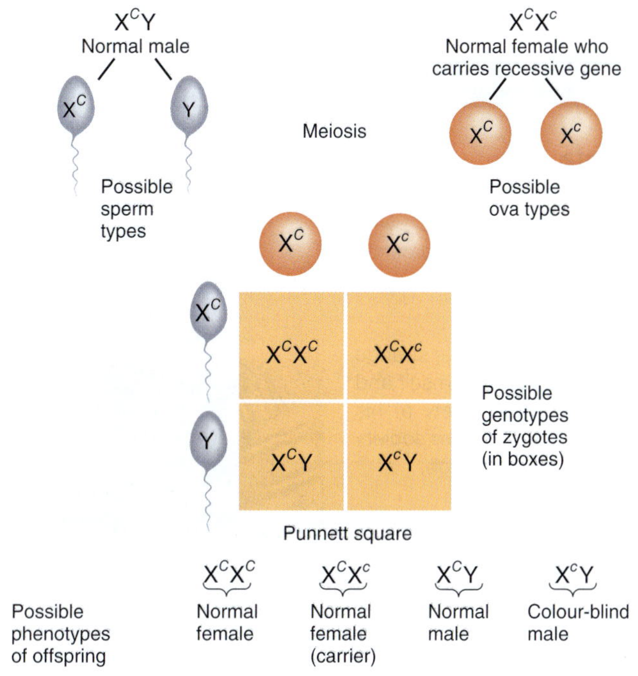

Source: Tortora and Derrickson (2009). Reproduced with permission of John Wiley & Sons.

3.6 Non-Mendelian (complex) inheritance

LEARNING OBJECTIVE 3.6 Describe the basics of non-Mendelian inheritance patterns.

This chapter is mainly concerned with understanding Mendelian inheritance patterns. However, there are many human traits and diseases that do not follow these simple inheritance patterns. We will not consider these in great detail but do need to be aware of them. One very well-known example is that of our blood groups. Our red blood cells have proteins on their surface that are antigenic, meaning that they will cause an immune response if introduced into the bloodstream of a person with a different blood group. This will cause the destruction of the red blood cells and severe illness or death. Blood transfusions can therefore only be from donors with compatible blood groups. Humans have one of four 'blood types', named A, B, AB and O. These types result from the different possible alleles of a single gene, so there is an A allele, a B allele and an O allele. Both A and B alleles are dominant over the O allele — so if you inherit an A and an O allele then you will have blood type A, just as if you inherited two A alleles. This is what we have seen previously with Mendelian inheritance. However, some people have blood type AB, having inherited an A and a B allele, and because these two alleles are co-dominant with each other, both are expressed in the phenotype of a person with this genotype.

Some genes have alleles that show incomplete dominance, in which case the phenotype is a mixture roughly halfway between the phenotype of one allele and the other; for example, the gene for flower colour might have a red allele and a white allele, which, if the alleles showed incomplete dominance, might result in a pink flower if they were both present.

Many of our traits are the result of not one but many genes, and are also influenced by our environment. With these complexities of inheritance, it is often much harder to determine a causative gene or genes for any disorder, which makes predicting inheritance risk much more difficult.

Xeroderma pigmentosum is an inherited condition that is strongly influenced by the environment. The condition is autosomal recessive and results in skin that is hypersensitive to ultraviolet light and its damaging effects. Sufferers are very prone to skin cancers and skin damage, and the disease shortens life expectancy considerably. If the sufferer can be completely protected from ultraviolet light from the sun, then the effects of the disease can be reduced or eliminated. The inherited disease phenylketonuria (PKU) is also environmentally influenced. In many countries, babies are screened for the mutant allele for this condition at birth, because if they can avoid phenylalanine in the diet from birth, they are spared the neurological degeneration that occurs with this condition (this is also why food and beverages have to clearly state if they contain phenylalanine). These conditions are also said to be 'modifiable' genetic diseases because the disease outcome can be modified by environmental changes.

CLINICALLY REASONED EPISODE OF CARE

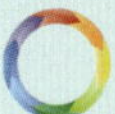

Schizophrenia

Consider the patient situation

Mark has recently been diagnosed with schizophrenia. He is brought into the emergency department by his wife.

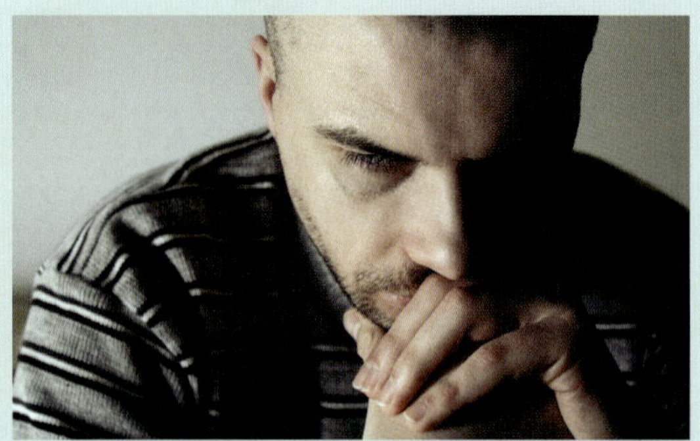

Collect cues and information

- Mental state assessment: Wife reports strange behaviour — Mark is mumbling to himself and expressing concerns about the safety of his family; he has been withdrawing from society and has had difficulty maintaining a job.
- Appearance: dishevelled.
- Family assessment: Mark's wife reports concerns that their children might develop schizophrenia.

Process information

Schizophrenia is a mental illness involving disorders of thought and mood, affecting about 1 per cent of the population. Individuals with schizophrenia experience periods of psychosis (delusions and hallucinations) as well as social withdrawal, poor self-care, and a range of cognitive impairments. The severity of any of these symptoms varies greatly between individuals. Therefore, not all patients will receive the same treatments, nor will they all respond the same way to these treatments. Unfortunately, many of the current treatments for schizophrenia also have severe side effects that greatly affect healthcare concordance. Although the exact cause of schizophrenia is still an area of intense research, it is clear that genetics plays a large role in its development. Schizophrenia is therefore considered a complex genetic disorder as it does not follow a simple Mendelian inheritance pattern. The identical twin of a schizophrenia sufferer has a 50–80 per cent chance of developing the condition also, but it is not a certainty, which highlights the complexity of its inheritance pattern. This makes it difficult to counsel individuals and families about their risk of inheriting this disorder as there are so many factors to consider. There is a slightly higher incidence of schizophrenia in males and onset is typically around puberty.

Nursing actions

1. Admission to psychiatric ward for medication review and specialist support.
   Rationale:
   - Appropriate medication and psychotherapy can help to mitigate the symptoms of schizophrenia.
   - Appropriate counselling about medications can help to mitigate the side effects and improve healthcare concordance.
2. Provide counselling for Mark and his wife about the inheritance of schizophrenia.
   Rationale:
   - Explain that schizophrenia is poorly understood and hard to determine, the family should look out for early signs as the best outcomes are achieved with early diagnosis and intervention, and there are some environmental triggers (such as illicit drug use) that can influence the development of schizophrenia in individuals who may have a genetic predisposition.
   - Appropriate support for the family of a person experiencing mental illness can contribute to mitigation of the symptoms of the illness, promoting independent living and reducing exacerbations.

Evaluate outcomes

Mark experiences a reduction in symptoms and is able to demonstrate appropriate self-care. Mark's wife reports a better understanding of Mark's illness and the factors of inheritance.

Source: Galletly et al. (2016); based on the Clinical Reasoning Cycle, Levett-Jones (2013).

Spontaneous mutation

There is another way for an unusual or abnormal gene to occur and cause genetic disorders. This is by spontaneous mutation. Because of the great speed and precision needed for replication of DNA, it is possible for mistakes to occur, and in this way genetic mutations arise. There is no way of predicting or preventing this, as the first sign will be disease manifestation. Sometimes, such mutations may lead to protein-altering changes towards the manifestation of a disease — this is called **spontaneous mutation disorder**.

Mutations that can cause disease due to their effects on various genes may also be brought about by trauma or environmental factors such as chemicals and ultraviolet radiation.

SKILLS IN PRACTICE

Genetic screening of newborns (heel prick or Guthrie test)

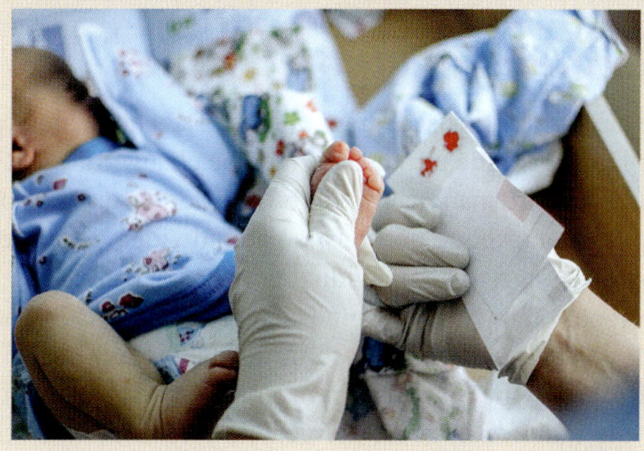

This is a genetic blood test that is performed on newborn babies at 2–5 days of age. Typically, the test is performed before the baby leaves hospital with the results provided on a subsequent visit with either the baby health nurse or the GP.

An explanation of the test procedure and purpose should be provided and consent obtained prior to the test. The procedure itself is quite straightforward, but it is essential that it is done in sterile conditions. The nurse should wear gloves to prevent any transfer of body fluids to the baby or to the test sample. The heel of the baby is cleaned with an appropriate agent and a small sharp needle (similar to those used for sampling blood glucose from a finger) is used to draw a drop of blood from the baby. Two blood drops are then squeezed onto a special piece of filter paper known as a Guthrie card. The blood is allowed to dry on the card and it is then packaged and sent to a pathology lab for testing. The infant may cry during this procedure, so it is important that the parents are on hand ready to cuddle and console the baby.

As consent is needed it is important that the purpose of the test is adequately explained. The blood taken by this test will be extracted from the Guthrie card and the DNA from the white blood cells extracted. An analysis of specific genes within the DNA will be conducted to identify if the baby has any of the alleles for a number of rare but serious genetic and metabolic conditions. The conditions screened for vary between countries, but will typically include cystic fibrosis, phenylketonuria (PKU), congenital hypothyroidism and galactosaemia. The reason these rare conditions are screened in this way is that prompt intervention provides the best outcome for individuals with these conditions. For PKU and galactosaemia, a simple early alteration to diet can prevent the onset of severe illness or fatality. Because they are inherited in a recessive fashion, the parents may not be aware of any family history of these conditions, so it is important to counsel them on the risks that they may be carriers of any of these conditions, based on your understanding of genetics and the incidence of the alleles involved in the population. It is also important to counsel them that this test is only a screening test, not a diagnostic test.

The conditions screened for in this test are continually being expanded. Australia added the genetic condition spinal muscular atrophy (SMA), one of Australia's leading causes of infant death, to the screening in 2018.

SKILLS IN PRACTICE

Congenital genetic defects — Duchenne muscular dystrophy

Genetic defects can affect 1–2 per cent of the population and are often undetected until the first recognisable symptoms develop. The paramedic dispatched to provide initial medical care for these genetic conditions may not realise the underlying problem until further medical examinations and diagnostic tests are undertaken.

For example, Duchenne muscular dystrophy (DMD) is an X-linked recessive genetic disorder with symptom onset occurring between ages 2 and 6, more often in boys than girls. The defective DMD gene is carried by the X chromosome, and is either inherited from parents or caused by a genetic change. Symptoms often start in mild forms, affecting the limbs such as preference walking on toes, waddling gait and usage of proximal muscles. Additionally, the arms are used to pull oneself into a standing position from a squatting position due to weakness of leg muscles. Within a few years, this progresses rapidly towards major mobility, and cardiac and respiratory problems. By the age of 20, 75 per cent of DMD patients will die, usually due to cardiac or respiratory failure. There are no current cures, but treatments are available which aim to manage symptoms and improve quality of life.

Special paramedic consideration

As a first medical responder, paramedics should be aware of the special care needs of a DMD patient. With impaired lung function and expansion, DMD patients should be transported in a position that helps to maximise lung expansion. Also, they are incapable of compensated hypovolaemia due to having a fixed cardiac output. Whenever possible, anaesthesia should not be used to avoid complications from some of the anaesthetic components, and polarising neuromuscular blocking agents should be avoided as they cause hyperkalaemia after rapid depolarisation of muscle cells.

Source: Muscular Dystrophy Australia (2018); Health Direct (2020); JEMS (2014).

Disorders of chromosomes

We have so far focused on mutations to a gene, which cause disease. A mutation represents a tiny change to our DNA (as little as one base may be changed), but it is also possible for large sections of a chromosome (and therefore many genes) to be affected through errors in the chromosome structure. These may involve duplication of large portions (so an individual has three alleles for all of the genes involved); deletions of large portions (so an individual only has one allele for many genes); rearrangements in which the order of the genes on the chromosome changes or a gene even moves between chromosomes; and also the addition or loss of an entire chromosome, as mentioned earlier in this chapter.

Rearrangements of chromosomes have varying effects, and typically do not cause serious problems for the individual, as all the genetic information is still present in their cells. However, the offspring of these individuals can be greatly affected, because of the separation of the homologous chromosomes into different gametes, which means that some gametes will not contain a complete set of genetic information or will contain too much. For example, if part of chromosome 21 had broken and attached to chromosome 14, when gametes are produced one of them will have a 'short' chromosome 21 that is missing information. The other gamete will have a chromosome 14 with some chromosome 21 attached plus a normal chromosome 21. A child produced from this gamete would end up with three alleles for genes on this segment of chromosome 21. This is one way in which a baby can end up with too many alleles for the genes of chromosome 21 resulting in Down syndrome.

CLINICALLY REASONED EPISODE OF CARE

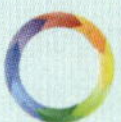

Acute lymphoblastic leukaemia (ALL)

Consider the patient situation

Casey is an 8-year-old girl who has been diagnosed with acute lymphoblastic leukaemia (ALL). Specifically, Casey has a form of ALL known as Ph+ALL, meaning that a rare genetic translocation between chromosomes creates a new chromosome known as Philadelphia (Ph+).

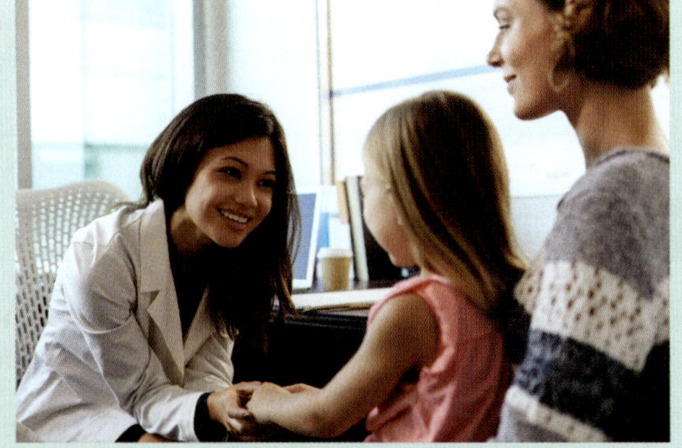

Collect cues and information

Casey has a diagnosis of Ph+ALL and has been commenced on a treatment which suppresses the activation of the protein causing her cancer. This has been successful in stopping the division of the ALL cells.

Casey has made a full recovery following treatment; however, her parents have some concerns and questions which should be addressed as part of the care provided. Casey's parents are understandably concerned about the diagnosis and treatment options, as well as her life expectancy, prognosis and the possibility of Casey passing on the abnormality to her future children.

Process information

The Philadelphia abnormality is the most common abnormality in leukaemia cells. Ph+ALL is the translocation of chromosomes 9 and 22 which creates a fusion gene, leading to the development of ALL. Improvements in modern medicine and medications have ensured that the prognosis for Ph+ALL today is promising. Young people, like Casey, have a more positive prognosis when it comes to ALL.

Significant research has occurred for ALL treatments in the past 10 years, and a more detailed understanding of how Ph+ALL occurs has led to improved treatments. Treatments for Ph+ALL include tyrosine kinase inhibitors (TKI) which block the BCR-ABL protein signals that form leukaemia cells. Other treatments are available if treatment regimens fail to work or lose their efficacy over time.

Casey's treatment has been successful; however, as with most cancers, there is always concern about relapse of cancer, treatment side effects and efficacy, and long-term side effects. Because of the way Ph+ALL occurs, it is unlikely that a person will pass down the trait to their future children.

Nursing actions

1. Build rapport with Casey's family.
   Rationale:
   - Building a rapport with patients and the family unit provides a conduit for effective communication and engagement.
   - Effective communication ensures the family are informed and empowered and anxiety is relieved.
2. Refer to a specialist nurse educator.
   Rationale:
   - While all nurses are required to educate, specialist educators are professionally and educationally prepared to provide specific and targeted education to families on the implications of Ph+ALL.
   - Specialist education will ensure that the family unit is adequately informed and empowered to participate in the treatment process.
   - Adequate education improves health literacy and health system knowledge, leading to improved understanding of treatments.
3. Coordinate follow-up appointments.
   Rationale:
   - Cancer treatment can be a highly stressful time for families and navigating the health system can be challenging and confusing. The coordination of appointments and treatments alleviates stress and anxiety while ensuring that the system is effectively navigated.

Evaluate outcomes

As a result of the nursing actions above, Casey's family report less stress, anxiety and confusion related to the diagnosis and treatment of her cancer, as well as more efficient navigation of the healthcare system.

Casey's parents can articulate understanding of their daughter's condition and prognosis and are able to keep all appointments for Casey's care. As a result, the family have improved their health system literacy and are able to be optimistic about the future.

Reflect on new processes and learning

Reflect on the scenario above and the clinical reasoning cycle. What role does the nurse play in improving patient/family education? How does this improve health literacy and navigation of the health system?

Source: Based on the Clinical Reasoning Cycle, Levett-Jones (2013).

SUMMARY

This completes the chapter on basic genetics. Although genetics may appear complicated, it is a very important subject because our genes not only make us what we are, but also leave us susceptible to certain diseases. Our genes have a say in how we respond to treatment for diseases, how we live our lives, work, develop relationships, and indeed survive in the world.

KEY TERMS

adenine (A) One of the four bases of DNA and RNA.

allele One of the possible DNA sequences that a particular gene can have.

amino acids The building blocks of proteins; there are 20 that are used for the synthesis of proteins as directed by the sequence of nucleotides.

anticodon A group of three bases on tRNA. The 20 amino acids have a particular anticodon so that it puts the right amino acid in the protein as identified by the DNA and mRNA sequence.

autosomal dominant disorder A medical disorder caused by a faulty version (allele) of dominant gene that is inherited from one of the parents.

autosomal recessive disorders A medical disorder caused when two faulty alleles for a gene are inherited: one from each parent.

autosomes Chromosomes that are not one of the two sex chromosomes. Humans have 22 pairs of autosomes.

base Component of nucleotides that form the code that specifies the cell's proteins. There are four bases used in DNA: A, C, T, G; and four in RNA: A, C, U, G. Bases from one DNA strand make complementary pairing with corresponding bases from another DNA strand to form a DNA double helix.

cell cycle The process by which a cell prepares for, and undertakes, cell growth and division.

centromere The point at which two chromatids are attached in a chromosome.

chromatids One of the DNA double helix strands of a replicated chromosome.

chromosomes Mixture of DNA and protein (chromatin) — contains our genetic makeup.

codon A triplet of bases on mRNA that encodes for a particular amino acid.

cytosine (C) One of the bases of DNA or RNA.

deoxyribose A major part of DNA, deoxyribose is derived from a sugar known as ribose but has lost an atom of oxygen.

diploid cells Cell that contains two of each chromosomes. See haploid cell.

DNA Deoxyribonucleic acid, found in the cell nucleus and is the molecule that houses the information in our genes.

dominant allele Allele of a gene that can exert its effects on the body on its own. In other words, it dominates a recessive allele at the same locus.

double helix Two strands of DNA joined together in a spiral formation.

elongation The continuation of protein synthesis process with the addition of corresponding amino acids according to the tRNA, allowing the nascent protein chain to grow.

equator of the cell The centre of the cell during cell division.

gametes A reproductive cell; spermatozoon (spermatozoa, sperm) or ovum (ova, egg).

genes A portion of DNA that codes for a protein. A unit of heredity in a living organism.

gene crossover Recombination; the process at the commencement of meiosis whereby genetic material may be transferred between chromatids of homologous chromosomes. Contributes to genetic diversity.

genotype The two particular alleles that an individual has for a gene. The genotype of a person will determine their phenotype.

guanine (G) One of the four bases of DNA or RNA.

haploid cells A cell that contains just one of each chromosome. See diploid cell.

hereditary The passing down of genes from generation to generation.

heterologous 'Different'. See homologous.

heterozygous A pair of dissimilar alleles for a particular gene locus. See homozygous.

histone protein Found in cell nuclei; it packages and orders the DNA into nucleosomes, making it possible for the chromosomes to fit into a cell without becoming tangled.

homologous 'Same'. See heterologous.

homozygous A pair of identical alleles for a particular gene locus. See heterozygous.

initiation The start of the protein synthesis process; occurs when the corresponding tRNA reaches the start codon, the first base triplet, AUG.

interphase The longest stage of the cell cycle, during which the cell is growing and preparing to divide.

locus A gene's position on a chromosome.

meiosis Process of cell division that allows for the production of haploid gametes from diploid cells, so ensuring the correct number of chromosomes are passed to the offspring.

Mendelian genetics The concepts of inheritance associated with characteristics (phenotypes) that are governed by a single gene (named after Gregor Mendel).

Mendel's law of independent assortment Members of different pairs of alleles are randomly sorted into the gametes.

Mendel's law of segregation Only one allele from each parent can be inherited by their child.

mitosis The process of cell division undertaken by somatic cells (not gametes) that ensures each cell obtained by this process has an exact copy of the chromosomes of the original cell.

mRNA Messenger ribonucleic acid; provides a means to get the information (genes) held in DNA out of the nucleus into the cytoplasm to provide the information to synthesise proteins.

nucleic acid A mixture of phosphoric acid, sugars, and organic bases, nucleic acids direct the course of protein synthesis (or production), so regulating all cell activities. DNA and RNA are nucleic acids.

nucleosome A unit of packaged DNA in a cell's nucleus; it consists of a segment of DNA wound around a histone.

nucleotides The building block of DNA and RNA, consisting of sugar (deoxyribose in DNA, ribose in RNA), phosphate and one of the four bases.

ova (ovum, eggs) Female reproductive cells, these cells are haploid.

peptidyl transferase An enzyme that catalyses peptide bond formation between adjacent amino acids allowing the growth of peptide chain during the translation process.

phenotypes The expressed features of a person, derived from the interaction of the genotype of a person with the environment.

poles Opposite ends of a cell during some stages of cell division.

purine A two-ringed structure present in DNA and RNA. Purines in DNA and RNA are the same — adenine and guanine.

pyrimidine A single-ringed structure present in DNA and RNA. Pyrimidines in DNA are cytosine and thymine, while within the RNA, they are present as cytosine and uracil.

recessive allele Requires another recessive allele at the same locus before it can have an effect on the body. In other words, it is not dominant over another allele of that gene.

ribosomes Small structures made from protein and ribosomal RNA involved in making proteins (see the chapter on cells, cellular compartments, transport systems, fluid movement between compartments).

RNA Ribonucleic acid; transcribed from DNA. (There are several types of RNA with mRNA, tRNA and rRNA essential for protein synthesis.)

RNA polymerase The main transcription enzyme required to make a complementary RNA molecule from a DNA template.

spermatozoa (spermatozoon, sperm) Male reproductive cells, these cells are haploid.

spontaneous mutation disorder A medical disorder caused by a new fault that has developed on a gene sequence; that is, neither of the parents carries the faulty version (allele) of that gene.

strands The long parts of the double helix, consisting of deoxyribose and phosphate.

termination The protein synthesis process in the ribosome is stopped at this point. No further addition of amino acids takes place from this point onwards, and subsequently the released protein sequence undergoes post-translation modification.

termination codon A triplet of bases (stop codon) that stops the joining of amino acids once the specified protein of that sequence has been produced.

thymine (T) One of the bases of DNA (not used in RNA).

transcription In genetics, the generation of RNA from DNA such that they hold the same information.

translation In genetics, the process by which information in the bases of mRNA is used to specify the amino acid sequence of a protein.

triplets Sequence of three DNA bases that code for an amino acid.

tRNA Transfer ribonucleic acid; important in the production of proteins as it decodes the message found in mRNA to provide the correct order of amino acids for the protein being produced.

uracil (U) One of the four bases of RNA (not used in DNA).

X-linked recessive diseases A medical disorder caused by a fault in a gene of the X chromosome (one of the sex chromosomes), inherited in a recessive pattern.

ACTIVITIES

TRUE OR FALSE

1 Males have 46 chromosomes, 22 pairs of autosomes an X and a Y.
2 A person with a heterozygous genotype would have a phenotype associated with the recessive allele.
3 Homologous chromosomes can exchange information between chromatids during meiosis.
4 The two strands of the double helix are held together by covalent bonds between complementary bases.
5 Having a blood group of AB is an example of non-Mendelian genetics.

CONDITIONS

The following is a list of common genetic conditions. Take some time and write notes about each of the conditions. You may make the notes taken from textbooks or other resources (e.g. people you work with in a clinical area), or you may make the notes as a result of people you have cared for. If you are making notes about people you have cared for, you must ensure that you adhere to the rules of confidentiality.

Motor neurone disease
Prader–Willi syndrome
Alzheimer's disease, early onset
Neurofibromatosis
Down syndrome
Turner syndrome

REFERENCES

Crespi, B. (2008) Turner syndrome and the evolution of human sexual dimorphism. *Evolutionary Applications* 1(3): 449–461.

Galletly, C., Castle, D., Dark, F., Humberstone, V. et al. (2016) Royal Australian and New Zealand College of Psychiatrists clinical practice guidelines for the management of schizophrenia and related disorders. *Australian and New Zealand Journal of Psychiatry* 50(5): 1–117.

Health Direct (2020) Duchenne muscular dystrophy. www.healthdirect.gov.au/duchenne-muscular-dystrophy (accessed February 2021).

JEMS (2014) Congenital genetic defects and the special considerations for prehospital care. www.jems.com/patient-care/congenital-genetic-defects-special-consi (accessed February 2021).

LeMone, P., Burke, K., Bauldoff, G. and Gubrud, P. (2015) *Medical–Surgical Nursing: Critical Thinking in Client Care*, 6th edn. Upper Saddle River, NJ: Pearson Prentice Hall.
Levett-Jones, T. (2013). *Clinical Reasoning: Learning to Think Like a Nurse.* Pearson Australia.
Muscular Dystrophy Australia (2018) Duchenne muscular dystrophy. www.mda.org.au/disorders/overview/dmd-bmd (accessed February 2021).
NSW Government, Centre for Genetics Education (2018) Fact sheet 40 — Turner syndrome. www.genetics.edu.au/publications-and-resources/facts-sheets/fact-sheet-40-turner-syndrome (accessed February 2021).
O'Sullivan, G.M., Velickovic, Z.M., Keir, M.W., MacPherson, J.L. and Rasko, J.E.J. (2019) Cell therapy and gene therapy manufacturing capabilities in Australia and New Zealand. *Cryotherapy* 21(12): 1258–1273.
Poulton, J. (2016) World's first three-parent baby raises questions about long-term health risks. *The Conversation*, 28 September. https://theconversation.com/worlds-first-three-parent-baby-raises-questions-about-long-term-health-risks-66189 (accessed February 2021).
Snustad, D.P. and Simmons, M.J. (2012) *Principles of Genetics*, 6th edn. Hoboken, NJ: John Wiley & Sons, Inc.
Tortora, G.J. and Derrickson, B.H. (2009) *Principles of Anatomy and Physiology*, 12th edn. Hoboken, NJ: John Wiley & Sons, Inc.
Tortora, G.J. and Derrickson, B.H. (2014) *Principles of Anatomy and Physiology*, 14th edn. Hoboken, NJ: John Wiley & Sons.

FURTHER READING

NEWBORN SCREENING

www.betterhealth.vic.gov.au/health/conditionsandtreatments/newborn-screening
www.health.gov.au/health-topics/pregnancy-birth-and-baby/newborn-bloodspot-screening

Every newborn child is offered genetic testing for several rare but serious medical conditions. These websites provide details and information for the tests available, how the tests are conducted, and the available support given for expecting Australian mothers or parents.

STUDIES ON IDENTICAL TWINS

https://blogs.biomedcentral.com/on-medicine/2018/09/06/how-identical-twins-are-helping-us-understand-epigenetic-factors-in-rheumatoid-arthritis

Information and updates on recent epigenetic studies conducted on identical twins.

GENE THERAPY

www.medicalresearch.nsw.gov.au/discovery-challenges-the-foundations-of-gene-therapy

Details of recent developments in the area of gene therapy conducted in world-leading medical research institutes based in Australia and of global collaborative partners.

https://theconversation.com/the-gene-therapy-revolution-is-here-medicine-is-scrambling-to-keep-pace-118329

Explores the past, current and possible future developments in gene therapy.

CRISPR

https://theconversation.com/what-is-crispr-gene-editing-and-how-does-it-work-84591

This link provides some details of the revolutionary gene-editing technology using CRISPR. The 2020 Nobel Prize in Chemistry was awarded to Professor Charpentier and Professor Doudna for the discovery of this innovative methodology.

Ph+ALL

www.stbaldricks.org/blog/post/what-is-philadelphia-chromosome-positive-all

Details of a rare subtype of the most common form of childhood cancer, Philadelphia Chromosome positive acute lymphoblastic leukaemia (Ph+ALL).

OTHER

Castillo-Fernandez, J., Spector, T.D. and Bell J.T. (2014) Epigenetics of discordant monozygotic twins: implications for disease. *Genome Medicine* 6: 60.
Ginn, S.L., Amaya, A.K., Alexander, I.E., Edelstein, M. and Abedi, M.R. (2018) Gene therapy clinical trials worldwide to 2017: an update. *J Gene Medicine* 20(5): e3015.
Lister Hill National Center for Biomedical Communications (2010) *Genetics Home Reference: Your Guide to Understanding Genetic Conditions*. Bethesda, MD. http://ghr.nlm.nih.gov.
Skirton, H. and Patch, C. (2013) *Genetics for Healthcare Professionals*. New York: Garland Science.
Vipond, K. (2013) Genetics: *A Guide for Students and Practitioners of Nursing and Health Care*, revised edn. Banbury: Scion Publishing Ltd.
Xiang, Z., Yang, Y., Chang, C. and Lu, Q. (2017) The epigenetic mechanisms for discordance of autoimmunity in monozygotic twins. *Journal of Autoimmunity* 83: 43–50.

ACKNOWLEDGEMENTS

Photo: © Elnur / Shutterstock.com
Photo: © Flickr Open / Getty Images
Photo: © Monkey Business Images / Shutterstock.com
Photo: © Themalni / Shutterstock.com
Photo: © Helen Sushitskaya / Shutterstock.com
Photo: © Monkey Business Images / Shutterstock.com

CHAPTER 4

Tissue

TEST YOUR PRIOR KNOWLEDGE

- List the four main types of body tissue.
- What are the main functions of epithelial tissue?
- Name the four types of connective tissue.
- Which types of muscle are involuntary?
- What are the main steps of tissue repair?

LEARNING OUTCOMES

After reading this chapter you will be able to:

4.1 describe the characteristics of epithelial tissue and list the classifications of epithelial tissue
4.2 discuss the functions of connective tissue and list the classifications of connective tissue
4.3 describe the structure of the three types of muscle tissue and their function
4.4 describe the types of nervous tissue cells
4.5 describe the process of tissue repair.

Introduction

The human body consists of around 50 trillion to 106 trillion individual structural working units called cells (Marieb & Hoehn 2018). Cells work together to ensure that homeostasis is maintained. Cells come in many different shapes, sizes and life spans; however, they can be categorised depending on their structure and functions. A group of cells that have a similar structure and function, working together as a unit, is called tissue, which unites to form organs for systems of the body (cells → tissue → organ → system). The study of tissue structure and function is called histology. Under a microscope, histologists describe tissues according to the physical features of the tissue, such as the shape and size of the cells, the pattern of cellular arrangement, the connections of cells to one another, and the amount of extracellular material present in the tissue.

Within the human body there are four distinct and primary types of tissue: 1) cells that provide a covering for organs and structures are referred to as **epithelial tissue**; 2) cells that provide support for structures are called **connective tissue**; 3) cells that govern body movement are muscle tissue; and 4) cells that help control homeostasis are nervous tissue. Most organs of the body contain a selection of all four tissue types. The heart, for example, contains muscle tissue, and is controlled by nervous tissue, lined by epithelial tissue and supported by connective tissue. Tissue also has the capacity to repair itself. This chapter examines all four types of tissue and the process of tissue repair.

4.1 Epithelial tissue

LEARNING OBJECTIVE 4.1 Describe the characteristics of epithelial tissue and list the classifications of epithelial tissue.

Epithelial tissue typically consists of one or more sheets of cells connected to each other with a layer of **extracellular matrix**, called the basement **membrane** (discussed later in the chapter). It forms boundaries between different environments and regulates the exchange of material between the internal and external environments. Epithelial tissue covers or lines body surfaces (i.e. skin), or it lines the walls and the organs within body cavities. The major role of epithelial tissue is to act as an interface; indeed, nearly all the substances absorbed or secreted by the body must pass through epithelial tissue. Broadly speaking, epithelial tissue has six main functions:

- absorption
- protection
- excretion
- secretion
- filtration
- sensory reception.

Not all epithelial tissue carries out all six functions. In many areas of the body, epithelial tissue specialises in just one or two functions. Epithelial tissue in the digestive system, for example, specialises in absorption of nutrients, whereas epithelial tissue within skin provides a protective layer.

Epithelial tissue cells are closely bonded together in continuous sheets, which have an apical and a **basal surface**. The **apical surface** faces outwards, towards the exterior of the organ it covers. Apical surfaces can be smooth, but most have hair-like extensions called microvilli. Microvilli dramatically increase the surface area of the epithelial tissue and therefore increase its ability for absorption and secretion. Some areas, within the respiratory tract, for example, possess larger hair-like extensions called cilia, which are also capable of propelling substances. Lying close to the basal surface is a thin sheet of **glycoproteins** that acts as a selective filter, governing which substances can enter epithelial tissue. Epithelial tissue is **innervated** by **neurones**, but it has no blood supply as such. Rather than being served by a network of capillaries, epithelial tissue receives a supply of nutrients from nearby blood vessels. Owing to its protective role, epithelial tissue needs to endure a great deal of abrasion and environmental damage, and epithelial cells need to be very hardy and tough. This hardiness is generated by their ability to divide and regenerate rapidly, resulting in the swift replacement of damaged epithelial cells. However, this regenerative capacity is reliant upon a plentiful supply of nutrients.

Epithelial tissue can be categorised into the following three distinct types:

- simple
- stratified
- glandular.

Simple epithelium consists of a single layer of cells bound into a continuous sheet. Stratified epithelium is also arranged into a continuous sheet but is thicker with numerous layers of cells. Glandular epithelium forms the **glands** of the body.

All epithelial cells have six sides; indeed, under a microscope, a cross-section of epithelial tissue looks like a honeycomb. Epithelial cells can be subdivided further into the following three different six-sided shapes:

- cuboidal
- columnar
- squamous.

As their names suggest, cuboidal and columnar epithelial cells are square and tall respectively, whereas squamous epithelial cells are rather flat and scaly (see figure 4.1). When examining the many different types of epithelial cell, it is easy to work out its size and shape by its name. For instance, simple squamous epithelium is thin, flat and scale-like.

FIGURE 4.1 Epithelial tissue is classified by shape and depth.

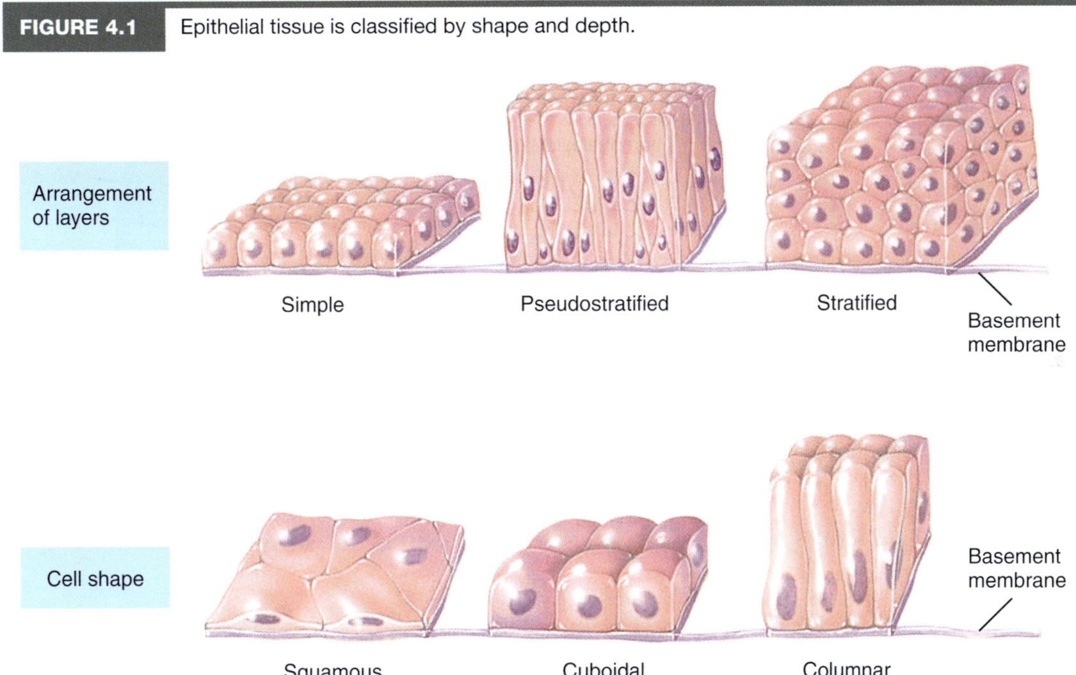

Source: Tortora and Derrickson (2017). Reproduced with permission of John Wiley & Sons.

Simple epithelium

Because simple epithelia consist of a single cellular layer they specialise in absorption, secretion and filtration rather than protection.

Simple squamous epithelium is quite often very permeable and is found where the **diffusion** of nutrients is essential. Capillary walls, the alveoli of the lungs and the glomeruli in the kidneys are all lined with simple squamous epithelium, which facilitates the rapid diffusion of nutrients. Simple squamous epithelium is also found within the heart and blood and lymph vessels. Simple squamous epithelium found within the heart and blood and lymph vessels is called endothelium (see figure 4.2).

Simple cuboidal epithelium specialises in secretion as well as absorption. Simple cuboidal epithelium is found in the lining of the ovaries, the kidney tubules and the ducts of smaller glands. It also forms part of the secretory portions of glands such as the thyroid and pancreas (see figure 4.3).

FIGURE 4.2 (a–c) Simple squamous epithelium forms the endothelial layer of blood vessels.

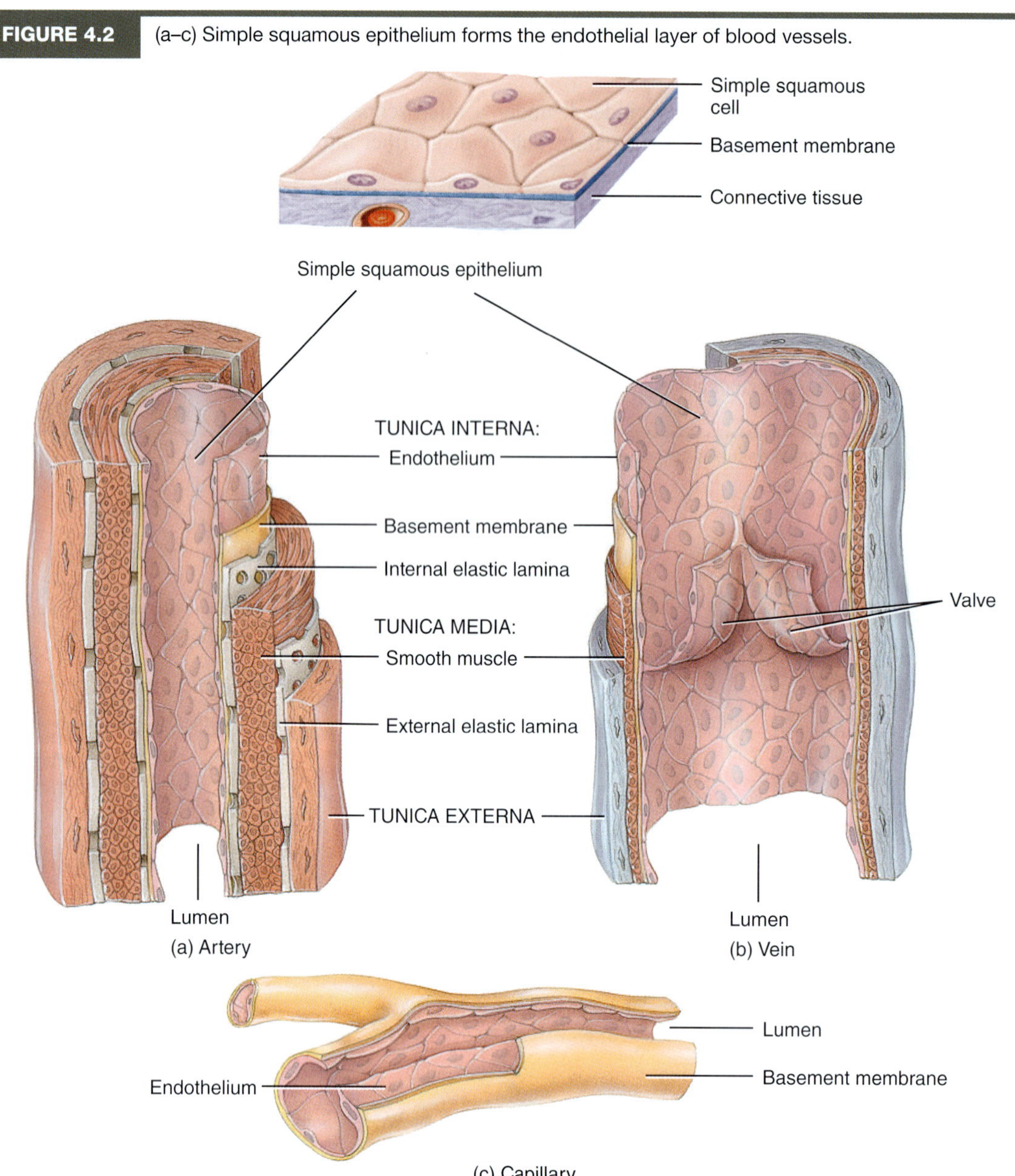

Simple squamous cell
Basement membrane
Connective tissue
Simple squamous epithelium
TUNICA INTERNA:
Endothelium
Basement membrane
Internal elastic lamina
TUNICA MEDIA:
Smooth muscle
External elastic lamina
TUNICA EXTERNA
Valve
Lumen
(a) Artery
Lumen
(b) Vein
Lumen
Basement membrane
Endothelium
(c) Capillary

Source: Tortora and Derrickson (2017). Reproduced with permission of John Wiley & Sons.

FIGURE 4.3 Simple cuboid epithelium forms part of the secretory portion of the pancreas.

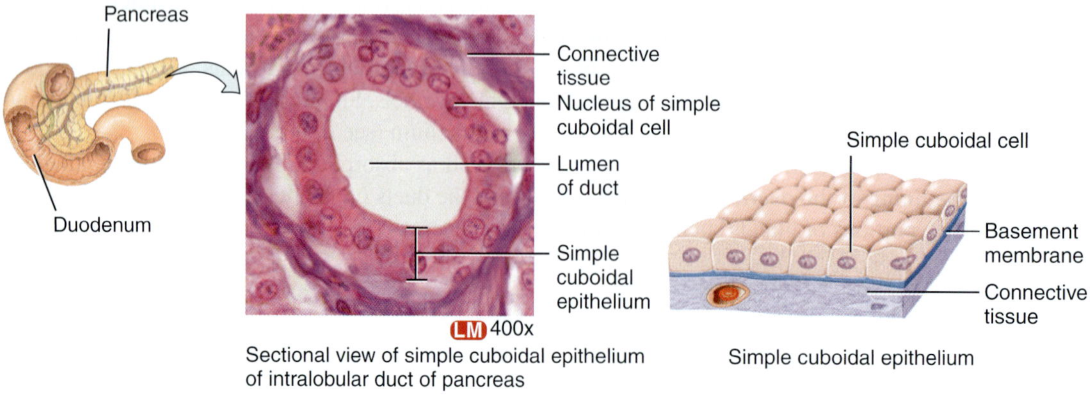

Pancreas
Duodenum
Connective tissue
Nucleus of simple cuboidal cell
Lumen of duct
Simple cuboidal epithelium
LM 400x
Sectional view of simple cuboidal epithelium of intralobular duct of pancreas
Simple cuboidal cell
Basement membrane
Connective tissue
Simple cuboidal epithelium

Source: Tortora and Derrickson (2017). Reproduced with permission of John Wiley & Sons.

Simple columnar epithelium can be ciliated or non-ciliated. As its name suggests, ciliated simple columnar epithelium has cilia on its apical surface. It is found in areas of the body where movement of fluids, mucus or other substances is required. Ciliated simple columnar epithelial tissue, for example, lines the passageways of the central nervous system and helps propel cerebrospinal fluid. It also lines the Fallopian tubes and helps move **oocytes** recently expelled from the ovaries (see figure 4.4). A common location for non-ciliated simple columnar epithelium is the lining of the digestive tract from the stomach to the rectum (see figure 4.5). Non-ciliated simple columnar epithelium performs two broad functions. Some possess microvilli, greatly increasing their surface area for absorption; others specialise in the secretion of mucus. Such cells are referred to as goblet cells owing to their cup-like shape. Simple columnar epithelial cells are generally of equal size. However, in some instances simple columnar epithelial cells vary in height, with only the tallest reaching the apical surface. This gives the illusion that the tissue has many layers, like stratified epithelium. Such examples of columnar epithelial tissue are called pseudostratified columnar epithelium. Pseudostratified columnar epithelium is found within the lining of the male reproductive system; however, the most common location is the lining of the respiratory tract (see figure 4.6).

FIGURE 4.4 Ciliated simple columnar epithelium lines the Fallopian tubes.

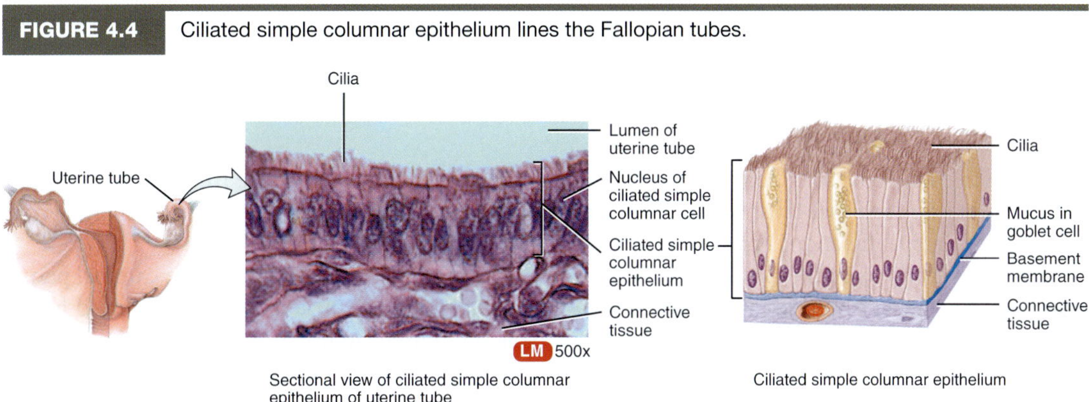

Source: Tortora and Derrickson (2017). Reproduced with permission of John Wiley & Sons.

FIGURE 4.5 Non-ciliated columnar epithelium lines the digestive tract.

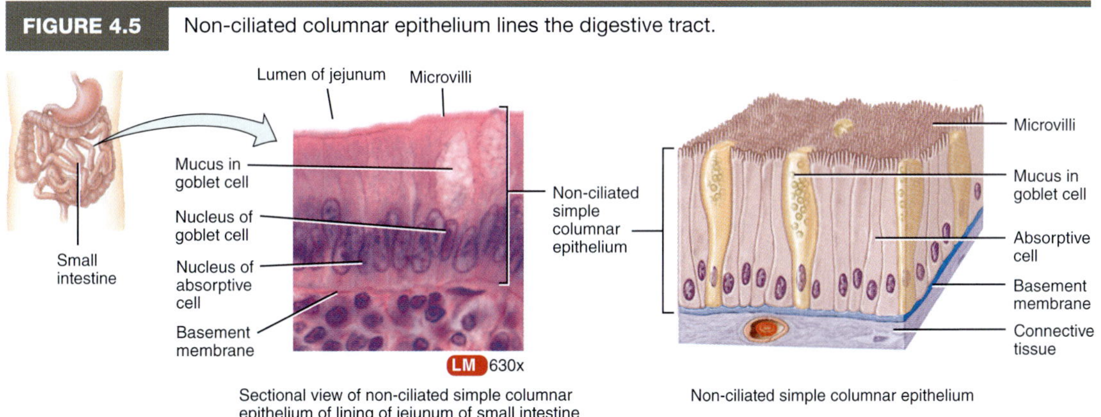

Source: Tortora and Derrickson (2017). Reproduced with permission of John Wiley & Sons.

FIGURE 4.6 Pseudostratified ciliated columnar epithelium lines the trachea.

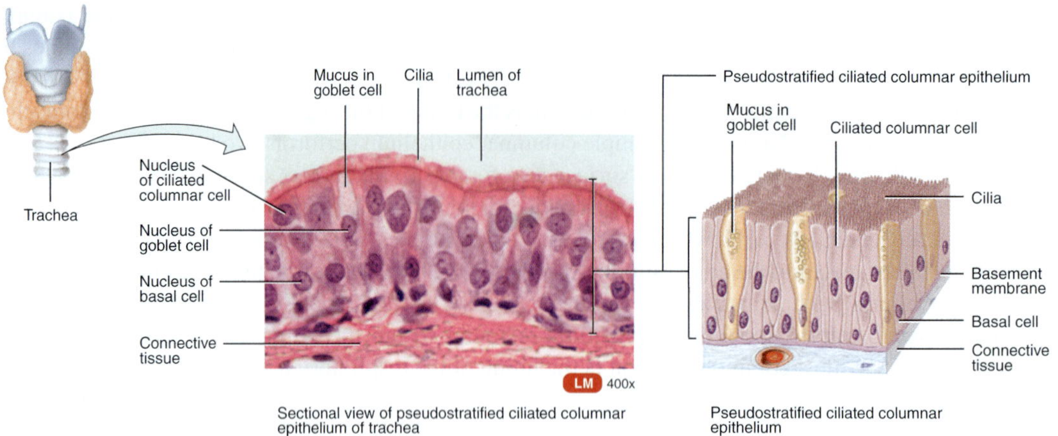

Source: Tortora and Derrickson (2017). Reproduced with permission of John Wiley & Sons.

Stratified epithelium

Unlike simple epithelia, stratified epithelia have many layers. The cells regenerate from below, with new cells dividing on the basal layer pushing the older cells towards the surface. As stratified epithelium is thicker, its principal function is protection.

Stratified squamous epithelium is the most common stratified epithelium and forms the external part of skin (see the chapter on the skin). Stratified squamous epithelial tissue is keratinised, toughened by the presence of **keratin**, a special tough fibrous protein. Non-keratinised stratified squamous epithelial tissue lines wet areas of the body — the mouth, the tongue and the vagina for example (see figure 4.7). Only the outer layers of stratified squamous epithelium are squamous in shape; the basal layers may be cuboidal or columnar.

FIGURE 4.7 Non-keratinised stratified squamous epithelial tissue lines the vagina.

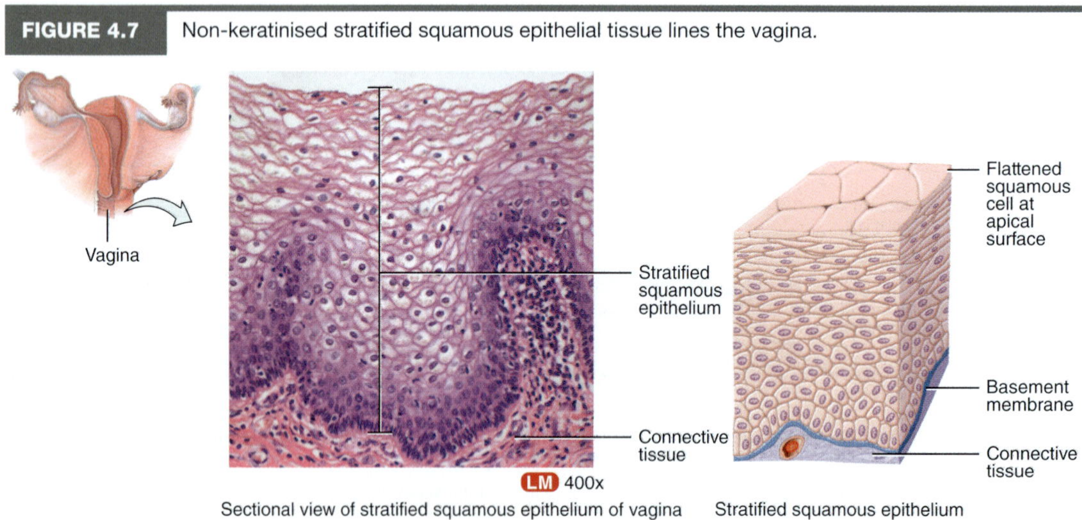

Source: Tortora and Derrickson (2017). Reproduced with permission of John Wiley & Sons.

Stratified cuboidal epithelium is found in the oesophagus, sweat glands and in the male urethra (see figure 4.8). Stratified columnar epithelium, however, is quite rare. Small amounts can be found in the male urethra and in the ducts of some glands. Another common example of stratified epithelium is transitional epithelium, which may have both squamous and cuboidal cells in its apical surface. The basal surface may contain both cuboidal and columnar cells. Transitional epithelium can withstand a great deal of stretch and is found in organs such as the bladder, which is subject to considerable distension (see figure 4.9).

FIGURE 4.8 Cuboidal epithelial tissue is found in the oesophagus.

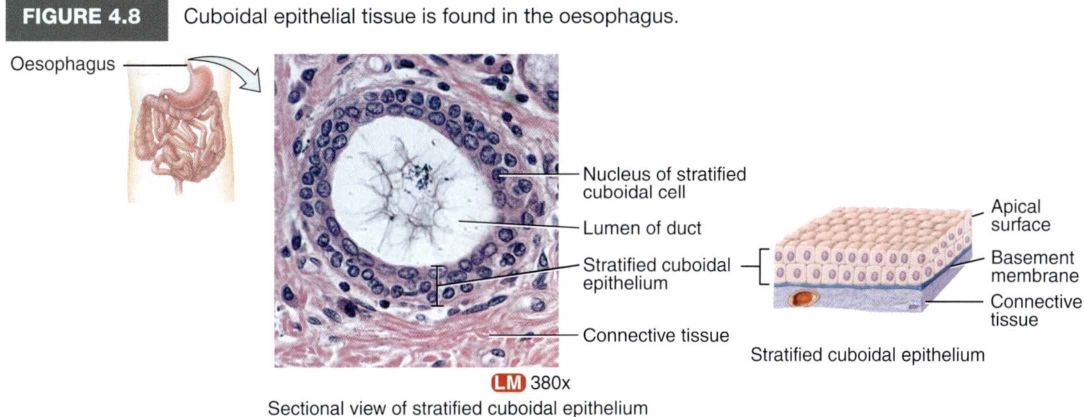

Sectional view of stratified cuboidal epithelium of the duct of an oesophageal gland

Source: Tortora and Derrickson (2017). Reproduced with permission of John Wiley & Sons.

FIGURE 4.9 Transitional epithelium lines the bladder and allows for distension.

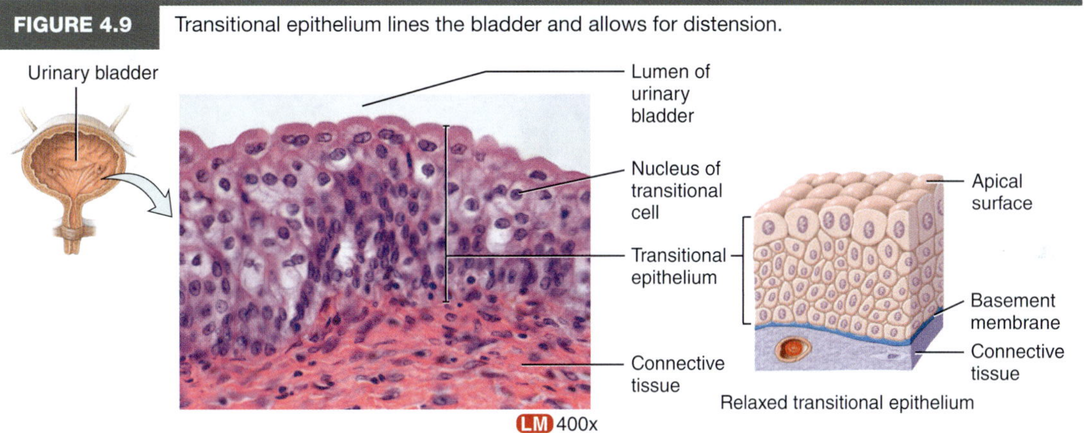

Sectional view of transitional epithelium of urinary bladder in relaxed state

Source: Tortora and Derrickson (2017). Reproduced with permission of John Wiley & Sons.

Glandular epithelia

The glands of the body are formed by glandular epithelia. All glands are classified as *endocrine* or *exocrine*. Glands that secrete their products internally are called **endocrine glands**. Endocrine glands release **hormones**, regulatory chemicals for use elsewhere in the body (see the chapter on the endocrine system). **Exocrine glands** release their products onto the surface of epithelial tissue. Exocrine glands are either *unicellular* or *multicellular*. Unicellular exocrine glands consist of a single cell type and the main example is the goblet cell, which releases a glycoprotein called mucin. Once dissolved in water, mucin forms mucus, which lubricates and protects surfaces. Multicellular exocrine glands are far more complex, coming in several shapes and sizes. Some exocrine glands are simple and consist of a single branched duct, whereas others are more complex with multibranched ducts (see figure 4.10). However, they all contain two distinct areas: an epithelial duct and secretory cells (acinus). Exocrine glands that are tubular in shape can be found within the digestive system and stomach. Other exocrine glands are spherical and referred to as alveolar or acinar. The oil glands within skin and mammary glands are two examples of spherical- or acinar-shaped exocrine glands. Glands that are both tubular and acinar are referred to as tubulacinar. The salivary glands, for example, are tubulacinar.

FIGURE 4.10 Exocrine glands classified by shape, with examples of location

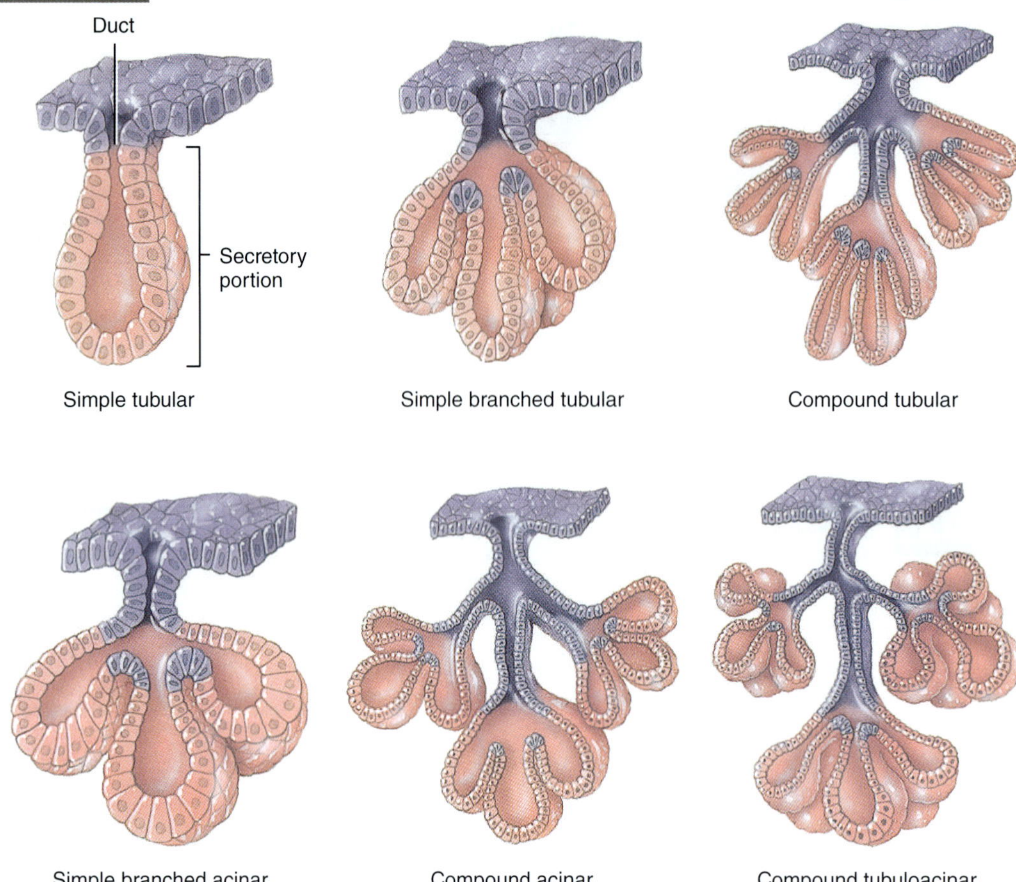

Source: Tortora and Derrickson (2017). Reproduced with permission of John Wiley & Sons.

CLINICAL CONSIDERATIONS

Burns

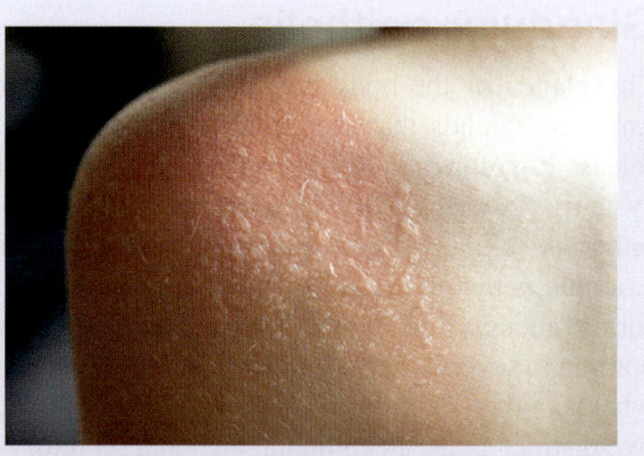

Burn injuries can arise from a variety of factors such as thermal (i.e. direct heat transfer from boiling liquid, fire or hot objects), chemicals, electricity or radiation (i.e. sunlight). In 2014, burn injuries made up 1 per cent of all Australian hospitalisation cases for injuries in a year period, with patients presenting with either partial-thickness (70%) or full-thickness (30%) burns (AIHW 2016). Indigenous Australians made up 9 per cent of all burns hospitalisation cases, or 0.6 per cent of the general Australian population compared with 0.2 per cent for the non-Indigenous population (AIHW 2016). The survival rates for burn patients have improved dramatically in the past five decades due to medical advances and burn management practices at specialised care centres.

Burns can be categorised into four types according to the depth of burnt tissue. Clinicians have to ascertain the type of burn according to the national guidelines for effective treatment and management plans (RCHM 2020).

1. *Superficial.* Only the outer epithelial layer or epidermis of the skin is damaged (e.g. sunburn). This is made up of four to five layers of epithelial cells. This type of burn leads to painful red skin, usually without blistering, and heals within days to a week, without scarring.

2. *Superficial partial thickness.* Both the epidermis and dermis layers are damaged. The dermis consists of blood capillaries and lymph vessels, nerves and hair follicles. This leads to painful episodes, usually with mild blisters which are sensitive to air. It takes 7 to 21 days to heal and may lead to permanent skin colour change.
3. *Deep partial thickness.* Damage to the deepest skin layer, known as, hypodermis or **subcutaneous** tissue. This layer is made up of blood vessels, adipose and connective tissue. Burns like these cause pain with deep pressure and formation of blisters. It takes longer than 21 days to heal and leaves severe scarring. It may require skin grafting to prevent infection and scarring.
4. *Full thickness.* Complete destruction of the skin with damage to underlying structures like nerves, muscles tendons and bones. This is painless due to loss of nerve endings with no blister formation. This type of burn appears waxy white to leathery grey or charred black, and needs surgical intervention to heal, resulting in severe scarring.

Hypothermia is a common complication for major burns when the burnt skin is unable to regulate body temperature. Severe burns can also lead to burn hypovolaemic shock (blood volume depletion) with loss of plasma from burnt surfaces and a rise in haematocrit levels producing severe haemoconcentration. This leads to low pulmonary artery occlusion pressure, respiratory/airway distress, increased vascular resistance and decreased cardiac output with overall complex metabolic changes. In addition to the aforementioned changes, a high chance of infection of burnt areas and kidney damage adds to the medical complexity, which requires a timely intervention to reduce long-term damage or mortality for patients with major burns — a high mortality rate presents when full-thickness burns cover more than 75 per cent of the body. The healthcare providers at various stages need to monitor for signs and symptoms indicating these complications very closely. Effective fluid resuscitation and/or airway management help to relieve the effect of rapid physiological changes.

4.2 Connective tissue

LEARNING OBJECTIVE 4.2 Discuss the functions of connective tissue and list the classifications of connective tissue.

Connective tissue is the most abundant and widely distributed tissue in the human body. Its main functions are to bind tissues together, reinforcement, insulation, protection, transport of substances within the body and support. All epithelial tissue is reinforced by the connective tissue base it rests upon (see figure 4.11). There are four types of connective tissue:

- connective tissue proper
- **cartilage**
- bone
- liquid connective tissue.

Connective tissue is not present on body surfaces and, unlike epithelial tissue, is highly vascular and receives a rich blood supply.

The following types of cell are present in connective tissue:

- adipocytes
- primary blast cells
- **macrophages**
- plasma cells
- mast cells
- leucocytes (white blood cells).

Adipose tissue is primarily made up of adipocytes, which are known as fat cells. Within connective tissue, adipocytes store triglycerides (fats). An adipocyte of white fat usually contains a single large liquid droplet that makes up the majority of the adult cell. The white fat makes up the most common type of adipose tissue and its function is to store energy in the form of lipids, as well as cushioning and insulating the body. The other type of fat is the brown version contained as multiple droplets within an adipocyte, which is usually present in infants for temperature regulation. Primary blast cells continually secrete ground substance and produce mature connective tissue cells. Each type of connective tissue contains its own unique primary blast cells (see table 4.1). Macrophages, plasma cells and white blood cells form part of the body's immune system. Their functions are as follows.

- Macrophages engulf invading substances and plasma cells produce antibodies.
- White blood cells are not normally found in significant numbers within connective tissue; however, they do migrate into connective tissue during inflammation.
- Mast cells produce histamine, which promotes vasodilatation during the body's inflammatory response.

FIGURE 4.11 Connective tissue reinforces epithelial tissue.

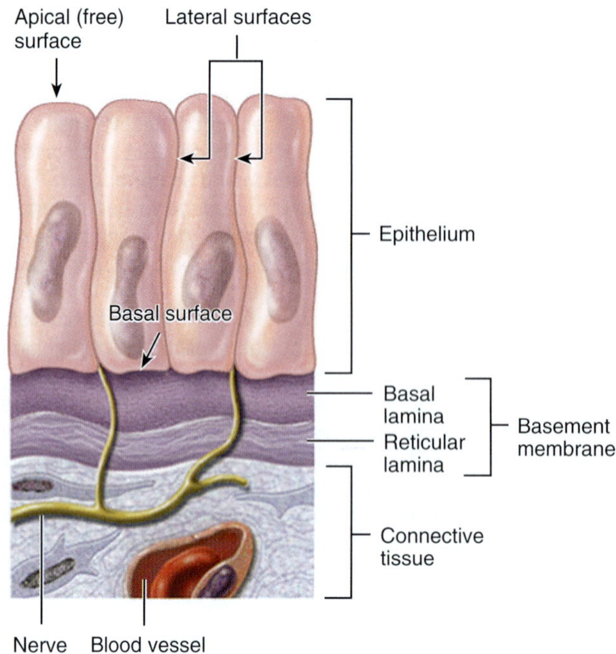

Source: Tortora and Derrickson (2017). Reproduced with permission of John Wiley & Sons.

TABLE 4.1 The major primary blast cells and their connective tissue type

Connective tissue type	Primary blast cell	Connective tissue cell
Connective tissue proper	Fibroblast	Fibrocyte
Cartilage	Chondroblast	Chondrocyte
Bone	Osteoblast	Osteocyte

Connective tissue cells are surrounded by a collection of substances referred to as the extracellular matrix. The function of the extracellular matrix is to ensure that connective tissue can bear weight and withstand tension, abuse and abrasion. As a result, connective tissue can cope with stresses and strains other tissues would not be able to tolerate. The two main elements of extracellular matrix are:

- ground substance
- fibres.

Ground substance

This consists of **interstitial fluid**, cell adhesion proteins and glycosaminoglycans. Cell adhesion proteins act as connective glue, keeping the tissue cells together. Glycosaminoglycans trap water and ensure ground substance has a jelly-like constitution. The higher the amount of glycosaminoglycans present, the harder the ground substance will be.

Fibres

There are three types of fibre found within extracellular matrix:

- collagen
- elastic
- reticular.

Collagen fibres are the most abundant fibre found within the extracellular matrix and are essentially the protein collagen. Collagen is very tough; indeed, collagen fibres are stronger than similar-sized steel fibres (Marieb & Hoehn 2018). Reticular fibres are much thinner but also contain bundles of collagen.

They provide support and strength and are found in greater numbers in soft organs such as the **spleen** and **lymph nodes**. Elastic fibres contain the rubberlike protein called elastin, which facilitates stretch and recoil. Elastic fibres are found in greater numbers in tissue that must endure stretch, such as skin and blood vessel walls (see figure 4.12).

FIGURE 4.12 Constituents of connective tissue

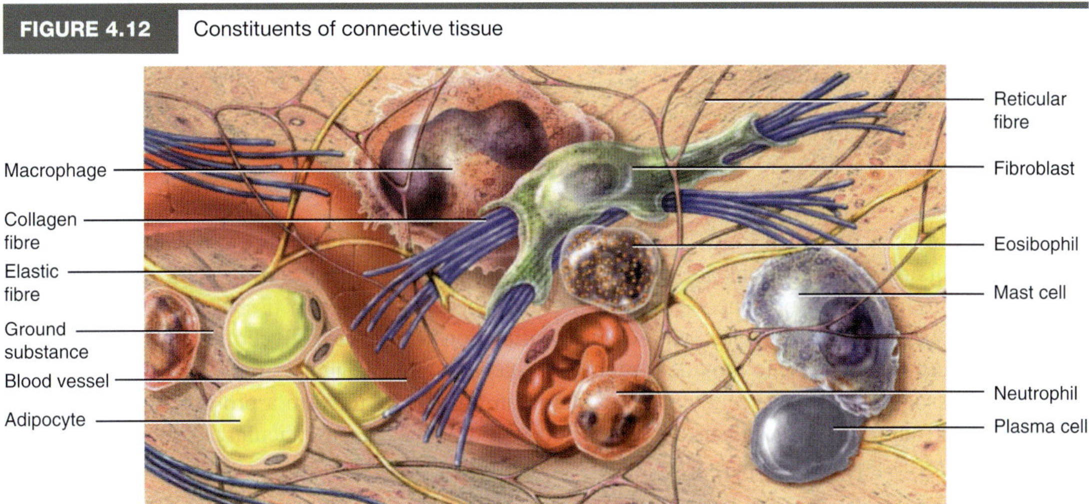

Source: Tortora and Derrickson (2017). Reproduced with permission of John Wiley & Sons.

Connective tissue proper

Aside from cartilage, bone and blood, all connective tissue belongs to this class. Connective tissue proper is subdivided further into:

- loose connective tissue
- dense connective tissue.

Loose connective tissue contains fewer fibres than dense connective tissue (see table 4.2).

TABLE 4.2 **Types of connective tissue proper, their main constituents, functions and locations**

Connective tissue	Main constituent	Functions	Main locations
Loose areolar	Collagen, elastic, reticular fibres	Strength Elasticity Support	Subcutaneous layer beneath skin
Loose adipose	Adipocytes	Insulation	Subcutaneous layer beneath skin
		Protection	Tissue surrounding heart and kidneys
		Energy store	Padding around joints
Loose reticular	Reticular fibres	Support	Liver
	Reticular cells	Filtration	Spleen Lymph nodes
Dense regular	Collagen fibres arranged in parallel	Strength	Tendons
		Support	Ligaments
Dense irregular	Collagen fibres arranged randomly	Strength	Skin
			Heart Tissue surrounding bone Tissue surrounding cartilage

(continued)

TABLE 4.2 *(continued)*

Connective tissue	Main constituent	Functions	Main locations
Dense elastic	Elastic fibres	Stretch	Lung tissue Arteries

Loose connective tissue

There are three types of loose connective tissue:

- areolar
- adipose
- reticular.

Areolar is the most abundant loose connective tissue. It contains all three fibres (collagen, elastic and reticular) and its primary functions are support, elasticity and strength. Areolar tissue is combined with adipose tissue to form the subcutaneous layer, which connects skin with other tissues and organs.

Adipose tissue contains adipocytes, whose primary function is to store triglycerides (fat). The primary functions of adipose tissue are to provide insulation, protection and an energy store.

Reticular tissue only contains reticular fibres. Its main function is to form a protective framework or **stroma** that surrounds the liver, spleen and lymph nodes. Within the spleen, reticular connective tissue can also filter blood, assisting with the removal of old blood cells.

Dense connective tissue

Dense connective tissue contains more collagen or elastic fibres. Dense connective tissue that is made primarily from collagen is said to be either regular or irregular depending on the organisation of the collagen fibres. Dense regular connective tissue contains collagen fibres that are arranged in parallel rows. It has a silvery appearance and is both tough and pliable. Dense, irregular connective tissue is found in ligaments and tendons. Its collagen fibres are randomly arranged but closely knitted together. Dense irregular tissue can withstand pressure and pulling forces and is found in skin and the heart as well as the membranes that surround cartilage and bone. Dense elastic connective tissue consists of elastic fibres. Dense elastic connective tissue is found in areas of the body that must withstand great amounts of stretch, such as arteries and lung tissue.

Cartilage

Cartilage contains a compact network of collagen fibres and is stronger than both loose and dense connective tissue. It is found in structures such as the nose, ears, knee, ankle, rib cage and windpipe. It is a flexible connective tissue that has the ability to return to its original shape after stress and movement. Its strength and resilience are provided by a gel-like substance called chondroitin sulphate, which is found in cartilage ground substance. Cartilage is surrounded by a layer of dense irregular tissue called perichondrium. Perichondrium is the only area of cartilage that is served by blood and nervous tissue. There are three types of cartilage:

- hyaline
- fibrocartilage
- elastic.

Hyaline cartilage is the most common cartilage in the human body. It mainly comprises collagen fibres with cartilage cells, with chondrocytes accounting for around 10 per cent of its volume. The collagen fibres are so fine they are almost invisible, giving hyaline cartilage a bluish appearance. Because hyaline cartilage is both strong and flexible it can act as a shock absorber, reducing friction around joints. Hyaline cartilage is also found in the rib cage and airways (e.g. nose, trachea and larynx).

Elastic cartilage is almost identical to hyaline cartilage. The major difference between hyaline and elastic cartilage is the greater presence of elastic fibres. Elastic cartilage can withstand greater movement and bending and is found in areas of the body where stretchability is required — the outer ear for example.

Fibrocartilage is the strongest of the three cartilages. Its strength is provided by rows of chondrocytes and collagen. Because it can withstand great pressure it is found where hyaline cartilage meets tendons or ligaments, between the discs of the **vertebrae** for example (see figure 4.13).

FIGURE 4.13 Where cartilage is found within the body

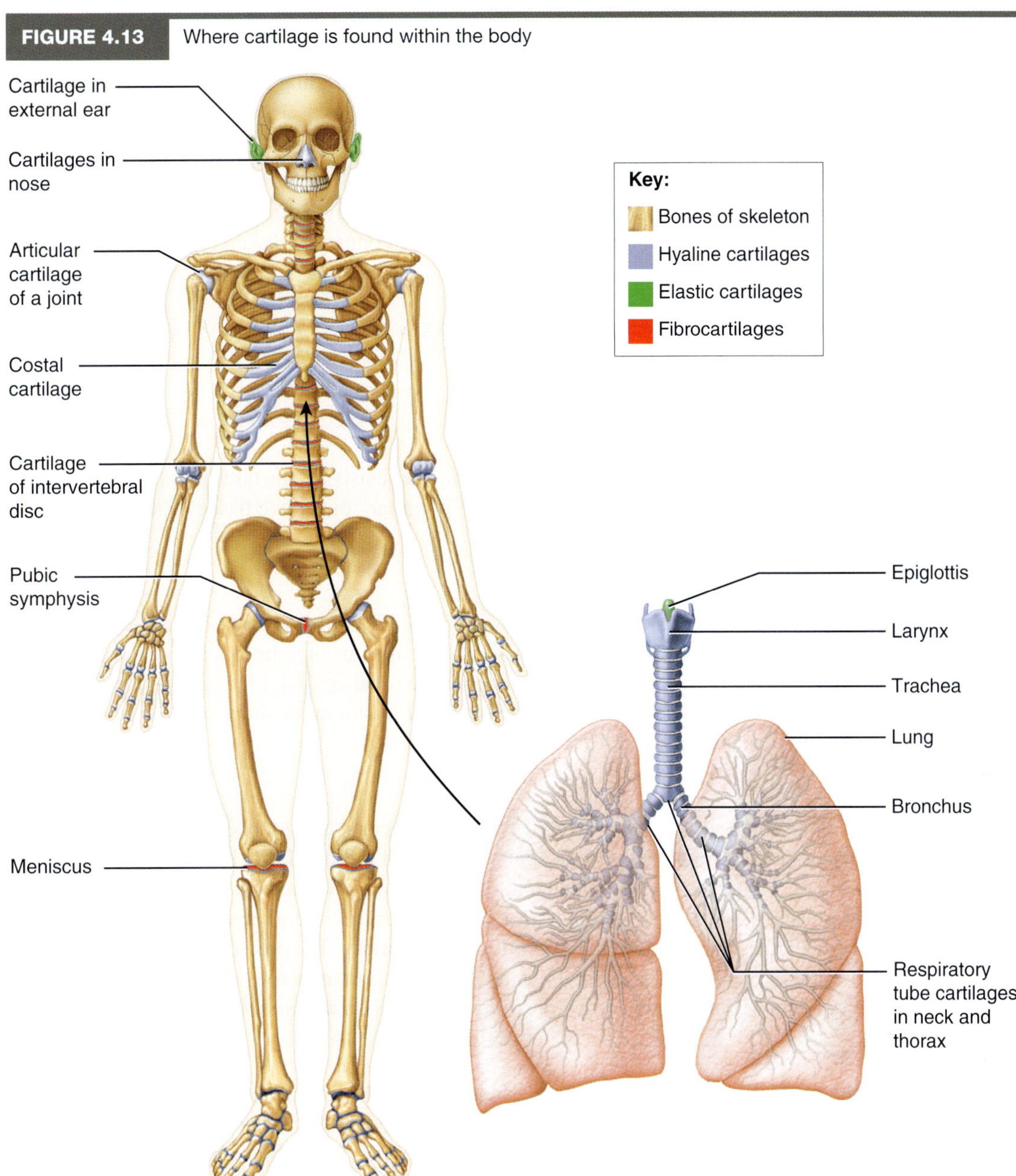

Source: Jenkins et al. (2009). Reproduced with permission of John Wiley & Sons.

Bone

Along with cartilage, bones make up the human skeletal frame. Bone is similar to cartilage but contains even greater amounts of collagen, and primarily contains calcium salts like calcium phosphate. For this reason, bone is harder and more rigid, facilitating greater protection and support for body structures. However, unlike cartilage, bone receives a rich supply of blood. Bone also stores fat and plays an important role in the production of blood cells. A more detailed examination of bones can be found in the chapter on the muscular system.

Liquid connective tissue

Connective tissue that has a liquid extracellular matrix includes:

- blood
- lymph.

Blood and lymph are said to be atypical connective tissues because, strictly speaking, they do not connect tissues or provide mechanical support. The extracellular matrix of blood is plasma. Blood cells include erythrocytes, leucocytes and platelets. Blood and plasma perform many important functions. For a detailed explanation of blood, see the chapter on the circulatory system. Lymph has a clear extracellular matrix very similar to plasma. The primary function of lymph is defence against invading pathogens. A more detailed exploration of lymph can be found in the chapter on the immune system.

Membranes

Membranes are sheets of tissue that cover or line areas of the human body. Structurally, membranes consist of an epithelial tissue layer that is bound to a basement layer of connective tissue. There are four major types of membrane:

- cutaneous
- mucous
- serous
- synovial.

Cutaneous membranes

The principal example of a cutaneous membrane is skin. It consists of an outer stratified squamous epithelial layer, which sits on top of a thick layer of dense irregular connective tissue. The functions and structure of skin are detailed in the chapter on the skin.

Mucous membranes

Mucous membranes line the external surfaces of body cavities. Examples include hollow organs of the digestive tract, the respiratory system and the renal system. All mucous membranes are wet or moist, but not all secrete lubricating mucus. The mucous membranes of the renal system, for example, are wet due to the presence of urine. Most mucous membranes contain stratified squamous or simple columnar epithelium supported by a layer of connective tissue referred to as lamina propria.

Serous membranes

Serous membranes or a serosa cover internal body cavities. They consist of areolar connective tissue that is covered by a special kind of simple squamous epithelium called mesothelium. Mesothelium secretes a watery substance referred to as serous fluid, which allows organs to slide against one another with ease. Serous membranes consist of an outer or parietal layer and an inner or visceral layer. The largest example is the peritoneum, which lines the organs of the **abdominopelvic cavity**. The protective lining of the lungs, the parietal and visceral pleura, provides another example of an important serous membrane. The parietal and visceral pleura glide over one another when the thorax expands on inspiration.

Synovial membranes

Unlike serous, mucous and cutaneous membranes, synovial membranes do not contain any epithelial tissue. Synovial membranes are mainly found in moving joints and consist of areolar connective tissue, adipocytes, and elastic and collagen fibres. They secrete synovial fluid, which bathes, nourishes and lubricates the joints. Synovial fluid also contains macrophages, which destroy invading microbes and remove debris from the joint cavity. Synovial membranes are also found in cushion-like sacs in the hands and feet that ease the movement of tendons (see figure 4.14).

FIGURE 4.14 Synovial membranes fill joint cavities.

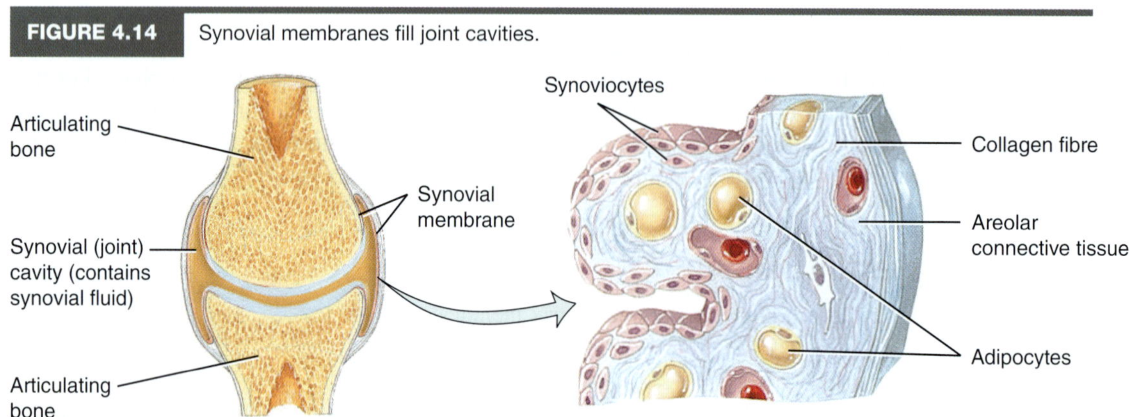

Source: Tortora and Derrickson (2017). Reproduced with permission of John Wiley & Sons.

CLINICAL CONSIDERATIONS

Peritonitis

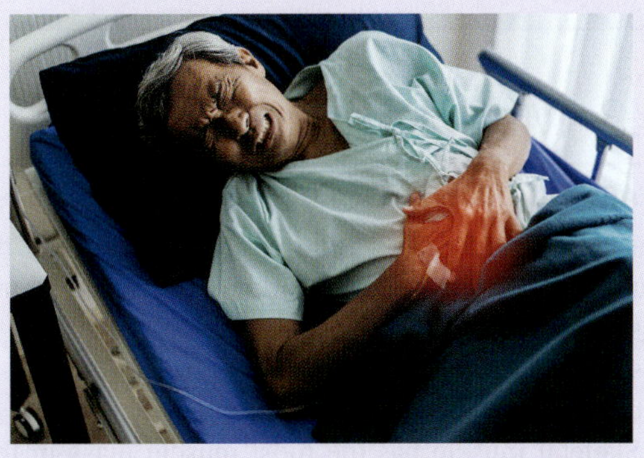

Peritonitis is a life-threatening inflammation of the peritoneum, the serous membrane that lines both the digestive organs and the wall of the abdominopelvic cavity. It may be classified as primary with spontaneous bacterial peritonitis, which is an infection of ascites due to liver or kidney disease. Conversely, peritonitis can be secondary due to inflammation or mechanical rupture in the gastrointestinal tract, genitourinary tract or a solid organ that causes the peritoneal cavity to be exposed to the resident flora, which may lead to bacterial infection. The causes of peritonitis are either chemical or bacterial. Chemical peritonitis occurs due to damage to neighbouring structures resulting in a mechanical break; that is, a piercing wound or ulcer that leaks digestive juices into the peritoneum without bacterial inoculation of the peritoneal cavity. Bacterial peritonitis results from the direct contamination of the peritoneum. If left unaddressed, chemical peritonitis will rapidly lead to bacterial peritonitis within 24 hours. Complications from peritonitis include loss of bowel movements and hypovolaemic shock.

Peritonitis can be a major complication of peritoneal dialysis as a result of technique failure. Australian research has shown that Indigenous patients receiving peritoneal dialysis are twice more likely to develop peritonitis than non-Indigenous Australians (Lim et al. 2005) due to higher technique failure, especially in rural areas (Marley et al. 2014).

Diagnoses for peritonitis involve physical examination, medical history collection, blood tests, X-ray or CT scans, and peritoneal fluid analysis (ANZGOSA n.d.). The treatment options include hospitalisation with fluid and electrolyte infusion, antibiotics, and surgery to drain and repair the area. Failure of timely intervention may lead to sepsis, multiorgan failure, or even death.

Peritonitis is an acute medical emergency and is associated with high mortality. Survival rates have increased since the use of **prophylactic antibiotics** (Hubert & VanMeter 2018).

CLINICAL CONSIDERATIONS

Pneumothorax

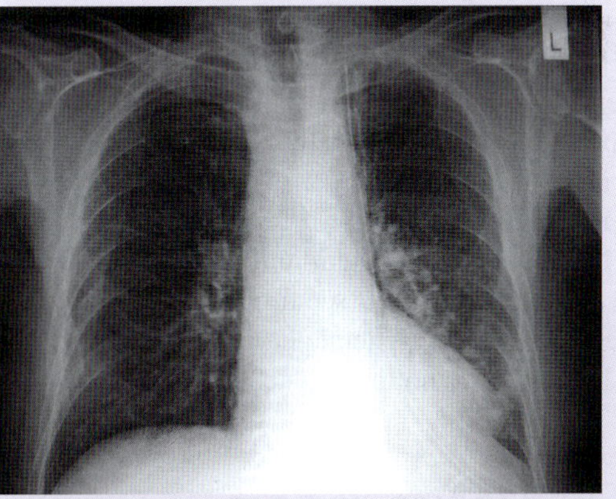

A pneumothorax or collapsed lung occurs when air accumulates in the pleural cavity, the small space between the visceral and parietal pleura. The most common form is the spontaneous or primary form that occurs in healthy people without an underlying cause, especially in those who are tall and thin or who undertake extreme activities such as scuba diving or high-altitude flying. The secondary form can occur due to complications from chronic lung diseases, especially chronic obstructive pulmonary disease (COPD), asthma and cystic fibrosis, and lung infections such as pneumonia and tuberculosis. Other forms include traumatic pneumothorax seen in accidents. In a small number of cases the pleura separates spontaneously due to a congenital defect. Diagnoses involve examinations of previous medical history, physical examinations (checking for breathing sounds) and chest X-rays or ultrasound imaging.

In a small pneumothorax, the lung may heal on its own by reinflating over time and can be treated with high-flow oxygen and frequent assessments. However, large pneumothorax cases are potentially life-threatening, and may require surgical interventions such as insertion of chest drains to remove the air (tension) from the pleura and allow the lungs to reinflate. In most cases, the correct placement of the chest tubes allows the lung to expand quickly and fully.

In the field, paramedics can diagnose pneumothorax with physical examinations for chest and breathing, and mobile ultrasound devices. The first line of medical intervention is an emergency chest decompression to reduce the progressive pressure build-up by trapped air in the pleural cavity (tension pneumothorax). Tension pneumothorax can cause respiratory compromise and haemodynamic instability, which may lead to morbidity or mortality if timely and adequate medical intervention is not provided (Raio et al. 2009).

4.3 Muscle tissue

LEARNING OBJECTIVE 4.3 Describe the structure of the three types of muscle tissue and their function.

Muscle tissue contains long muscle fibres whose primary function is to generate force. Muscle tissue is found where there is a need for movement and maintenance of posture. Muscle is classified in three ways:

- skeletal
- smooth
- cardiac.

Skeletal muscle has the most muscle mass in the body and is found adjacent to the skeleton and its function is twofold: the movement of the skeleton and the maintenance of body posture. It is attached to bones via tendons made up of collagen. The structure of the muscle fibres within skeletal muscle gives a striped or striated appearance. These fibres are bound with connective tissue and arranged in parallel with their long axes. Skeletal muscle is also voluntary, meaning its movement can be controlled by conscious control (see figure 4.15).

Smooth muscle, on the other hand, is both involuntary and non-striated. Smooth muscle is found in hollow internal structures (organs or tubes) where fluid or solid substances need to be propelled from one area to another. This allows the repeated contractions to change the shape of the structure. Smooth muscle is the primary muscle of internal organs, and is found in blood vessels, where blood is propelled through the vascular system, the gastrointestinal tract, where **chyme** is moved from the stomach through the intestines towards the rectum, and the urinary bladder to store and release urine. The smooth muscle contracts and relaxes much slower than either skeletal or cardiac muscle, uses less energy to create a given amount of force, and can sustain the force for longer periods of time.

Cardiac muscle is striated, but it is also involuntary. As its name suggests, cardiac muscle is only found in the heart and provides the driving force of contraction. A more detailed examination of muscle can be found in the chapter on the skeletal system.

4.4 Nervous tissue

LEARNING OBJECTIVE 4.4 Describe the types of nervous tissue cells.

Nervous tissue is found within the nervous system (see the chapter on the nervous system). There are two types of nervous tissue cells:

- neurones
- **neuroglia**.

Neurones are the functioning unit of the nervous system. They consist of three basic parts: the cell body, an axon and dendrites (see figure 4.16). Their primary function is the propagation of nerve signals within the central and peripheral nervous systems.

Neuroglia do not propagate nerve signals; rather, they nourish, protect and support neurones.

4.5 Tissue repair

LEARNING OBJECTIVE 4.5 Describe the process of tissue repair.

Tissue repair occurs in order to replace cells that are damaged, worn out or dead. Each of the four tissue types has the capacity to regenerate and replace cells injured by trauma, disease or other events. However, the tissue types have differing success rates. Because epithelial cells have to withstand large amounts of wear and tear, they have great capacity for renewal. Epithelial tissue often contains immature cells called stem cells, which can divide and replace lost cells easily. Most connective tissue also has great capacity for renewal; however, owing to the lack of blood supply, cartilage can take a long time to heal.

FIGURE 4.15 The major muscle types with examples of their location: (a) skeletal muscle; (b) cardiac muscle; (c) smooth muscle

(a)

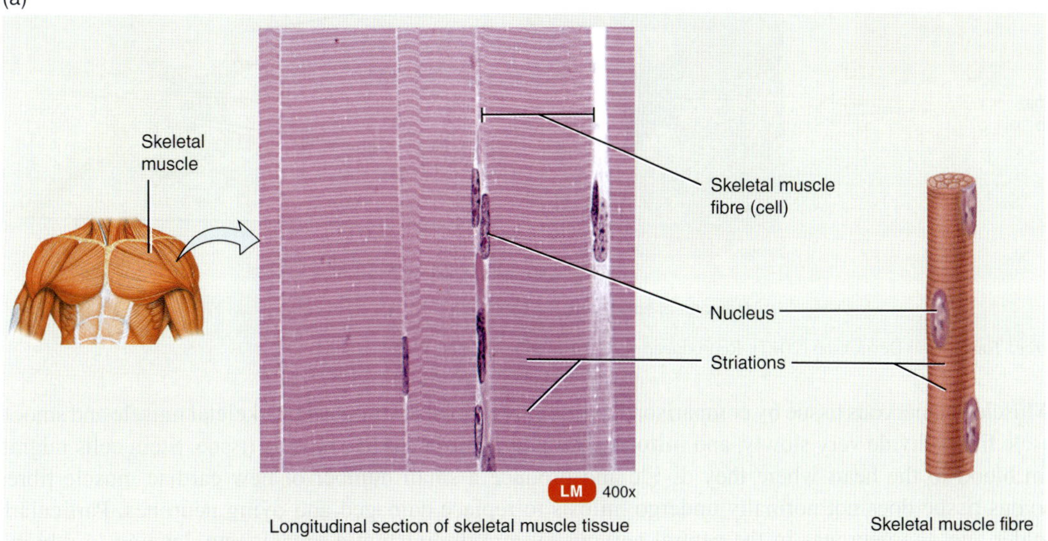

(b)

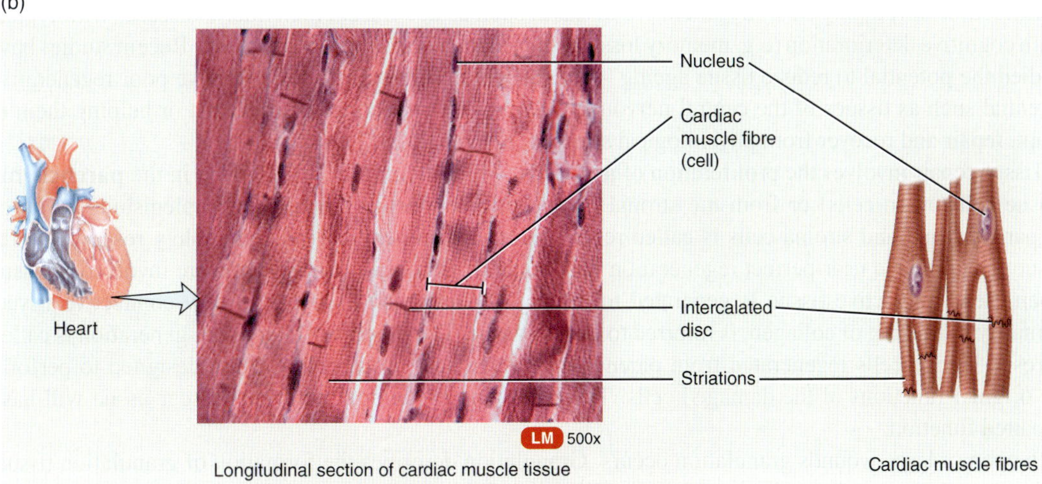

(c)

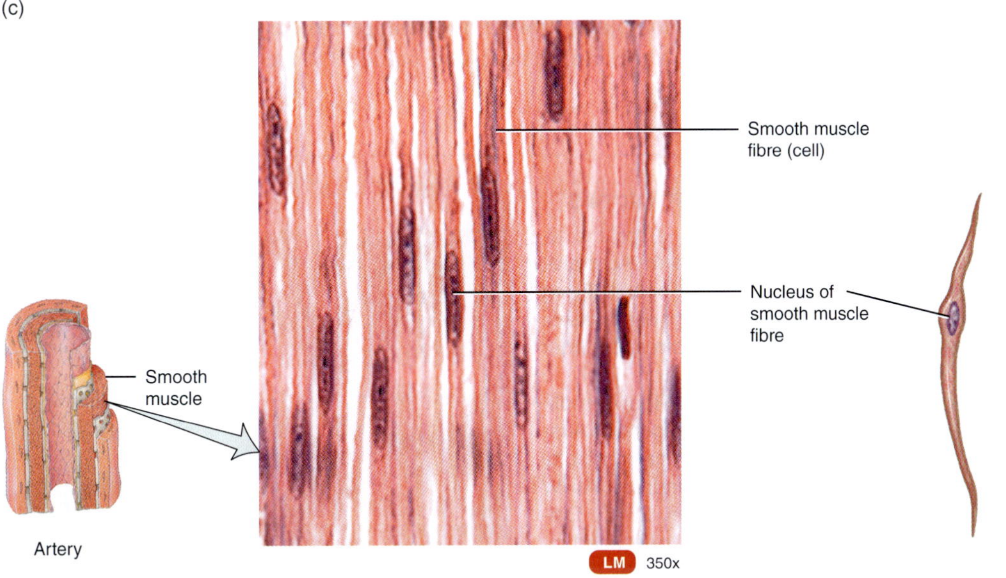

Source: Tortora and Derrickson (2017). Reproduced with permission of John Wiley & Sons.

FIGURE 4.16 An example of nervous tissue

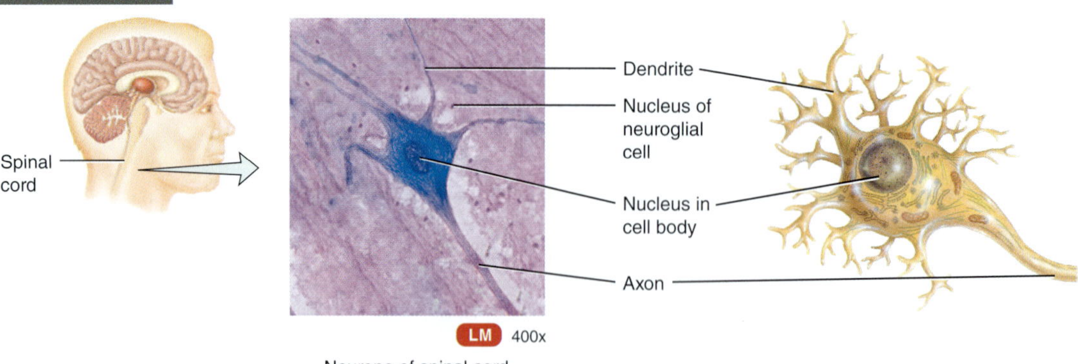

Source: Tortora and Derrickson (2017). Reproduced with permission of John Wiley & Sons.

Muscle and nervous tissue by comparison have poor regeneration properties. Skeletal muscle and smooth muscle fibres divide very slowly, and **mitosis** does not occur in cardiac muscle tissue. Stem cells migrate from blood to the heart where they divide and produce a small number of new cardiac muscle fibres. Nervous tissue does not normally undergo mitosis to replace damaged and dying neurones. Particularly in older age, the neurones in the central nervous system diminish at a greater rate, leading to a higher likelihood of developing neurodegenerative diseases such as age-onset Alzheimer's disease, with typical brain cognitive deterioration (e.g. memory loss; see the chapter on the nervous system). Recent studies have studied the potential to reduce tissue ageing — in particular, for tissues known to have poor regenerative potential such as tissues of the central nervous system — by protecting them against or helping them to adapt, repair and recover from physiological stresses (Kim et al. 2017).

Tissue repair involves the proliferation of new cells, which stem from cell division in the **parenchyma** (tissue cells/organ cells) or from the stroma (supporting connective tissue). The replenishing of tissue by parenchymal and stroma cells is called regeneration. If parenchymal cells are solely responsible for tissue repair, then a near-perfect regeneration may occur. If fibroblasts from stroma are involved in tissue repair, new connective tissue is generated to replace the damaged tissue. This new connective tissue, primarily consisting of collagen, is referred to as scar tissue. The process of scar tissue generation is called fibrosis. Unlike cells regenerated from parenchymal cells, scar tissue cells are not designed to perform the original functions of the damaged cells. Therefore, any organ or structure with scar tissue will have impaired function.

In open or large wounds granulation occurs. Granulation describes the formation of granulation tissue, which covers the healing tissue and secretes bacterial fluid. During this process both parenchymal and stromal cells are active in the repair. Fibroblasts provide new collagen tissue to strengthen the area, and new blood capillaries sprout new buds and bring the necessary nutrients to the area.

CLINICAL CONSIDERATIONS

Diabetes and diabetic foot ulcers

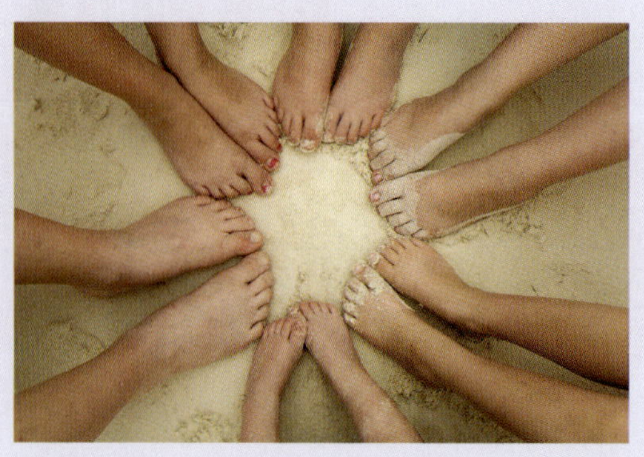

Diabetes is a condition that presents a great challenge to global healthcare systems. In Australia, there are approximately 1.7 million people living with diabetes, with a number of undiagnosed cases. Australians with Aboriginal and Torres Islander background are three to six times more likely to develop diabetes and diabetes-related foot complications and amputations than non-Indigenous Australians, contributing significantly to the morbidity and mortality associated with the condition (AIHW 2020b; Chuter et al. 2019; West et al. 2017). Diabetic foot is a condition frequently experienced by patients with diabetic peripheral neuropathy (figure 4.17). In these instances, the foot is often deformed and becomes insensitive, leading to pain, tingling, weakness or reduced sensation, and the patient may develop an unusual walking gait. Diabetes-related foot problems are a major healthcare burden that is estimated to cost over $1.6 billion annually (with approximately $2.7 billion attributed to diabetes) (AIHW 2020a; Chuter et al. 2019).

FIGURE 4.17 Diabetic foot ulcer

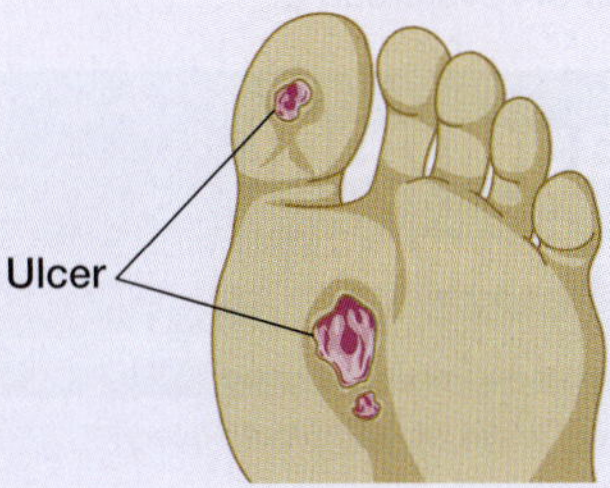

Source: James (2017).

Between 12 and 25 per cent of patients with diabetes develop leg and foot ulcers over their lifetime (Jeyaraman et al. 2019). This is because diabetes can cause macroangiopathy, which obstructs blood flow in large arteries. The slower flow of blood through the arteries in the legs results in the development of leg and foot ulcers, which usually starts with a minor trauma such as a small break (ulceration) to the skin of the foot. Patients with diabetes also experience lengthy recovery times from leg and foot injuries, and are also unlikely to notice any mild injuries to the foot due to a lack of sensation and inadequate inflammatory response required for wound healing. The lack of blood flow causes tissue ischaemia and also reduces the tissue's ability to fight off the infection following improper wound healing. Those patients with diabetes are therefore at increased risk of developing gangrene and amputation (Hubert & VanMeter 2018). Scientists believe that 85 per cent of diabetes-related amputations are avoidable if the diabetes is managed with proper medical care (Diabetes Australia 2019). Moreover, Jeyaraman and colleagues (2019) found that the death rate of patients with diabetic foot ulcers compared with patients with diabetes but without diabetic foot ulcers is more than twofold. In fact, diabetic foot ulcers are internationally known to be the main cause of diabetes-related hospital presentations, prolonged hospitalisations, foot amputations, and even death (Diabetic Foot Australia 2017).

SKILLS IN PRACTICE

Nursing and paramedic practice for burns

Nursing practice

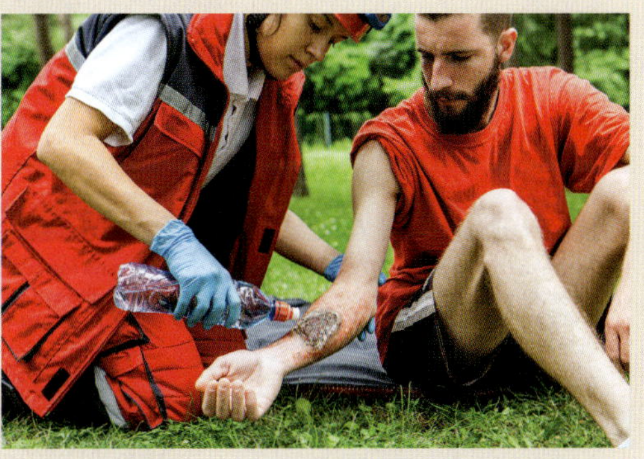

Depending on the complexity, the capacity for survival and recovery of burn patients may involve several multidisciplinary groups working together with complementary skills, such as emergency, plastics, respiratory, orthopaedics, infectious disease, intensive care and psychiatry. For severe burns (according to the national guidelines), the patient may be admitted into a specialised burns unit for effective wound management and undergo an adequate rehabilitation process to increase survival rate. In particular, a burns nurse who specialises in wound care, skin graft care and intensive care assists in the rehabilitation process by working together with other therapists for various rehabilitation aspects — physical (physiotherapist, occupational therapist), diet (dietician) and psychosocial (psychologist, psychiatrist, social and chaplain workers).

Paramedic practice

The safety of the attending paramedics is paramount and appropriate precautions need to be taken. Paramedics attending to burn victims should understand and apply the standard initial management criteria (ANZBA criteria) (figure 4.18) and wound care for severe burns. During a retrieval, one of the earliest interventions is to activate cooling of the affected area with running water for 20 to 60 minutes, protecting the patient from hypothermia, and initiating early airway assessment and management when necessary. Subsequently, appropriate care with 100 per cent oxygen delivery, analgesia, sedative and intravenous fluid may be administered while undertaking frequent airway assessment. Finally, burns may be covered with clean plastic cling wrap to contain the moisture (minimising wound dessication), and to reduce likelihood of infection and heat loss (Queensland Ambulance Service 2020).

FIGURE 4.18 Initial management of severe burns

Initial Management of Severe Burns

For burn injuries in adults >20% TBSA and children >10% TBSA or who meet the ANZBA transfer criteria, consider early consultation with retrieval service and burn centre

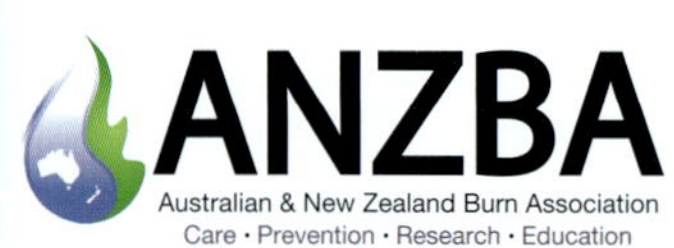

Specific points to note in the primary survey with respect to burn injury:

PRIMARY SURVEY	
AIRWAY 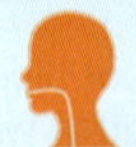	Assess for history of burn in enclosed space, signs of upper airway oedema, sooty sputum, facial burns, respiratory distress (dyspnoea, stridor, wheeze, hoarse voice). If any of the above present, airway is at risk. Consider need for intubation and secure airway as required. Maintain spinal precautions as required especially with explosion or electrical burns.
BREATHING 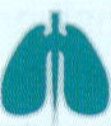	Assess breathing and support as required. Assess adequacy of breathing where circumferential burns on chest wall — consider escharotomy. Administer humidified 100% FiO2. Establish baseline ABGs and SaO2 (goal: >95%).
CIRCULATION 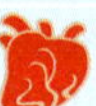	Assess circulation: colour, refill, HR, BP. Insert 2 large bore peripheral IV lines. If unable consider central or intraosseous access.

Specific points to note in the secondary survey and initial management of burn injury:

FLUID RESUSCITATION	Guide fluid resuscitation with Parkland formula/Ambulance protocol. Insert urinary catheter. Titrate fluid resuscitation to urine output goals: **Adults:** 0.5–1.0 ml/kg/hr (30–50 ml/hr) **Paediatrics <30 kg:** 1 ml/kg/hr Maintain accurate fluid balance chart.
ANALGESIA	Assess pain score to determine analgesic requirements. **Adults:** 2–5 mg morphine IV repeat every 5 minutes **Paediatrics:** IV morphine 0.1 mg/kg repeat every 5 minutes. Maximum 0.3 mg/kg Re-assess pain score (goal: Adult VAS pain score <4) and adjust analgesia accordingly. Consider morphine infusion for ongoing pain relief.
MANAGING WOUND	Assess extent of burn using Rule of Nines. Clean then cover the wound (see below).
CIRCUMFERENTIAL BURNS	Elevate limbs where circumferential burns present. Assess perfusion distal to burn: capillary refill, pulse, warmth, colour. Liaise with burn service if escharotomy required (cool to touch, weak or no pulse distally).
OTHER	Cover the patient to prevent heat loss. Insert nasogastric tube for burns >20% TBSA adults and 10% TBSA paediatrics. Keep nil orally. Administer tetanus immunoglobulin if required. Investigative tests as indicated.

Wound care for transit	Fluid resuscitation	Transfer checklist
First aid: cool running H2O ≥20 mins **Clean the wound:** Normal saline or 0.1% chlorhexidine Remove small loose dermis or blisters **Assess:** Extent and depth of burn injury and for circumferential injury **Cover:** Cling wrap longitudinally if immediate transfer (<8 hr). Paraffin gauze or silver dressing if T/F delayed	**Parkland formula:** **3–4 mL IV fluid x %TBSA x kg/24 hr** ½ fluid in 8/24 post injury ½ fluid in 16/24 post injury Hartmann's solution Paediatric maintenance fluids: 5% dextrose in ½ normal saline Up to 10 kg: 100 mL/kg/day 10–20 kg: 1000 mL + 50 mL/kg >10 kg/day 20–30 kg: 1500 mL + 20 mL/kg >20 kg/day	✓Airway secure ✓O2 insitu ✓IV access established and secure ✓Fluid resuscitation commenced ✓Urinary catheter inserted and secure ✓Pain controlled ✓Wounds are covered and patient is warm ✓Elevate burnt area as appropriate ✓Tetoxid if indicated ✓Nasogastric insitu as necessary ✓Retrieval services aware ✓N.O.K. aware ✓History and relevant documentation copied

Source: Australian and New Zealand Burn Association (ANZBA) (2019).

SUMMARY

All human cells can be categorised into four classifications: epithelial tissue, connective tissue, muscle tissue and nervous tissue. Epithelial tissue covers or lines structures and organs. It specialises in absorption, secretion, protection, excretion, filtration and sensory reception. Almost every substance that passes in and out of the body travels through epithelial tissue. Connective tissue not only connects tissues, but also protects, supports and insulates them. Connective tissue is dense and strong; examples include cartilage and bone. Muscle tissue provides movement and posture, whereas nervous tissue forms the major part of the nervous system. Tissue has the ability to regenerate and renew itself; however, epithelial and connective tissues have a greater capacity for repair than other tissues.

KEY TERMS

abdominopelvic cavity Body cavity that encompasses the abdominal and pelvic cavities. The abdominal cavity contains the stomach, intestines, spleen, liver and other associated digestive organs. The pelvic cavity contains the bladder and some reproductive organs.

apical surface Surface of body organ that faces outwards, towards the surface.

basal surface Surface that forms the base of a body organ.

cartilage Strong form of connective tissue that contains a dense network of collagen and elastic fibres.

chyme A fluid substance consisting of partially digested food and digestive enzymes, which is found travelling through the digestive tract.

connective tissue Tissue that binds, reinforces, insulates, protects and supports structures.

diffusion The movement of particles from areas of high concentration to low concentration.

endocrine glands Glands that release hormones.

epithelial tissue Tissue that lines or covers body surfaces.

exocrine glands Glands that secrete their products externally (i.e. mucus, sweat).

extracellular matrix A collection of largely non-living substances that separate the living cells of connective tissue.

glands Structures that manufacture a product (e.g. hormones, mucus, sweat).

glycoproteins Special proteins that contain simple sugar chains. Glycoproteins play an important role in cell-to-cell communication.

hormones Regulatory chemicals released by endocrine glands for use elsewhere in the body (e.g. thyroxine, insulin).

innervated Stimulated by nerve cells.

interstitial fluid The fluid that bathes cells.

keratin A special tough fibrous protein found in skin.

lymph nodes Small lymphatic structures that filter lymphatic fluid.

macrophages White blood cells that specialise in the destruction and consumption of invading pathogens.

membrane A sheet of tissue that covers or lines an area of the body.

mitosis The division and replication of cells.

neuroglia Cells of the nervous system that support and nourish neurones.

neurones A nerve fibre.

oocytes Female reproductive cell.

parenchyma The cells that constitute the function part of an organ.

prophylactic antibiotics Antibiotics prescribed to prevent infection.

spleen Large lymph organ, responsible for production of lymphocytes, immune response and the cleansing of blood.

stroma The internal framework of an organ.

subcutaneous Underneath the skin.

vertebrae The disc-shaped bones that make up the spinal column.

REFERENCES

Australian and New Zealand Burn Association (ANZBA) (2019) Severe burns. https://anzba.org.au/care/severe-burns (accessed January 2021).

Australian and New Zealand Gastric and Oesophageal Surgery Association (ANZGOSA) (n.d.) Peritonitis. www.anzgosa.org/peritonitis.html (accessed January 2021).

Australian Institute of Health and Welfare (AIHW) (2016) Hospitalised burn injuries Australia 2013–14. www.aihw.gov.au/reports/injury/hospitalised-burn-injuries-australia-2013-14/contents/summary (accessed January 2021).

Australian Institute of Health and Welfare (AIHW) (2020a) Diabetes. www.aihw.gov.au/reports/diabetes/diabetes (accessed January 2021).

Australian Institute of Health and Welfare (AIHW) (2020b) Data tables: diabetes 2020. www.aihw.gov.au/reports-data/health-conditions-disability-deaths/diabetes/data (accessed January 2021).

Chuter, V., West, M., Hawke, F. and Searle, A. (2019) Where do we stand? The availability and efficacy of diabetes related foot health programs for Aboriginal and Torres Strait Islander Australians: a systematic review. *Journal of Foot and Ankle Research* 12: 17.

Diabetes Australia (2019) Severe burns. www.diabetesaustralia.com.au/wp-content/uploads/4400-facts-and-figures.pdf (accessed January 2021).

Diabetic Foot Australia (2017) Australian diabetes-related foot disease strategy 2018–2022: the first step towards ending avoidable amputations within a generation. www.diabeticfootaustralia.org/wp-content/uploads/National-Strategy-to-end-avoidable-amputations-in-a-generation-final-1.pdf (accessed January 2021).

Hubert, R.J. and VanMeter, K.C. (2018) *Gould's Pathophysiology for the Health Professions*, 6th edn. St Louis, MO: Elsevier.

James, A. (2017) Diabetic foot ulcers left untreated can lead to amputation. *Scripps Local Media*. www.wmar2news.com/news/health/gbmc/diabetic-foot-ulcers-left-untreated-can-lead-ot-amputation (accessed February 2021).

Jenkins, G.W., Kemnitz, C.P. and Tortora, G.J. (2009) *Anatomy and Physiology from Science to Life*. Hoboken, NJ: John Wiley & Sons, Inc.

Jeyaraman, K., Berhane, T., Hamilton, M., Chandra, A.P. and Falhammar, H. (2019) Mortality in patients with diabetic foot ulcer: a retrospective study of 513 cases from a single Centre in the Northern Territory of Australia. *BMC Endocrine Disorders* 19(1): 1.

Kim, B., Brandli, A., Mitrofanis, J., Stone, J., Purushothuman, S. and Johnstone, D.M. (2017) Remote tissue conditioning — an emerging approach for inducing body-wide protection against diseases of ageing. *Ageing Research Reviews* 37: 69–78.

Lim, W.H., Johnson, D.W. and McDonald, S.P. (2005) Higher rate and earlier peritonitis in Aboriginal patients compared to non-Aboriginal patients with end-stage renal failure maintained on peritoneal dialysis in Australia: analysis of ANZDATA. *Nephrology (Carlton)* 10(2): 192–197.

Marieb, E. and Hoehn, K. (2018) *Human Anatomy and Physiology — Global Edition*, 11th edn. Harlow: Pearson Education.

Marley, J.V., Moore, S., Fitzclarence, C., Warr, K. and Atkinson, D. (2014) Peritoneal dialysis outcomes of Indigenous Australian patients of remote Kimberley origin. *Australian Journal of Rural Health* 22(3): 101–108.

Queensland Ambulance Service (2020) Clinical practice guidelines: trauma/burns. www.ambulance.qld.gov.au/docs/clinical/cpg/CPG_Burns.pdf (accessed January 2021).

Raio, C.C., Modayil, V., Cassara, M., Dubon, M., Patel, J., Shah, T., Chun, P., Nelson, M., Chiricolo, G., Sama, A.E. and Liu, Y.T. (2009) Can emergency medical services personnel identify pneumothorax on focused ultrasound examinations? *Critical Ultrasound Journal* 1, 65–68.

The Royal Children's Hospital Melbourne (RCHM) (2020) Burns — acute management. www.rch.org.au/clinicalguide/guideline_index/Burns (accessed January 2021).

Tortora, G.J. and Derrickson, B.H. (2017) *Principles of Anatomy and Physiology*, 15th edn. Hoboken, NJ: John Wiley & Sons, Inc.

West, M., Chute, V., Munteanu, S. and Hawke, F. (2017) Defining the gap: a systematic review of the difference in rates of diabetes-related foot complications in Aboriginal and Torres Strait Islander Australians and non-Indigenous Australians. *Journal of Foot and Ankle Research* 10: 48.

FURTHER READING

Queensland Ambulance Service (2020) Clinical practice procedures: respiratory/emergency chest decompression — pneumodart®. www.ambulance.qld.gov.au/docs/clinical/cpp/CPP_Emergency%20chest%20decompression_Pneumodart.pdf (accessed January 2021).

ACKNOWLEDGEMENTS

Photo: © Irishasel / Shutterstock.com
Photo: © WHYFRAME / Shutterstock.com
Photo: © iStockphoto / Getty Images
Photo: © Alan Poulson Photography / Shutterstock.com
Photo: © Microgen / Shutterstock.com
Figure 4.17: © 2017 Scripps Media, Inc.
Figure 4.18: © The Australian and New Zealand Burn Association

CHAPTER 5

Embryology

TEST YOUR PRIOR KNOWLEDGE

- What are the processes which produce the gametes?
- What anatomical features develop during the embryonic period?
- At what stage is an embryo considered a foetus?
- Define the range of gestational weeks that characterise each trimester.
- List three complications of pregnancy.

LEARNING OUTCOMES

After reading this chapter you will be able to:

5.1 describe the maturational processes involved in making gametes fertilisation competent
5.2 outline pre-implantation embryo development
5.3 discuss implantation and early placental development
5.4 provide an overview of post-implantation embryogenesis and foetal development
5.5 describe common pregnancy complications and their symptomology.

Introduction

Embryo is derived from the Greek word 'ἔμβρυον' or 'embryon' meaning the unborn. Embryology encompasses the development of **gametes** (eggs and sperm), the events surrounding **fertilisation** of the egg by a sperm cell, as well as the subsequent development of a genetically unique embryo and later foetus (figure 5.1). In this chapter we will investigate these processes, and you will see the human embryo progress from a **zygote** (fertilised egg) through the various stages of development before becoming a foetus after the ninth week of conception.

FIGURE 5.1 The early embryo develops from a simple group of cells into complex shapes and structures in the early weeks.

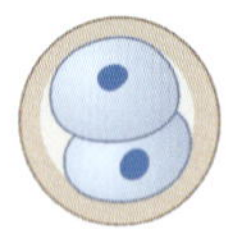
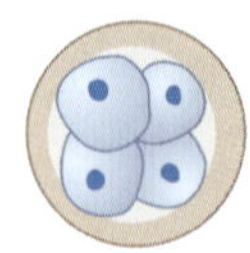
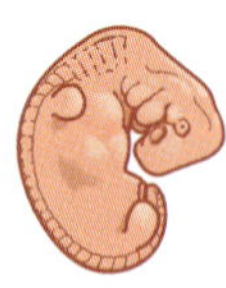
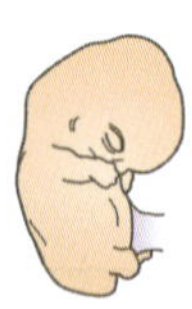
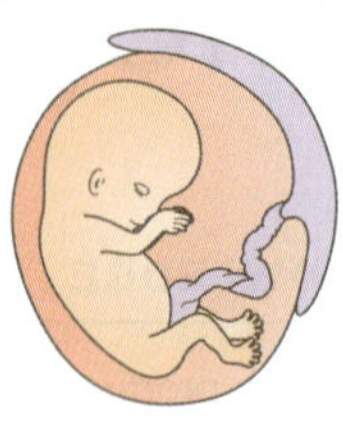
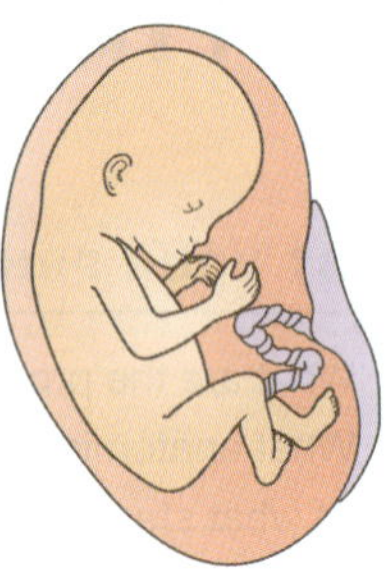

Source: Webster and de Wreede (2016). Reproduced with permission of John Wiley & Sons.

A note on timings

When following the development of an embryo, the date of fertilisation gives us the start of embryonic development, while for clinical care purposes, gestational stage is based on a woman's last menstrual period. Since this would be approximately two weeks prior to fertilisation, there is a two-week disparity between embryonic age and gestational age. We have attempted to clarify these two scales used throughout.

5.1 Final maturation of the oocyte and sperm

LEARNING OBJECTIVE 5.1 Describe the maturational processes involved in making gametes fertilisation competent.

Oocyte maturation and ovulation

We will detail the process of oogenesis (the production of a mature egg) further in the chapter on the reproductive system, but it is important to know that follicle growth occurs within the ovary and that mature follicle development is controlled by gonadotropic hormones; this process is specifically mediated by **follicle stimulating hormone (FSH)** and **luteinising hormone (LH)** (figure 5.2).

During oogenesis, a number of follicles develop; however, only one is recruited to become the 'dominant follicle'. This process occurs when **oestrogen** levels peak towards the end of the follicular phase causing a surge in levels of LH and FSH (24–36 h). An LH-induced signalling cascade results in secretion of proteolytic enzymes that break down the follicle lining (blister), forming a hole called the stigma where the oocyte (egg) within the cumulus–oocyte complex is released. This complex describes a mature oocyte surrounded by specialised somatic cells called cumulus cells. All remaining recruited yet un-ovulated follicles break down — a process called follicular **atresia**. Upon **ovulation**, the cumulus–oocyte complex is released from the ruptured follicle and moves out into the peritoneal cavity through the stigma, where it is caught by the long, finger-like fimbriae at the end of the **Fallopian tube** (also known as the uterine tube or oviduct) and pushed along by cilia towards the uterus, where it is then available to be fertilised. Ovulation marks the end of the follicular phase of the ovarian cycle and the start of the luteal phase (figure 5.2). The process of ovulation occurs in one ovary only each month, with a slightly increased occurrence in the right ovary compared with the left ovary.

During recruitment/development and ovulation, the oocyte completes a special type of cell division known as meiosis; occurring in stages, the oocyte completes meiosis I and commences meiosis II where it will pause in the metaphase (see the chapter on the reproductive system). If fertilisation does not occur, the oocyte will degenerate between 12 and 24 h after ovulation. In the ovary, having released the oocyte, the remaining follicle will fold inward on itself, transforming into the **corpus luteum (CL)**. The CL then becomes responsible for the ongoing production of oestrogen and **progesterone**. These hormones signal to the endometrial glands, beginning the production of the proliferative and secretory **endometrium** in preparation for **implantation** of a fertilised embryo and pregnancy maintenance (figure 5.2).

FIGURE 5.2 Hormones of the menstrual cycle

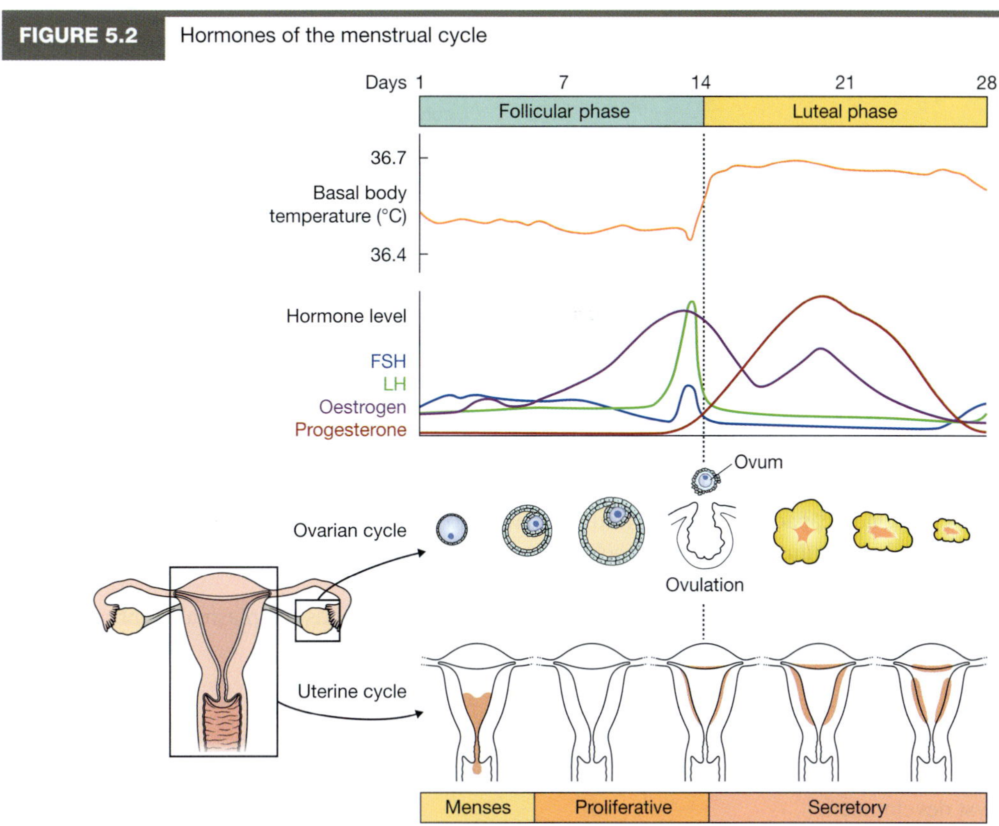

Source: Webster et al. (2018). Reproduced with permission of John Wiley & Sons.

Sperm maturation

While the events of sperm and egg maturation initially occur independently, they converge and synchronise in the female reproductive tract prior to fertilisation. The chapter on the reproductive system covers the process of sperm production in the testes, but when sperm exit the testes, they still have several maturation steps to complete as they travel through the **epididymis** and female reproductive tract towards the site of fertilisation.

During epididymal transit the protein and lipid architecture of the sperm is altered, after which the sperm acquire the potential for forward progressive motility and zona pellucida binding — effectively, this is where they learn to swim! Sperm can also be stored in the epididymis for 2–4 days (Sullivan & Mieusset 2016). Once sperm completely transverse the epididymis to the vas deferens in readiness for ejaculation, they are mixed with diluting fluids from the seminal vesicles and other accessory glands to form the semen (sperm and seminal plasma). At this stage, the sperm remain largely immobile until the mechanical and chemical stimulation by ejaculation and the glandular secretions stimulate the physiological activation of the sperm cells, readying them for the subsequent maturational phases of capacitation, hyperactivation and acrosome reaction which occur during the accession of the female reproductive tract.

Capacitation/hyperactivation is the penultimate step in the maturation of human sperm required to enable them to fertilise an oocyte (egg). Capacitation involves the removal of steroids and epididymal/seminal glycoproteins, resulting in a more fluid membrane with an increased permeability to calcium (Ca^{2+}). The resultant influx of Ca^{2+} into the sperm then increases the intracellular cAMP levels, and subsequently motility (Aitken & Nixon 2013). Hyperactivation (a specialised type of motility) coincides with the onset of capacitation and is also the result of increased Ca^{2+} levels. Specifically, hyperactivation is characterised by large whipping movements of the tail together with larger sideways swinging movements of the head.

The destabilisation of the acrosomal sperm head membrane by a process known as the acrosome reaction is the final stages of sperm maturation (Zhou et al. 2017). The acrosome reaction allows the penetration and fusion of the sperm with the plasma membrane of the oocyte for fertilisation (Bromfield & Nixon 2013) (figure 5.3).

FIGURE 5.3 Sperm approaching the ovum

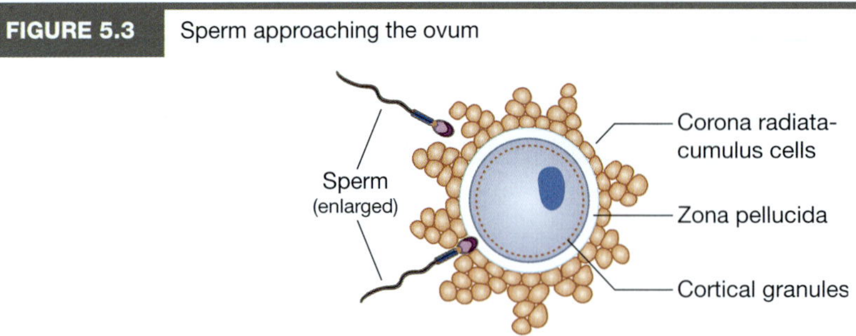

***Source*:** Webster and de Wreede (2016). Reproduced with permission of John Wiley & Sons.

Day 1: Fertilisation

Fertilisation or 'conception' involves the union of an egg and a sperm, usually occurring in the ampulla (midsection) of the Fallopian tube. The result of this merger is the production of a single cell zygote, or fertilised egg. Once capacitated sperm find their way to the cumulus–oocyte complex, they must penetrate through the cumulus cell mass to reach the zona pellucida (and subsequently the oocyte within); hyperactivation and the acrosome reaction aid these processes.

The zona pellucida is a specialised glycoprotein matrix which surrounds the plasma membrane of the oocytes with important roles in:

- oocyte development
- protection
- species-specific binding
- prevention of polyspermy (more than one sperm fertilising)
- blastocyst development
- precluding premature implantation.

Once through the zona pellucida, the sperm must bind and fuse with the plasma membrane (or oolemma) of the oocyte. Fusion of sperm with the oolemma is still poorly understood, but is believed to require the presence of membrane proteins on both the sperm and the oocyte (see figure 5.4). Once the spermatozoon has 'docked' onto the oolemma (1), the two membranes coalesce, enabling the transfer of the paternal nucleus, centrosomes (an organelle which organises microtubules and regulates the cell division), paternal mRNA, protein and the mitochondria (which are later eliminated) (2–5).

FIGURE 5.4 (a, b): Spermatozoon (motile sperm) passing through cumulus cells and meeting the zona pellucida

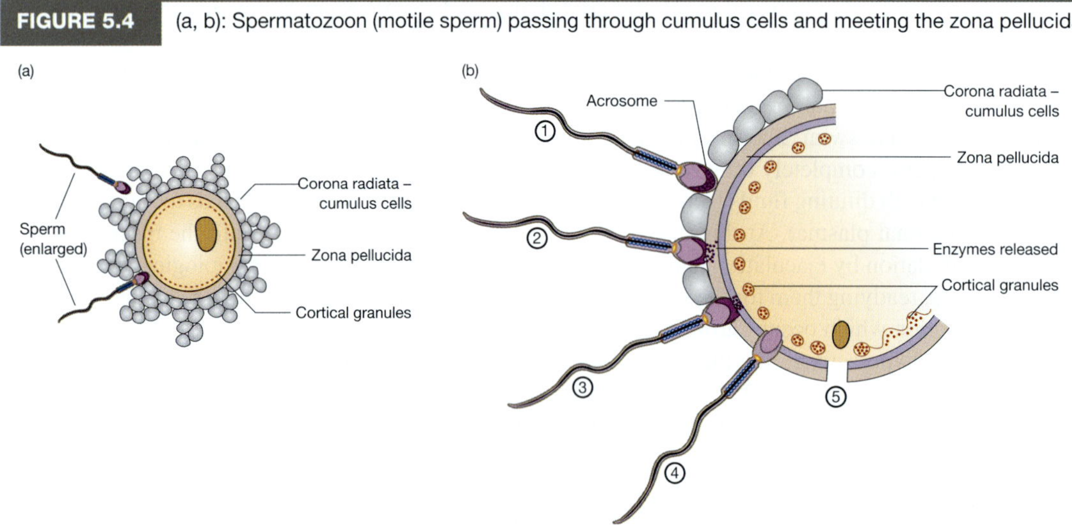

***Source*:** Webster et al. (2018). Reproduced with permission of John Wiley & Sons.

The paternal nucleus within the sperm contains highly condensed genetic material. Following fusion, the paternal nucleus is 'unpacked' (or decondensed) and reorganised into the paternal pronucleus. Meanwhile, following meiosis II, the maternal genome in the oocyte is simultaneously enclosed by its own nucleic membrane and decondensed to form the maternal pronucleus. Both pronuclei undergo DNA duplication (12–18 h) and migrate towards the cell middle and their nuclear membranes break down. The centrosome, delivered by the spermatozoa, plays an important role in the convergence of the two pronuclei for nuclei fusion (known as syngamy). Syngamy enables haploid chromosomal pairing (of maternal and paternal chromosomes), DNA replication and the first mitotic division resulting in a two-cell embryo.

5.2 Days 2–5: Pre-implantation development

LEARNING OBJECTIVE 5.2 Outline pre-implantation embryo development.

As the embryo (now called a zygote — that is, a fertilised egg) develops, it travels through the Fallopian tube into the uterine cavity, carried by the currents created by the cilia of the epithelium lining the Fallopian tubes and the contractions of its layer of smooth muscle. Some 24 hours after fertilisation the zygote begins its first cell division, to produce the two-cell embryo. For the next 5 days, the cells of the developing embryo divide approximately every 24 hours (often with distinct names for the embryo at stages of development), doubling the number of cells each time (figure 5.5).

FIGURE 5.5 The continuation of meiosis II and a zygote becoming a morula and then a blastocyst

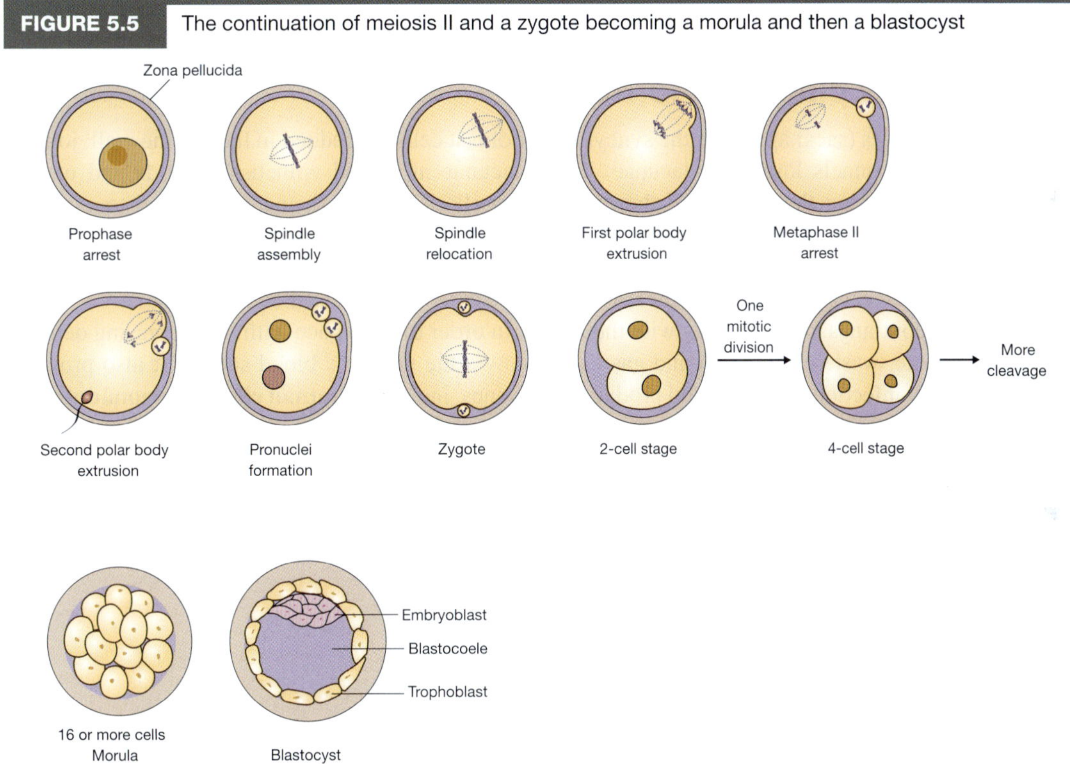

Source: Webster and de Wreede (2016). Reproduced with permission of John Wiley & Sons.

Approximately 3 days after fertilisation, the ball of cells reaches the uterus and begins to undergo a shape change, to produce the 'mulberry-shaped' embryo, known as a morula (figure 5.5). The cells begin to secrete fluid into an internal cavity, around which the cells then organise themselves around a fluid-filled cavity. Following this, the embryo is known as a blastocyst; at this stage it contains 70–100 cells.

At the blastocyst stage, cells delineate into two distinct cell lines: one that gives rise to the extraembryonic structures, the chorionic sac and foetal portion of the placenta (trophoblast cells) and one (the inner cell mass, or embryoblast) that constitutes the embryonic tissues (Morris et al. 2012; Niakan et al. 2012).

The trophoblast cells secrete enzymes that degrade the zona pellucida in readiness for the 'hatching' required for implantation. The zona pellucida has acted as a protective immunological barrier until now, preventing premature implantation. Once hatched, the embryo is free to adhere to the uterine lining, access the uterine secretions for nutrition, and grow. The term '**conceptus**' includes all structures that develop from the zygote (both the embryo and appendages such as the placenta).

5.3 Day 6: Implantation

LEARNING OBJECTIVE 5.3 Discuss implantation and early placental development.

At the end of the sixth day of development, the embryo will embed in the endometrium of the uterus in a process known as implantation. The time during which this can occur — the 'implantation window' — is a relatively short time frame during which the uterus is receptive to the blastocyst as a result of the action of oestrogen and progesterone on the endometrium. Implantation usually takes place in the top $\frac{1}{3}$ of the uterus during the secretory phase of the menstrual cycle while levels of these hormones are high.

There are three main stages of implantation (figure 5.6). First, the blastocyst reaches the uterus and loosely adheres to the endometrium. The outer trophoblast cells of the blastocyst then interact with the endometrial cells in the adhesion stage. Finally, the blastocyst embeds itself in the uterine lining via the actions of specialised trophoblast cells which secrete enzymes and other factors to erode the endometrial cells away, allowing the embryo to penetrate down into the endometrium. These specialised trophoblast cells then rapidly divide and completely surround the embryo by the time it is fully embedded in the endometrium. Implantation signals the end of the pre-embryonic stage of development and the beginning of placenta formation. A significant percentage (50–75%) of blastocysts will fail at this stage for a variety of reasons. When this occurs, the blastocyst is shed along with the endometrium during menstruation. The high rate of implantation failure explains why a pregnancy is unlikely to be achieved in a single ovulation cycle.

Week 2: Early placental formation

Extracellular vacuoles (sacs) appear in the syncytiotrophoblast cells embedded in the uterine wall, joining together to form channels known as lacunae. These lacunae are filled with tissue fluids and uterine secretions and, following the erosion of the maternal capillaries, fill with maternal blood to establish early uteroplacental circulation. Implantation ends at the second week of development. At this stage the 'embryonic bud' consists schematically of two hemispheric cavities that lie on one above the other. These include the amniotic cavity and the umbilical vesicle and can be easily identified in figure 5.7.

The placenta continues to grow along with the foetus, in order to keep pace with the increasing demand for nutrient uptake, waste elimination and gas exchange via the mother's blood supply. It also provides protection against infectious particles and produces hormones, including **human chorionic gonadotropin (hCG)**. Specifically, hCG is secreted by the trophoblast cells of the implanted embryo and is responsible for the maintenance of the corpus luteum to ensure it continues to secrete progesterone and oestrogen to sustain pregnancy (and maintain the endometrial lining). The hCG accumulates in the maternal bloodstream, increasing exponentially in the first 7–10 weeks of pregnancy and peaking by 10–12 weeks (Korevaar et al. 2015). The presence of hCG in the urine is used as an indicator of pregnancy in most pregnancy tests.

FIGURE 5.6 Implantation

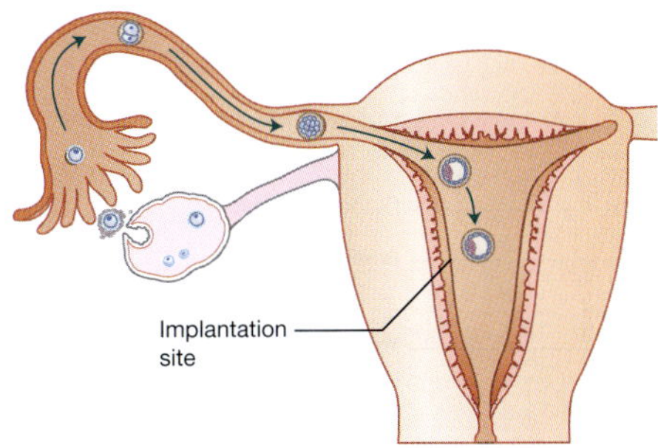

Normal implantation commonly occurs in the superior parts of the uterus, but can occur at a number of sites

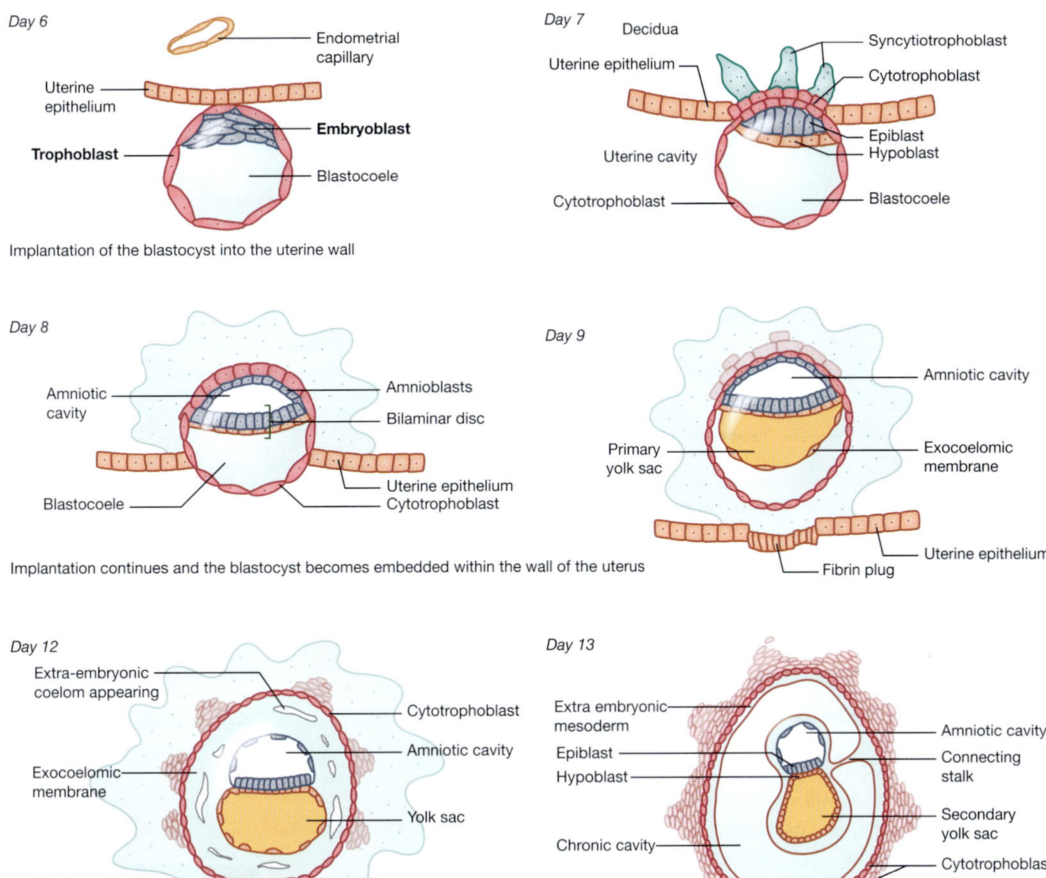

Implantation of the blastocyst into the uterine wall

Implantation continues and the blastocyst becomes embedded within the wall of the uterus

The development of the chorionic cavity between the amniotic cavity, yolk sac and the chorion leaves a connecting stalk between the embryo and the developing placenta

Source: Webster and de Wreede (2016). Reproduced with permission of John Wiley & Sons.

FIGURE 5.7 The placenta

Maternal spiral arteries of the endometrium

Extra-embryonic coelom appearing

Exocoelomic membrane

Uterine epithelium

Cytotrophoblast

Amniotic cavity

Yolk sac

The blastocyst has implanted into the endometrium and the cells of the trophoblast invade the maternal tissue. (End of week 2)

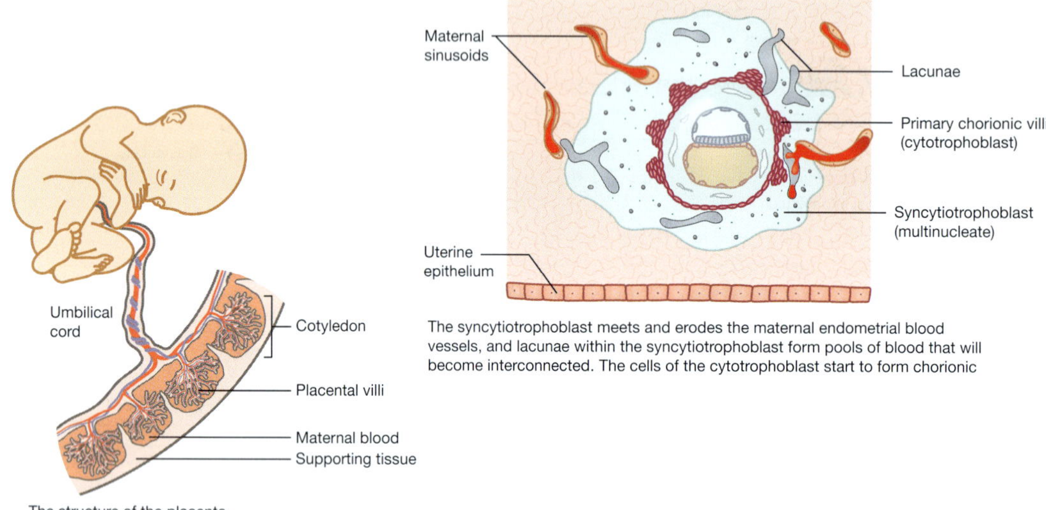

The syncytiotrophoblast meets and erodes the maternal endometrial blood vessels, and lacunae within the syncytiotrophoblast form pools of blood that will become interconnected. The cells of the cytotrophoblast start to form chorionic

The structure of the placenta

Source: Webster and de Wreede (2016). Reproduced with permission of John Wiley & Sons.

CLINICAL CONSIDERATIONS

Pregnancy tests

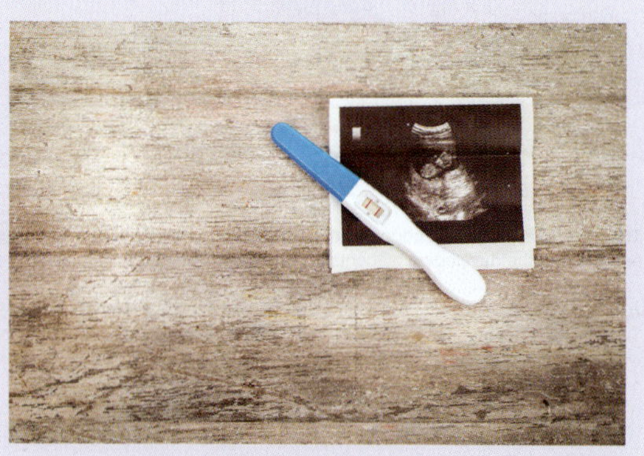

A pregnancy is confirmed by the presence of human chorionic gonadotropin (hCG) in the mother's urine or blood. Beginning at embryo implantation, hCG can first be detected in a blood sample approximately 11 days after conception.

Tests for blood hCG are more sensitive than those for urine levels (99.5–100%) and enable the time of pregnancy to be determined. Additionally, an hCG blood test can distinguish between normal progressing and abnormal pregnancies (e.g. molar pregnancies or ectopic pregnancies). Venous blood must be collected by a health professional and sent away for laboratory analysis.

Early diagnosis of pregnancy enables early preventative interventions to ensure maternal and foetal health (e.g. antenatal care, avoidance of alcohol and nicotine) and is also beneficial for women who do not wish to proceed with their pregnancy, as it enables the pregnancy to be terminated in the early stages.

5.4 Weeks 3–8: Post-implantation embryonic development

LEARNING OBJECTIVE 5.4 Provide an overview of post-implantation embryogenesis and foetal development.

The embryonic period is the developmental phase which occurs during the first eight weeks after fertilisation. The key feature of this period is the complex differentiation occurring, which establishes the basic body form as cells change to specialist types of cell and the embryo starts to form (**embryogenesis**).

Differentiation of embryonic or germ layers

During the latter stage of embryonic development, the cells begin to form the three primary cell lineages that give rise to all adult tissues. This process is known as **gastrulation** and occurs shortly after implantation following the differentiation of the inner cell mass into a two-layered plate of cells called the bilaminar embryonic disc, the 'epiblast' and the 'hypoblast' (figure 5.8). The hypoblast forms extraembryonic tissues, while the epiblast progresses to form the embryo proper.

FIGURE 5.8 Gastrulation

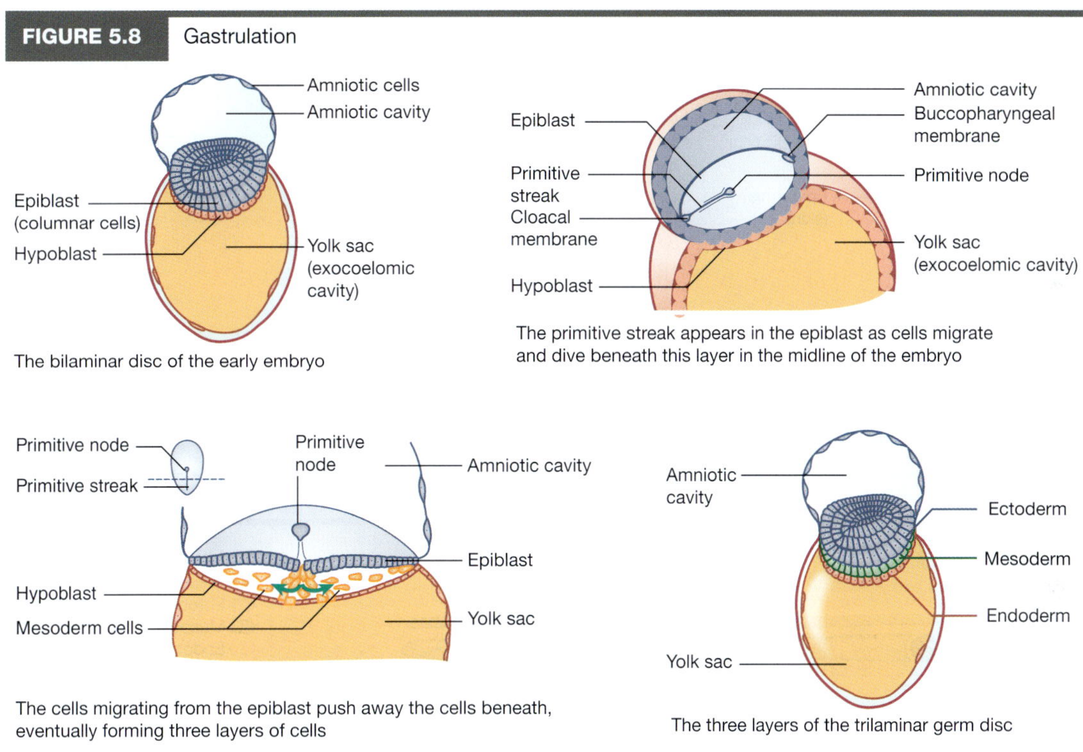

Source: Webster and de Wreede (2016). Reproduced with permission of John Wiley & Sons.

Through gastrulation, the epiblast splits into the three germ layers: the **ectoderm**, **mesoderm** and **endoderm**. The cells of each germ layer differentiate and specialise to form tissues, organs and organ systems. Differentiation occurs when the form and function of cells change to reflect a distinct function or developmental fate.

The ectoderm gives rise to the skin and nervous system. The endoderm becomes the lining of digestive and respiratory tracts, parts of the liver and the pancreas, and the bladder lining. The mesoderm develops into the muscles, skeleton, circulatory system, excretory system (except the bladder lining), gonads and the inner layer of skin (dermis) (figure 5.9).

Gastrulation is of clinical importance as it is a period highly susceptible to damaging factors — such as alcohol, caffeine and tobacco — known as teratogens (any agent causing foetal abnormality). Exposure to teratogens during this period can result in significant developmental consequences to the embryo and may result in spontaneous abortion.

Neurulation is another critical event occurring in early embryonic development. It is the formation of the neural tube from a layer of ectoderm cells. This tube will develop into the brain, spinal cord and retina.

The three-layered embryonic disc curls under with the ectoderm on the outside, resulting in the formation of the neural tube (figure 5.10).

FIGURE 5.9 The fate of the three germ layers

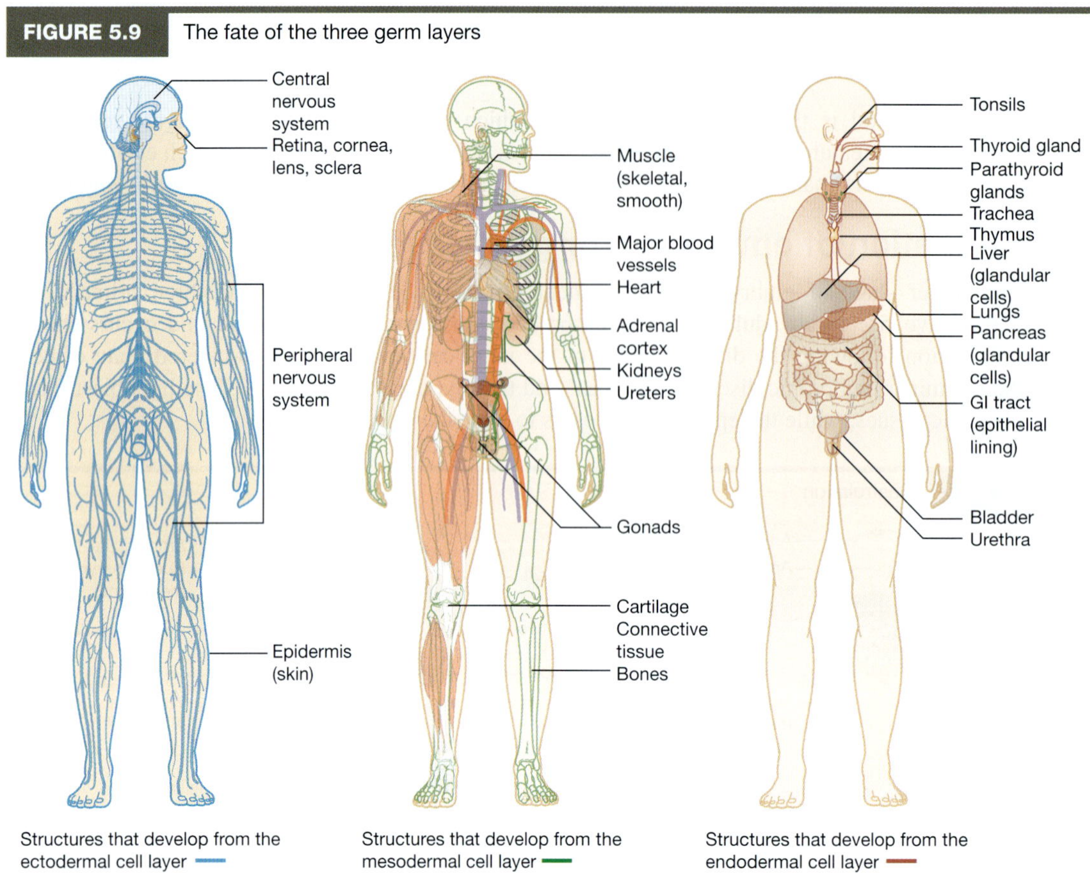

Source: Webster and de Wreede (2016). Reproduced with permission of John Wiley & Sons.

FIGURE 5.10 Neurulation

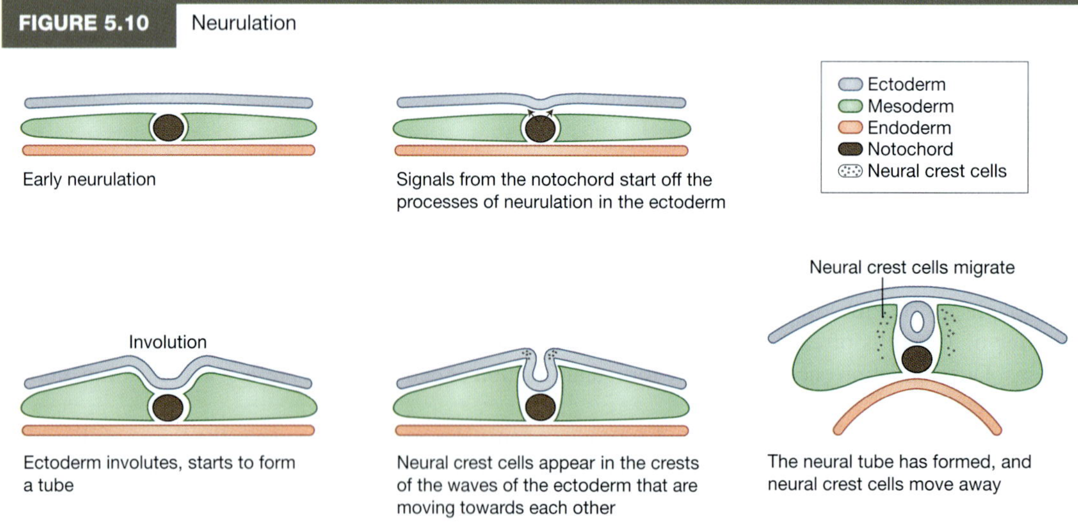

Source: Webster and de Wreede (2016). Reproduced with permission of John Wiley & Sons.

Week 3

During week 3, after neurulation, the brain enlarges at the site of the future head and somites develop from the mesoderm, appearing first as lumps on either side of the neural tube and developing into the vertebrae and ribs (figure 5.11). At the same time, the epidermis is developing from the ectoderm.

FIGURE 5.11 Fourth week embryo: lateral aspect of the fourth week embryo with visible pharyngeal arches

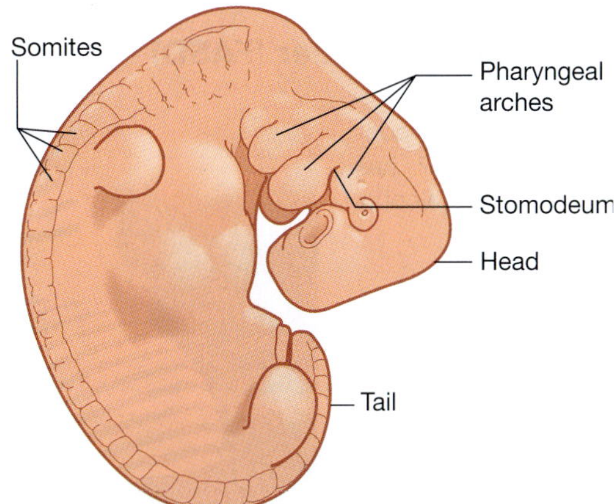

Source: Webster and de Wreede (2016). Reproduced with permission of John Wiley & Sons.

Week 4

By the beginning of the fourth week, the embryo is approximately 2 mm in length. The head and tail ends begin to curl inwards, forming a C-shape. The head develops primitive eyes and the future inner ear canal. Pharyngeal arches, the future jaw and ears, develop as lumps in the neck region (figure 5.11). The heart develops from a tube of mesoderm and begins to beat, forming the earliest functioning organ. In addition, the arm and leg buds appear, arising from both the ectoderm and mesoderm.

Week 5

Rapid brain growth characterises this stage, where distinct brain areas and cranial nerves also begin to develop. The arm buds flatten and become 'paddle-like'. Heart chambers develop, and the primitive gonads form at the genital ridge. By the end of this week the embryo is 1 cm in length.

Week 6

The embryonic eyes gain pigment and the external ears form. There is also brain and head expansion, while the hand buds form finger rays. The heart further develops, and circulation is established as the liver begins to produce blood cells. The primordial germ cells also complete their migration to the gonads and a distinct tail can be observed.

Weeks 7 and 8

The final two-week period of the embryonic development phase is marked by distinct facial, organ system (especially the gastrointestinal tract) and neuromuscular development. The development of mouth, tongue and palate is also completed during this time. The eyelids grow and fuse together (they will not open until the 25th week) and the fingers and toes develop. The differentiation of the early gonads into testes or ovaries commences based on genetic sex and the tail bud disappears. The end of week 8 marks the end of the embryonic period and the beginning of the foetal period. Foetal movement is now visible on ultrasound.

The embryonic period is the most susceptible to major congenital complications and embryo loss or **miscarriage**. This is perhaps not surprising, given the extraordinary complexity of development that occurs in these first eight weeks. Embryonic loss can occur because of intrinsic errors in the developing embryo, including chromosomal anomalies and genetic defects, as well as through environmental factors, such as exposure to teratogens, or uterine anomalies. Consequently, the earlier a woman is aware of a pregnancy, the sooner certain interventions, such as folate and iron supplementation and reducing alcohol consumption, can be introduced to support healthy embryo development.

CLINICALLY REASONED EPISODE OF CARE

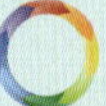

Foetal alcohol spectrum disorder (FASD)

Consider the patient situation

Isabella's mother, Natalie, reported alcohol consumption during pregnancy, and a GP has now diagnosed Isabella with foetal alcohol spectrum disorder.

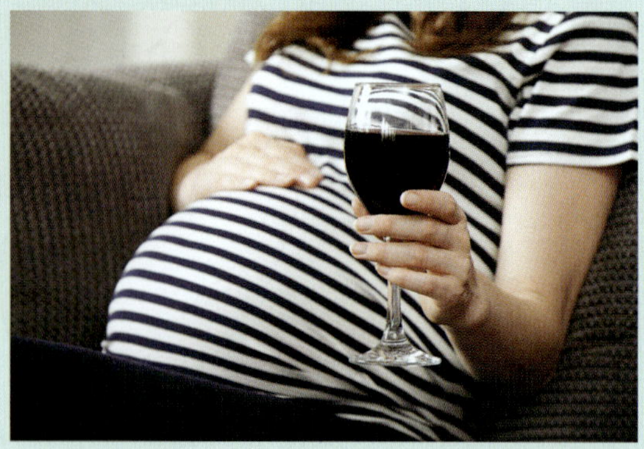

Collect cues and information

Isabella is a school-aged girl who has been diagnosed with foetal alcohol spectrum disorder. Isabella has small eyes, a thin upper lip, a short and upturned nose, and a smooth philtrum. Isabella displays some behaviours which are consistent with FASD, including hyperactivity and mood changes.

As part of the general practice team, the practice nurse has been included in Isabella's care to ensure that care is coordinated and effective. There is no cure for FASD; however, early intervention and support is important for individuals and families.

Process information

Foetal alcohol spectrum disorder (FASD) is a diagnostic term used to describe the impacts on a developing foetus that has been exposed to alcohol during **gestation**. Alcohol is able to cross the placenta in pregnancy into the bloodstream of the foetus. Because the foetus metabolises alcohol at a much lower rate than adults, the foetus is exposed to higher alcohol levels. The development of FASD is dependent on factors including the amount and frequency of alcohol used, parent age, health of the mother (nutrition, tobacco use, mental health), and environmental factors such as stress.

Most children and adults who have FASD live with cognitive, behavioural, health and learning difficulties, including problems with memory, attention, cause and effect reasoning, impulsivity, receptive language and adaptive functioning difficulties. These difficulties are lifelong and have an impact on behaviour. Positive outcomes can be achieved when parents are appropriately supported to understand their child's behaviour as a symptom of neurological impairment.

The treatment and management of FASD include evidence-based behavioural intervention programs, occupational therapy, speech therapy, physiotherapy, impulse and memory processing interventions, and help with sleeping and eating.

Identify problems/issues

1. Behavioural and learning issues, which are common for those living with FASD
2. Coordination of appointments for specialists and allied health
3. Ongoing management and support for Isabella and Natalie

Nursing actions

1. Provide education to school staff about the behavioural and learning concerns associated with FASD.
   Rationale:
   - FASD is associated with behavioural and impulse control issues. Nurses are well placed to provide education and support to professional staff.
   - Education and information sharing can facilitate additional support mechanisms to support Isabella at school.
2. Coordination of referrals and appointments for specialists and allied health interventions.
   Rationale:
   - It can be difficult for consumers and families to navigate the health system, particularly when there are multiple disciplines and health professionals involved in care. Having a central point of contact and care coordination can ensure that consumers and families are able to manage appointments and treatments effectively.
   - Nurses, particularly those part of the general practice team, are well placed to act as care coordinators.
3. Provide ongoing support and management to Isabella, Natalie and their family.
   Rationale:
   - A diagnosis of FASD can be an ongoing challenge for individuals and families.
   - Nurses work within a holistic framework of planning, assessment, implementation and evaluation in caring for individuals and their families.

Reflect on new processes and learning

Reflect on the role of the general practice in the coordination of care from a primary healthcare perspective. What role can the nurse play in care coordination and management within the general practice setting?

Source: Based on the Clinical Reasoning Cycle, Levett-Jones (2013).

Late gestation and birth: gestational weeks 13–40 (embryonic weeks 11–38)

Human pregnancy is divided into trimesters (three-month periods). The first trimester extends from conception to about the twelfth week of pregnancy (embryo week 10). The second trimester extends from weeks 13 to 27, and the third trimester from 28 weeks until birth. A typical pregnancy spans a total of 40 weeks from the first day of the last menstrual period to the birth of the baby (see figure 5.12). Birth occurring earlier than 37 weeks is considered '**pre-term**' birth and carries considerable risk for the foetus.

FIGURE 5.12 Embryonic and foetal periods: the scale, in weeks, shows how gestation is dated clinically and embryonically. The LMP refers to the date of the 'last menstrual period' from which the clinical period of gestation is determined. Embryologically, development begins with fertilisation.

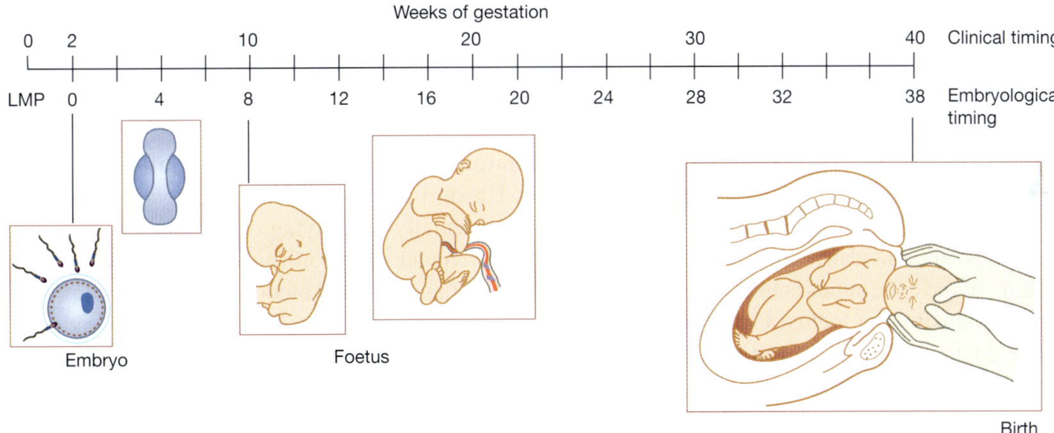

Source: Webster and de Wreede (2016). Reproduced with permission of John Wiley & Sons.

The first trimester (also see post-implantation development)

During the first trimester, elevated progesterone levels and other hormonal changes can affect almost every organ in the mother's body. Women may suffer from extreme fatigue, morning sickness, food cravings or aversions, mood swings and constipation, among other problems.

By the end of first trimester all major systems and organs of the baby have developed and are functioning, including the circulatory, nervous, digestive and urinary systems. The embryo is taking on a 'human shape', although the head is larger in proportion to the rest of the body. After eight weeks, the embryo is now referred to as a foetus (which means offspring). It is important to note that even though the organs and body systems are fully formed by the end of 12 weeks, the foetus cannot survive independently.

The second trimester (13–27 weeks gestation)

Nausea and fatigue may be reduced or entirely eliminated, while physical signs of a baby such as the 'baby bump' will start to manifest as the women's abdomen expands to house the growing baby. During this time, it is possible, through testing and ultrasound, to determine the baby's sex. In the later stages of this trimester, the pregnant woman may also begin to feel the foetus moving.

By week 13 the baby has begun to produce urine and release it into the amniotic sac, making amniotic fluid. Its bones are beginning to harden. By weeks 15 and 16 the baby's scalp pattern develops, and its eyes begin to move. The baby's limb movements also become coordinated and can be detected during ultrasound exams. During weeks 17, 18 and 19 the baby's toenails develop, it gains the ability to hear, it becomes more active (rolling and flipping) and the vernix caseosa (a protective coating against abrasions, chapping and hardening that can result from exposure to amniotic fluid) begins to cover the baby. For female babies, the uterus and vaginal canal are also forming during this time.

In the final weeks of the second trimester the baby is completely covered with a fine, downy hair called 'lanugo'. The lanugo helps hold the vernix caseosa on the skin. In addition, the sucking reflex is also developing, and the baby's hair becomes visible, so too are the foot and fingerprints. For males, the testes will also have begun to descend. Importantly, during week 26, the baby's lungs develop, beginning to produce surfactant, the substance that allows the air sacs in the lungs to inflate — and keeps them from collapsing and sticking together when they deflate. At week 27, the second trimester ends.

CLINICAL CONSIDERATIONS

Prenatal monitoring

Brenda, 30, is in the final trimester of her second pregnancy. During a routine antenatal visit, her midwife performs an ultrasound and measures the baby's heart rate. Brenda's baby has 130 beats per minute, within the normal range of 120–160 beats per minute.

An abnormal foetal heart rate or rhythm can indicate a problem, such as inadequate oxygen to the foetus. An abnormal foetal heart rate very late in pregnancy may indicate the need for an emergency caesarean delivery. Foetal heart rate may be monitored during labour, particularly for high-risk pregnancies. Short-lasting accelerations in the foetal heart rate during labour are a sign of a healthy foetus, and stimuli such as moving the mother's abdomen or gently pressing the baby's head as it is passing through the cervix should provoke these accelerations in heart rate.

The third trimester and birth

An expectant mother may experience significant discomfort in this trimester, as the significant growth of the baby places more pressure on the internal organs. Upward pressure of the foetus on the diaphragm may make breathing difficult, and create gastric reflux, especially when lying down, whereas downward pressure on the bladder reduces its capacity and makes frequent urination (polyuria) a feature. Further swelling of the extremities is likely, due to the combination of an increased blood volume and compression of more veins by the foetus. **Colostrum** may leak from breasts, which are also likely to be tender, and uterine contractions may be felt, which can indicate real or false labour.

In readiness for birth, the baby will reposition itself in the lower abdomen/pelvis and the cervix will thin and soften in a process called '**effacement**'. After week 37, the baby is considered 'full term', and at this point the baby's organs are fully functional. The normal birth weight of a newborn ranges from 2500 g to 4000 g (5 pounds 5 ounces to 8 pounds 8 ounces), with an average length of around 50 cm (approximately 20 inches).

MEDICINES MANAGEMENT

Pain relief during labour

During the initial stage of labour, a woman will experience pain caused by the contraction of the uterus and dilation/stretching of the cervix. Towards the end of the first stage and into the second stage of labour, more intense pain is caused by pressure on the birth canal, vulva and perineum.

Pain perception is influenced by a variety of factors and will determine the maternal physiologic responses to the pain. If labour pain causes maternal anxiety, it is likely to manifest as muscular tension which may impair uterine contractility. There are non-medical and medical options for pain relief during labour, depending upon maternal preference, intensity of pain and the anticipated length of labour. Non-medical methods of pain relief include relaxation, active birth, massage, heat and water, transcutaneous electrical nerve stimulation (TENS) and sterile water injections. The medical methods used most commonly are nitrous oxide gas (administered in a 50/50 mix with oxygen), opioid analgesic intravenous injection and local anaesthetic epidural administration (table 5.1).

TABLE 5.1 Pharmacological methods of pain relief during labour (informed by Grant 2020)

Drug	Method	Indication for use	Effectiveness	Side effects	Duration
Oxygen/nitrous oxide	Inhalation 50/50 mixture of oxygen and nitrous oxide	First and second stages of labour	Mild	Faint, nausea and vomiting	Short-acting during inhalation
Opioid analgesic (e.g. pethidine/ meperidine, morphine)	Intravenous or intramuscular	First stage (most effective in early active labour)	Dependent on specific opioid administered	Nausea and vomiting; respiratory depression in newborn — naloxone used to reverse this effect	2–4 hours
Pudendal nerve block	Infiltration of right and left pudendal nerves (S2–S4) just below ischial spines (reduced sensation from perineum/ vagina)	For operative vaginal delivery (in second-stage labour)	Moderate/- good analgesia		45–90 minutes
Perineal infiltration	0.5% lidocaine at posterior fourchette (rear of vaginal opening)	To facilitate episiotomy and/or before suturing tears/epi-siotomies	Effective local analgesia within 5 minutes		45–90 minutes
Remifentanil PCA (patient-controlled analgesia)	Intravenous (powerful opiate)	For patients in whom epidural is contraindi-cated or who wish a less complete analgesic block	Good	Respiratory depression (Maternal and neonatal)	Ultra short (1–5 min)
Epidural anaesthesia	Injection of 0.25–0.5% bupivacaine via catheter into extradural space (L3–L4)	First- and second-stage caesarean section (CS)	Complete pain relief in >95% within 20 minutes	Transient hypotension (preload with IV fluids); decreased mobility; dural puncture <1/100; increased length of second-stage labour	Continuous infusion with top-ups every 3–4 hours
Spinal anaesthesia	0.5% bupi-vacaine into subarachnoid space	Operative delivery (e.g. forceps or CS manual removal of placenta)	Complete pain relief within few minutes	Respiratory depression	Single injection — wears off after 3–4 hours

5.5 Complications of pregnancy

LEARNING OBJECTIVE 5.5 Describe common pregnancy complications and their symptomology.

Complications of pregnancy may include 'implantation abnormalities' or problems associated with gestation. Some common pregnancy complications include the following.

Ectopic pregnancies

Usually an embryo implants within the body of the uterus. However, in 1–2 per cent of cases, the embryo implants outside the uterus leading to an ectopic pregnancy or an extra-uterine pregnancy. Abnormal implantation sites may include the Fallopian tubes or the external surface of the uterus, ovary, bowel, gastrointestinal tract, mesentery or peritoneal wall. Almost all (99%) of ectopic pregnancies are tubal pregnancies, with all other sites combined representing only 1 per cent of ectopic pregnancies. These pregnancies can result in haemorrhages and sterility (e.g. if the Fallopian tube ruptures).

Pregnancy loss/miscarriage and stillbirth

Pregnancy loss can occur at any stage of gestation. Miscarriage is the loss of a baby before 20 weeks gestation. Approximately 20 per cent of confirmed pregnancies end in miscarriage, although it is likely that some women miscarry without knowing they are pregnant. Signs that a miscarriage has occurred include cramping, abdominal pain and vaginal spotting/bleeding.

Later-term pregnancy loss, or **stillbirth**, occurs when a baby is lost after 20 weeks gestation or during birth. A stillbirth may occur due to congenital anomalies, chromosomal abnormalities or premature birth.

There is no evidence that exercising, stress, working or having sex causes pregnancy loss and most women who have lost a pregnancy will go on to successfully carry a subsequent pregnancy to term. However, in rare instances, usually due to chromosomal abnormalities, some women may experience recurrent miscarriages (3 or more in a row); in these cases, assisted reproductive strategies, such as use of donor eggs or embryos, may be used to overcome infertility.

CLINICAL CONSIDERATIONS

Pre-eclampsia

Pre-eclampsia usually affects pregnant women during the second half of pregnancy or immediately after delivery of their baby. A combination of elevated blood pressure, protein in the urine and oedema in the extremities suggest pre-eclampsia. Untreated, the condition can have serious complications for mother and child and can be life-threatening for both.

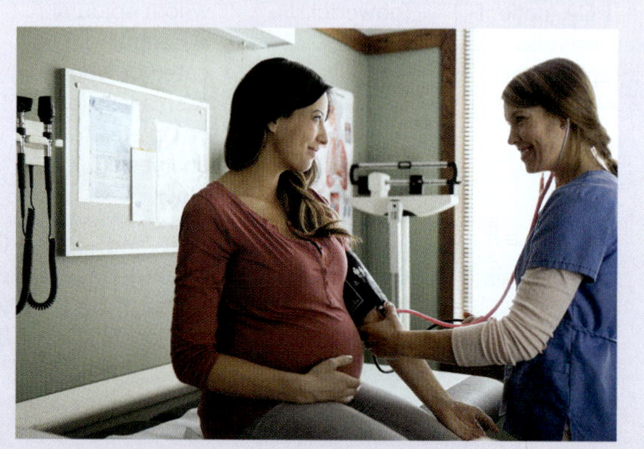

During routine antenatal appointments, the mother's blood pressure will be monitored. If readings of 140 mmHg systolic and/or 90 mmHg diastolic are observed on two or more occasions, and accompanied by one or more of the following organ system features, the mother may be diagnosed with pre-eclampsia. Protein in the urine, as indicated by a urine protein to creatinine ratio of ≥ 30 mg/mmol, is common in pre-eclampsia, but this feature is not mandatory in making a diagnosis. In more severe cases, the patient may also exhibit renal insufficiency (serum creatinine ≥ 0.09 mmol/L), liver disease, neurological problems (including convulsions) and haematological disturbances (thrombocytopenia or placental insufficiency). While pre-eclampsia can be managed until the baby is mature enough to be delivered, by administration of antihypertensive medication for example, the only cure for pre-eclampsia is delivery of the baby. For more information see the Australian Government Department of Health (2020).

CLINICALLY REASONED EPISODE OF CARE

Gestational diabetes

Consider the patient situation

Naomi is pregnant with her first child and has recently been diagnosed with gestational diabetes.

Naomi has been referred to the diabetes nurse educator for education and support related to the management of her gestational diabetes.

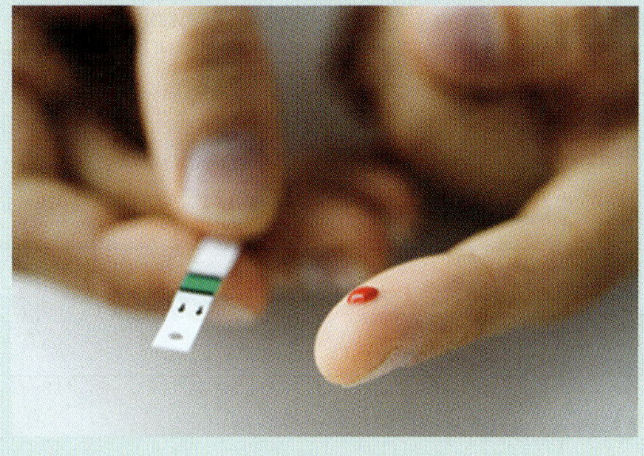

Collect cues and information

Naomi is a 31-year-old female who is currently 26 weeks pregnant. Naomi has a body mass index (BMI) of 30, which is in the obese category. Naomi has attended a routine oral glucose tolerance test (GTT). The GTT is conducted on all pregnant women between 24 and 28 weeks of pregnancy. An oral glucose solution is ingested by the woman and a series of fasting blood tests are collected. A result of >7 mmol when fasting, or a result of >11.1 mmol after two hours of ingestion, determines a diagnosis of gestational diabetes.

Naomi has a family history of type 2 diabetes, with her mother and brother both living with the condition.

Process information

The hormones that occur in the body during pregnancy can have an effect on other hormones such as insulin, leading to higher than normal blood glucose levels. If not controlled, gestational diabetes can lead to premature birth, high birth weight (macrosomia), and ongoing issues for mother and baby.

Approximately 12–14 per cent of women will develop gestational diabetes. Women who have a high BMI and who have family members with type 2 diabetes are at increased risk of developing gestational diabetes.

Gestational diabetes poses a greater risk of induction of birth and caesarean section, and some babies will require additional support after birth, including management of blood glucose levels and feeding support. For these reasons it is important to effectively monitor and manage gestational diabetes during pregnancy.

Establish goals

1. Nutritional and exercise control of gestational diabetes
2. Education on monitoring blood glucose levels
3. Education on injecting insulin

Nursing actions

1. Educate Naomi and her family on gestational diabetes, including risks to mother and baby.
   Rationale:
   - Many people are unaware of the risks that gestational diabetes poses to pregnancy and to both the mother and baby.
   - Educating individuals provides the avenue to communicate risks, and how and when to seek help.
2. Provide education and support materials for nutrition and exercise during pregnancy.
   Rationale:
   - Adequate nutrition and exercise are essential elements when managing gestational diabetes.
   - Education and support materials, such as nutritional charts and exercise guidelines, are an important part of the diabetes nurse educator role.
   - Nurse educators are well placed to provide immediate and ongoing education to individuals and families.
3. Provide education on how and when to monitor blood glucose levels and inject insulin.
   Rationale:
   - Managing diabetes can be a challenge for individuals. Given the nature of the illness, knowing how to monitor and manage blood glucose levels and insulin in different situations (such as hypoglycaemia or hyperglycaemia) is important.
   - Monitoring blood glucose levels takes commitment and practice.
   - One-on-one education and training provides the avenue for nurses to ensure that the person understands and can utilise the equipment effectively.
   - Including family members ensures that Naomi will have support when managing her diabetes at home.

Evaluate outcomes

As a result of the nursing actions above, Naomi welcomed a baby girl, Matilda. Matilda was born within a normal weight range. Naomi has regular follow-up tests for diabetes and continues to maintain a healthy lifestyle with her family.

Reflect on new processes and learning

Including family members in the education and management of gestational diabetes may help to ensure the success of its management and have benefits to the whole family unit. Reflect on the scenario and consider how including family members in the education and management of Naomi's gestational diabetes may prove beneficial to her mother and brother.

Source: Based on the Clinical Reasoning Cycle, Levett-Jones (2013).

SKILLS IN PRACTICE

Ultrasound

Obstetric ultrasound is a diagnostic imaging tool used for foetal screening during pregnancy. Ultrasound uses high-frequency, non-audible soundwaves which, when reflected off internal structures, create a real-time image. It does not expose patients to ionising radiation, as occurs with X-ray imaging.

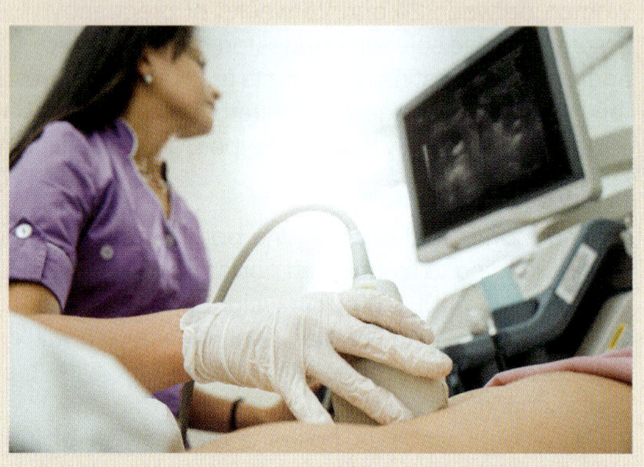

Most obstetric ultrasounds performed after 10 weeks of pregnancy are abdominal. A transducer is moved over the mother's abdomen to visualise the foetus. Ultrasound can identify severe abnormalities that may be incompatible with life or cause significant morbidity, in addition to milder anomalies amenable to antenatal intervention.

A routine obstetric ultrasound is recommended for all pregnant women at 18–22 weeks gestation. This scan can confirm the timing of the pregnancy by measurement of the foetus and identify any abnormalities (Salomon et al. 2011). At this stage the foetus is at a size and developmental stage that allows detailed examination of the skull, central nervous system, heart, thorax, gastrointestinal tract, urogenital systems and skeleton as well as the placenta and amniotic fluid.

Additionally, when possible, it is recommended that pregnant women have an obstetric ultrasound between 11 and 13.9 weeks gestational age, known as the nuchal or dating scan. An ultrasound performed at this earlier stage provides a more accurate estimate of the timing of the pregnancy and can also identify multiple foetuses and major congenital abnormalities. Nuchal translucency (figure 5.13) measures the space (fluid) between the cervical spine and skin and this measurement can be correlated to a number of chromosomal anomalies (e.g. Trisomy 21 or Down syndrome — instances where **aneuploidy**, or abnormal numbers of chromosomes, occurs).

The sensitivity and accuracy of ultrasound is reduced in women with a high body mass, or low amniotic fluid. Drinking a few glasses of water prior to the ultrasound may achieve a clearer image by enlarging the bladder and pushing the foetus up out of the pelvis.

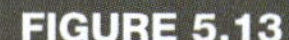

FIGURE 5.13 Antenatal screening: nuchal translucency describes the space between the cervical spine and the skin that is measured during an ultrasound. The collection of fluid here increases in some developmental anomalies.

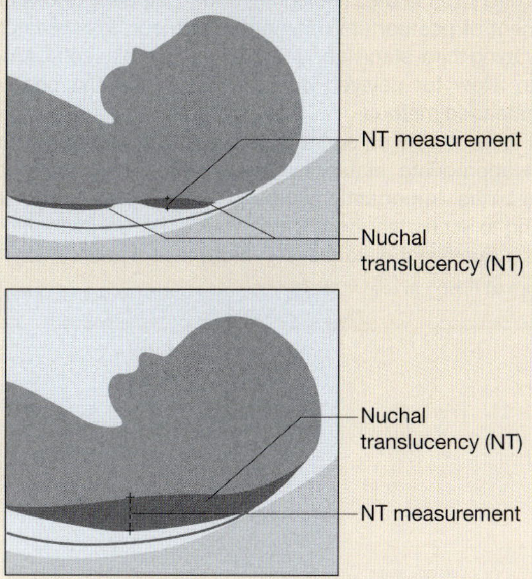

Source: Webster and de Wreede (2016). Reproduced with permission of John Wiley & Sons.

SKILLS IN PRACTICE

Unplanned out-of-hospital births

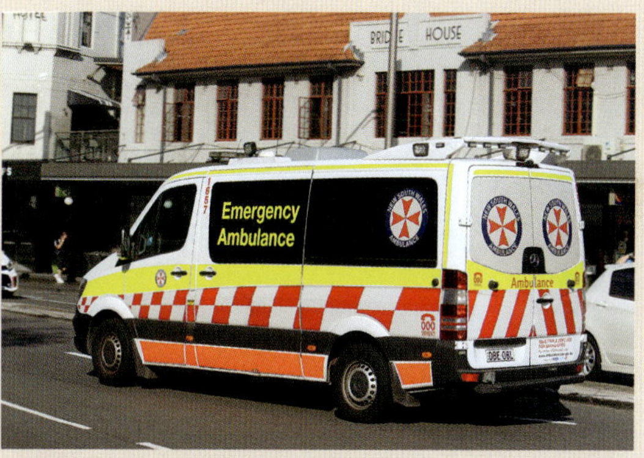

Although most births in Australia occur in hospitals, around 0.5 per cent of births occur prior to arrival at hospital (excluding pre-planned homebirths). Paramedics attending such births are faced with increased risks of pregnancy complications and/or managing adverse effects to the health of both mother (postpartum haemorrhage, postnatal anaemia, perineal tears) and baby (low birth weight, prematurity, hypothermia and hypoglycaemia), with the risk of perinatal mortality up to threefold higher compared with an in-hospital delivery (Gutvirtz et al. 2020).

While many out-of-hospital births occur without complication, paramedics attending unplanned out-of-hospital births must be able to identify and accurately manage pregnancy-related conditions using evidence-based guidelines to provide safe and effective care. Knowledge and skills around the following are key.

- *Foetal wellbeing*. If the birth has not yet occurred, steps to assessing the wellbeing of a foetus prior to birth should include assessment of normal foetal movements, foetal heart rate and abdominal palpation to confirm presentation. Awareness of less than 10 foetal movements over two hours requires review. If auscultation of the foetal heart rate is performed, a Doppler may be used from 12 weeks; alternatively, a stethoscope may be used after 20 weeks gestation. It is important to take a maternal pulse at the same time to ensure you are able to differentiate between a foetal pulse and maternal pulse. The stethoscope should be placed over the anterior shoulder of the foetus as located by the abdominal palp.

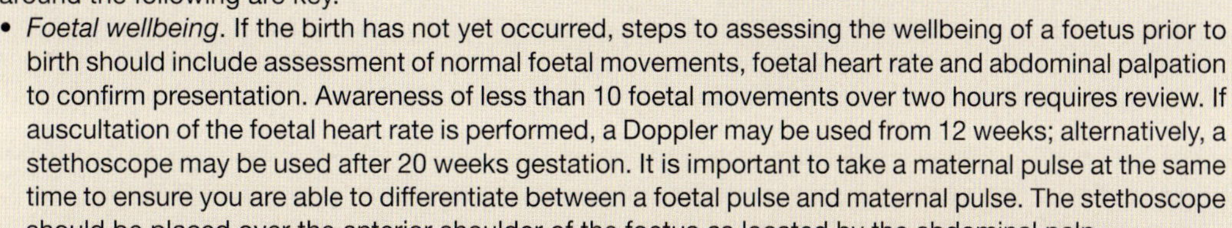

- *Continuing care: newborn*. In the first minutes and hours post birth, the key care objectives of the newborn are to: 1) establish and maintain effective respiration; 2) prevent hypothermia (via skin-to-skin contact and appropriate wrapping); and 3) initiate the first feed within the first 30 minutes of life. To monitor newborn health, the APGAR score is used immediately after birth (at 1 and 5 minutes), with the paramedic allocating points to five simple criteria: colour (**A**ppearance), heart rate (**P**ulse), reflex irritability (**G**rimace), muscle tone (**A**ctivity) and breathing (**R**espiration). At the 5-minute interval,

APGAR scores less than 7 are indicative of neonatal problems requiring further medical attention and investigation of abnormal vital signs. Vital signs should continue to be monitored every 15 minutes during transport.

- *Continuing care: mother*. Immediate care objectives of the mother in the hours post birth include: 1) the monitoring of vital signs every 15 minutes (including fundal palpation and vaginal loss during transport); 2) monitoring/management of postpartum haemorrhage (blood loss greater than 500 mL in the first 24 hours); and 3) encouraging third-stage labour (birthing of the placenta). Modified active management of third-stage labour to allow for delayed cord clamping and the use of uterotonic medications (oxytocics) is the recommended method.

If birth is imminent it is safer to stay on scene to manage complications in a controlled environment; however, transport to an appropriate maternity facility is a primary care objective when attending unplanned out-of-hospital births. Importantly, although complications associated with such births are low, they can be challenging to accurately identify and manage when occurring in the community setting, particularly if the setting is a significant distance (e.g. more than 4 hours away) from specialist care.

Sources: Gutvirtz et al. (2020); and Flanagan et al. (2017).

SUMMARY

Embryology encompasses much more than the early stages of a pregnancy; it includes all the factors responsible for a healthy and successful pregnancy. From the maturation of gametes to the birth of a healthy baby, there are numerous stages where medical monitoring and/or interventions are applicable. Consequently, there are many important roles for health professionals to play throughout this process and a robust knowledge of fertilisation, conception, embryo development, gestation and birth are essential attributes for anyone specialising in this field.

KEY TERMS

aneuploidy The presence of an abnormal number of chromosomes in a cell.
atresia Degeneration process of the ovarian follicles that do not ovulate.
colostrum First secretion from the mammary glands after birth.
conceptus Denotes the embryo and its associated extraembryonic structures (i.e. placenta).
corpus luteum (CL) A hormone-secreting structure that develops in an ovary at the sight of ovulation.
ectoderm The outermost of the three primary germ layers of an embryo.
effacement Process by which the cervix prepares for delivery (soften, shorten and become thinner) after the baby has repositioned itself in the lower in the abdomen/pelvis region.
embryogenesis The formation and development of an embryo.
endoderm The innermost of the three primary germ layers of an embryo.
endometrium The inner epithelial layer and mucous membrane of the mammalian uterus.
epididymis Highly convoluted which connects the testis to the vas deferens.
Fallopian tube (also known as an oviduct or uterine tube). Uterine appendages leading from the ovaries into the uterus.
fertilisation The union of the male and female gamete (sperm and oocyte).
follicle stimulating hormone (FSH) Sex hormone produced by the pituitary gland.
gametes Haploid sex cells (eggs and called sperm).
gastrulation Phase of early embryonic development during which the single-layered blastula is reorganised into a multilayered structure known as the gastrula.
gestation The period of development between conception and birth.
human chorionic gonadotropin (hCG) Hormone secreted by the placenta which forms the basis of pregnancy tests.
implantation The process of attachment and invasion of the uterus endometrium by the blastocyst.
luteinising hormone (LH) Hormone produced in the anterior pituitary gland which triggers ovulation and corpus luteum development.
mesoderm The innermost layer of the three primary germ layers of an embryo.
miscarriage Pregnancy loss before 20 weeks of pregnancy.
oestrogen Steroid hormones which promote the development and maintenance of female characteristics of the body.
ovulation A phase of the female menstrual cycle that involves the release of an egg (ovum) from one of the ovaries.
pre-eclampsia A serious condition of pregnancy, usually characterised by high blood pressure, protein in the urine and severe swelling.
pre-term Labour delivery before 37 completed weeks of pregnancy.
progesterone Hormone released by the corpus luteum in the ovary.
stillbirth Loss of a foetus or baby after 20 weeks gestation or during birth.
zygote A fertilised egg.

REFERENCES

Aitken, R.J. and Nixon, B. (2013) Sperm capacitation: a distant landscape glimpsed but unexplored. *Molecular Human Reproduction* 19: 785–793.

Australian Government Department of Health (2020) 26 Risk of pre-eclampsia. www.health.gov.au/resources/pregnancy-care-guidelines/part-d-clinical-assessments/risk-of-pre-eclampsia (accessed February 2021).

Bromfield, E.G. and Nixon, B. (2013) The function of chaperone proteins in the assemblage of protein complexes involved in gamete adhesion and fusion processes. *Reproduction* 145: R31–42.

Flanagan, B., Lord, B. and Barnes, M. (2017) Is unplanned out-of-hospital birth managed by paramedics 'infrequent', 'normal' and 'uncomplicated'? *BMC Pregnancy Childbirth* 17: 436.

Grant, G.J. (2020) Pharmacologic management of pain during labor and delivery. www.uptodate.com/contents/pharmacologic-management-of-pain-during-labor-and-delivery (accessed December 2020).

Gutvirtz, G., Wainstock, T., Landau, D. and Sheiner, E. (2020). Unplanned out-of-hospital birth-short and long-term consequences for the offspring. *Journal of Clinical Medicine* 9(2): 339.

Korevaar, T.I., Steegers, E.A., de Rijke, Y.B. et al. (2015). Reference ranges and determinants of total hCG levels during pregnancy: the Generation R Study. *European Journal of Epidemiology* 30: 1057–1066.

Levett-Jones, T. (2013). *Clinical Reasoning: Learning to Think Like a Nurse*. Pearson Australia.

Morris, S.A., Grewal, S., Barrios, F., Patankar, S.N., Strauss, B., Buttery, L., Alexander, M., Shakesheff, K.M. and Zernicka-Goetz, M. (2012) Dynamics of anterior-posterior axis formation in the developing mouse embryo. *Nature Communications* 3: 673.

Niakan, K.K., Han, J., Pedersen, R.A., Simon, C. and Pera, R.A. (2012) Human pre-implantation embryo development. *Development* 139: 829–841.

Salomon, L.J., Alfirevic, Z., Berghella, V. et al. (2011) Practice guidelines for performance of the routine mid-trimester fetal ultrasound scan. *Ultrasound in Obstetrics and Gynaecology* 37: 116–126.

Sullivan, R. and Mieusset, R. (2016) The human epididymis: its function in sperm maturation. *Human Reproduction Update* 22(5): 574–587.

Webster, S. and de Wreede, R. (2016) *Embryology at a Glance*, 2nd edn. Wiley-Blackwell.

Webster, S., Morris, G. and Kevelighan, E. (2018) *Essential Human Development*, Wiley-Blackwell.

Zhou, W., Anderson, A.L., Turner, A.P., De Iuliis, G.N., McCluskey, A., McLaughlin, E.A. and Nixon, B. (2017) Characterization of a novel role for the dynamin mechanoenzymes in the regulation of human sperm acrosomal exocytosis. *Molecular Human Reproduction* 23: 657–673.

FURTHER READING

BIRTHS IN AUSTRALIA

www.abs.gov.au/statistics/people/population/births-australia/latest-release

This ABS data includes information about births, fertility and infertility rates in Australia.

PREGNANCY CARE GUIDELINES: PRE-ECLAMPSIA

https://beta.health.gov.au/resources/pregnancy-care-guidelines/part-d-clinical-assessments/risk-of-pre-eclampsia

This link from the Australian Government Department of Health outlines the pregnancy care guidelines to identify and manage the risk of pre-eclampsia.

DIABETES AUSTRALIA

www.diabetesaustralia.com.au

Diabetes Australia is the national body for people affected by all types of diabetes and those at risk. Working in partnership with diabetes health professionals and educators, researchers and healthcare providers, Diabetes Australia is committed to reducing the impact of diabetes on the Australian community.

NATIONAL DIABETES SERVICES SCHEME

https://pregnancyanddiabetes.com.au

The National Diabetes Services Scheme is an initiative of the Australian government administered with the assistance of Diabetes Australia. This website provides information on pregnancy and diabetes.

GESTATIONAL DIABETES FACT SHEET

http://gd.ndss.com.au/Global/GD/Understanding%20Gestational%20Diabetes%20-%20high%20res.pdf

STILLBIRTH FOUNDATION OF AUSTRALIA

https://stillbirthfoundation.org.au/stillbirth

The mission of the Stillbirth Foundation of Australia is to significantly reduce the incidence of stillbirth through research, education and advocacy.

WORLD HEALTH ORGANIZATION (WHO): SEXUAL AND REPRODUCTIVE HEALTH

www.who.int/reproductivehealth/en

With regard to reproduction, the WHO gathers information about abortion, adolescents, reproductive cancers, sexually transmitted and reproductive tract infections, contraception, infertility, maternal and perinatal health, sexual health, stillbirths and violence against women.

ACKNOWLEDGEMENTS

Photo: © Pikul Noorod / Shutterstock.com
Photo: © SpeedKingz / Shutterstock.com
Photo: © Hero Images / Getty Images
Photo: © Syda Productions / Shutterstock.com
Photo: © Roman Zaiets / Shutterstock.com
Photo: © Rose Makin / Shutterstock.com

CHAPTER 6

The muscular system

TEST YOUR PRIOR KNOWLEDGE

- List the functions of the muscular system.
- Name the different types of muscles found in the human body.
- Describe the energy sources that enable muscles to contract.
- List the stages involved in muscle contraction.
- List the different types of body movement.

LEARNING OUTCOMES

After reading this chapter you will be able to:

6.1 describe the structure and functions of the muscular system, and the different types of muscles in the human body

6.2 describe how a muscle contracts

6.3 describe the energy sources that muscles use

6.4 name the major muscles of the body and their functions.

Body map

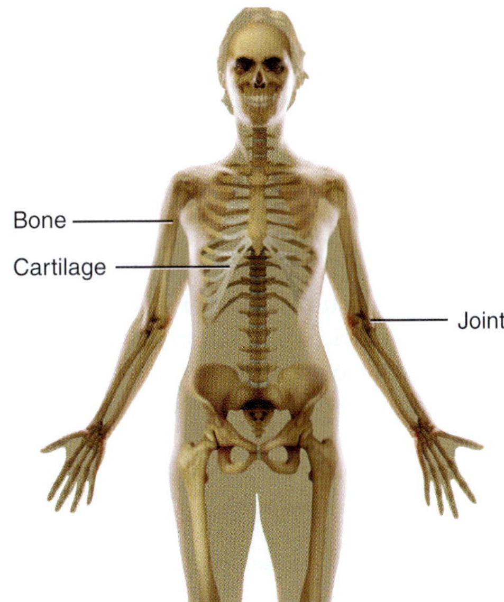

Introduction

All physical function of the body involves muscular activity, and as muscles are responsible for all body movement, they can be considered the 'machines' of the body. This chapter will discuss the structure and function of the muscular system.

6.1 Types of muscle tissue

LEARNING OBJECTIVE 6.1 Describe the structure and functions of the muscular system, and the different types of muscles in the human body.

The body contains three types of muscle tissue: smooth, cardiac and skeletal. Table 6.1 provides a summary of the different types of muscle tissue.

TABLE 6.1 Different types of muscle tissue

Skeletal muscle	Smooth muscle	Cardiac muscle
Attached to bones or the skin (facial muscles only)	Found in the walls of hollow visceral organs and blood vessels	Located in the walls of the heart
Single, long cylindrical cells	Single, narrow, rod-shaped cells	Branching chains of cells
Striated, multinucleated cells	Non-striated, uninucleated cells	Striated, uninucleated cells
Under voluntary control	Involuntary control	Involuntary control

Smooth or visceral muscle

Smooth or visceral muscle is located in the walls of hollow internal organs and blood vessels of the body; for example, the small intestine, blood vessels (arteries, arterioles, venules and veins), bronchioles of the respiratory tract, urinary bladder and ureters, uterus and uterine tubes, but not the heart. Smooth muscle fibres have a single nucleus, are usually arranged in parallel lines and are not striated. Smooth muscles are involuntary, do not fatigue easily and are controlled by the medulla oblongata in the brain, which is responsible for controlling involuntary action throughout the body. Smooth muscle is discussed in more detail in the chapter on the digestive system.

Cardiac

Cardiac muscle, found only in the heart, is also a form of involuntary muscle and forms the walls of the heart. Its main function is to propel blood into the circulation by making the right atrium contract. Cardiac muscles also have a single nucleus, are striated, branched and tubular. Cardiac muscle is discussed in more detail in the chapter on the cardiac system.

Skeletal

The skeletal muscles make up the muscular system of the body (composed of over 600 muscles) and account for 40–50 per cent of the body weight in an adult. The skeletal muscles are the only voluntary muscles of the body (i.e. are consciously controlled) and are the muscles involved in moving bones and generating external movement. Skeletal muscle is also referred to as striped or striated muscle because of the banded patterns of the cells seen under the microscope.

The rest of this chapter will focus on skeletal muscle only as both smooth and cardiac muscle are discussed in more detail elsewhere.

Functions of the muscular system

The muscular system plays five important roles in the body:

- maintains posture
- produces movement
- stabilises joints
- protection
- generates heat.

Maintenance of body posture

Despite the continuous downward pull of gravity, the body is able to maintain an erect or seated posture because of the continuous tiny adjustments that the skeletal muscles make.

Production of movement

The body's ability to mobilise is a result of skeletal muscle activity and muscle contraction, as when muscles contract they pull on the **tendons** and bones of the skeleton to produce movement.

Stabilisation of joints

Muscle tendons play a vital role in stabilising and reinforcing the joints of the body. During movement, skeletal muscles pull on the bones and stabilise the joints of the skeleton.

Protection and control of internal tissue structures/organs

Skeletal muscle plays an important role in protecting the internal organs, as the visceral organs and tissues contained within the abdominal cavity are protected by layers of skeletal muscle tissue within the abdominal wall and floor of the pelvic cavity. Similarly, the orifices contained within the digestive and urinary tracts are encircled by skeletal muscle, and this allows for voluntary control over swallowing, urination and defecation (Martini & Bartholomew 2017).

Generation of heat

Heat generation is vital in maintaining normal body temperature, and skeletal muscles, which account for 40 per cent of the body's mass, are the muscle type mostly responsible for the body's heat generation. During muscle contraction, **adenosine triphosphate (ATP)** is hydrolysed to release the stored energy, with nearly three-quarters of this energy escaping as heat.

Composition of skeletal muscle tissue

As muscles contain other types of tissues, such as blood vessels and connective and nervous tissue, they are considered to be organs (Logenbaker 2017). Each cell in skeletal muscle tissue is also referred to as a single muscle fibre, which, owing to its large size, contains hundreds of nuclei (i.e. are multinucleate). A skeletal muscle consists of individual muscle fibres that are markedly different from a 'typical' cell (not least by their size) bundled into fascicles and surrounded by three layers of connective tissue.

CLINICAL CONSIDERATIONS

Rhabdomyolysis

Rhabdomyolysis is a serious syndrome that can occur following damage to a muscle. This may result in part of the muscle tissue dying and the contents entering the bloodstream which can lead to complications such as renal failure.

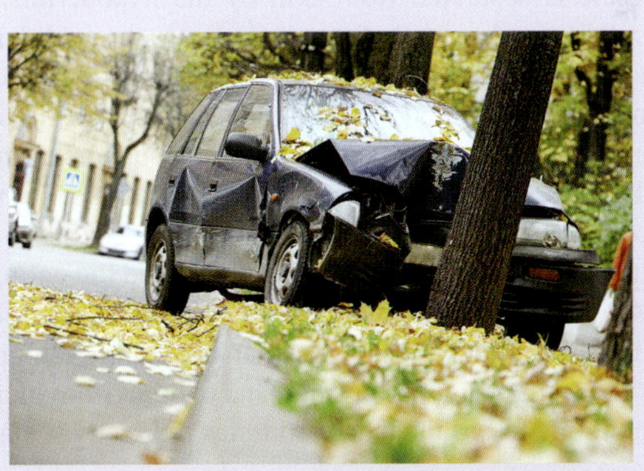

Traumatic causes of rhabdomyolysis include:

- a crush injury such as from a traffic collision, fall or building collapse
- long-lasting muscle compression such as that caused by prolonged immobilisation after a fall or lying unconscious on a hard surface during illness or while under the influence of alcohol or medication
- electrical shock injury, lightning strike or third-degree burn
- venom from a snake or insect bite.

Non-traumatic causes of rhabdomyolysis include:

- the use of alcohol or illegal drugs such as heroin, cocaine or amphetamines
- extreme muscle strain, especially in someone who is an untrained athlete; this can happen in elite athletes too, and it can be more dangerous as there is more muscle mass to break down
- the use of medications such as antipsychotics or statins, especially when given in high doses
- a very high body temperature (hyperthermia) or heat stroke
- seizures or delirium tremens

- a metabolic disorder such as diabetic ketoacidosis
- diseases of the muscles (myopathy) such as congenital muscle enzyme deficiency or Duchenne muscular dystrophy
- viral infections such as the flu, HIV or herpes simplex virus
- bacterial infections leading to toxins in tissues or the bloodstream (sepsis).

A previous history of rhabdomyolysis also increases the risk of having rhabdomyolysis again.

The 'classic triad' of rhabdomyolysis symptoms are muscle pain in the shoulders, thighs or lower back; muscle weakness or trouble moving arms and legs; and dark-red or brown urine or decreased urination. However, half of patients with the condition may have no muscle-related symptoms. The clinical presentation and a raised level of creatinine kinase (a by-product of muscle breakdown) in the blood may assist with diagnosis. Treatment aims to support the kidneys and reverse the symptoms of renal failure; in rare cases this may require haemodialysis.

HOMEOSTATIC IMBALANCE

Muscle cramping

Muscle cramps are involuntary muscle spasms that can result in an over-shortening of the muscle and are accompanied by mild to severe pain. While typically lasting only a few seconds they can persist for several hours in some cases and occur at a rate of 50–60 per cent in the healthy adult population (Giuriato et al. 2018). While there are many factors that influence cramping, there are three broad categories of causative factors: 1) cramping related to exercise; 2) idiopathic nocturnal cramps, where cramps occur during sleep but have no identifiable cause; and 3) cramping associated with a pathology such as neuropathy and metabolic disturbances. However, in many cases the exact source of the muscle excitation is yet to be fully determined.

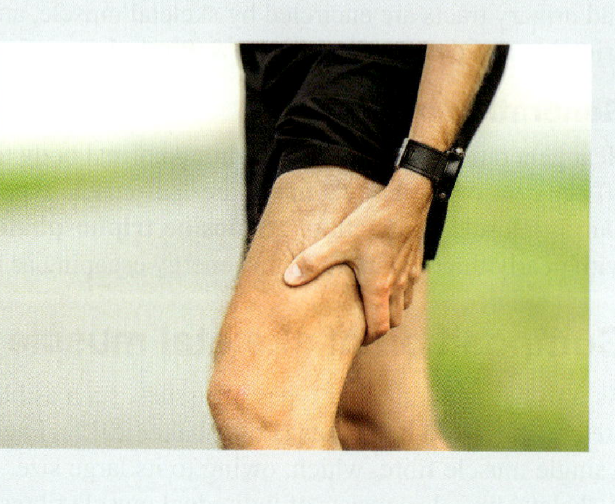

Gross anatomy of skeletal muscles

Muscle is separated from skin by the hypodermis, which consists of adipose tissue (which provides insulation and protects the muscle from physical damage) and a dense, broad band of connective tissue known as fascia, which supports and surrounds muscle tissue and provides a pathway for nerves and the lymphatic and blood vessels to enter and exit a muscle. Extending from the fascia are three layers of connective tissue that also play a role in supporting and protecting the muscle and are necessary to ensure that the force of contraction from each muscle cell is transmitted to its points of attachment to the skeleton (see figure 6.1). These are:

- the *epimysium*, which is wrapped around the entire muscle
- the *perimysium*, which surrounds bundles of muscle fibres known as fascicles
- the *endomysium*, which is wrapped around each individual muscle cell.

The epimysium, perimysium and endomysium blend into either strong, cord-like tendons or into sheet-like **aponeuroses** that attach muscles indirectly to bones, cartilages or connective tissue.

SKILLS IN PRACTICE

Intramuscular injection

An intramuscular (IM) injection is given directly into a selected muscle. While there are several sites on the body that are suitable for IM injections, the most common areas used are:

- the deltoid muscle of the upper arm
- the vastus lateralis muscle, which forms part of the quadriceps muscle group of the upper leg
- the gluteus medius (ventrogluteal site) muscle, which runs beneath the gluteus maximus from the ilium to the femur.

IM injections are used for the delivery of certain drugs that (for various reasons) cannot be given via an oral, intravenous or subcutaneous route. The IM route enables a large amount (up to 5 mL) of drug to be introduced at one time, minimises tissue irritation and provides faster absorption than subcutaneous/intradermal injections.

FIGURE 6.1 Gross anatomy of a skeletal muscle

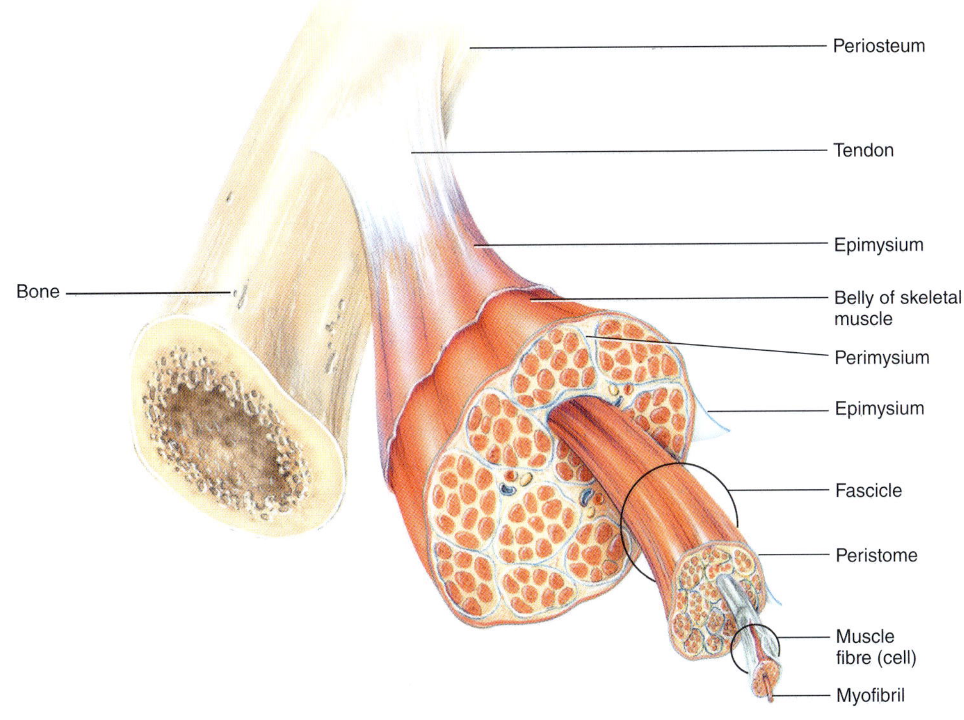

Source: Tortora and Derrickson (2009). Reproduced with permission of John Wiley & Sons.

Microanatomy of skeletal muscle fibre

When examined microscopically, skeletal muscle cells appear cylindrical in shape, have a distinctive banded appearance of alternate light and dark stripes and lie parallel to each other (see figure 6.2). Table 6.2 provides a summary of the cellular components of a muscle fibre.

TABLE 6.2 **Cellular components of a muscle fibre**

Name	Function
Sarcolemma	Plasma membrane of a muscle fibre that forms **T tubules**
Sarcoplasm	Cytoplasm of the muscle fibre that contains **myofibrils**
Myofibril	Consists of bundles of myofilaments and plays a key role in muscle contraction
Myofilament	Consists of thick and thin filaments that give muscle tissue its striated appearance and plays a role in muscle contraction
Myoglobin	A reddish-brown pigment (gives muscle tissue its dark-red colour) that stores oxygen for muscle contraction
T tubule	Fluid-filled tubular structure that releases calcium from the sarcoplasmic reticulum
Sarcoplasmic reticulum	Storage site for calcium ions

FIGURE 6.2 Diagram showing a skeletal muscle fibre

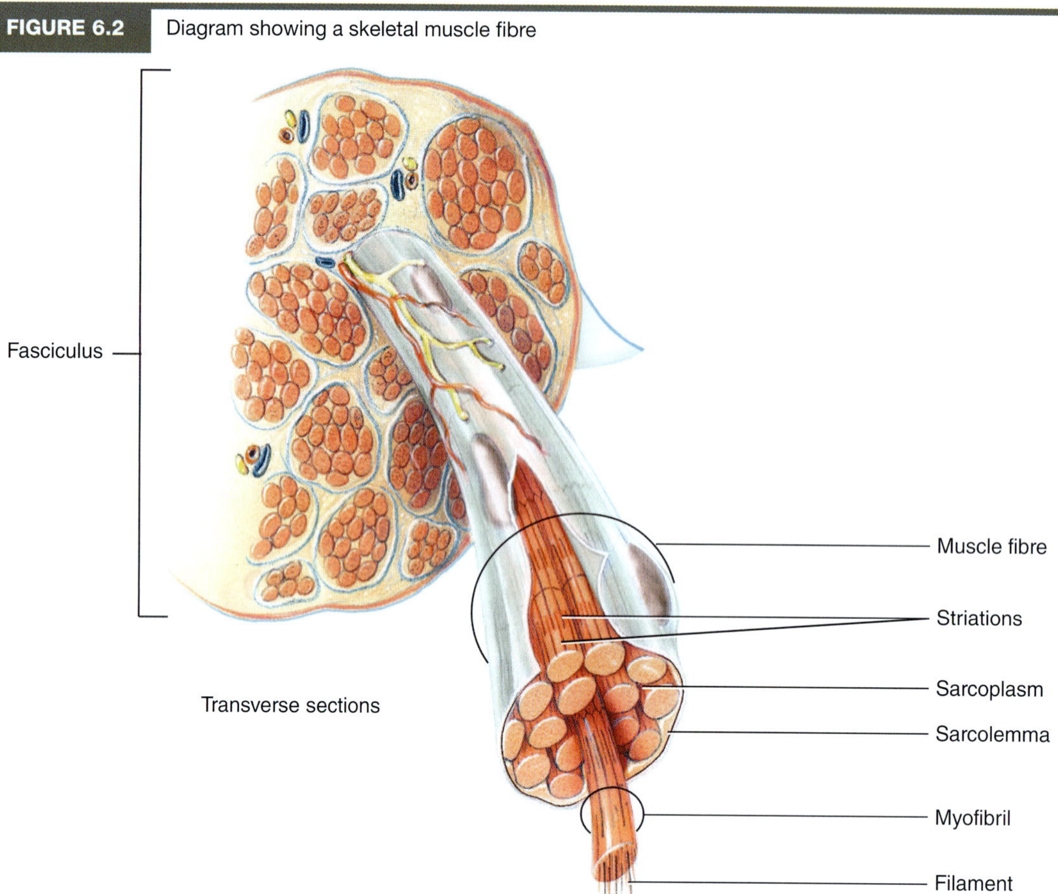

The sarcolemma and transverse tubules

Each muscle fibre is covered by a plasma membrane called the sarcolemma and contains cylindrical structures called myofibrils suspended in a matrix called the sarcoplasm (cytoplasm), which extends along the entire length of the muscle fibre. The surface of the sarcolemma is scattered with openings that lead into a network of narrow tubules called transverse or 'T' tubules that are filled with extracellular fluid and form passageways through the muscle fibre (Martini & Bartholomew 2017).

The sarcoplasm

The sarcoplasm contains multiple mitochondria, which produce large amounts of ATP during muscle contraction (Tortora & Derrickson 2017) and it is here that the T tubules make contact with a membrane-bound structure known as the sarcoplasmic reticulum (SR). The SR stores calcium ions (essential for muscle contraction) in structures called cisternae and myoglobin (a reddish-brown pigment that is similar to haemoglobin), which stores oxygen until required for ATP generation.

The myofibrils

Myofibrils (which are bundles of myofilaments) are thread-like structures found abundantly in the sarcoplasm. The myofibrils play a key role in the muscle contraction mechanism and contain two types of protein filaments: thick filaments composed of myosin; and thin filaments composed of **actin** and two other proteins, tropomyosin and troponin. These filaments form compartments know as sarcomeres, which are the basic functional units of striated muscle fibres (Tortora & Derrickson 2017). Each myofibril contains approximately 10 000 sarcomeres arranged end to end. The sarcomeres are separated from each other by dense zigzagging protein-based structures called Z discs.

The sarcomeres

Extending across each of the thick filaments found within the sarcomere is a dark area known as the A band in the centre of which is a narrow H zone. On either side of the A band there is a lighter coloured area consisting of thin filaments called the I band. The alternating A and I bands give skeletal muscles their striated (striped) appearance.

CLINICALLY REASONED EPISODE OF CARE

Muscular dystrophy

Consider the patient situation

Siobhan is a newborn baby. At birth, Siobhan had decreased tone and was weak. She is now being cared for in the neonatal unit.

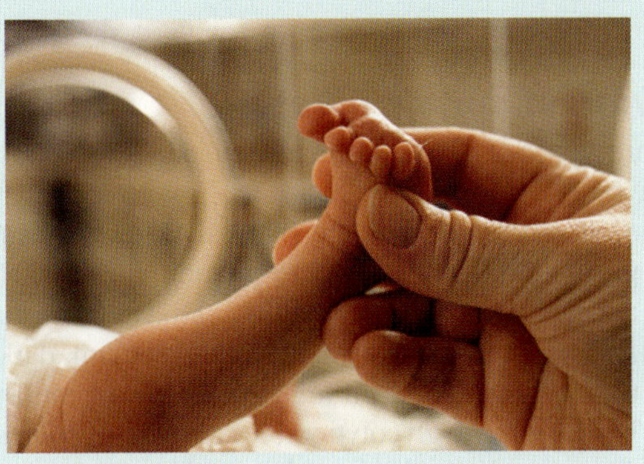

Collect cues and information

Siobhan has been transferred to the neonatal unit. She has since been subjected to a number of tests and procedures, including a lumbar puncture; blood tests; and observations of hands, stature and flexibility.

A geneticist comes to see Siobhan and takes note of a range of symptoms, which are run through a database of genetic disorders. Siobhan is subsequently diagnosed with congenital myotonic dystrophy.

Process information

Muscular dystrophy is a broad term applied to an inherited group of disorders that destroy the muscles by causing muscle fibres to degenerate, shrink in size and eventually die. The muscle fibres that die are replaced with fat and connective tissue.

Newborns with congenital muscular dystrophy have problems controlling their muscles. The first sign is often weak muscles and difficulty holding their heads up. Children with muscular dystrophy are late developers, and are late to crawl and walk. Muscular dystrophy can affect breathing and cause stiff and frozen joints. Some children with congenital muscular dystrophy have intellectual disabilities.

Muscular dystrophy is diagnosed through a series of tests. It can take some time to form a diagnosis and to ensure that the correct diagnosis is made. Myotonic dystrophy is caused by gene mutations in the DMPK and CNBP genes. Myotonic dystrophy is inherited. Treatments for myotonic dystrophy vary between individuals and may include physiotherapy, pain management and mobility aids.

Muscular dystrophy is a progressive, life-limiting disease.

Identify problems/issues

1. Management of a newborn undergoing multiple tests and procedures
2. Care for a newborn and family pending diagnosis
3. Provision of information, education and appropriate referral to various teams post diagnosis

Nursing actions

1. Prepare the patient and family for procedures and tests.
   Rationale:
   - To ensure seamless diagnosis and treatment, nurses can assist in procedures and tests; for example, blood tests and preparing for and assisting with lumbar puncture.
   - Nurses are well placed to inform individuals and family members about pending procedures and tests, including how and where the procedure will take place.
2. Provide care and support to newborn.
   Rationale:
   - Children with muscular dystrophy will often require respiratory and physical support, including oxygen therapy and feeding support.
   - Clinical observations and care such as pressure injury prevention are tasks undertaken by the nurse, and are particularly important to caring for a child with muscular dystrophy.
3. Refer to a nurse specialist for education and learning resources.
   Rationale:
   - A diagnosis of muscular dystrophy can be a challenging time for parents and families. A specialist nurse educator is well placed to provide detailed and targeted information and education as well as ongoing care support to parents and families.

Evaluate outcomes

As a result of the immediate nursing management and care, Siobhan receives a diagnosis. Siobhan is now 8 years old; she has mobility problems and is unable to speak as other 8-year-olds do. However, she makes known her needs and plays with other children and her sibling.

Reflect on new processes and learning

Consider the implications to the family unit. What role can nurses play in the diagnosis, management and ongoing support of families with a diagnosis of muscular dystrophy?

Source: Based on the Clinical Reasoning Cycle, Levett-Jones (2013).

Types of muscle fibres

Three types of muscle fibres are found in skeletal muscles and are found in varying proportions throughout the body.

- *Slow oxidative fibres* are small, dark-red fibres (due to containing large amounts of myoglobin) that generate ATP by **aerobic** respiration; they make up approximately 50 per cent of skeletal muscle and are capable of slow, prolonged contractions and are not easily fatigued.
- *Fast oxidative–glycolytic fibres* are medium, dark-red fibres that also generate ATP by aerobic respiration but, owing to their high **glycogen** content, are also able to generate ATP by **anaerobic** glycolysis. Fast oxidative–glycolytic fibres are able to contract and relax more quickly than slow oxidative fibres.
- *Fast glycolytic fibres* are large white fibres (low myoglobin content) that generate ATP mainly by anaerobic glycolysis and provide the most rapid and powerful muscle contractions, but fatigue easily.

Blood supply

Skeletal muscles have a very extensive blood supply and receive a total of 1 L of blood each minute, which equates to 20 per cent of the resting cardiac output. This increases to 15–20 L min^{-1} when exercising intensively. As a general rule, each skeletal muscle is supplied by an artery and one or two veins, and each muscle fibre is in close contact with a network of microscopic capillaries within the endomysium.

CLINICAL CONSIDERATIONS

Acute compartment syndrome

In the limbs the connections between the muscle fibres and the skeleton are robust; consequently, muscles are commonly isolated in dense collagen-based compartments. These compartments are where the blood vessels and nerves that supply a specific muscle enter.

When an injury to a limb occurs, if the resulting oedema develops within a compartment where there is little room for tissue expansion, the interstitial pressure will increase. As pressure within the compartment becomes higher than that within the capillaries, blood flow, and hence tissue perfusion, slows and may ultimately stop (Harris & Hobson 2015). This can result in tissue ischaemia and muscle death, with the contents of the affected muscle fibres potentially entering the bloodstream (rhabdomyolysis). Common causes of compartment syndrome include limb fractures, crush injuries, vascular compromise and drug overdose involving heroin or cocaine.

Early diagnosis of compartment syndrome is essential to avoid long-term disability. Nurses and other members of the multidisciplinary team must have an awareness and understanding of the condition. They must also be aware of the signs and symptoms and initiate immediate appropriate action once compartment syndrome is suspected. Being able to identify patients who are at greatest risk and offer appropriate analgesia while monitoring them is a key element of care.

6.2 Skeletal muscle contraction and relaxation

LEARNING OBJECTIVE 6.2 Describe how a muscle contracts.

The ability of skeletal muscle to contract is controlled by the body's nervous system, and each muscle fibre is controlled by a motor neurone (nerve cell), which may stimulate a few muscle cells or several hundred depending on the particular muscle and the work it does. Skeletal muscle contracts in response to stimulation by an electrical signal (muscle action potential) delivered by the motor neurone, which is found halfway along the muscle cell, where it terminates at the neuromuscular junction. Here, the sarcolemma is specialised to form a motor end plate.

Although a muscle fibre normally has a single motor end plate, the densely branched motor neurone axons (see figure 6.3) mean that one motor neurone axon can connect and control many muscle fibres. The motor neurone and the muscle fibres it controls are known as a motor unit.

FIGURE 6.3 Motor unit

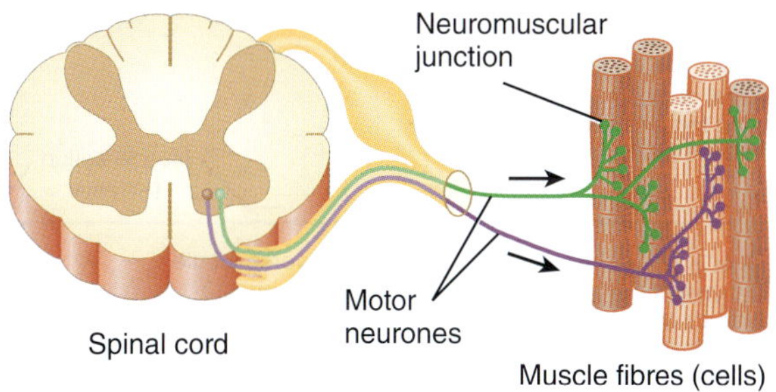

Source: Tortora and Derrickson (2009). Reproduced with permission of John Wiley & Sons.

When a nerve impulse reaches the axon terminals, the neurotransmitter **acetylcholine (ACh)** that stimulates skeletal muscle is released into the synaptic cleft, which is a small gap that separates the membrane of the nerve cell from the membrane of the muscle fibre (Shier et al. 2018). The synaptic cleft and motor end plate contain **acetylcholinesterase (AChE)**, which breaks down molecules of ACh. The release of ACh results in changes to the sarcolemma that trigger the contraction of the muscle fibre.

CLINICAL CONSIDERATIONS

Botulism

Botulism can arise from the consumption of contaminated or smoked food and is caused by ingestion of spores from the bacterium *Clostridium botulinum*, which is commonly found in soil and water. One of the toxins released from the bacterium prevents the release of ACh at the synaptic terminals of muscle cells and prevents an action potential in the sarcolemma from occurring. If not treated quickly this can result in potentially fatal muscular paralysis. Treatment is with an anti-toxin and the use of mechanical ventilation if the respiratory system is affected (Public Health England 2019).

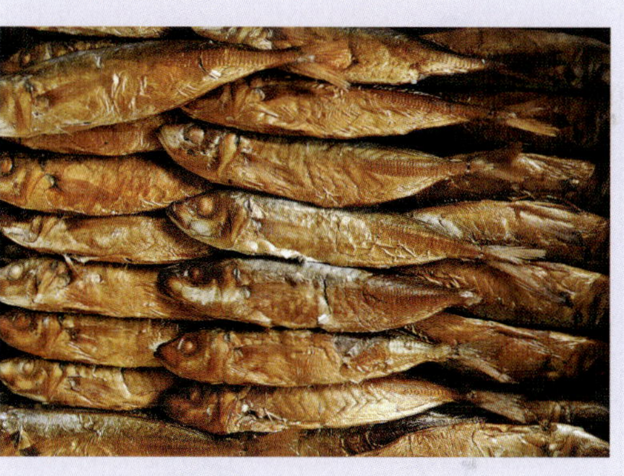

Skeletal muscle fibres are stimulated by neurones that control the production of an action potential (electrical impulse) in the sarcolemma by the following.

- *The release of ACh.* An action potential travels along a motor neurone until it reaches the synaptic terminal where vesicles contained within the synaptic terminal release ACh into the synaptic cleft between the motor neurone and the motor end plate.
- *The binding of ACh at the motor end plate.* The ACh molecules diffuse across the synaptic cleft and bind to ACh receptors on the sarcolemma. This changes the permeability of the membrane and allows sodium ions (Na^+) into the sarcoplasm, which triggers the production of a muscle action potential in the sarcolemma.
- *The conduction of action potentials by the sarcolemma.* The action potential spreads across the entire surface of the sarcolemma and then travels down the transverse tubules to the cisternae which encircle the sarcomeres of the muscle fibre. As a result of the action potential travelling across it, the cisternae release significant amounts of calcium ions (Ca^{2+}) which leads to the initiation of a muscle contraction. Each nerve impulse normally results in one muscle action potential and stages 2 and 3 are repeated if more ACh is released by another nerve impulse.
- *Muscle relaxation.* Action potential generation ceases as ACh is broken down by AChE and the concentration of calcium ions in the sarcoplasm declines. Once calcium ions return to normal resting levels, muscle contraction will end and muscle relaxation occurs.

Figure 6.4 provides a summary of the steps involved in skeletal muscle contraction and relaxation.

FIGURE 6.4 Summary of muscle contraction and relaxation

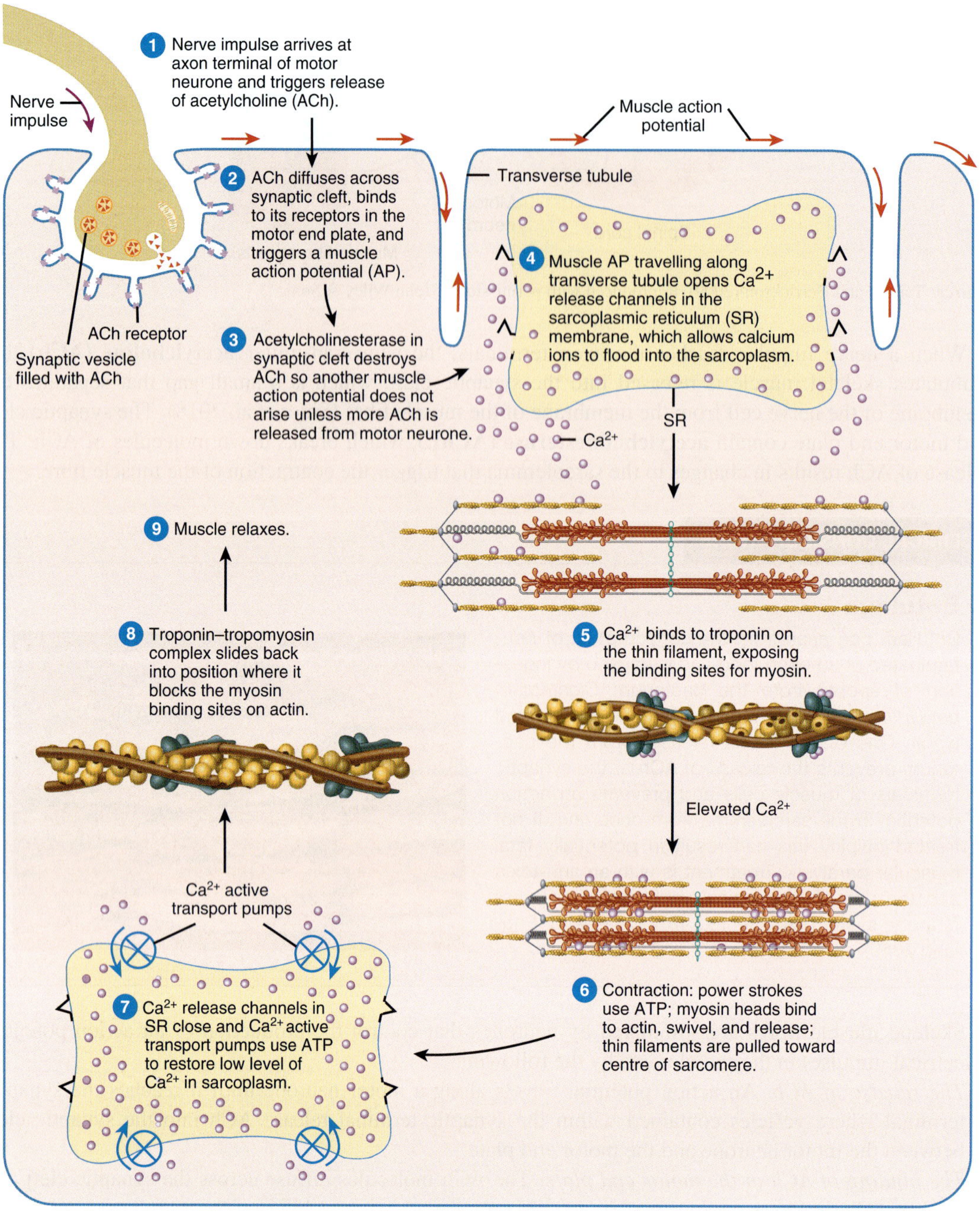

Source: Tortora and Derrickson (2009). Reproduced with permission of John Wiley & Sons.

MEDICINES MANAGEMENT

Pyridostigmine

Pyridostigmine is an anticholinesterase agent or AChE inhibitor and is used mainly to enhance neuromuscular transmission and improve muscle strength in voluntary and involuntary muscles of patients with **myasthenia gravis**. AChE inhibitors inhibit AChE, raising the concentration of ACh at the neuromuscular junction. In so doing they prolong the action of ACh by inhibiting the action of the enzyme AChE (Joint Formulary Committee 2018).

Cautions and contraindications

The drug should be used with caution in patients who have asthma, heart disease, epilepsy, Parkinsonism, thyroid disease or stomach ulcer. AChE inhibitors should not be given to patients with intestinal or urinary obstruction.

Adverse effects of pyridostigmine include nausea, vomiting, abdominal cramps, diarrhoea, excessive salivation, sweating, bradycardia and bronchospasm. Adverse effects of the drug may be minimised by precise dosage adjustment.

SKILLS IN PRACTICE

Electromyography (EMG)/nerve conduction studies

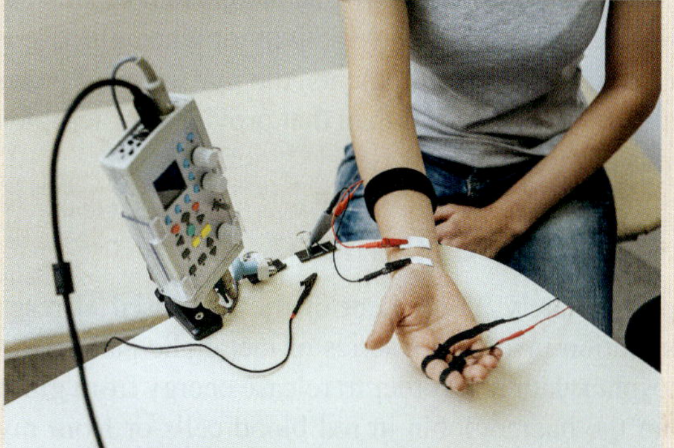

This routine test is performed in specialist hospitals; patient details and consent are required before the procedure. The EMG records the electrical impulses that the muscles produce. The nerve conduction test measures the speed at which impulses travel along a nerve. These tests help to determine how well the nerves and muscles are functioning.

Before the test the patient should:

- remove any jewellery
- wear clothing with short sleeves and/or loose clothing
- avoid using lotions and creams before the test
- eat and take any medication as normal.

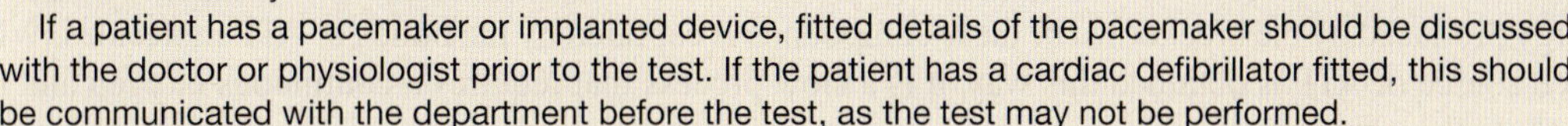

If a patient has a pacemaker or implanted device, fitted details of the pacemaker should be discussed with the doctor or physiologist prior to the test. If the patient has a cardiac defibrillator fitted, this should be communicated with the department before the test, as the test may not be performed.

The appointment for the test is around 45 minutes. There are three parts to the test and these are described below. The patient may not need all three parts; this depends on the clinical problem and the findings during the test.

Part 1: Sensory nerve testing

The skin is cleaned with an alcohol wipe.

Then the nerves, which supply sensation, are tested using ring electrodes on the fingers or button electrodes on all other parts of the body. For a short time during the test the patient will feel a repetitive tapping/tingling sensation.

Measurements are made between the electrodes using a tape measure and a marker pen; small dots are made on the skin, but these will wash off.

Part 2: Motor nerve testing

This test provides a check of the nerve supply to the muscles. There is a tapping/tingling sensation similar to that felt during part 1, caused by a muscle being stimulated. Measurements are taken.

Part 3: EMG testing

A small needle is inserted into the muscles to be tested and is specifically designed to carry a fine recording wire; the patient may feel a sharp scratch. Any electrical activity while the muscle is at rest is examined. The patient is asked to use the muscles so that they can be observed in their pattern of activity. The activity is displayed on a screen and can also be heard on a speaker as a crackling sound. The test may be repeated for different muscles.

The results are available usually within two days of the test being performed. A report is sent to the healthcare professional who made the referral.

The muscles tested may feel sore for a short time after the examination. The patient is able to continue their activities as normal, including driving after the test.

The nurse may be required to assist the patient before, during or after the test.

6.3 Energy sources for muscle contraction

LEARNING OBJECTIVE 6.3 Describe the energy sources that muscles use.

Muscle fibres require an energy source to enable them to contract as and when needed. This is provided initially in the form of ATP, which is stored in the muscle fibre. However, as only small amounts of ATP are stored in the muscle fibre, it is quickly depleted when the muscle is used and needs to be continuously available to power muscles. Therefore, working muscles require additional pathways to produce ATP, including the following.

- *Creatine phosphate.* This is broken down into creatine, phosphate and energy and is the energy that is used to synthesise more ATP. Most of the creatine formed is used to resynthesise creatine phosphate and the creatine not used is converted to the waste product creatinine, which is excreted by the kidneys.
- *Anaerobic respiration.* Glycogen is the most abundant energy source found in muscle fibres and is broken down into glucose when it is needed to provide energy for muscle contraction. Glucose is initially broken down into pyruvic acid without the need for oxygen — a process known as glycolysis — and the small amounts of energy that are created by this process are captured by the bonds of ATP molecules.

During intensive muscle activity or when glucose and oxygen delivery are (temporarily) insufficient to meet the muscle requirements, the pyruvic acid generated during glycolysis converts to lactic acid. This pathway is much faster than that provided by aerobic respiration and can provide sufficient ATP for short spells of intensive exercise.

Aerobic respiration

Approximately 95 per cent of the ATP used at rest and during moderate exercise comes from aerobic respiration involving a series of metabolic pathways that use oxygen — collectively known as oxidative phosphorylation. In order to release energy from glucose, oxygen is necessary; muscles receive this either from the haemoglobin in red blood cells or from myoglobin, a protein that stores some oxygen within the muscle cells. During aerobic respiration, glucose is broken down into carbon dioxide and water. The energy produced by the breakdown of these compounds is captured by the bonds of ATP molecules. While a rich source of ATP is obtained this way, it is a slow process that requires a continuous oxygen and fuel supply to the muscles.

Figure 6.5 provides an overview of the different ATP sources available for muscles.

Oxygen debt

When the body is moderately active or at rest, the cardiovascular and respiratory systems of the body can usually supply sufficient oxygen to skeletal muscles to support the aerobic reactions of cellular respiration (Shier et al. 2018). However, when more strenuous activity is undertaken and a muscle relies on anaerobic respiration to supply its energy needs, it incurs an oxygen debt (Longenbaker 2017), which requires the body to dispose of lactic acid and replenish creatinine phosphate in order to repay the debt.

MEDICINES MANAGEMENT

Anabolic steroids

Anabolic steroids are synthetic substances related to testosterone that promote the growth of skeletal muscle (anabolism) by increasing protein within cells, particularly skeletal muscles, and which promote the development of male sexual characteristics (androgenic) — for example, the growth of the vocal cords, testicles (primary sexual characteristics) and body hair (secondary sexual characteristics). Anabolic steroids can be legally prescribed to treat conditions resulting from steroid hormone deficiency, such as delayed puberty, and, owing to their ability to stimulate muscle growth and appetite, diseases that result in loss of lean muscle mass, such as cancer and AIDS. However, some athletes, bodybuilders and others abuse these drugs in an attempt to enhance performance and/or improve their physical appearance. Doses taken by users may be 10 to 100 times higher than the doses prescribed to treat medical conditions, with the abuse of anabolic steroids potentially leading to aggression and other psychiatric problems, including extreme mood changes, paranoid jealousy, manic-like symptoms and anger ('roid rage') that may lead to violence. Furthermore, steroid abuse may lead to serious, and even irreversible, health problems, including kidney impairment or failure, damage to the liver and cardiovascular problems, including enlargement of the heart, high blood pressure and changes in blood cholesterol that can lead to an increased risk of stroke and heart attack (National Institute on Drug Abuse 2019).

FIGURE 6.5 (a–c) Sources of ATP for muscle energy

ATP
Creatine
ATP
Energy for muscle contraction
ADP
Creatine phosphate
ADP
P
Relaxed muscle
Contracting muscle

(a) ATP from creatine phosphate

Muscle glycogen
From blood
Glucose
Glycolysis
2 ATP (net gain)
2 Pyruvic acid
2 Lactic acid
Into blood

(b) ATP from anaerobic glycolysis

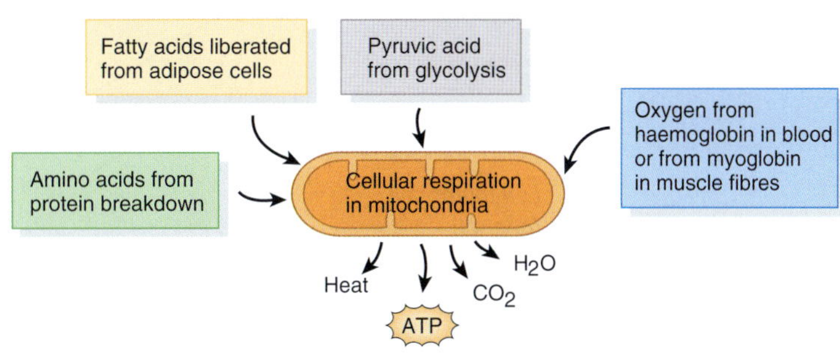

(c) ATP from aerobic cellular respiration

Source: Tortora and Derrickson (2009). Reproduced with permission of John Wiley & Sons.

Muscle fatigue

Muscle fatigue occurs when a muscle fibre can no longer contract despite continued neural stimulation and occurs as a result of the oxygen debt that occurs during prolonged muscle activity.

CLINICALLY REASONED EPISODE OF CARE

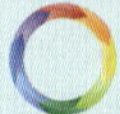

Fibromyalgia: a generalised pain disorder

Consider the patient situation

Claire is a 42-year-old mother of three and a registered nurse who stopped working three years ago due to disabling pain. 'If I told you about all of my aches and pain, you'd think I was nuts,' she told her new doctor. 'I've had so many tests for my pain, fatigue, bowel problems and numbness. Everything always comes back normal and doctors always tell me I'm just stressed, and I need to relax. I don't really want to talk about any of those other problems. I'm just here to get the medications for my migraines and for my depression.'

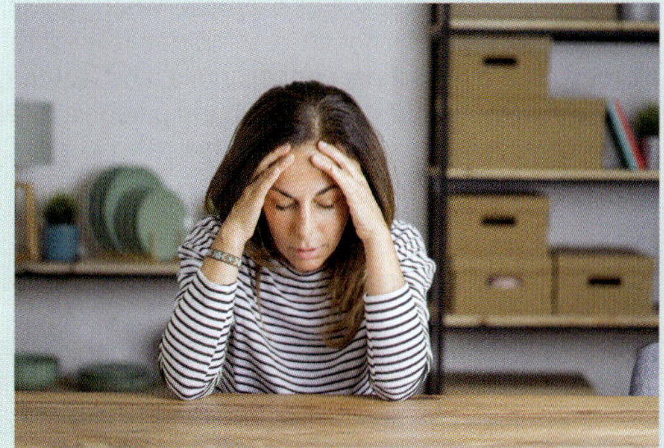

Collect cues and information

Health and lifestyle history: Given that Claire is presenting to a new doctor, a thorough health history would be appropriate. This needs to be done with respect and acceptance as Claire clearly feels that she is not being heard.

Pain assessment: A number of spots on the body have been shown to be very sensitive to pressure in fibromyalgia patients. These areas are called tender points. Healthcare providers diagnosing fibromyalgia will typically perform a tender point examination. The possible tender points tested are shown in figure 6.6. The control points are normally relatively insensitive to pressure in healthy people. With treatment, the number and pain severity of these tender points often decrease.

General physical assessment: This includes genitourinary, abdominal, reproductive, neurological and cardiovascular assessments.

FIGURE 6.6 Sites which are commonly tender for people experiencing fibromyalgia. In healthy people, the control points are normally relatively insensitive to pressure.

Low cervical
Second rib
Lateral epicondyle
Knee
Mid-forehead (control)
Left thumbnail (control)
Occiput
Trapezius
Supraspinatus
Dorsum right forearm (control)
Gluteal
Greater trochanter

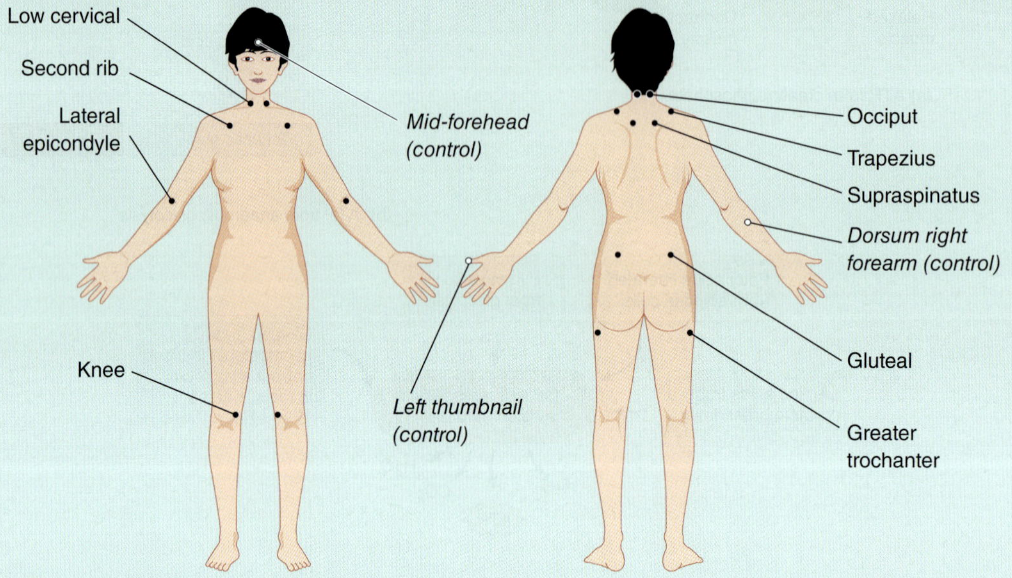

Process information

Most people with fibromyalgia experience a variety of symptoms; this often causes healthcare providers, and even patients, to wonder if there really is something wrong or if the patient is exaggerating. Patients are often told that their symptoms are make-believe, or signs of anxiety or stress.

Fibromyalgia is a chronic pain condition in which people experience aches and pain throughout much of their body as well as a number of other physical and emotional complaints, including headaches. Symptoms include widespread body pain, fatigue, morning stiffness, sleep disturbance, numbness, headaches, anxiety, depression, dry eyes, irritable bowel syndrome (constipation and diarrhoea), urinary urgency, menstrual problems and Raynaud's syndrome (a vascular disorder in which blood circulation is restricted in the fingers and toes).

Research studies now show that the increased pain experienced by people with fibromyalgia is not imaginary, but the result of a lower pain threshold and increased sensitivity to painful stimulation. Those with fibromyalgia feel non-painful sensations the same as other people, but they perceive painful sensations more acutely. For example, when touching a hot object, a person with fibromyalgia detects the heat as painfully hot at a temperature several degrees lower than people without fibromyalgia. Fibromyalgia affects 2 per cent of adults, and women are more likely to have fibromyalgia than men. Some people think of fibromyalgia as a young person's disease, but fibromyalgia affects people throughout their adult years, including elderly patients.

Nursing actions

1. Provide reassurance and engage in respectful, active listening to promote trust and treatment concordance. Reassure Claire that with time her symptoms and need for medication will decrease.
   Rationale:
   - Some people, such as Claire, decide that it is best to stop mentioning their problems. Unfortunately, not getting a definitive diagnosis usually results in a lack of effective treatment, persistent symptoms, frustration and mental health illness. To improve Claire's outcomes, trust needs to be developed.
2. Discuss and educate on proposed therapies and targeted pain management techniques; for example, stress management and distraction techniques, aerobic exercise, a nutritionally dense diet (food high in nutrients but relatively low in kilojoules) and antidepressant medication.

Rationale:

- Treatment for fibromyalgia attempts to ease symptoms and improve quality of life, but there is no known cure at present.

Evaluate outcomes

Claire reports a reduction in symptoms and increased satisfaction with life.

Source: Based on the Clinical Reasoning Cycle, Levett-Jones (2013); Arthritis Australia (2017); Musculoskeletal Australia (2020).

HOMEOSTATIC IMBALANCE

Sarcopenia

Sarcopenia is an age-related muscle disease that is characterised by reductions in muscle quality, muscle mass and muscle strength. Sarcopenia is a progressive disorder that can be defined as either primary (age-related sarcopenia) or secondary (where sarcopenia is caused by factors other than, or in addition to, ageing). Primary sarcopenia can begin from age 25 and is exacerbated by physical inactivity or immobility, poor nutrition, nutrient malabsorption and anorexia (Cruz-Jentoft et al. 2019). Sarcopenia is clinically significant as it is associated with increased risk of metabolic syndrome, increased fall risk, poorer outcomes in cancer treatment, cirrhosis of the liver, increased risk of hospitalisation/readmission, and functional impairments related to decreased strength and muscle mass (Zanker et al. 2019). Sarcopenia is largely diagnosed by assessing patient strength through the measurement of grip strength or using the chair stand test, which is the time taken to rise five times from a seated position in a chair. Additionally, muscle mass can also be measured using either dual-energy X-ray absorptiometry (DEXA) or bioelectrical impedance analysis (BIA). While sarcopenia inevitably occurs as a result of ageing, its effects can be slowed through regular exercise and appropriate nutrition.

Sarcopenia is a major contributor to health and healthcare considerations in ageing populations and is closely linked to several of Australia's national health priorities. Sarcopenia greatly increases the risk of falls and injury in the elderly and contributes to disordered skeletal muscle metabolism, which gives rise to the development of metabolic syndrome, insulin resistance, and ultimately type 2 diabetes. Additionally, the decreased mobility and quality of life experienced by sufferers has an enormous impact on mental health. Given sarcopenia's widespread clinical implications, there is a pressing need for early detection and treatment strategies to limit the burden of disease in elderly Australians.

6.4 Organisation of the skeletal muscular system

LEARNING OBJECTIVE 6.4 Name the major muscles of the body and their functions.

Every one of the body's skeletal muscles is attached at a minimum of two points to bone or other connective tissue. When one part of the skeleton is moved by muscle contraction, related parts have to be steadied by other muscles for the movement to be effective. The origin of a muscle is on the stationary bone where it begins, and the muscle ends at an insertion on the bone that moves (Logenbaker 2017).

Muscles can be named according to size, shape, location and number of origins, associated bones and the action of the muscle. Table 6.3 provides examples of the criteria used to name muscles.

TABLE 6.3 Muscle names

Character/term	Definition	Example
	Direction	
Transverse	Across	Transversus
Oblique	Diagonal	Abdominis
Rectus	Straight	External oblique Rectus abdominis

(continued)

TABLE 6.3 *(continued)*

Character/term	Definition	Example
	Shape	
Trapezius	Trapezoid	Trapezius
Deltoid	Triangular	Deltoid
Obicularis	Circular	Obicularis oculi
Rhomboid	Diamond-shaped	Rhomboideus
Platys	Flat	Platysma
	Size	
Major	Larger	Pectoralis major
Minor	Smaller	Pectoralis minor
Maximus	Largest	Gluteus maximus
Minimus	Smallest	Gluteus minimus
Longus	Longest	Adductor longus
Latissimus	Widest	Latissimus dorsi
	Number of origins	
Biceps	Two origins	Biceps brachii
Triceps	Three origins	Triceps brachii
Quadriceps	Four origins	Quadriceps femoris

The body's skeletal muscles can be divided into four areas:

- head and neck muscles
- muscles of the upper limbs (shoulder, arm, forearm)
- trunk (thorax and abdomen)
- muscles of the lower limbs (hip, pelvis/thigh, leg).

The major muscles of the body are listed according to body area in tables 6.4, 6.5, 6.6 and 6.7 and illustrated in figures 6.7, 6.8, 6.9 and 6.10.

TABLE 6.4 **Muscles of the head and neck**

Muscle	Origin	Insertion	Function
Frontalis	Skin and muscles around eye	Skin of eyebrow and bridge of nose	Wrinkles forehead Raises eyebrows
Occipitalis	Occipital bone	Galea aponeurotica (tendinous sheet)	Tenses and retracts scalp
Obicularis oculi	Maxillary and frontal bones	Skin around eye	Closes eye
Buccinator	Maxillary bone and mandible	Fibres of orbicularis oris	Compresses cheeks
Zygomaticus	Zygomatic bone	Obicularis oculi	Raises corner of mouth

Obicularis oris	Muscles near the mouth	Skin of central lip	Closes and protrudes lips
Masseter	Zygomatic arch/mandible	Lateral surface of mandible	Closes jaw
Temporalis	Temporal bone		Closes jaw
Pterygoids (medial and lateral)	Sphenoid and maxillary bones	Medial and **anterior** surface of mandible	Elevates and depresses mandible Moves mandible from side to side
Platysma	Fascia in upper chest	Lower mandible	Draws mouth downward
Stylohyoid	Temporal bone	Hyoid bone	Depresses hyoid bone and larynx
Mylohyoid	Mandible	Hyoid bone	Depresses mandible Elevates floor of mouth
Sternocleidomastoid	Margins of sternum of clavicle	Mastoid region of skull	Flexes the neck Rotates head

TABLE 6.5 **Muscles of the upper limbs (shoulder, arm and hand)**

Muscle	Origin	Insertion	Function
Levator scapulae	Transverse processes of cervical vertebrae	Scapula	Elevates scapula
Trapezius	Occipital bone and cervical and thoracic vertebrae	Clavicle, spine and scapula	Help to extend the head Adduct the scapulae when shoulders are shrugged or pulled back
Rotator cuff muscles • supraspinatus • infraspinatus • subscapularis • teres minor • teres major	**Posterior** surface above and below scapula	Humerus	A group of muscles that are responsible for angular and rotational movements of the arm
Pectoralis major	Clavicle, sternum and upper ribs	Humerus	Flexes and adducts the arm
	Muscles that move the forearm		
Biceps brachii	Between the scapula and forearm	Radius	Flexes and supinates the forearm
	Between the scapula and forearm	Ulna	Extends the elbow/forearm
Brachialis	Between humerus and ulna	Ulna	Flexes forearm
	Muscles that move the hand and fingers		
Flexor and extensor carpi	Base of second and third metacarpal bones	Base of second and third metacarpals	Flexion, extension abduction and adduction at wrist
Flexor and extensor digitorum	Posterior and distal phalanges	Base and surface of phalanges in fingers 2–5	Flexion and extension at finger joints and wrist
Palmaris longus	Distal end of humerus	Fascia of palm	Flexes the wrist

TABLE 6.6 Muscles of the trunk (thorax and abdomen)

Muscle	Origin	Insertion	Function
Internal intercostals	Superior border of each rib	Inferior border of preceding rib	Depress the rib cage and contract during forced expiration
External intercostals	Inferior border of each rib	Superior border of next rib	Elevate the ribs during inspiration
Diaphragm	Ribs 4–10, lumbar vertebrae	Tendon near to centre of diaphragm	Contracts to allow inhalation Relaxes to allow exhalation
Internal and external obliques	Between the lower ribs and pelvic girdle	Lower ribs, iliac crest and crest of pubis	Compress the abdominal cavity and protect and support the abdominal organs Rotation of the trunk
Transversus abdominis	Lower ribs, iliac crest and inguinal ligament	Extend horizontally across the abdomen from sternum to crest of pubis	Compress the abdominal cavity, protect and support the abdominal organs Rotation of the trunk
Rectus abdominis	Crest of pubic bone and symphysis pubis	Sternum and ribs	Compress the abdominal cavity, protect and support the abdominal organs Assists with flexing and rotating the lumbar spine

TABLE 6.7 Muscles of the lower limbs (hip, pelvis/thigh and leg)

Muscle	Origin	Insertion	Function
Psoas major	Lumbar vertebrae	Femur	Flexes thigh
Gluteus maximus	Sacrum, coccyx and surface of Ilium	Femur and fascia of thigh	Extends thigh at hip
Gluteus medius and minimus	Surface of Ilium	Femur	Abducts and rotates thigh
Adductor group	Pubic bone and ischial tuberosity	Posterior surface of femur	Adducts, flexes, extends and rotates thigh
Quadriceps femoris group • rectus femoris • vastus lateralis • vastus medialis • vastus intermedius • sartorius	Ilium, acetabulum and femur Ilium	Patella Tibia	Extends leg at knee Flexes, abducts and rotates thing to allow crossing of legs
Hamstring group • biceps femoris • semitendinosus • semimembranosus	Femur, ischial tuberosity, iliac spine	Tibia and head of fibula	Flexes and rotates leg, abducts, rotates and extends thigh
Posterior compartment • gastrocnemius • soleus • tibialis posterior	Femur Fibula and tibia Tibia and fibula	Calcaneus (by means of the Achilles tendon) Second, third and fourth metatarsals	Flexes foot and leg at knee joint Flexes foot Flexes and inverts foot
Anterior compartment • tibialis anterior • extensor digitorum longus	Tibia Tibia and fibula	First metatarsal Middle and distal phalanges of each toe	Dorsiflexes and inverts foot Dorsiflexes and everts foot, extends toes
Lateral compartment • fibularis longus	Fibula and tibia	First metatarsal	Flexes and everts foot

FIGURE 6.7 (a, b) Head and neck muscles

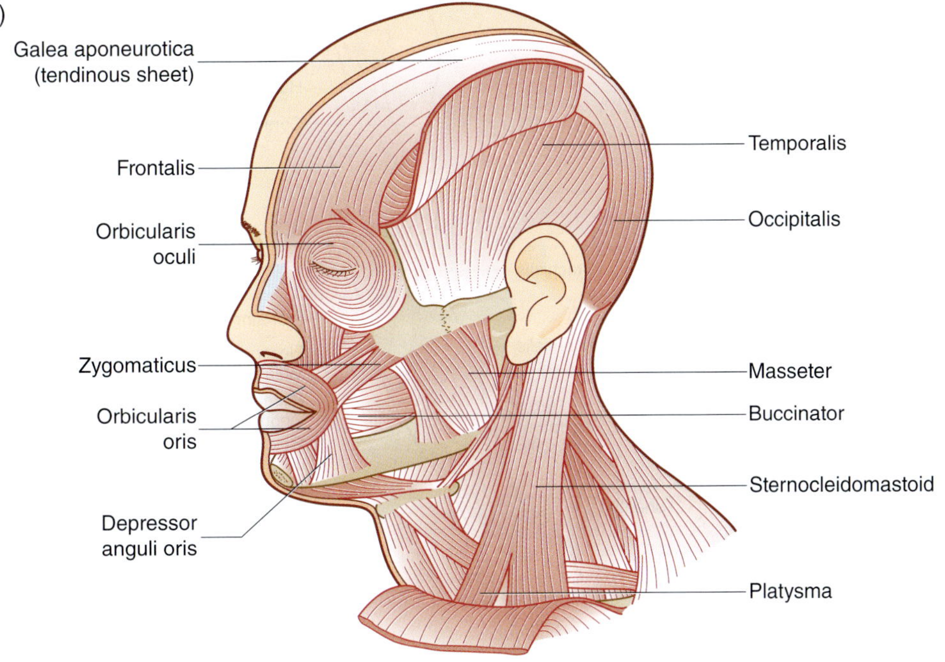

An anterior and lateral view

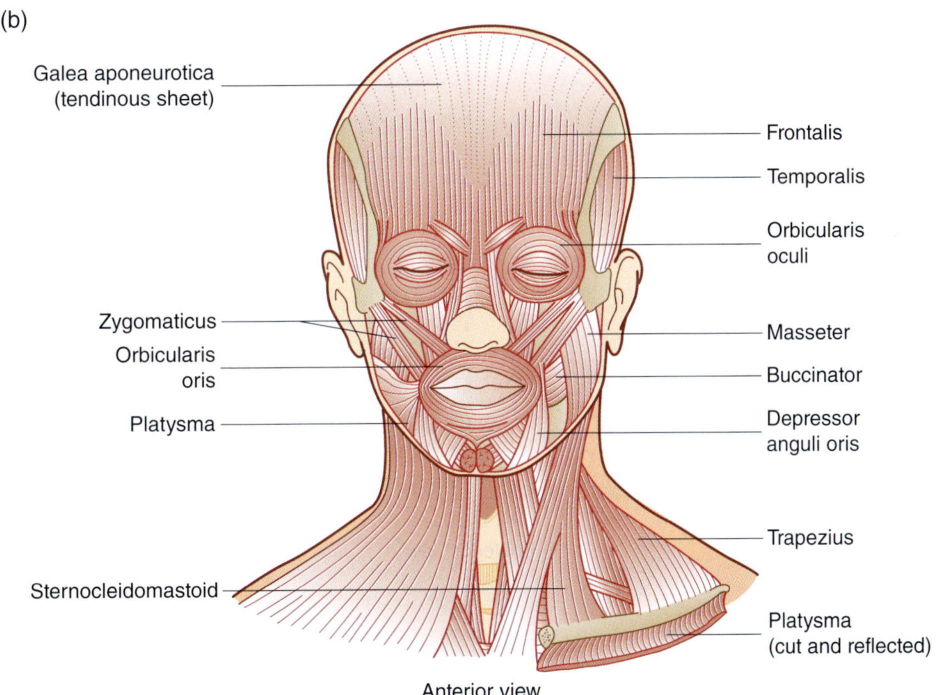

Anterior view

Source: Tortora and Derrickson (2009). Reproduced with permission of John Wiley & Sons.

FIGURE 6.8 (a–g) Muscles of the upper limbs (shoulder, arm and hand)

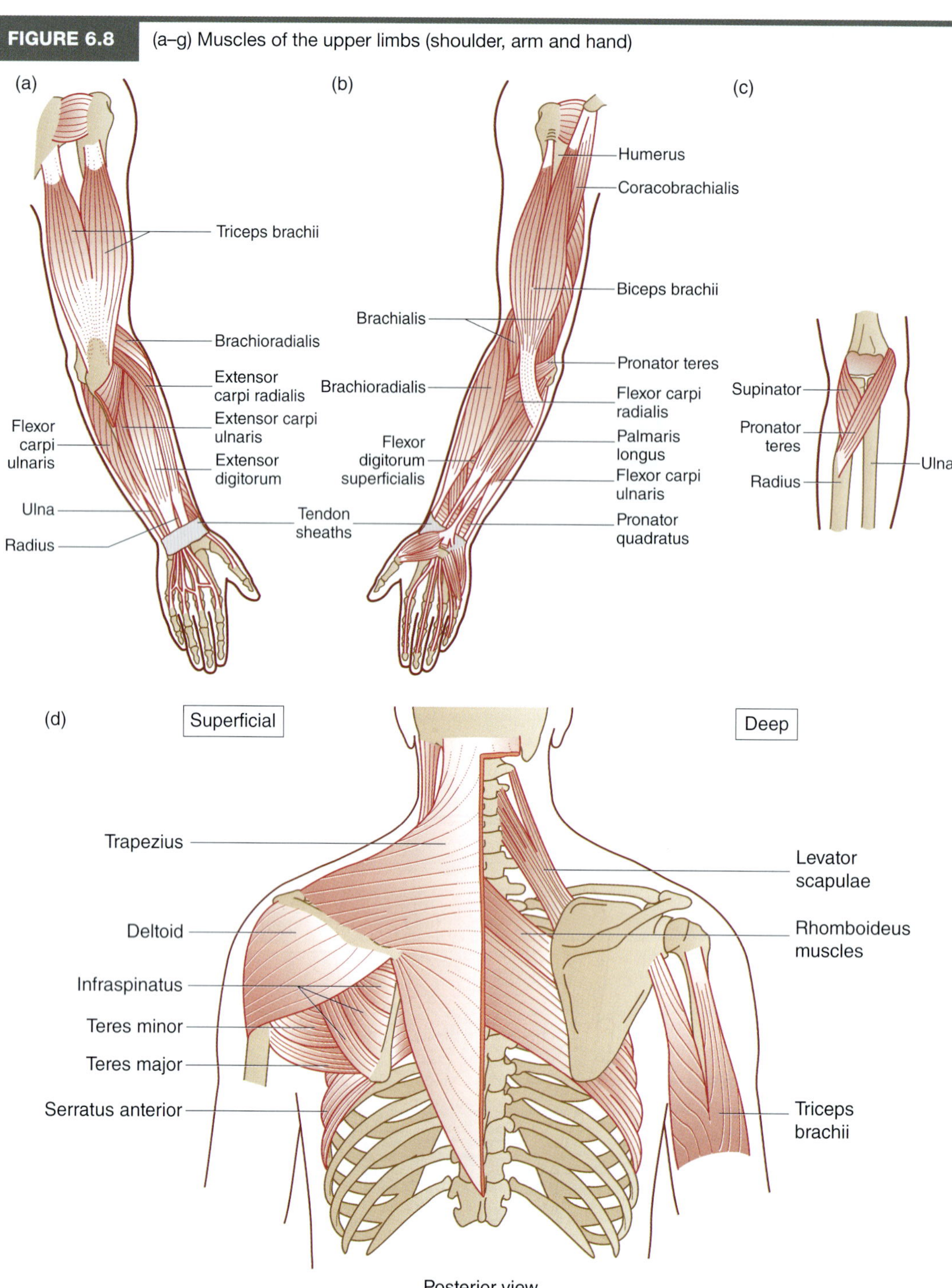

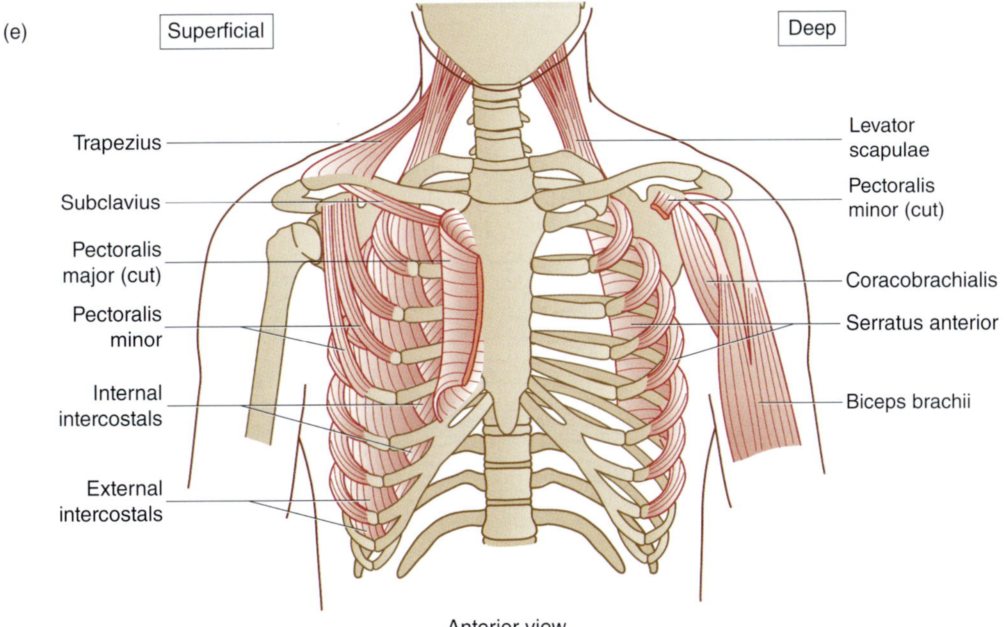
(e)
Superficial
Deep
Trapezius
Subclavius
Pectoralis major (cut)
Pectoralis minor
Internal intercostals
External intercostals
Levator scapulae
Pectoralis minor (cut)
Coracobrachialis
Serratus anterior
Biceps brachii
Anterior view

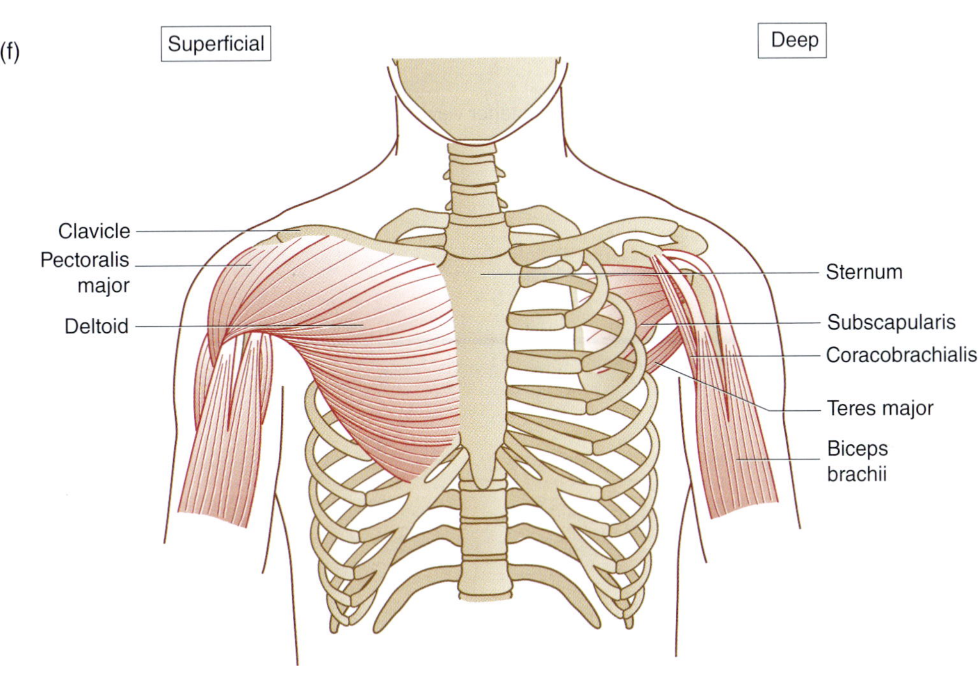
(f)
Superficial
Deep
Clavicle
Pectoralis major
Deltoid
Sternum
Subscapularis
Coracobrachialis
Teres major
Biceps brachii
Anterior view

FIGURE 6.8 *(continued)*

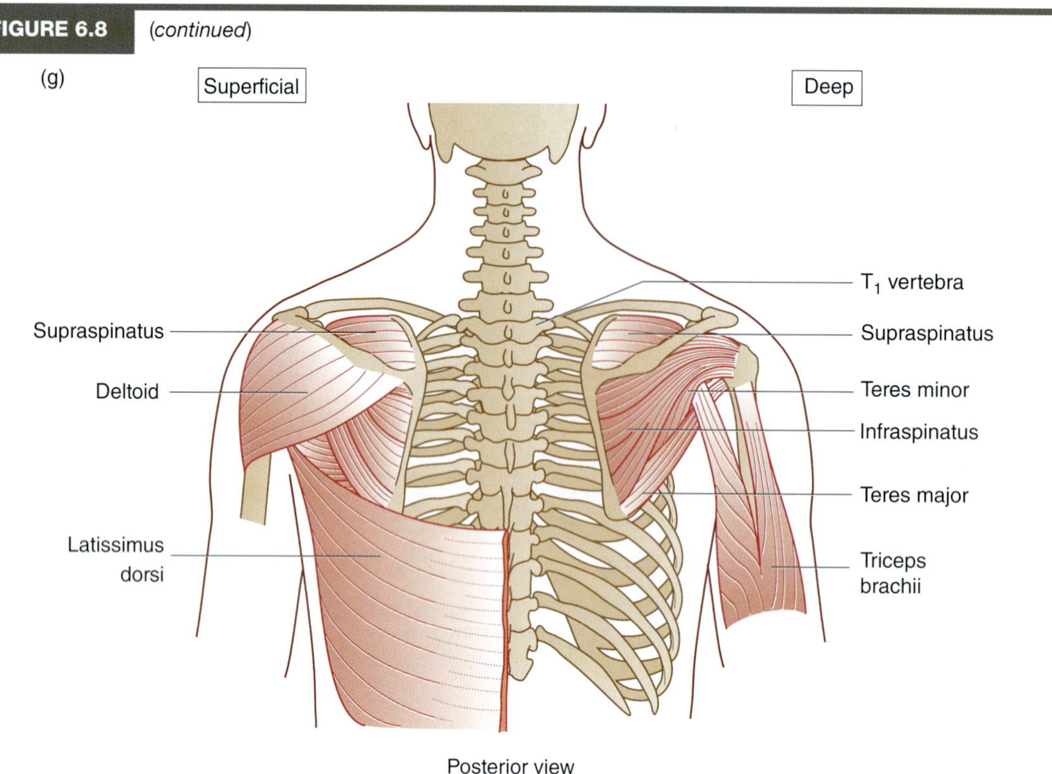

FIGURE 6.9 Trunk (thorax and abdomen)

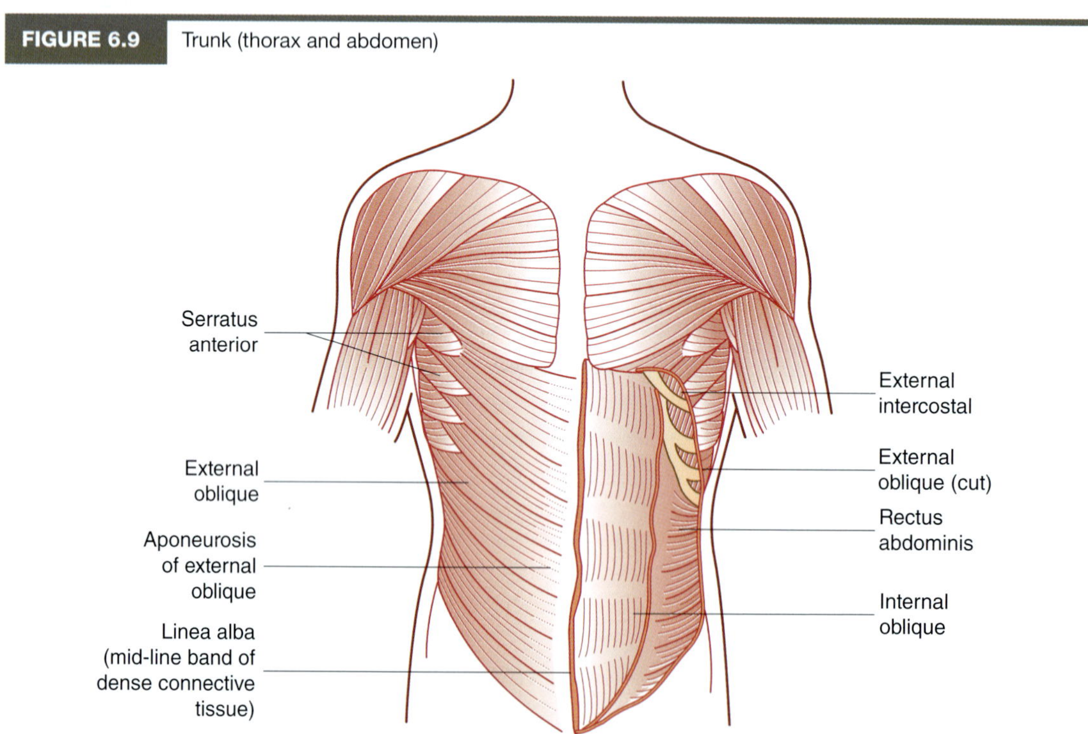

FIGURE 6.10 (a–f) Muscles of the lower limbs (hip, pelvis/thigh and leg)

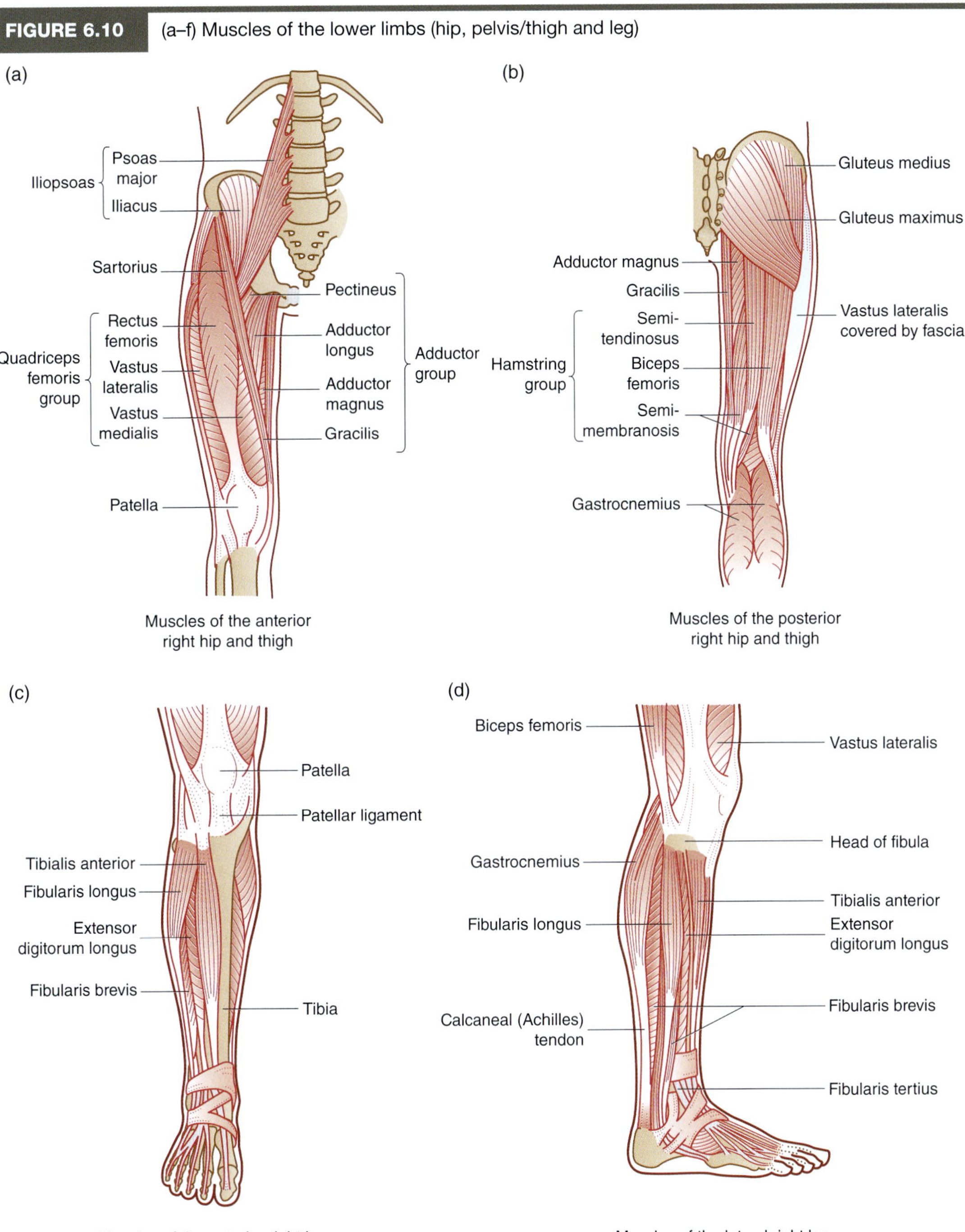

FIGURE 6.10 *(continued)*

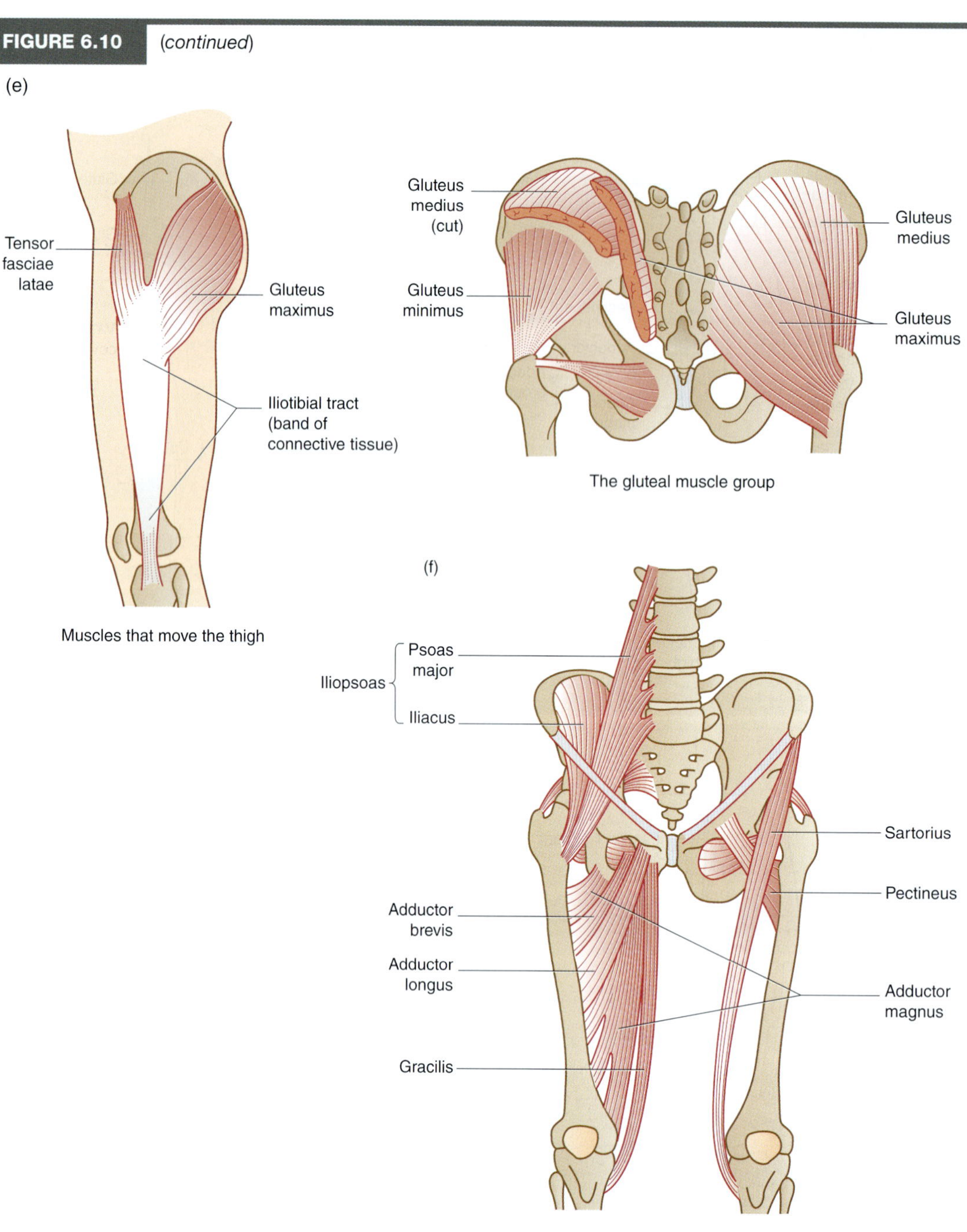

Muscles that move the thigh

The gluteal muscle group

The iliopsoas muscle and the adductor group

Figures 6.11 and 6.12 provide an overview of the major muscles of the body.

FIGURE 6.11 Anterior view of the major muscles of the body

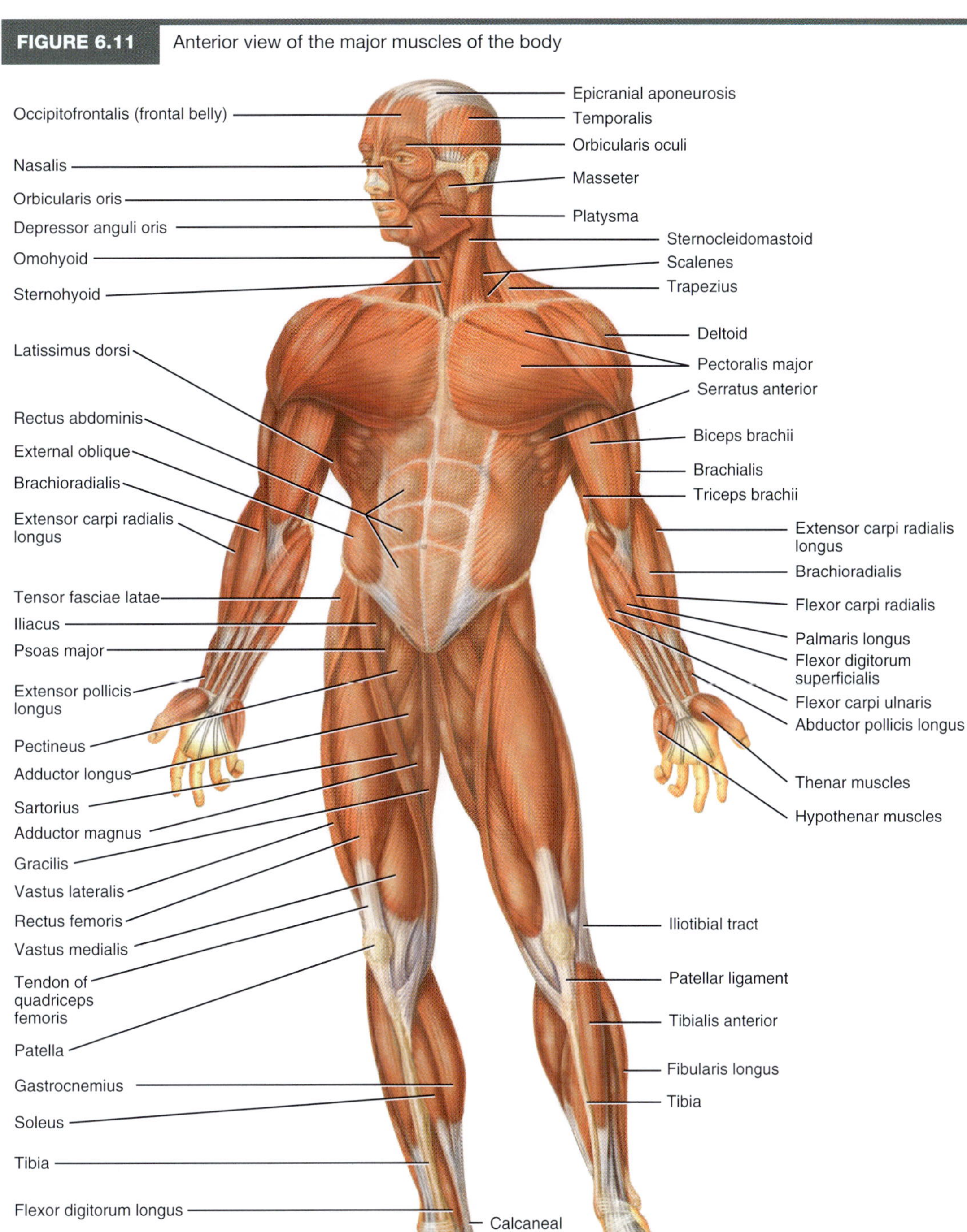

Source: Tortora and Derrickson (2009). Reproduced with permission of John Wiley & Sons.

FIGURE 6.12 Posterior view of the major muscles of the body

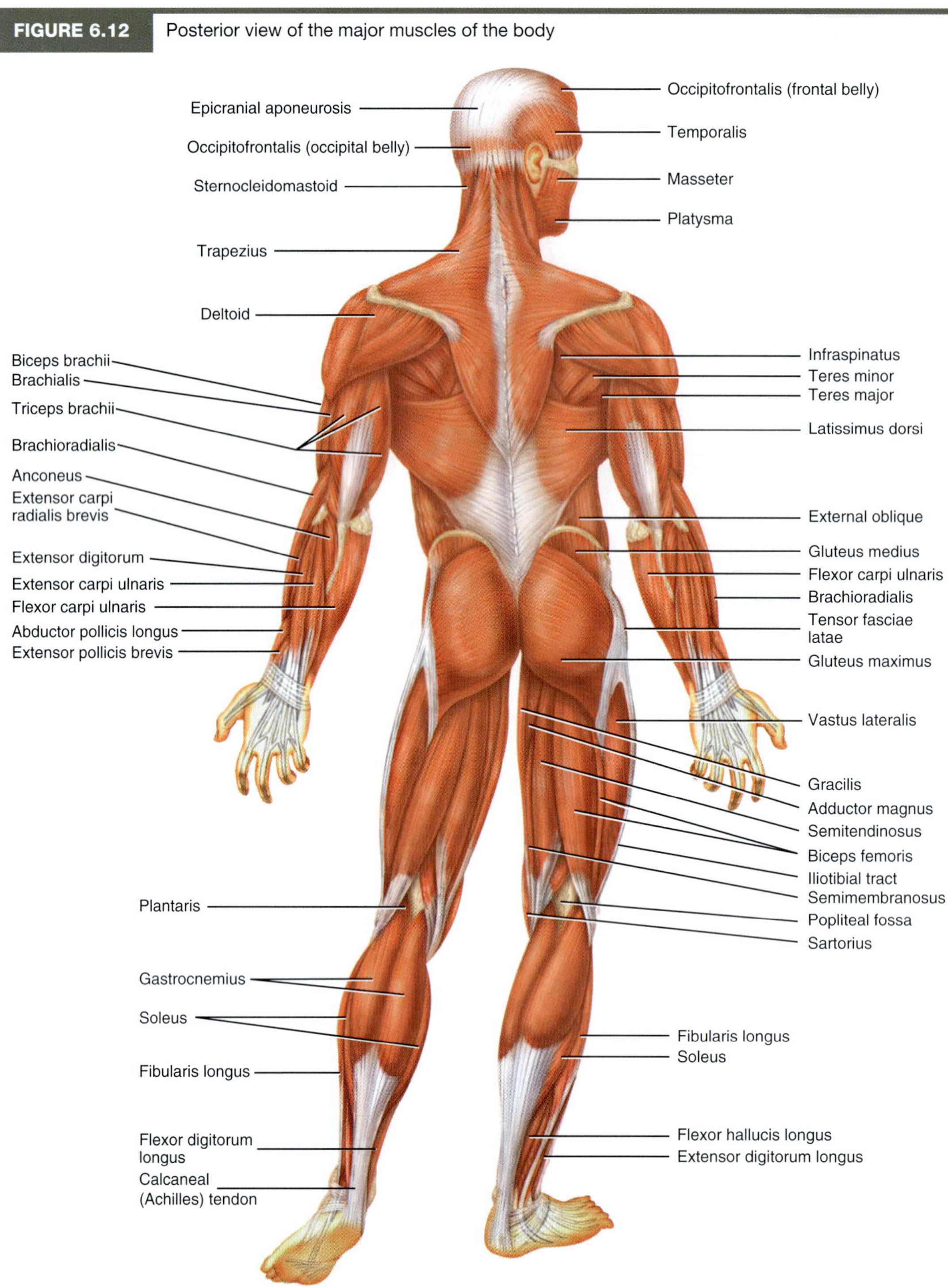

Source: Tortora and Derrickson (2009). Reproduced with permission of John Wiley & Sons.

Skeletal muscle movement

Skeletal muscle movement occurs as a result of more than one muscle moving, as muscles invariably move in groups. As a general rule, when a muscle contracts at a joint, one bone remains fairly stationary and the other one moves. The origin of a muscle is on the stationary bone and the insertion of a muscle is on the bone that moves. The action of each muscle is dependent upon how the muscle is attached to either side of a joint and also the kind of joint it is associated with. When a muscle contracts it produces a specific action. However, muscles can only pull; they cannot push, as when a muscle contracts it becomes shorter. Usually, there are at least two opposing muscles (agonist and **antagonist**) acting on a joint that bring about movement in opposite directions. An agonist or prime mover is a muscle primarily responsible for producing an action, while an antagonist of a prime mover causes muscle movement in the opposite direction; for example, an agonist may cause an arm to bend, while the antagonist will cause it to straighten.

Common types of body movements include:

- extension — a movement that increases the angle or distance between two bones or parts of the body
- hyperextension — an extension angle greater than 180°
- flexion — the opposite of extension, in that it is a movement that decreases the angle or distance between two bones and brings the bones closer together and is a common movement of hinge joints (e.g. bending the elbow or knee)
- abduction — moving a limb away from the midline of the body
- adduction — (the opposite of abduction) the movement of a limb towards the midline of the body
- rotation — a movement common to ball-and-socket joints and is the movement of a bone around its longitudinal axis
- circumduction — a combination of abduction, adduction, extension and flexion.

Table 6.8 provides a summary of the different actions of muscle movement.

TABLE 6.8 Types of muscle movement

Action	Definition
Extension	Increases the angle or distance between two bones or parts of the body
Flexion	Decreases the angle of a joint
Abduction	Moves away from the midline
Adduction	Moves closer to the midline
Circumduction	A combination of flexion, extension, abduction and adduction
Supination	Turns the palm up
Pronation	Turns the palm down
Plantar flexion	Lowers the foot (point the toes)
Dorsiflexion	Elevates the foot
Rotation	Moves a bone around its longitudinal axis

CLINICALLY REASONED EPISODE OF CARE

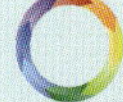

Sprained ankle

Consider the patient situation

Emily is an 8-year-old girl who has presented to the emergency department complaining of pain to her ankle.

Collect cues and information

Emily's mother reports to the triage nurse that Emily was at gymnastics and landed awkwardly on her ankle. Upon examination, Emily's ankle is swollen and bruised and she is reluctant to weight bear because it is painful. After seeing the medical officer and undergoing examination, Emily is diagnosed with a sprained ankle.

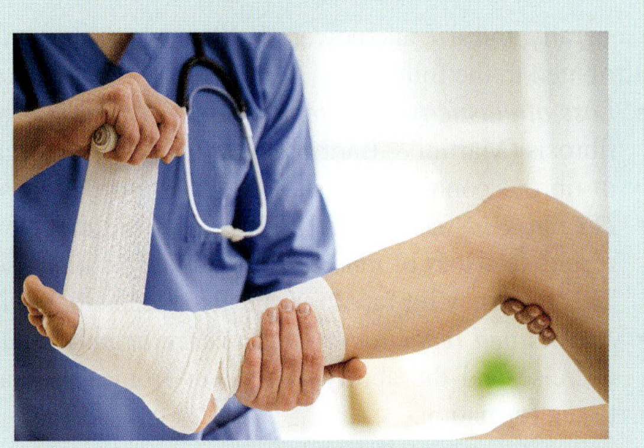

Process information

Ankle sprains are common in children, and result from a sudden movement, roll or twist at the ankle. The ligaments surrounding the ankle joint are overstretched beyond their normal movement. Most sprained ankles will involve the ligament on the outer side of the ankle.

Symptoms of a sprained ankle include pain when weight bearing, swelling, bruising and restricted range of movement. Risk factors for a sprained ankle include sports of high activity (such as jumping), uneven surfaces, prior injuries and improper shoes. If not treated appropriately, a sprained ankle can result in chronic pain and ongoing tendon issues.

Given the clinical context and mechanism of injury, Emily is likely to be experiencing a sprained ankle and her subsequent diagnosis supports this.

Establish goals

1. Pain management
2. RICE
3. Education for Emily and her parents

Nursing actions

1. Administer pain relief.
   Rationale:
   - A sprained ankle can be very painful, therefore the comfort of the individual should be a priority.
   - Appropriate pain management is required to assess , bandage and manage the ankle in the emergency department.
2. Treat following the RICE management method.
   Rationale:
   - Management of a sprained ankle includes the following:
     - **R**est the limb
     - **I**ce the affected area to reduce inflammation
     - **C**ompression bandage to immobilise the limb and to reduce inflammation
     - **E**levate the limb above the heart to reduce blood flow, which reduces inflammation and pain.
3. Educate Emily and her family on the ongoing management of sprains.
   Rationale:
   - Emily and her family will need to continue to RICE the limb to reduce pain and inflammation.
   - Education involves discussion on the use of pain relief/non-steroidal anti-inflammatories, the application of an icepack to the ankle every 2–4 hours, keeping limbs elevated when lying down, and exercises to stretch the ankle and minimise stiffness.

Evaluate outcomes

Due to the nursing actions above, Emily makes a recovery from her ankle injury after two weeks and can return to gymnastics at her full capacity.

Reflect on new processes and learning

Consider the patient situation and the role of the emergency department nurse. How can the nurse ensure the streamlining of services through the department in cases such as Emily's? Consider nurse-initiated pain relief and RICE management.

Source: Based on the Clinical Reasoning Cycle, Levett-Jones (2013).

The effects of ageing

Generally, the size and power of all muscle tissues within the body decrease as the body ages. This can be attributed to the following.

- *Loss of elasticity to skeletal muscle.* As muscles age they lose their elasticity due to a process called fibrosis (Martini & Bartholomew 2017). Fibrosis causes ageing muscles to develop increasing amounts of fibrous connective tissue, which results in a loss of flexibility, movement and circulation.
- *Decrease in size of muscle fibres.* As the muscle ages, the number of myofibrils decreases and this results in a loss of muscle strength and an increased tendency for the muscle to fatigue more quickly. This tendency for rapid fatigue also means that, with age, there is a lower tolerance for exercise.
- *Age-related reduction in cardiovascular performance.* Blood flow to muscles does not increase with exercise and the ability to recover from muscular injuries decreases and is likely to result in scar tissue formation.

SUMMARY

Muscular tissue is either smooth, cardiac or skeletal and is a specialised tissue that is structured to contract. In so doing, it causes movement of bones at a joint or in soft tissues. Through its ability to sustain partial contraction of muscle, the muscular system also plays an important role in maintaining body posture for a long period of time. Skeletal muscle also plays an important role in heat production and is able to adjust heat production in extremes of environmental temperatures.

KEY TERMS

acetylcholine (ACh) Neurotransmitter responsible for the transmission of a nerve impulse across a synaptic cleft.
acetylcholinesterase (AChE) Enzyme that breaks down acetylcholine.
actin One of the two major proteins of muscle that make up the myofibrils of muscle cells.
adenosine triphosphate (ATP) Molecule used by cells when energy is needed.
aerobic With oxygen.
anaerobic Without oxygen.
antagonist Muscle that acts in opposition to a prime mover.
anterior Pertaining to the front.
aponeuroses Membranous sheet connecting a muscle and the part it moves.
glycogen A polysaccharide that stores energy for muscle contraction.
ligament Strong connective tissue that connects bone.
myasthenia gravis Muscle weakness due to an inability to respond to the neurotransmitter ACh.
myofibrils A bundle of myofilaments that contracts.
myoglobin A red pigment that stores oxygen for muscle contraction.
posterior Pertaining to the back.
sarcolemma Plasma membrane of a muscle fibre that forms T tubules.
sarcoplasm Cytoplasm of a muscle fibre that contains organelles, including myofibrils.
tendons Tissue that connects muscle to bone.
T tubules Extensions of the sarcolemma that extend into the muscle fibre.

FIND OUT MORE

1. Name and describe the three forms of human muscle tissue and list where they are found in the body.
2. Outline how ATP is supplied to muscles.
3. Describe the processes that enable a muscle to contract.
4. Explain how ageing affects skeletal muscle.
5. Describe a neuromuscular junction.
6. Why does skeletal muscle appear striated when looked at under the microscope?
7. What role does calcium play in the muscle?
8. What do anabolic and catabolic mean?
9. What does myalgia mean?
10. What is the other name for the collarbone?

CONDITIONS

The following is a list of conditions that are associated with the muscular system. Take some time and write notes about each of the conditions. You may make the notes taken from textbooks or other resources (e.g. people you work with in a clinical area), or you may make the notes as a result of people you have cared for. If you are making notes about people you have cared for, you must ensure that you adhere to the rules of confidentiality.

Muscular dystrophy

Myasthenia gravis

Fibromyalgia

Tetanus

Rigor mortis

Muscle cramps

Poliomyelitis

Rhabdomyolysis

Sarcoma

Fibrosis

Botulism

REFERENCES

Arthritis Australia (2017) Fibromyalgia. https://arthritisaustralia.com.au/types-of-arthritis/fibromyalgia (accessed February 2021).

Cruz-Jentoft, A.J., Bahat, G., Bauer, J., Boirie, Y., Bruyère, O., Cederholm, T., Cooper, C., Landi, F., Rolland, Y., Sayer, A.A., Schneider, S.M., Sieber, C.C., Topinkova, E., Vandewoude, M., Visser, M., Zamboni, M.; Writing Group for the European Working Group on Sarcopenia in Older People 2 (EWGSOP2), and the Extended Group for EWGSOP2. (2019) Sarcopenia: revised European consensus on definition and diagnosis. *Age Ageing* 48(1): 16–31.

Giuriato, G., Pedrinolla, A., Schena, F. and Venturelli, M. (2018) Muscle cramps: a comparison of the two-leading hypothesis. *Journal of Electromyography and Kinesiology* 41: 89–95.

Harris, C. and Hobson, M. (2015) The management of soft tissue injuries and compartment syndrome. *Orthopaedics II: Spine and Pelvis* 33(6): 251–256.

Joint Formulary Committee (2018) *BNF 75*. London: Pharmaceutical Press.

Levett-Jones, T. (2013) *Clinical Reasoning: Learning to Think Like a Nurse*. Frenchs Forest, NSW: Pearson Australia.

Logenbaker, S.N. (2017) *Mader's Understanding Human Anatomy and Physiology*, 9th edn. London: McGraw-Hill.

Martini, F.H. and Bartholomew, E.F. (2017) *Essentials of Anatomy and Physiology*, 7th edn. Upper Saddle River, NJ: Pearson Education.

Musculosketal Australia (2020) Fibromyalgia. www.msk.org.au/fibromyalgia (accessed February 2021).

National Institute on Drug Abuse (2019) Drug facts: anabolic steroids. www.drugabuse.gov/publications/drugfacts/anabolic-steroids (accessed May 2019).
Public Health England (2019) Botulism. www.gov.uk/government/publications/botulism-clinical-and-public-health-management (accessed May 2019).
Shier, D., Butler, J. and Lewis, R. (2018) *Hole's Human Anatomy and Physiology*, 15th edn. Maidenhead: McGraw-Hill.
Tortora, G.J. and Derrickson, B.H. (2009) *Principles of Anatomy and Physiology*, 12th edn. Hoboken, NJ: John Wiley & Sons, Inc.
Tortora, G.J. and Derrickson B.H. (2017) *Principles of Anatomy and Physiology*, 15th edn. Hoboken, NJ: John Wiley& Sons, Inc.
Zanker, J., Scott, D., Reijnierse, E.M., Brennan-Olsen, S.L., Daly, R.M., Girgis, C.M., Grossmann, M., Hayes, A., Henwood, T., Hirani, V., Inderjeeth, C.A., Iuliano, S., Keogh, J.W.L., Lewis, J.R., Maier, A.B., Pasco, J.A., Phu, S., Sanders, K.M., Sim, M., Visvanathan, R., Waters, D.L., Yu, S.C.Y. and Duque, G. (2019) Establishing an operational definition of sarcopenia in Australia and New Zealand: Delphi method based consensus statement. *The Journal of Nutrition, Health and Aging*. 23(1): 105–110.

FURTHER READING

BRAIN FOUNDATION AUSTRALIA

https://brainfoundation.org.au/about-us

The Brain Foundation is a nationally registered charity dedicated to funding world-class research Australia-wide into neurological disorders, brain disease and brain injuries.

TALK TO FRANK

www.talktofrank.com

Provides friendly confidential information about drugs.

ACKNOWLEDGEMENTS

Photo: © Dmitry Kalinovsky / Shutterstock.com
Photo: © Blazej Lyjak / Shutterstock.com
Photo: © Photodisc / Gett Images
Photo: © Antonio V. Oquias / Shutterstock.com
Photo: © Roman Zaiets / Shutterstock.com
Photo: © Shift Drive / Shutterstock.com
Photo: © VGstockstudio / Shutterstock.com

CHAPTER 7

The skeletal system

TEST YOUR PRIOR KNOWLEDGE

- What are the main functions of the skeletal system?
- Which minerals are particularly important with respect to bone?
- What functions does bone perform?
- What makes bones strong?
- What makes bones flexible?

LEARNING OUTCOMES

After reading this chapter you will be able to:

7.1 describe all the functions of the skeletal system

7.2 discuss the composition and function of bone as a tissue, and outline the factors that impact bone density and explain how they do this

7.3 describe the other connective tissues associated with the skeleton and their roles

7.4 list the various types of bone and joints.

Body map

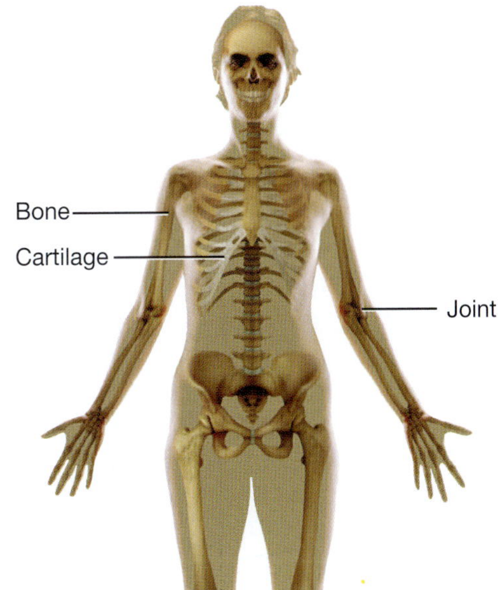

Introduction

Viewing a skeleton in the laboratory often creates the impression that bone is a solid, dry, inert material. In fact, in a living organism, bone is a very metabolically active tissue that has a large blood supply and is remodelled constantly. Bones are always in the process of adjusting and readjusting themselves to be able to respond optimally to the stresses placed on them, and the **remodelling** also plays an important role in calcium homeostasis.

The skeleton provides us with shape, protection for delicate organs, and a system of levers, which, along with muscles, give us the power of movement. This system of levers against which muscles can exert forces, includes joints, which maximise the range of movements we can make. When considering the skeleton as a whole, therefore, it is useful to consider not only the bone, but also the other connective tissues that hold the bone together, form joints and connect muscle to bone to enable movement. These tissues are the **cartilage**, **ligaments** and tendons that are found closely associated with bone, and which will also be included in this chapter.

7.1 The functions of the skeletal system

LEARNING OBJECTIVE 7.1 Describe all the functions of the skeletal system.

Bone is an engineering wonder; it is a living tissue and yet it has the tensile strength of steel and the compressive strength of concrete while being light enough to allow us to move around with ease.

While bones are strong enough to protect underlying tissue and support our body weight, they are not solid — only the outer edges of bones consist of dense, solid bone, known as compact bone; the interior of the bone contains lighter bone that forms a meshwork rather than a solid mass; this is known as spongy or trabecular bone. Spongy bone, while not as strong as compact bone, is much lighter, due to the many spaces in the bone, avoiding an excessively heavy skeleton. However spongy bone still adds interior strength to a bone; the columns of spongy bone act as 'struts', which stabilise and strengthen the bone structure internally. In the centre of the bones there is a cavity, known as the medullary cavity, which houses the blood vessels supplying the bone, and the bone **marrow**, responsible for blood cell production. Surrounding the outside of most bones is a fibrous membrane called the **periosteum** (figure 7.1).

FIGURE 7.1 Compact and spongy bone, and their blood supply

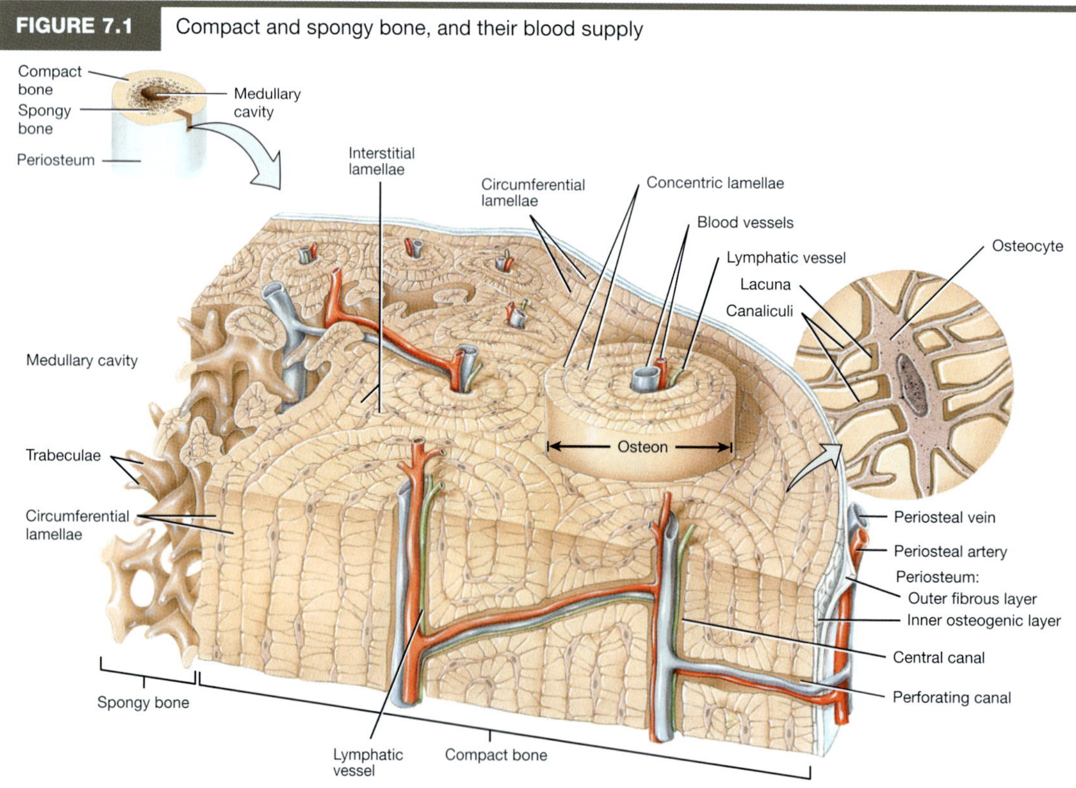

Source: Tortora and Derrickson (2009). Reproduced with permission of John Wiley & Sons.

In addition to these functions, bone represents a huge storage depot for minerals such as calcium and phosphate and is involved in the homeostatic regulation of these minerals in the blood. Therefore, bones perform the following physiological roles.

- *Support and protection.* Bones are vital for providing support and form for soft tissues of the body. Since bone is an incompressible tissue, the skeleton provides the overall body shape, with soft tissues attached to the bones and around the bones. Without this support and form, we'd be a mass of soft tissue!

  Bone also provides excellent protection for delicate organs; the skull completely encases the delicate brain, the sternum and ribs protect the lungs and heart, and the vertebrae protect the spinal cord. In the lower body, the pelvis protects the abdominal and reproductive organs. Since bone must also enable movement, some compromises have to be made in the bony protection that encases our organs. So, the organs of the chest are protected by a 'cage' formed by ribs, which allows the chest cavity to expand and contract during breathing and allows for a range of movement around the chest. Similarly, the vertebral column, rather than being a rigid bony tube, consists of 26 vertebrae with movable joints between, which allow bending and stretching while still protecting the spinal cord.
- *Enabling efficient movement.* The bones enable purposeful movement, either of the whole body, or just parts of it. Bones of the limbs act as rigid levers which the muscles pull on to move. Without bone to anchor them, the movements produced by muscle would not be able to move the body very far. Other bones form the basis of supportive platforms which, when pulled on by the muscles, maintain body position and posture. Our tendency to walk on two legs instead of four creates a great deal of additional stress for the bones and muscles of the back that keep us in that upright position. The movements that are possible, from tiny, precise finger movements, to whole body movements, are enabled by the moving **articulations** between bones, known as joints, and the pulling action of the skeletal muscles on the bones that form the joints (in tandem with the relaxation of opposing muscles to enable this movement; see the chapter on the muscular system).
- *Haemopoiesis.* Bones also produce our blood cells — a process known as **haemopoiesis**. Haemopoiesis occurs only in red bone marrow (also known as myeloid tissue), which in adults fills the internal cavity of the vertebrae, pelvis, ribs, skull and the ends of the long bones. These bones are therefore the source of our red and white blood cells during adult life.

  Red bone marrow contains multipotent stem cells. These are cells that are not yet committed to being a particular type of cell, and can still develop to become any of the blood cells. These stem cells give rise to the various white blood cells which are vital for our immune response, and the red blood cells, which are vital for carrying oxygen through the blood to all our tissues. The blood cells need to be regularly re-supplied, as they only last for a limited time in circulation (around 90 days in the case of red blood cells). Failure of the bone marrow to produce enough blood cells can result in immune deficiency and increased risk of infections if white cells are deficient, or severe anaemia if red cells are deficient. An illustration of the production of blood cells from the red bone marrow stem cells is shown in figure 17.1 in the chapter on the immune system. Not all bones in the adult contain red marrow — some bones, such as the shafts of long bones, are filled with yellow marrow, which is mainly fat.
- *Calcium homeostasis.* Bone is a huge store of the minerals calcium and phosphate, and has the ability to release stored minerals in response to the body's demands. For example, when the level of calcium in the blood decreases, the bones can release calcium into the bloodstream. This release is part of the homeostatic control of plasma calcium levels, which is necessary because calcium ions are so physiologically active, being essential for processes such as nervous communication, muscle contraction and blood clotting; parathyroid hormone is the main controller of this system.

A healthy skeleton is therefore vital for many aspects of our normal function.

CLINICAL CONSIDERATIONS

Gout

Gout is an acute and very painful arthritic condition caused by a problem with uric acid metabolism, resulting in small crystals of uric acid forming in the joints and causing inflammation and pain, which can be severe. Single joints may be affected (often the metatarsophalangeal joint of the big toe), or multiple joints. The big toe is affected more often because uric acid will crystallise more readily at lower temperatures, and the joints of the toe are more likely to get cold.

The condition is related to the metabolism of compounds known as purines, which are part of the molecules that carry the genetic code, DNA and RNA. Found naturally in the body and in many of the foods you eat, uric acid is produced when purines are metabolised, so an abnormally high level of purine metabolism or an inadequate excretion of uric acid by the kidney can cause gout. In most sufferers, the problem is an inability to excrete adequate amounts of uric acid in the urine.

Overproduction of uric acid occurs in disorders that result in a high cell turnover, as purines are released from the dead cells. Cell death caused by chemotherapy can raise uric acid levels, as can excessive exercise and obesity.

An excessive intake of purines due to a diet rich in high-purine foods such as anchovies, sardines, sweetbreads, kidney, liver, meat extracts and alcohol is also associated with an increased risk of gout.

For further information see Arthritis Australia, https://arthritisaustralia.com.au/types-of-arthritis/gout.

7.2 Bone as a tissue

LEARNING OBJECTIVE 7.2 Discuss the composition and function of bone as a tissue, and outline the factors that impact bone density and explain how they do this.

Bone is a connective tissue, and, in common with all connective tissues, consists of specialised cells embedded in an extracellular matrix. The specialised cells in bone are of three types: **osteoblasts**, **osteoclasts** and **osteocytes**, each performing their own specific roles. The extracellular matrix of bone consists of an organic framework made of the protein **collagen**, onto which an inorganic 'cement' of calcium salts is laid in successive layers. The result is a material that is hard, rigid and strong (due to the calcium salts), but also flexible (due to the collagen). These properties result in a bone which has very good tensile strength (this can be tested by trying to snap a long bone along its length), good compressive strength (this can be tested by trying to compress a bone by placing weight on top of it) and good flexibility (this can be tested by observing how much a bone will bend before it snaps). Healthy bone will contain collagen and calcium salts in the correct proportions and will display all these characteristics. Diseases which affect the production of normal collagen in the bone will result in bones which lack the normal flexibility and therefore break more easily when large forces are placed on them. An example of this is the inherited disorder brittle bone disease (osteogenesis imperfecta). Conversely, a lack of calcium salts in the bone will result in bones that are softer than normal and will bend when large forces are placed on them (see the homeostatic imbalance box on rickets). Perhaps the most common disorder, though, is one where the balance of collagen to calcium salts is normal, but the density of bone is low; the bones are not as compact and dense as they should be — a disorder known as osteoporosis. It is important to understand that in osteoporosis the bone composition is normal (unlike diseases such as brittle bone disease or rickets), but there is not enough bone present to resist all the stresses placed on the skeleton, and so **fractures** become more of a risk.

HOMEOSTATIC IMBALANCE

Rickets

The childhood disease rickets is an example of a condition caused by a homeostatic imbalance in the body. Also known as osteomalacia, this disease occurs as a result of inadequate active vitamin D, with symptoms including stunted growth, bowed legs and bone pain. Because of the key role that activated vitamin D plays in the absorption of dietary calcium (helping it to travel across the small intestine into circulation), vitamin D deficiency can lead to subsequent disturbances in calcium homeostasis (in particular, low calcium levels in the blood, which is termed hypocalcaemia). To restore these levels, and thus allow calcium to carry out its plethora of essential physiological roles, the breakdown of bone is increased to release stored calcium into the bloodstream, resulting in the aforementioned symptoms.

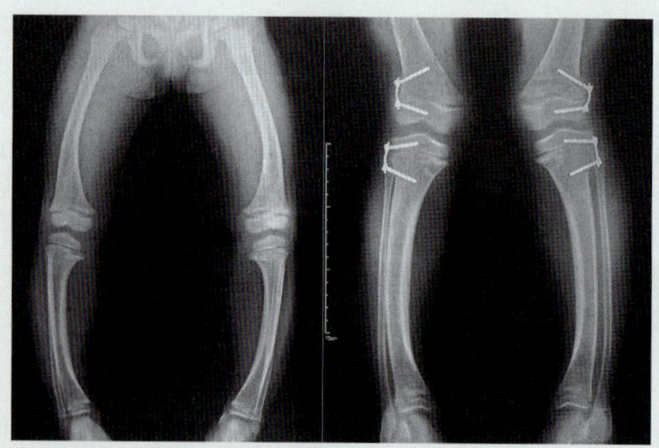

Bone is not simply an impressively strong and flexible material — it is also a dynamic and responsive tissue, which is constantly being broken down and renewed (a process known as bone remodelling). This turnover of bone is mainly as a result of another unique feature of bone — its piezoelectric properties. Materials which show a piezoelectric effect can generate charge, and therefore electricity, in response to mechanical stress. When a mechanical stress is placed on a bone, therefore, the bone generates charge along the lines of greatest stress, or load. This charge stimulates the building of more bone along those stress lines. In this way, each bone strengthens itself to meet the loads that are being placed on it; this process is commonly known as Wolff's law, which was first described by German surgeon Julius Wolff in the late nineteenth century. This adaptation to stress is the reason why loading bones by taking regular weight-bearing exercise is so important for bone health — the load on the bones is what generates the signals which maintain bone integrity and lead to stronger bones. Consider, for example, how recovery from breaking a bone in your leg would include physical therapy to return strength to the leg — this is not only important to restore muscle but also to strengthen the bone(s). Removing any kind of weight-bearing exercise, through long periods of physical inactivity such as enforced bed rest, leads to a rapid reduction in bone density (and increased risk of fracture).

The functions of bone are carried out by the three bone cell types.

Osteoblasts

Osteoblasts synthesise the organic matrix of bone (the collagen) and then they control the deposition of calcium salts onto the collagen to create hardened bone. These cells are therefore responsible for the creation of new bone and the repair of fractured bone. As such, you can think of these cells as being the 'bone builders' (hint: remember B for 'blast' and 'build').

Osteoclasts

Osteoclasts are large cells which seal themselves onto an area of bone and secrete enzymes and acid onto the bone to dissolve it. The action of osteoclasts therefore removes bone and releases minerals from the bone into the bloodstream. These are the cells responsible for the breaking down, or **resorption**, of bone (hint: think C for 'clast' and the 'crunching' of bone). Importantly, osteoclast action is also the first step in bone renewal and repair; first the osteoclasts pass over the bone to be repaired and take away the surface, and then osteoblasts follow in their wake, creating new bone on the freshly cleaned surface.

The density of bone therefore depends on the balance of osteoblast and osteoclast activity; if osteoclasts are more active than osteoblasts, there will be a loss of bone density, and if osteoblasts are more active than osteoclasts, there will be an increase in bone density. Various factors are known to influence the activity of one or other of these cells, and therefore the bone density, and more are being discovered as research on bone physiology progresses. The most important factors are shown in table 7.1.

TABLE 7.1 Factors affecting bone density

Cause building of bone, either due to increased osteoblast or decreased osteoclast activity	Cause resorption of bone, either due to decreased osteoblast or increased osteoclast activity
Adequate oestrogen level	Decreased oestrogen level (including the onset of menopause)
Sufficient mechanical stress (weight-bearing activities)	Insufficient weight-bearing activities
Sufficient dietary calcium intake	Insufficient dietary calcium intake
Sufficient vitamin D	Insufficient vitamin D
Growth hormone	Parathyroid hormone

Osteocytes

These cells start off as osteoblasts, but, during the formation of compact bone, they begin to change their form and develop long, finger-like processes. They then become sealed into the compact bone, as new bone is laid down around them, and their cell processes extend through small canals in the bone and connect with those of other osteocytes. Osteocytes can be seen in figure 7.1, positioned along the concentric rings of the compact bone, with their cell processes extending to contact one another. Osteocytes therefore form a living network that extends throughout compact bone, capable of detecting and signalling changes in the bone. The functions of osteocytes are still not fully understood, but they are believed to be the cells which convert mechanical stress on the bone into electrical signals. The cells, sealed inside the bone matrix, are ideally positioned to detect the size and direction of the forces placed on the bone, making osteocytes the source of the piezoelectric properties of bone.

MEDICINES MANAGEMENT

Bisphosphonates

Fractures, particularly of the hip and the vertebrae, are much more common in post-menopausal women and older men with osteoporosis. The drugs known as bisphosphonates, which include alendronate and zoledronate, can reduce the occurrence of these fractures drastically. The drugs can be taken orally (e.g. alendronate) or given as an infusion once a year (e.g. zoledronate). They act by inhibiting the actions of bone-resorbing osteoclasts, attaching to the calcium salts in the matrix of bone tissue. When osteoclasts start to resorb the bone, the drug is absorbed by the osteoclast and interferes with its function by stopping it from sealing itself onto the bone and also shortening the life of the osteoclasts. This tips the balance in favour of osteoblast activity, meaning more bone is built than is broken down, helping to increase bone density. Because osteoclast activity is important in bone remodelling, there is a lower rate of remodelling in the bone when these drugs are used.

Bisphosphonates are also used in post-menopausal women who have been treated for breast cancer as they have been found to reduce the spread of the cancer to bone.

In common with all drugs, the bisphosphonates have side effects, including osteonecrosis of the jaw, a condition in which the bone of the jaw starts to die, with the loss of teeth and need for dental supportive therapy. Although rarely reported, this side effect is more likely with high-dose infusion. Anyone due to start bisphosphonate therapy is advised to get any required dental work completed before starting on the drug. The most common side effect of infusion of these drugs, however, is flu-like symptoms occurring within 24 hours of the infusion and resolving after a day or two. For more information see The Royal Australian College of General Practitioners and Osteoporosis Australia (2017).

7.3 Other connective tissues closely associated with the skeletal system

LEARNING OBJECTIVE 7.3 Describe the other connective tissues associated with the skeleton and their roles.

Connective tissues are characterised by specialised cells embedded in an extracellular matrix. The matrix gives the connective tissue its strength and resilience and the cells make and repair the matrix. Besides bone, the connective tissues that are intimately associated with the skeleton are cartilage, ligaments and tendons, and an examination of the function of the skeleton would be incomplete without these connective tissues. The protein collagen features strongly in the extracellular matrix of each of these tissues — closely packed collagen fibres providing the strength required for these tissues to resist the forces they are subjected to, and to provide a certain amount of elasticity too. These tissues do not have their own blood supply (they are avascular), which slows healing when they are damaged. They receive nutrients by diffusion from blood vessels supplying nearby structures, and from joint fluid, in the case of the cartilage found in joints.

Cartilage

This tissue forms various structures in the body (e.g. the outer ear and tip of the nose), and it also provides vital protection and cushioning between bones at numerous joints. Roughening and erosion of cartilage that occur with wear and tear in the later years of life is the first step in the joint inflammation and deterioration that we recognise as osteoarthritis.

There are three types of cartilage.

- *Hyaline cartilage.* This cartilage is adapted for protecting bones from the effects of friction as they move against each other or other structures. Hyaline cartilage has a surface that is smooth and glassy. This greatly reduces friction during movement, as it allows the cartilage-covered surfaces to slide over each other easily. Hyaline cartilage is found covering the ends of bones at each movable joint, at the tips of the ribs, the tip of the nose and forming most of the foetal skeleton.

- *Elastic cartilage.* This cartilage is similar in appearance to hyaline cartilage, but under a microscope, fibres of the protein elastin can be seen in the extracellular matrix. The elastin gives the cartilage the ability to snap back to its original position when it is pulled out of shape. This cartilage is vital to maintain the shape of structures which are regularly bent or stretched in some way as part of their function, such as the epiglottis — a flap of cartilage located above the larynx that folds down to cover the larynx whenever swallowing occurs. This prevents food from entering and blocking the airways. The outer ear of humans and other mammals consists of elastic cartilage, maintaining the shape of the ear.
- *Fibrocartilage.* This form of cartilage forms a transition between cartilage and ligament. It contains a high proportion of collagen, which while present in many connective tissues, is at a higher concentration and in two forms (type I and type II) in fibrocartilage. This makes this cartilage strong, reasonably elastic and resistant to compression. It is found forming the outer edge of the intervertebral discs (known as the annulus fibrosus) and the menisci in the knee joint. In these locations this cartilage forms a spongy pad, cushioning joints which take a great deal of weight. Fibrocartilage also forms the pubic symphysis — the anterior joint between the pelvic bones.

Ligaments

These are the strong 'straps' that connect bones together. They can be seen wrapping across a joint between the bones that form the joint. The number and tightness of the ligaments at a movable joint will determine both its stability and its range of motion. A more stable joint will have many ligaments holding the bones in position but will have a more limited range of motion for the same reason. People who have unusually lax, stretchable ligaments will have the ability to 'hyper-extend' their joints, a property commonly referred to as double-jointedness.

Tendons

Tendons are the dense connective tissue structures that anchor muscles to bone, enabling the contraction of a muscle to result in the movement of a bone, and the bending or straightening of a joint. Tendons are also slightly elastic, so that sudden strong muscle contractions are less likely to damage the tendon or the bone, but they are also strong enough to endure the powerful forces that muscles can generate, and transmit those forces into movement of the bones.

CLINICALLY REASONED EPISODE OF CARE

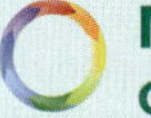

Musculoskeletal injury

Consider the patient situation

Folomi is a 36-year-old with two children under the age of 8. She works as a care assistant for a large residential care home. Five months ago, she sustained a back injury at work and since then has been unable to work due to the pain and restricted mobility. Folomi sees the practice nurse and tells her the pain is nonstop and that she feels down and tired all the time. She says there are days that she does not even want to get out of bed, and if it were not for her children she would not bother. Folomi is tearful and tells the nurse she feels she cannot go on anymore as it is all too much.

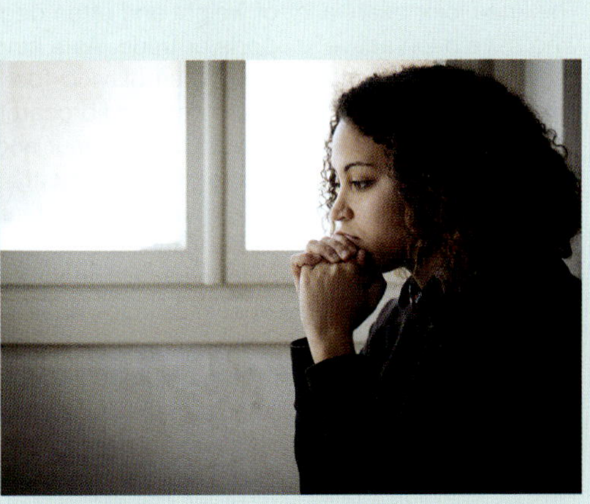

Collect cues and information

- Health history: review previous information and confirm with Folomi that the information is correct.
- Physical assessment: all systems, but with particular attention to neurological and musculoskeletal assessment.
- Pain assessment: utilise a validated assessment tool used by the health organisation.
- Medication review: assess risks and benefits of all medications being taken by Folomi; ask about all prescribed, over-the-counter, complementary, legal and illicit drug consumption.
- Mental state assessment: utilise the appropriate assessment tool used by the health organisation.

Process information

Musculoskeletal disorders, particularly when they are painful and disabling, can induce or exacerbate mental health disorders. Pain comes with an element of negative emotion as part of the experience and, combined with the limitation of normal activities, this can be very depressing for the sufferer. This can feed a vicious cycle, in which lowered mood intensifies the pain and reduces motivation for the sufferer to follow rehabilitation regimes. A musculoskeletal disorder lasting longer than 12 weeks is considered chronic. People who suffer from chronic pain symptoms often report feelings of fatigue, being 'fed up' with their symptoms, and a sense that their pain is never going to end. All of this has the potential to further exacerbate low mood and increase the risk of the injury becoming a long-term disability.

Nursing actions

1. Use reassurance and respectful, active listening to promote trust and treatment concordance.
   Rationale:
   - To improve Folomi's outcomes, trust needs to be developed.
2. Gain consent for referrals to a physiotherapist, a social worker and community mental health teams.
   Rationale:
   - Folomi's situation is complex as physical health issues have impacted her mental health. Achieving good outcomes with Folomi will require interprofessional collaboration. However, regardless of the person's situation, consent is required.
3. Develop a pain management plan with interprofessional collaboration — a GP management plan and Team Care Arrangements (Pain Management Network 2021).
   Rationale:
   - A plan facilitates communication between health professionals and the patient, and can assist with encouraging treatment concordance (Chapman 2018).
4. Provide details for a local support group.
   Rationale:
   - There is strong evidence that support groups are an effective component of support for a person living with chronic illness or disability (Worrall et al. 2018; Connect Groups n.d.).

Evaluate outcomes

Folomi reports a reduction in symptoms and increased satisfaction with life.

Source: Based on the Clinical Reasoning Cycle, Levett-Jones (2013).

CLINICAL CONSIDERATIONS

Knee reconstruction

The knee joint bears a lot of weight and often degenerates in the later years of life, particularly in people who have been active in sports or trade. As a hinge joint, the knee is damaged by twisting actions such as those that can often occur when playing football, when forcing the knee joint to twist can tear the ligaments which hold it in place and the fibrocartilage pads in the joint (the menisci). Over time and use, the articular cartilage at the ends of the femur and tibia can wear away, the menisci (cartilage within the knee) can tear, and one or more of the ligaments that stabilise the joint (the collateral ligaments and the anterior and posterior cruciate ligaments) can tear. There are now surgical options to repair the joint and its associated ligaments and cartilage.

- The articulating surfaces of the femur and tibia can be replaced with metal, or some other hardwearing material, in a procedure known as knee replacement surgery.
- Meniscal injuries, if not too severe, may heal on their own, but bigger tears, particularly in the inner portion of the meniscus without a blood supply, can be surgically trimmed or repaired.
- Injury to the cruciate ligaments of the knee can be surgically repaired by taking a graft from the tendon of nearby muscle. These knee reconstruction procedures are performed by keyhole surgery in the joint, known as arthroscopy, and can be done quite quickly. The post-surgical recovery, however, may be prolonged, due to the slow healing rate of cartilage, tendons and ligaments.

Bone formation

The template for the bones forms **in utero**, in the form of hyaline cartilage 'models' of the bones. By the end of the third month of pregnancy, the template for the skeleton is completely formed, but consists almost entirely of hyaline cartilage (itself formed from **mesenchyme**, or embryonic connective tissue). This cartilage is gradually replaced by bone, a process known as **ossification**, which begins with **calcification** of the cartilage, followed by osteoblast invasion and bone creation to replace the cartilage. Because it occurs inside a cartilage template, this process is known as endochondral ossification (figure 7.2) and is the way in which most of our bones are formed. During the ossification process, which starts at the centre of the cartilage and moves out, blood vessels grow into the cavity of the bone. In the case of a long bone, as shown in figure 7.2, by the time the bone is fully developed, the only remaining cartilage is at the two bone ends, and a narrow strip between the end and the shaft of the bone. The cartilage covering the ends of the bone becomes the articular cartilage, reducing friction and protecting the bone end at the joint, and the strip of cartilage that separates the bone end from the shaft acts as a growth point, allowing the bone to elongate from this point as the person grows. This strip is called the growth plate or the epiphyseal plate (see image 6 in figure 7.2).

FIGURE 7.2 Endochondral ossification of the tibia

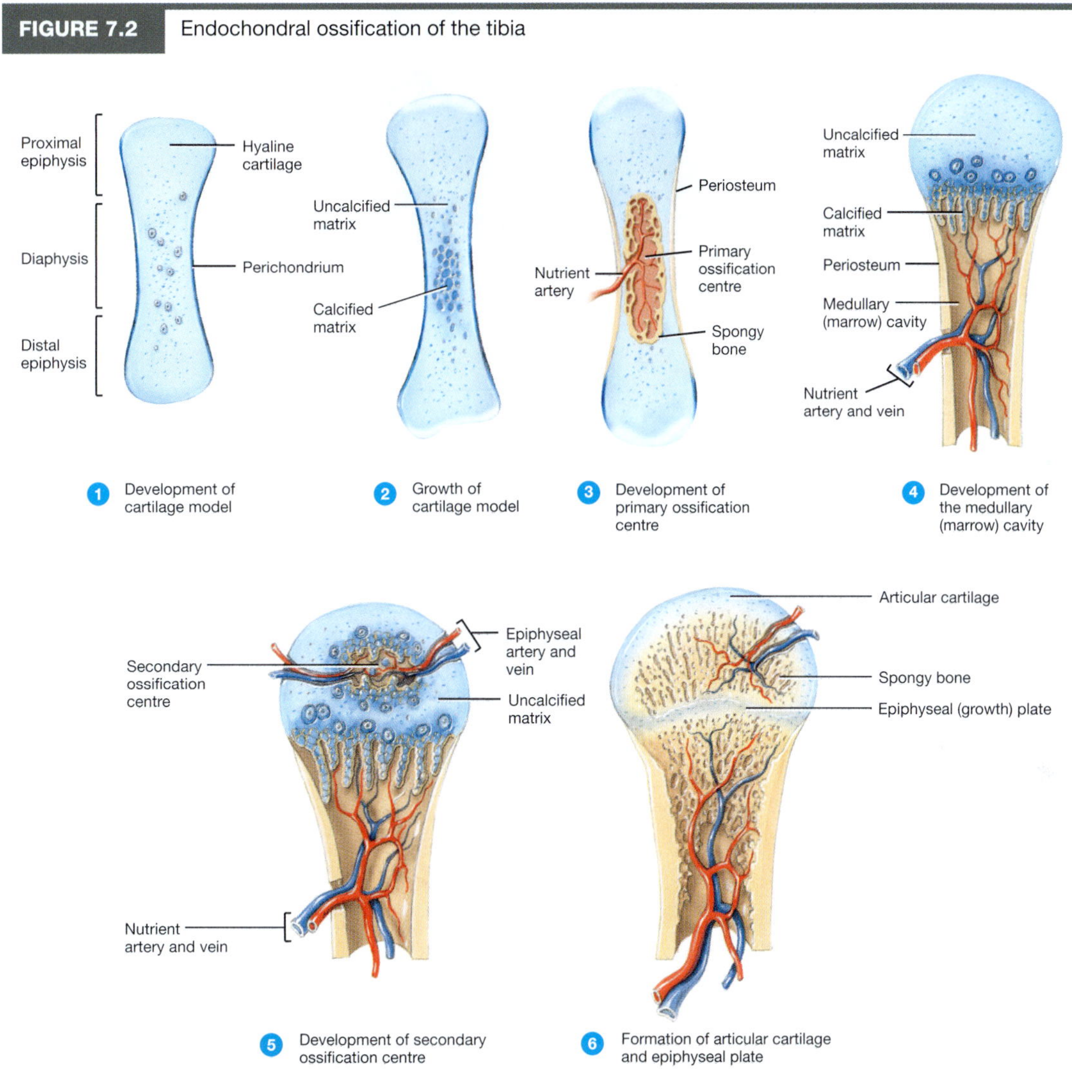

Source: Tortora and Derrickson (2009). Reproduced with permission of John Wiley & Sons.

Because the ossification of the entire skeleton is not complete by birth, infants are born with large amounts of cartilage (important for birthing and to allow for ongoing growth and development). They also have a greater number of bones than adults, but many of these bones fuse together during maturation, resulting in the normal number of bones by adulthood. The bones of babies and children are softer and more porous than an adult's, but become harder and denser with age, reaching their peak density at age 20–30.

Bone growth

Growth in stature comes about because the bones of the limbs grow in length. This longitudinal growth is accompanied by an increase in the thickness of bones, so the body proportions are maintained as an individual grows.

Growth in bone length occurs at the cartilage of the epiphyseal plate (at each end of the bone, within the **epiphysis**). In early puberty, the chondrocytes (cartilage cells) in the cartilage divide continuously, creating new cartilage on the side of the epiphyseal plate closest to the end of the bone, while osteoblasts invade the cartilage from the shaft side of the plate, ossifying the tissue. In this way, the cartilage plate advances towards the bone end, while the bone grows in length as the trailing edge of the epiphyseal plate ossifies — to this end, the new bone 'chases' the existing cartilage along the bone (figure 7.3).

FIGURE 7.3 Long bones grow in length from the cartilaginous epiphyseal plates.

(a) Radiograph showing the epiphyseal plate of the femur of a 3-year-old

(b) Histology of the epiphyseal plate

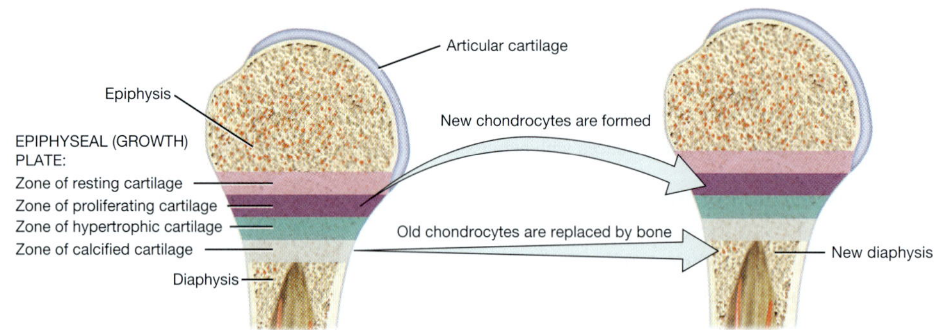

(c) Lengthwise growth of bone at epiphyseal plate

Source: Tortora and Derrickson (2014). Reproduced with permission of John Wiley & Sons.

Growth of the long bones ceases when the division of chondrocytes in the leading edge of the plate slows down and eventually stops, towards the end of puberty. The ossification of the epiphyseal growth plate continues, and the plate finally becomes fully ossified when the cartilage front stops advancing. Both the growth spurt that occurs during puberty and the closure of the epiphyseal plate at the end of puberty are driven by the sex hormones; oestrogen in women and testosterone in men (Weise et al. 2001).

Growth of bone width (across the circumference) occurs on the outer surface of the bone. Osteoblasts lay down new bone on the outer bone surface in the concentric layers seen in compact bone. Meanwhile, osteoclast activity on the inner surface of the bone (in the bone cavity) removes bone. In this way, the size of cavity increases with the overall circumference of the bone, preserving the proportions and helping to regulate bone mass (figure 7.4).

FIGURE 7.4 Bones increase in width but maintain the same proportion of compact bone to medullary cavity.

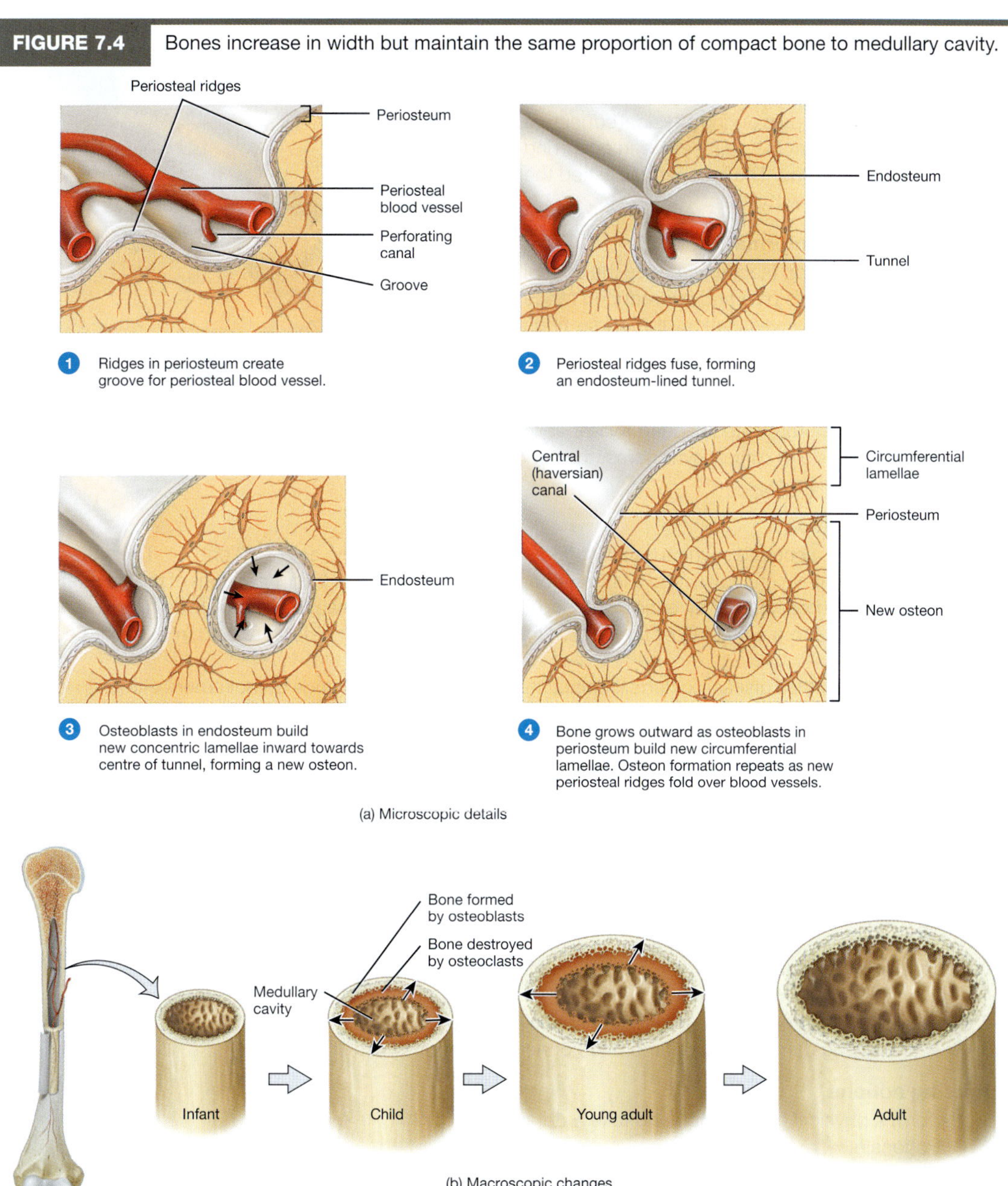

Source: Tortora and Derrickson (2014). Reproduced with permission of John Wiley & Sons.

Bone remodelling

The removal and renewal of the bone (remodelling) continues throughout adult life. Whether this remodelling process results in loss of bone or maintenance and strengthening of bone will be determined by the conditions the body is exposed to, many of which are within our control (table 7.1). Lifestyle choices are important when it comes to ensuring a healthy skeleton into old age.

CLINICALLY REASONED EPISODE OF CARE

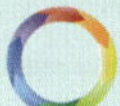

Perthes disease

Consider the patient situation

Kylie is an 8-year-old female who is currently attending school. Kylie has complained of right groin, thigh and knee pain during physical education class, and reports that the pain has been occurring for a number of months. The teacher has asked the school nurse to review Kylie.

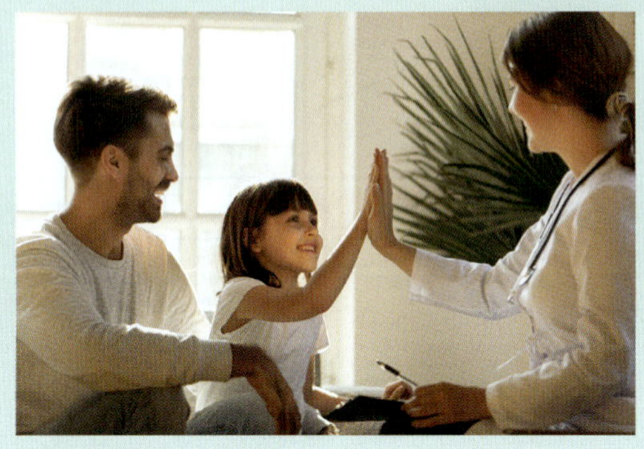

Collect cues and information

The physical education teacher engages the school nurse to assess Kylie's pain and her reduced range of movement. Upon investigation, the nurse finds that Kylie has been experiencing pain for a number of months and has reduced range of movement in her right hip and muscle wastage of the gluteal muscle. These symptoms are affecting Kylie's ability to participate in physical education lessons.

Given Kylie's age and clinical symptoms, the school nurse suspects it is Perthes disease and proceeds with this nursing diagnosis.

Process information

Perthes disease is a condition which usually affects children between the ages of 3 and 11. The causes of Perthes disease remain unknown, and it is a rare condition, affecting less than 1 per cent of the population. The condition is characterised by a lack of blood flow to the femoral head in one or both hips. The lack of blood flow leads to a softening of the bone, which can then lead to deformity, and in extreme cases, bone death.

Symptoms of Perthes disease include limping; stiffness and reduced range of movement of the hip joint; pain in the knee, thigh and groin; and myopenia (muscle wastage). Diagnosis of Perthes disease occurs via a thorough history, physical examination and X-ray.

In most cases, the head of the femur bone will regenerate. However, in some cases, additional treatment and support is required to ensure that there are no ongoing issues such as bone degeneration or death, muscle constriction and wastage, or gait performance. Treatment options for Perthes disease depend on the severity of the condition and include rest, physiotherapy, a brace or splint, and in some cases, surgery.

Kylie is currently in the correct age group for Perthes disease and is displaying some symptoms typical of the condition. The nurse understands that early diagnostics and treatments will lead to better outcomes for Kylie.

Identify problems/issues

1. Pain and reduced range of motion of hip joint
2. Reduced ability to participate in physical school activities
3. Risk of ongoing damage and deterioration of head of femur

Nursing actions

1. Perform a physical examination and take a detailed history.

   Rationale:
   - This details the physical and historical characteristics of pain and decreased range of motion.
   - This provides clear and appropriate information for referral to a general practitioner.
   - This allows for the immediate management of pain (under appropriate nursing protocols and procedures).

2. Refer to a general practitioner.
   Rationale:
   - A general practitioner is the most appropriate person for coordination of assessment, diagnosis, specialist care and ongoing management of care.
   - Perthes disease requires specialist input and treatment.
   - Referral to specialist care and treatment will enable the best outcomes for Kylie and her family.
3. Provide ongoing support to Kylie and her family, as well as school educators.
   Rationale:
   - Nurses are well placed to provide ongoing support and education to individuals and their families.
   - The school nurse can monitor Kylie's condition in the future.
   - Nurses are well placed to provide support and information to educators, which may inform adjustments at school to support recovery.

Evaluate outcomes

As a result of the actions above, Kylie's general practitioner refers her to an orthopaedic specialist. A physiotherapy program is commenced to strengthen and stretch the muscles of the affected area. This is beneficial in improving Kylie's range of movement. Kylie attends the orthopaedic clinic every 4 months for ongoing care and X-rays. After 12 months of physiotherapy and follow-up, Kylie's condition improves, and she is not suffering any pain in her hip or leg. The femoral head appears larger and more regularly shaped on X-ray, and Kylie is discharged from specialist care.

Reflect on new processes and learning

What role could the school nurse play in providing ongoing assessment and support to the multidisciplinary team in the management of Kylie's Perthes disease?

Source: Based on the Clinical Reasoning Cycle, Levett-Jones (2013).

CLINICALLY REASONED EPISODE OF CARE

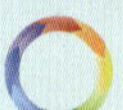

Osteomyelitis

Consider the patient situation

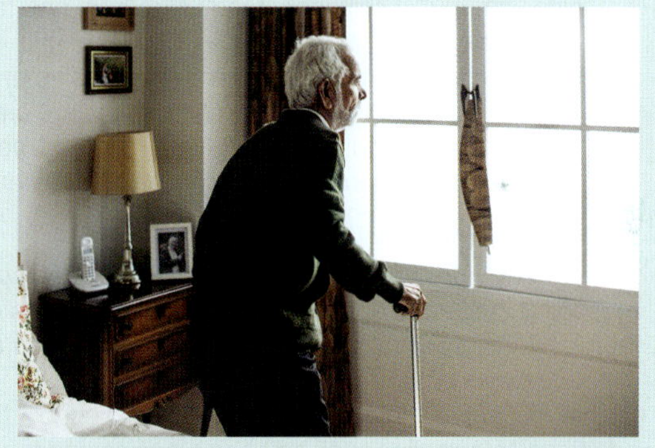

After years of pain and difficulty walking, Mr Singh, a 75-year-old male, has recently undergone replacement hip surgery. The head of Mr Singh's femur was removed and replaced with a metal ball which was attached by a shaft extending down into the medullary cavity of the femur. The socket of the ball-and-socket joint was also lined with metal. This is also known as a total hip replacement.

After an initial uncomplicated recovery, Mr Singh returned home under the care of his wife and daughter. However, 7 days after his surgery, Mr Singh started to experience pain and fever.

His general practitioner referred Mr Singh back to the hospital. A subsequent bone scan confirmed a diagnosis of osteomyelitis and he has been admitted to the ward for antibiotic treatment pending further surgical intervention.

Collect cues and information

Mr Singh is reporting pain within the hip and fever. On arrival to the ward, Mr Singh's temperature is 37.9 °C. Given the context of Mr Singh's recent hip replacement, it is reasonable to presume the presence of an infection.

A bone scan has been performed and a diagnosis of osteomyelitis has been made. Mr Singh's medical team has prescribed antibiotics and are currently assessing the need for further surgical intervention.

He has been admitted to the orthopaedic ward to commence treatment. Given the likelihood of a *Staphylococcus aureus* infection, antimicrobial agents to treat this have been chosen. Identifying the infectious organism would require a bone biopsy; however, this will take time and treatment should not be delayed.

Process information

Osteomyelitis is a bone infection that can occur after trauma (particularly open fractures) or surgery on bones and joints. Implant-related bone infections, occurring after joint prosthesis (e.g. the hip, knee, shoulder or ankle) or osteosynthesis (e.g. plates, screws, nails implant for fractures or osteotomies), are one of the most challenging complications in orthopaedic surgery. Fortunately, it is a relatively rare occurrence with around 1 per cent of people developing the infection post operatively.

If left untreated, osteomyelitis can lead to osteonecrosis (bone death), arthritis and, more acutely, sepsis. Osteomyelitis is painful and can lead to a chronic condition with complicated management and ongoing issues. Therefore, timely management of the condition is a priority.

Identify problems/issues

1. Treatment and management of acute osteomyelitis
2. Pain and symptom management of osteomyelitis
3. Liaison between individual, family and multidisciplinary team on treatment options and priorities of care

Nursing actions

1. Conduct physical examination and observations of Mr Singh.
   Rationale:
   - A nursing assessment begins with a thorough physical examination and history taking, including the completion of clinical observations (e.g. respiratory rate, oxygen saturations, heart rate, blood pressure, blood glucose level, pain).
   - Initial assessment allows nurses to assess the efficacy of interventions as well as monitor for clinical deterioration of condition.
2. Administer antimicrobial/antibiotic treatment.
   Rationale:
   - The early administration of antibiotics is a priority to mitigate the risk of deterioration and sepsis.
   - While further tests and treatments are pending, initiation of antibiotics commences treatment for the condition.
3. Provide pain management.
   Rationale:
   - Osteomyelitis is often a painful condition, and associated symptoms such as fever and swelling can be uncomfortable for patients.
   - Pain and symptom management is a priority for nurses and patients to ensure comfort.
4. Liaise with multidisciplinary team, Mr Singh and family.
   Rationale:
   - Ensure that the treatment regime is inclusive of the wants and needs of the individual and family.
   - Ensure that results and treatments plans are clearly communicated with the individual and family.
   - Ensure that the individual and family are informed of choices and treatments, and that care providers are adequately communicating with the individual.

Evaluate outcomes

As with any nursing intervention, the above nursing management will be completed within the clinical reasoning cycle and subject to constant processes of planning, assessment and evaluation. Mr Singh's interventions, such as clinical observations, will be evaluated at regular intervals (usually a minimum of 4-hourly depending on clinical guidelines).

The efficacy of treatment will be assessed by the multidisciplinary team and will be informed by additional information such as bone biopsies and the ongoing clinical information collected by the nursing team; this includes vital signs, wound assessment, and range of movement and pain, among other clinical markers.

Reflect on new processes and learning

How do you think the nursing actions for Mr Singh's care would change if a decision was made to surgically remove the prosthetic hip?

Source: Based on the Clinical Reasoning Cycle, Levett-Jones (2013).

Bone fractures

Bone is one of the few tissues with the capacity to heal completely, replacing damaged tissue with new, fully functional bone rather than with scar tissue. It is therefore able to regenerate itself after a fracture in a way similar to the initial formation of bone during development. The copious blood supply to bone is essential in fracture healing, bringing phagocytic white blood cells to the area to 'tidy up', removing any bone fragments and dead and dying cells, and to protect against infection. The regrowth of any blood vessels that were damaged is also vital for complete healing to occur (Marsell & Einhorn 2011). The steps of the healing process after a fracture of the bone are outlined in figure 7.5.

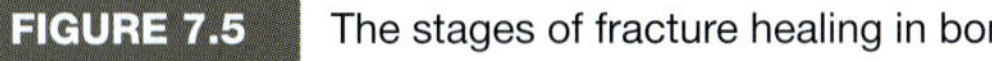
FIGURE 7.5 The stages of fracture healing in bone

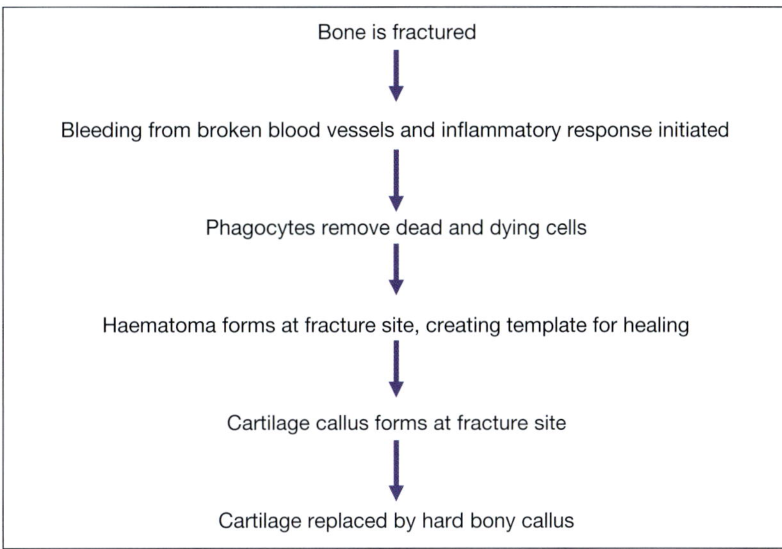

The broken bone ends will be stabilised somewhat by the formation of a natural splint known as the cartilaginous callus, and later fully stabilised with the formation of the hard, **osseous** (bony) callus. At this point the bone will be able to start bearing weight again. The remodelling of bone from the rather disorganised bone of the hard callus to the organised **lamellar** arrangement of normal compact bone with spongy bone in the interior will occur gradually, stimulated by the loading of the bone during weight-bearing activities — hence the need for physical therapy to assist with recovery. A completely healed fracture will show no evidence of the repair, and no scar tissue. The same is not true after injury to ligaments, cartilage or tendons, all of which lack regenerative capacity. In these tissues, an injury may be repaired, but the replacement tissue will be fibrous scar tissue rather than normally functioning tissue, and the structure will be permanently weakened unless surgical repair or replacement is carried out.

CLINICALLY REASONED EPISODE OF CARE

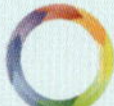

Colles' fracture

Consider the patient situation

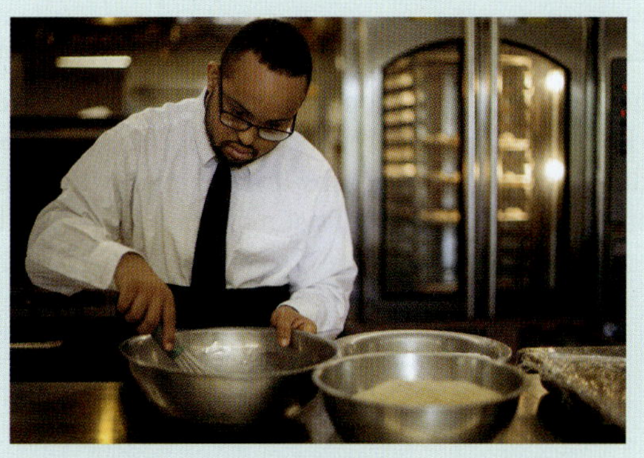

Bob is a 45-year-old man who has learning disabilities. He lives in supported accommodation and works in a local café for two days a week. On the way to work one morning, Bob slipped over, landing on his outstretched right hand. Although it was painful, he continued his journey and went in to work.

Over the next week it was noticed that Bob was not using his right hand normally and he kept dropping items at the café. There were episodes when Bob would cry for no apparent reason and he would tell staff his hand was sore. He would be given two paracetamol, which seemed to help him. This went on for another week until Bob was strongly encouraged to go and see his GP.

Collect cues and information

Nurses need to have a good understanding of the needs of people with learning disabilities across the life span in order to ensure they offer the right support and make reasonable adjustments.

- Health history and pain assessment: use language and assessment tools which are respectful and appropriate for Bob.
- X-ray as requested by GP: a Colles' fracture is diagnosed.
- Social assessment: determine Bob's living and working circumstances and level of support available.

Process information

A Colles' fracture is a fracture of the end of the radius and is typically produced after a fall when a person has broken their fall with their arm outstretched. The broken end of the radius is bent upwards and needs realigning (known as reducing the fracture), to prevent permanent deformation of the wrist. There is also a risk of nerve damage with this fracture, since the median nerve, which supplies the muscles of the hand, travels down the radius. This fracture can take 1–2 years to completely heal.

Nursing actions

1. Administer prescribed pain relief and provide reassurance during reduction of fracture and application of plaster cast.
   Rationale:
   - Access to pain management is a fundamental human right and manipulation of a fracture and application of the plaster cast can be very painful. Adequate pain relief and reassurance will also enable Bob to assist with the process.
2. Provide education to Bob and his support person about potential complications from the fracture, plaster cast and pain management.
   Rationale:
   - Any fracture can result in complications such as nerve damage or compartment syndrome. Education will minimise risk of these complications.
3. Assess need for interprofessional support (e.g. physiotherapist, occupational therapist) and gain consent from Bob and/or his guardian as needed.
   Rationale:
   - Achieving good outcomes with Bob may require interprofessional collaboration. Regardless of the person's situation, consent is required.
4. Organise follow-up care with the nurse and GP.
   Rationale:
   - Follow-up care is essential to determine patient progress to recovery and detect any complications or deterioration.

Evaluate outcomes

Bob reports no complications from the fracture or plaster cast and reports adequate pain relief. He is able to return to work and resume his usual activities with minimal limitation and adequate support.

Source: Based on the Clinical Reasoning Cycle, Levett-Jones (2013).

7.4 The axial and appendicular skeleton

LEARNING OBJECTIVE 7.4 List the various types of bone and joints.

There are 206 named bones in the adult human skeleton (figure 7.6).

For classification purposes, the skeleton is divided into two parts: the axial skeleton, consisting of the skull, vertebral column, ribs and sternum, which form the central axis of the body (table 7.2); and the appendicular skeleton, consisting of the 126 bones that form the limbs (table 7.3).

FIGURE 7.6 The human skeleton (a) anterior view, (b) posterior view; axial skeleton blue and appendicular skeleton white

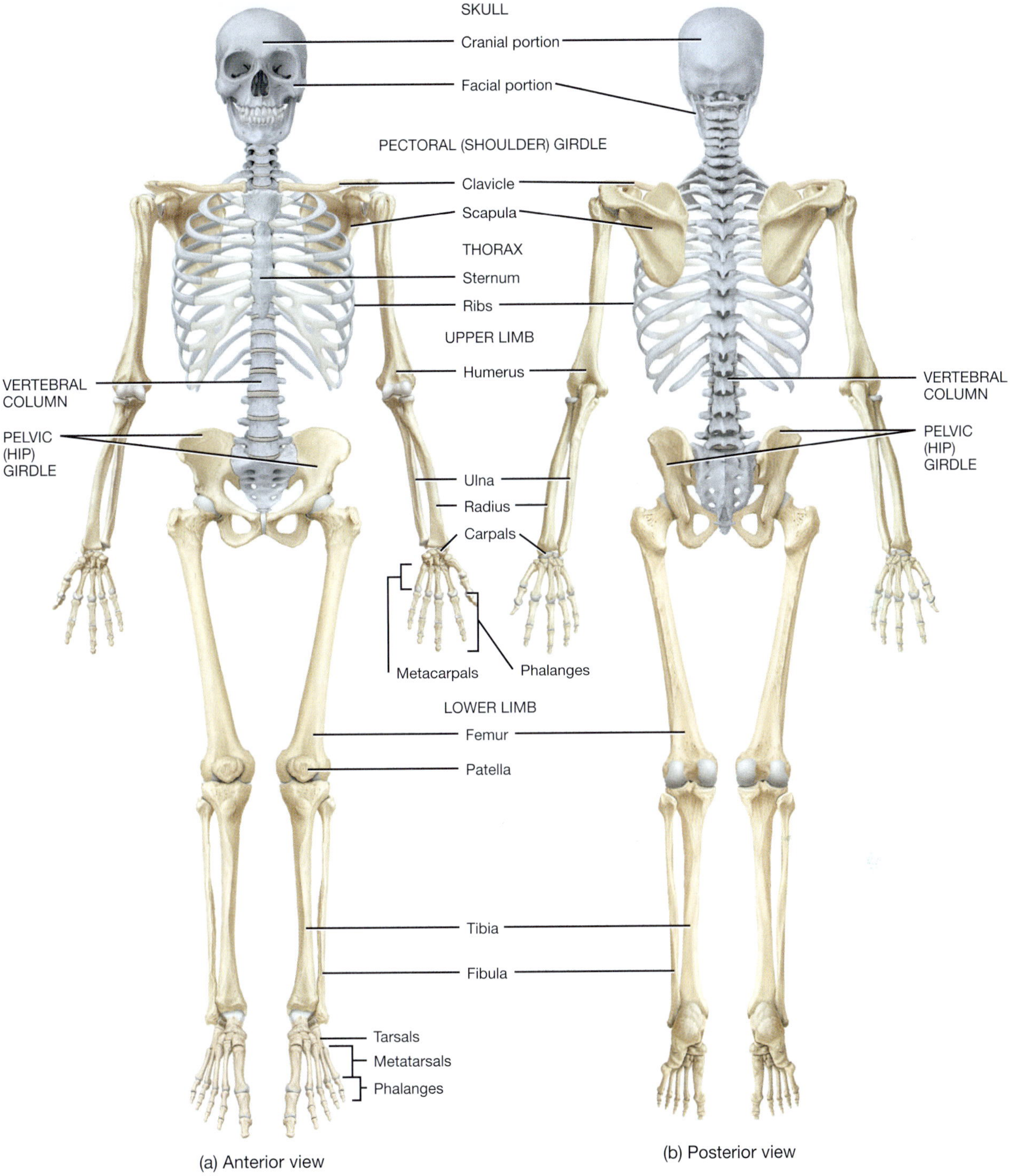

Source: Tortora and Derrickson (2009). Reproduced with permission of John Wiley & Sons.

TABLE 7.2 The bones of the axial skeleton

Structure	Number of bones
Skull	
Cranium	8
Face	14
Hyoid	1
Auditory ossicles	6
Vertebral column This number counts the sacrum and coccyx as single vertebrae. They are actually formed from fused vertebrae (5 sacral and 4 coccygeal). Some sources give the number of vertebrae as 33 for this reason.	26
Thorax	
Sternum	1
Ribs	24
Total number of bones in the axial skeleton	**80**

TABLE 7.3 The bones of the appendicular skeleton

Structure	Number of bones
Pectoral girdle	22
Clavicle	
Scapula	
Upper limbs	
Humerus	2
Ulna	2
Radius	2
Carpals	16
Metacarpals	10
Phalanges	28
Pelvic girdle	2
Pelvic bone	
Lower limbs	
Femur	2
Patella	2
Fibula	2
Tibia	2
Tarsals	14
Metatarsals	10
Phalanges	28
Total number of bones in the appendicular skeleton	**126**
Total number of bones in the adult human skeleton	**206**

Bone shapes

As can be readily seen by looking at an entire skeleton, bones can take a variety of shapes depending on their position and function. A number of bone shapes are recognised, and these bones are often collectively referred to by their shapes.

Long bones

These bones are longer than they are wide and include the humerus, femur, radius, ulna, tibia and fibula. The clavicles, metacarpals, metatarsals and phalanges are also long bones despite their shortness. These bones allow limb movement.

Long bones consist of a shaft (**diaphysis**) composed primarily of compact bone and ends (epiphyses) composed mainly of **spongy (cancellous) bone**. Between the two is an intermediate region known as the **metaphysis**, also containing spongy bone (figure 7.7).

The compact bone in the shafts forms supportive pillars of bone, which are thickest at the point where the forces applied to the bone are greatest (figure 7.7).

FIGURE 7.7 Parts of a long bone

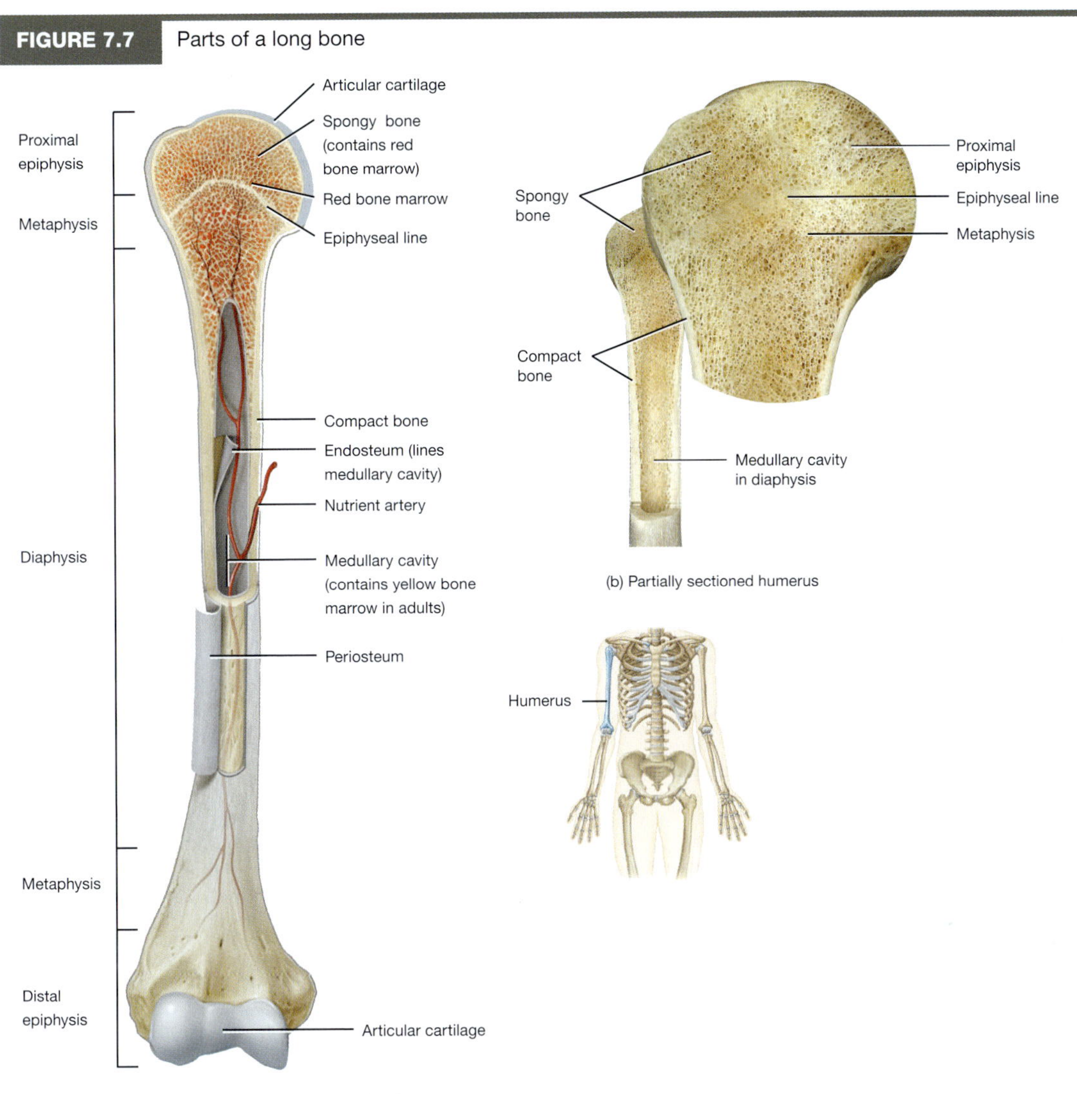

(a) Partially sectioned humerus (arm bone)

(b) Partially sectioned humerus

Source: Tortora and Derrickson (2009). Reproduced with permission of John Wiley & Sons.

Short bones

These bones are usually roughly as wide as they are long. They tend to be found at locations in the limbs where only limited movement is required, such as the wrists and ankles. Examples include the carpals of the wrist and the tarsals of the foot (figure 7.8). These bones have a thin layer of compact bone over predominantly spongy or cancellous bone.

Flat bones

These are thin bones that are found encasing and protecting delicate tissue (such as the skull), or where there is a need for a broad surface for extensive muscle attachment (such as the scapula, or shoulder blade). Other examples include the sternum, ribs and some bones of the pelvis (figure 7.9).

FIGURE 7.8 The tarsal bones — short bones

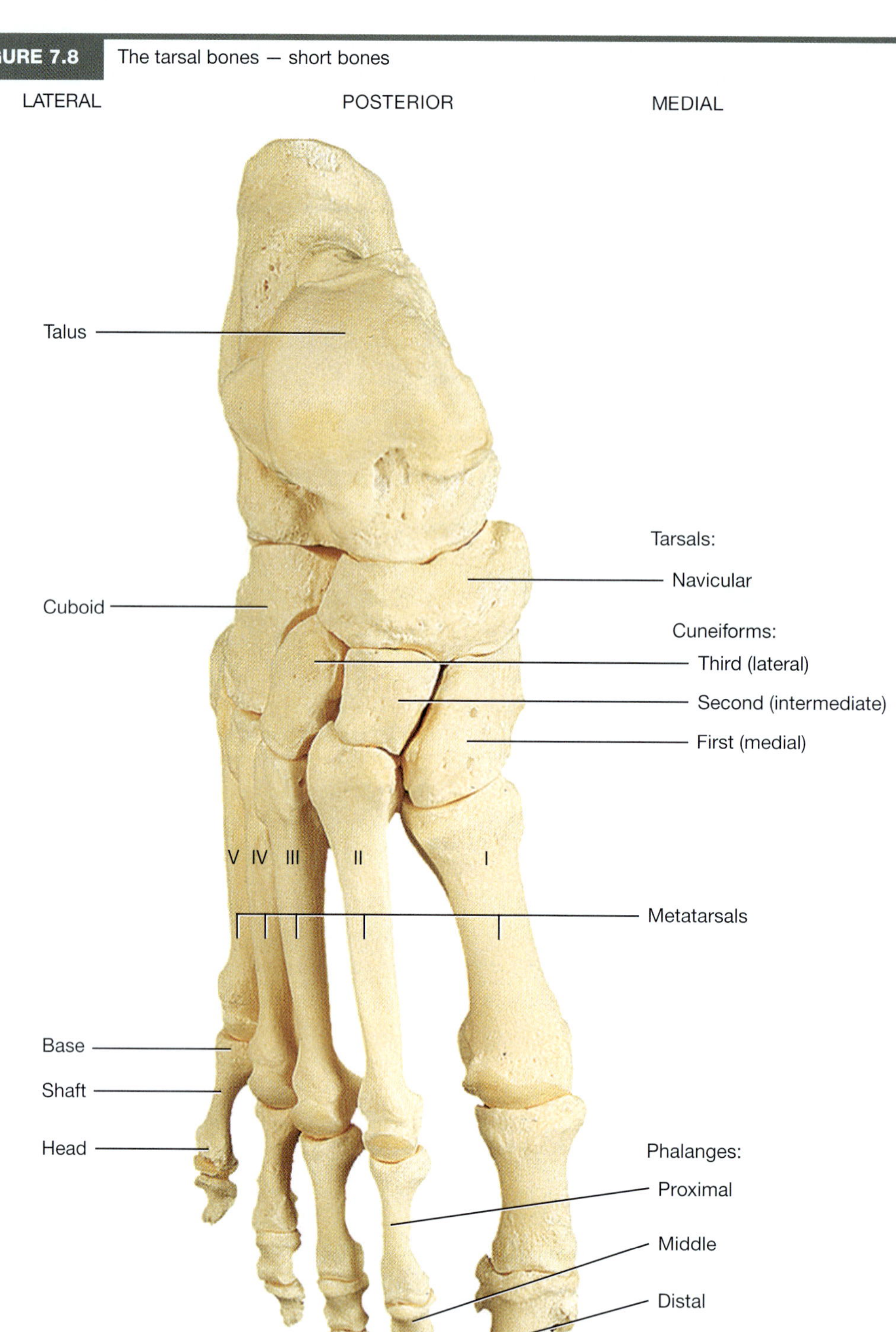

Source: Tortora (2008). Reproduced with permission of John Wiley & Sons.

FIGURE 7.9 Examples of flat bones: in (a) the sternum and in (b) the scapula and ribs

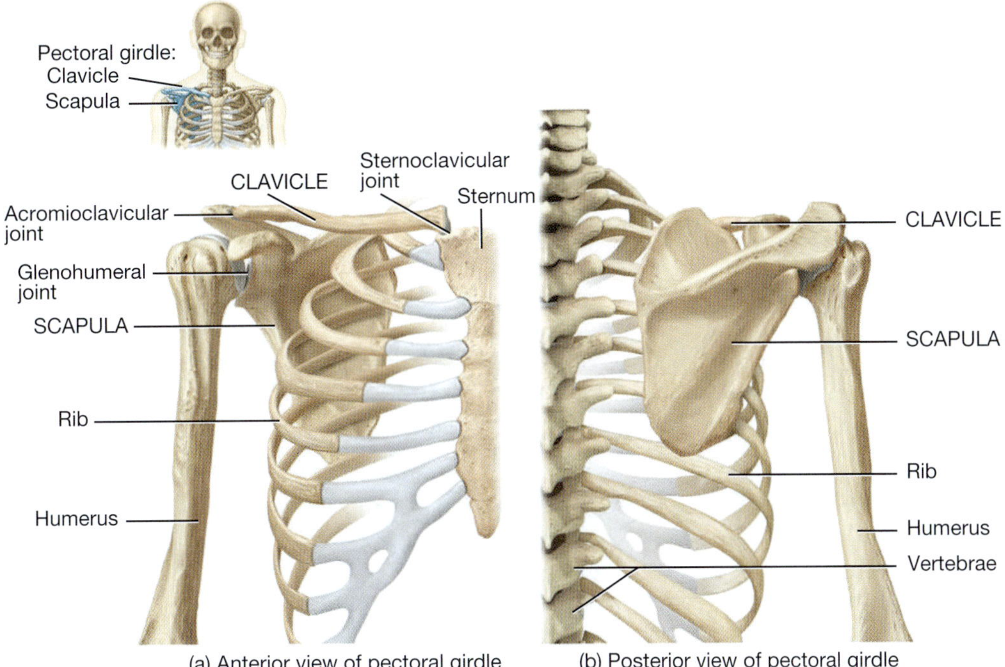

(a) Anterior view of pectoral girdle (b) Posterior view of pectoral girdle

Source: Tortora and Derrickson (2014). Reproduced with permission of John Wiley & Sons.

Irregular bones

These are bones that, because of their irregular shapes, do not fit into any of the categories already described. They also consist of spongy bone enclosed by thin layers of compact bone. These specialised bones include the vertebrae (figure 7.10), the sphenoid and zygomatic bones of the skull and the ossicles of the ear.

FIGURE 7.10 (a, b) The vertebrae — irregular bones

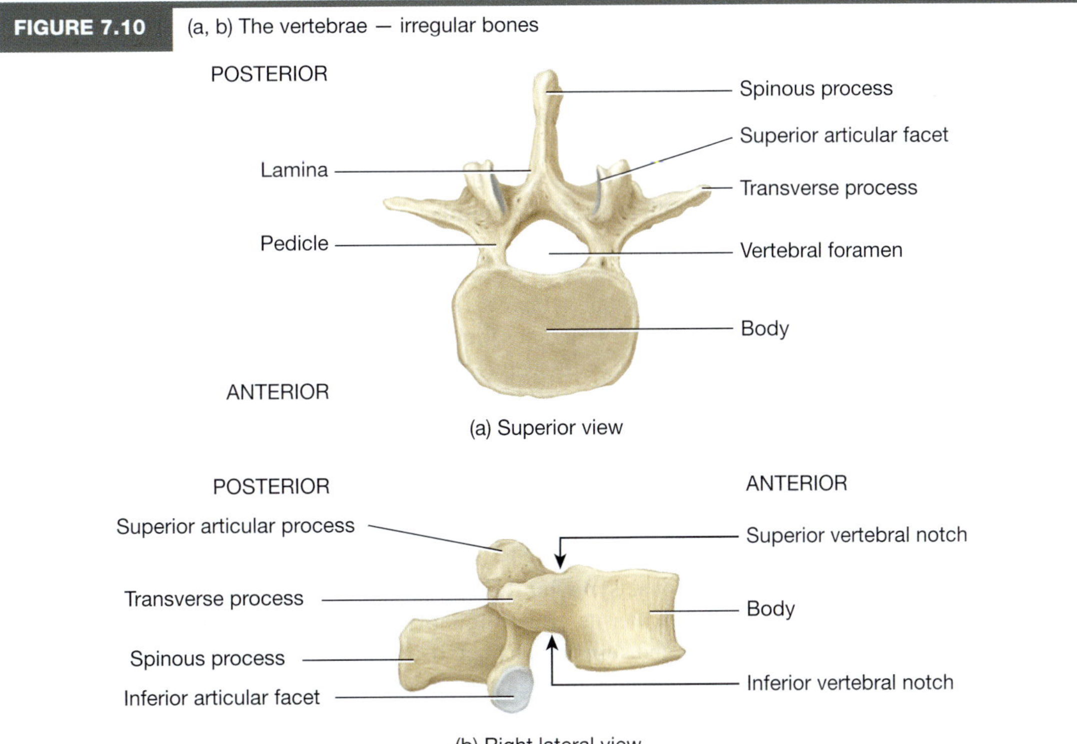

Source: Tortora and Derrickson (2009). Reproduced with permission of John Wiley & Sons.

Sesamoid bones

Sesamoid bones are bones that develop within tendons at points where a tendon passes close to a joint and their role seems to be to protect the tendon from friction and rubbing at that point. They are small and round and take their name from the fact that their appearance reminded early anatomists of sesame seeds. The main example of this type of bone is the patella (figure 7.11).

FIGURE 7.11 A sesamoid bone, the patella — shown in lateral view, in the tendon of the quadriceps muscle, positioned to protect the tendon from friction when the knee joint bends

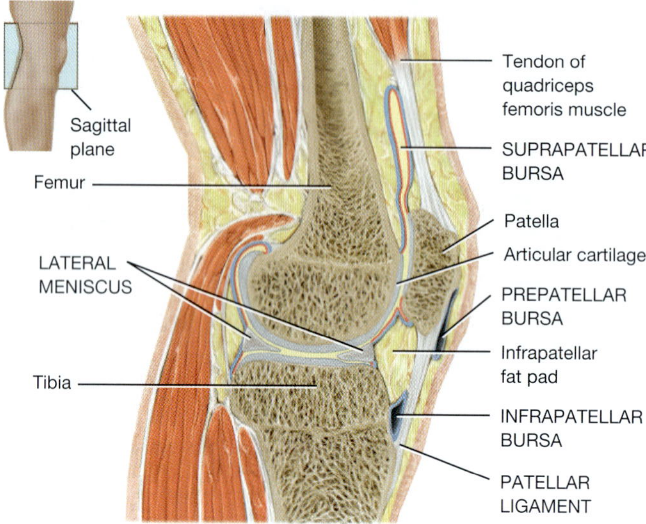

Source: Tortora and Derrickson (2014). Reproduced with permission of John Wiley & Sons.

Joints

A joint is the point at which two or more bones meet. There are three major types of joints: fibrous, cartilaginous and synovial.

Fibrous joints

These joints, also called synarthrodial joints, are held together by only a ligament which fills the space between the bone ends. Examples of synarthrodial joints are the connection between the teeth and their bony sockets, the joint between the radius and the ulna, the joint between the tibia and fibula, and the sutures (joints) between bones in the skull. Most **fibrous joints** are fixed (with no movement).

Cartilaginous joints

These joints are also called symphyses (singular symphysis). They occur where the connection between the articulating bones is made up of cartilage. Examples include the intervertebral joints in the spine and the pubic symphysis, between the two halves of the pelvis. **Cartilaginous joints** allow for some limited movement and are sometimes termed amphiarthrodial joints.

Synovial joints

Synovial joints, also known as diarthrodial joints, are by far the most common type of joint. They are extremely movable and adapted to allow free movement while minimising friction and the resultant heating caused by repeated movements. These joints are enclosed in a fluid-filled capsule, the lining of which produces a thick, lubricating fluid known as **synovial fluid**. Filling the space between bones in the joint (the **synovial cavity**), this fluid is named after its visual similarity to the white of an egg ('*syn*', like; and '*ovum*', egg), and it is similarly viscous and slippery; characteristics which reduce friction in the joint, by keeping the bone ends apart so that they do not move against one another, but against a cushion of slippery synovial fluid. The fluid also supplies nutrients to the cartilage and removes waste products. If the joint becomes immobile for a period of time the fluid becomes more gel-like, returning to its normal consistency when the joint begins to move again. Hyaline cartilage covers the ends of the articulating bones at the joint, and the smooth glassy surface of this cartilage further reduces friction.

There are six types of synovial joints, and these are classified by the shape of the joint and the movement available (see table 7.4).

TABLE 7.4 Six types of joints

Type of joint	Movement at joint	Examples	Structure
Hinge	A convex portion of one bone fits into a concave portion of another bone. The movement reflects the movement of a household hinge and bracket; movement is limited to **flexion** and extension as the joint opens and closes. These joints therefore move in one plane only.	Elbow, knee (shown below) 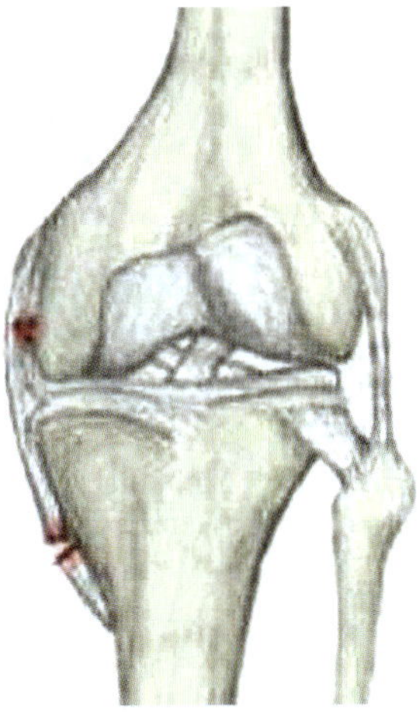	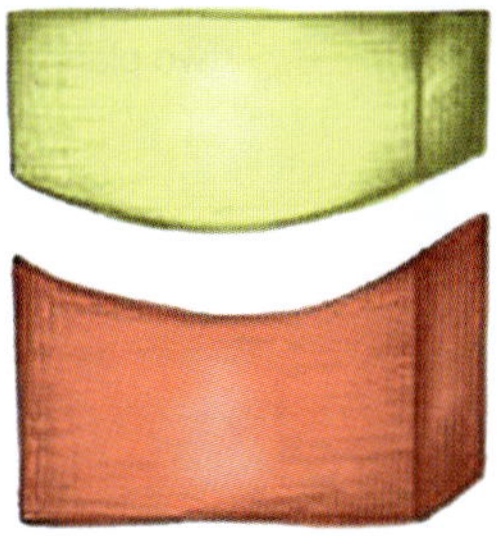
Pivot	A rounded part of one bone fits into the groove of another bone. These joints permit a rotation movement of one bone around another.	Radius and ulna, atlas and axis (shown below) 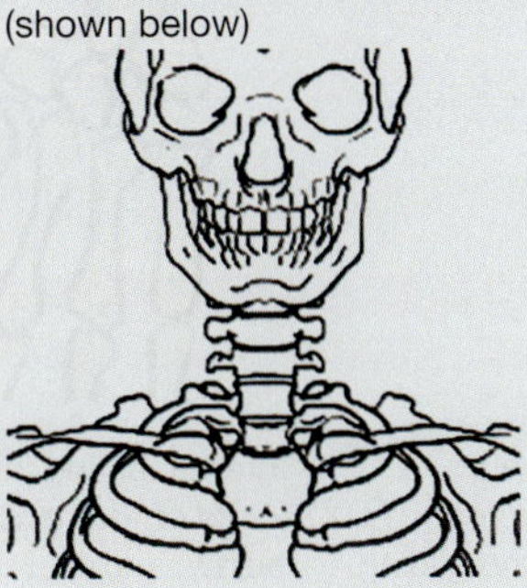	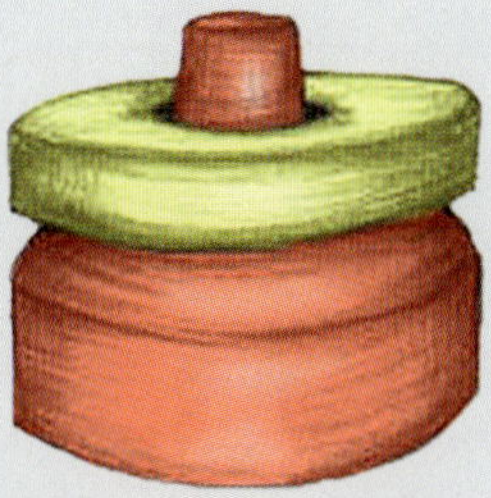
Ball and socket	The spherical end of one bone (the ball) fits into a concave socket of another bone. Movement can occur in several planes, including **abduction** and **adduction**.	Hip (shown below), shoulder 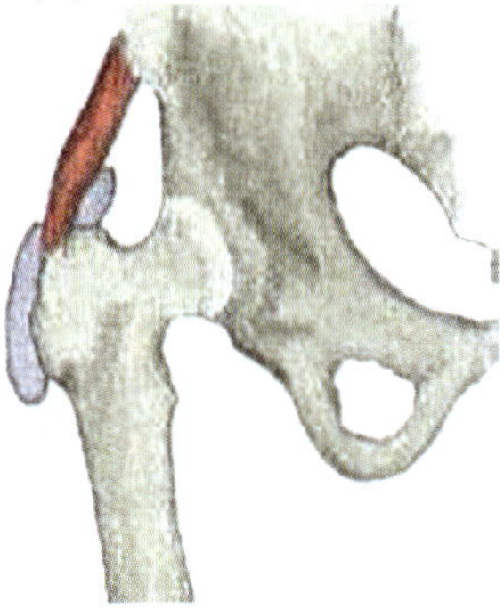	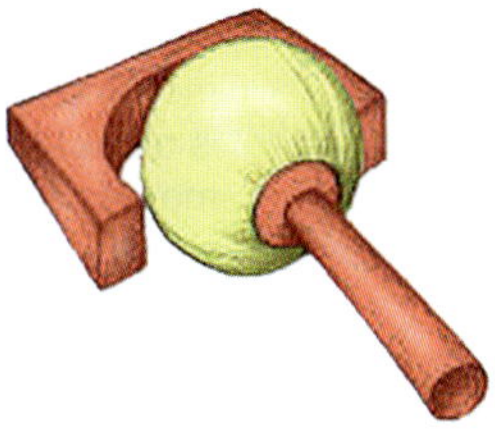

(continued)

TABLE 7.4 *(continued)*

Type of joint	Movement at joint	Examples	Structure
Condyloid	An oval surface of one bone fits into a concavity of another bone. Movement can occur in two planes.	Radiocarpal and metacarpophalangeal joints of the hand (shown below)	
Saddle	Similar to **condyloid joints**, but these joints permit greater movement. Movement can occur in three planes.	Carpometacarpal joints of the thumb (shown below)	
Gliding (plane)	These joints have a flat or slightly curved surface, permitting gliding movements. The joints are bound by ligaments, and movement in all directions is restricted. The joint moves back and forth and side to side.	Intertarsal and intercarpal joints of the hands (shown below) and feet	

CLINICAL CONSIDERATIONS

Osteoarthritis: a national health priority

The millions of movements that occur over a lifetime of movement inevitably result in wear and tear on the joints, particularly joints which bear a lot of weight and are involved in very basic movements like walking, often resulting in the degenerative condition osteoarthritis. It is estimated that 1 in 11 Australians have osteoarthritis (i.e. 9.3% of the population, or approximately 2.2 million people). While osteoarthritis affects people of all ages, it is thought that 1 in 3 Australians over the age of 75 have the condition. It is more prevalent in females, with the detrimental health effects most pronounced in those aged 45 and over (Australian Institute of Health and Welfare 2020).

The joint damage characterised by osteoarthritis is a roughening of the surface of the normally smooth and glassy hyaline articular cartilage, followed by inflammation in the affected joint as a result of the increased friction on movement. This process is quite gradual and can lead to the development of **osteophytes** (bone spurs) and eventually the complete wearing away of the articular cartilage. If the joint is one of the major weight-bearing joints, and particularly if the person is overweight, the bones ends can be forced together until they are rubbing directly against each other when the joint moves. The result is pain and stiffness in the joint; this is often worse after a period of rest, but reduces after activity.

The impact of osteoarthritis will differ from person to person; the care of those with osteoarthritis will depend on the assessment of individual needs. There is no cure for osteoarthritis, but there are many interventions that can be implemented to help improve the health and wellbeing of the person being cared for.

A multidisciplinary approach to care is required, be this in a hospital setting or in the person's own home. Adjustments to lifestyle — for example, an increase in exercise and the modification of footwear — can help. The administration of medicines to control pain and inflammation can also help the person carry out their activities of living in a more effective way, allowing the person to remain independent and continue with their normal activities as much as possible (see the medicines management box on diclofenac).

For the cases in which mobility is severely affected due to pain, there is also a surgical option; hip and knee replacements are now very common — the damaged bone ends can be replaced and/or resurfaced by metal or other resistant materials. This procedure is very effective and often gives osteoarthritis sufferers a new lease of life.

MEDICINES MANAGEMENT

Diclofenac

Skeletal conditions such as osteoarthritis, rheumatoid arthritis and gout often require both pharmacological and non-pharmacological therapies, with medication used to help manage symptoms such as inflammation and pain. Diclofenac is a commonly available non-steroidal anti-inflammatory drug (available in Australia under brand names such as Voltaren and Dencorub); it can be administered topically, orally, or via injection or suppository. Diclofenac has its action by reducing the production of prostaglandins that are involved in producing the inflammatory response and the associated pain, thus relieving the patient's pain.

Non-steroidal anti-inflammatory drugs such as diclofenac, however, are notorious for causing ulceration of the stomach due to the loss of protective prostaglandins. The concurrent use of drugs such as misoprostol, a synthetic prostaglandin, can help reduce such risks in patients who are at high risk for developing gastric or intestinal ulcers (e.g. patients with previous gastrointestinal bleeding or chronic renal failure). Misoprostol has a number of actions, including increasing the production of thick mucus in the stomach which protects the stomach wall, and reducing the production of stomach acid. The effects of misoprostol therefore counteract some of the side effects of the non-steroidal inflammatory drug.

Pharmacological management of these conditions is complicated by the presence of various comorbidities and possible adverse effects. For example, misoprostol should not be used by pregnant women as the misoprostol may cause premature labour or uterine rupture (miscarriage). This is because the prostaglandin is very important in the initiation of labour, and taking a drug containing it may initiate early labour. Likewise, those who have active gastric or intestinal bleeding should not use this medication. Furthermore, diclofenac can increase the risk of fatal heart attack or stroke; this risk is increased if the medication is used long term or if the person has heart disease. For these reasons, the use of such drugs are limited to the lowest dose required to control symptoms on an as-needed basis.

Prior to administering this medicine, the nurse must determine if the person is allergic to diclofenac or misoprostol, or if there is active gastric or intestinal bleeding. The drug should not be given until after a detailed medical history has been taken as it is contraindicated in some conditions (Australian Medicines Handbook 2020).

SUMMARY

The human skeleton is a dynamic, living structure that is constantly readjusting itself to perform optimally. It provides a supportive and protective framework for our body form, with its incredible strength and flexibility, and its ability to regenerate itself after damage. The skeleton also provides the levers which can be worked by the action of muscles to produce movements, from the tiniest flick of a fingertip to the powerful impulse that propels a sprinter out of the blocks when the starting gun fires. Impressive as this is, it is not all that our skeleton does for us. The red marrow inside some of our bones is the source of all our blood cells, which provide us with immunity and with the ability to transport oxygen around the body to the tissues. And because the skeleton represents such a huge store of deposited calcium, bones are also central to the homeostatic control of plasma calcium level, and act as a source of calcium to 'top up' plasma calcium when necessary, thus ensuring that all the myriad functions that calcium ions trigger are not disrupted by abnormal calcium concentrations in the blood.

KEY TERMS

abduction Movement away from the body's midline.
adduction Movement towards the body's midline.
articulations The meeting point for two bones at a joint.
ball and socket A synovial joint in which the rounded surface of one bone fits within the cup-shaped depression of the socket of the other bone.
calcification Deposition of mineral salts in a framework formed by collagen fibres.
cartilage Strong, tough material on the bone ends that helps to distribute the load within the joint; the slippery surface allows smooth movement between the bones; a type of connective tissue.
cartilaginous joints A joint where the bones are held together tightly by cartilage; little movement occurs in this joint. This joint does not have a synovial cavity.
collagen A protein that makes up most of the connective tissue.
condyloid joints A synovial joint that allows one oval-shaped bone to fit into an elliptical cavity of another.
diaphysis The shaft of a long bone.
epiphysis The end of long bone.
fibrous joints A type of joint that allows little or no movement.
flexion Movement at a joint which produces a decrease in the angle formed between the two bones.
fractures Breaks in a bone.
gliding A synovial joint whose articulating surfaces are usually flat, allowing only side-to-side or back-and-forth movement.
haemopoiesis The formation and development of blood cells in the bone marrow.
in utero Within the uterus.
lacuna A small, hollow space found in any tissue.
lamellar A concentric ring of hard, calcified matrix found in compact bones.
ligaments Tough, fibrous bands of connective tissue that hold the bones together at a joint.
marrow A sponge-like material found in the cavities of some bones. Red bone marrow, found in short, flat and irregular bones and the epiphyses of long bones, produces blood cells.
mesenchyme Embryonic connective tissue from which nearly all other connective tissue arises.
metaphysis The narrow transitional section of a long bone that lies between the diaphysis (bone shaft) and the epiphysis (bone end).
osseous Bony.
ossicle A small bone of the middle ear — the malleus, the incus, the stapes.
ossification The formation of bone; sometimes called osteogenesis.
osteoblasts Cells that are responsible for the formation of bone.
osteoclasts Large cells that are responsible for absorption and removal of bone.
osteocytes Cells that started as osteoblasts but become trapped within the bony matrix and serve a monitoring function.
osteon The basic unit of structure in adult compact bone.
osteophytes Overgrowth of new bone around the side of osteoarthritic joints; also known as spur growth.

periosteum Membrane covering bones, which consists of connective tissue, osteogenic cells and osteoblasts. This is vital for bone growth, repair and nutrition.
pivot A joint where a rounded or conical-shaped surface of a bone articulates with a ring formed partly by another bone or ligament, permitting a rotational movement; for example, shaking the head.
remodelling Replacement of old bone by new.
resorption Removal of existing tissue.
saddle A synovial joint articulates the surface of a saddle-shaped bone on the other bone that is said to be shaped like the legs of the rider.
spongy (cancellous) bone A type of bone recognisable by its 'holey' or spongy appearance, due to the latticework of bone struts. It is found in the middle of most bones, between the outer compact bone and the inner cavity. It helps to provide some strength while keeping weight down.
synovial cavity The space between the articulating bones of a synovial joint, filled with synovial fluid.
synovial fluid A clear pale yellow, viscous fluid that lubricates and cushions joints.

ACTIVITIES

TRUE OR FALSE

1. The skeleton is a living organism.
2. There are more bones in adults than in babies.
3. Bone stores and releases calcium.
4. The ribs protect the pancreas.
5. Yellow bone marrow produces red blood cells.
6. There is no difference between the weight and size of male and female bones.
7. The patella is located in the humerus.
8. Osteoblasts forms new bone.
9. Replacement of old bone by new is called remodelling.
10. The axial skeleton has more bones than the appendicular skeleton.

MATCH EACH BONE TO ITS CORRECT SHAPE

Shape	Bone
Irregular bone	Sternum
Long bone	Zygomatic
Flat bone	Metacarpal
Short bone	Hyoid
	Tarsal
	Femur
	Ethmoid
	Scapula

FIND OUT MORE

1. Why do healthy bones require exercise?
2. Describe the composition of bone.
3. How does the skeletal system help to maintain homeostasis?
4. In bone remodelling, how do osteoblasts and osteoclasts work together?
5. What happens to bone as we age?
6. What is synovial fluid?
7. Describe the healing that occurs after a fracture has been sustained.

8 Discuss intramembranous ossification.
9 What factors are essential for bone remodelling?
10 Where in the body are the two sesamoid bones and what are they called?

CONDITIONS

The following is a list of conditions that are associated with the skeletal system. Take some time and write notes about each of the conditions. You may make the notes taken from textbooks or other resources, or you may make the notes from patients you have cared for. If you are doing this, you must ensure that you adhere to the rules of confidentiality.

Fractured neck of femur
Osteoarthritis
Osteoporosis
Gout
Osteomyelitis
Osteosarcoma
Rheumatoid arthritis

REFERENCES

Australian Institute of Health and Welfare (2020) Osteoarthritis. www.aihw.gov.au/reports/chronic-musculoskeletal-conditions/osteoarthritis (accessed 13 January 2021).

Australian Medicines Handbook (2020) Diclofenac. https://amhonline.amh.net.au/chapters/rheumatological-drugs/drugs-other-musculoskeletal-conditions/nsaids/diclofenac?menu=vertical (accessed 13 January 2021).

Chapman, H. (2018) Nursing theories 4: adherence and concordance. *Nursing Times* [online] 114(2): 50. www.nursingtimes.net/roles/nurse-educators/nursing-theories-4-adherence-and-concordance-15-01-2018 (accessed January 2021).

ConnectGroups (n.d.) https://connectgroups.org.au (accessed February 2021).

International Association for the Study of Pain (2018) Declaration of Montréal. www.iasp-pain.org/DeclarationofMontreal (accessed January 2021).

Levett-Jones, T. (2013). *Clinical Reasoning: Learning to Think Like a Nurse*. Pearson Australia.

Marsell, R. and Einhorn, T.A. (2011) The biology of fracture healing. *Injury* 42(6): 551–555.

Pain Management Network (2021) Assessment. www.aci.health.nsw.gov.au/chronic-pain/health-professionals/assessment (accessed January 2021).

The Royal Australian College of General Practitioners and Osteoporosis Australia (2017) *Osteoporosis Prevention, Diagnosis and Management in Postmenopausal Women and Men Over 50 years of Age*, 2nd edn. East Melbourne, Vic: RACGP.

Tortora, G.J. (2008) *A Brief Atlas of the Human Skeleton, Surface Anatomy and Selected Medical Images*. New York: John Wiley & Sons, Inc.

Tortora, G.J. and Derrickson, B.H. (2009) *Principles of Anatomy and Physiology*, 12th edn. Hoboken, NJ: John Wiley & Sons, Inc.

Tortora, G.J. and Derrickson, B.H. (2014) *Principles of Anatomy and Physiology*, 15th edn. Hoboken, NJ: John Wiley & Sons, Inc.
Weise, M., Stacy De-Levi, S., Barnes, K.M., Gafni, R.I., Abad, V. and Baron, J. (2001) Effects of estrogen on growth plate senescence and epiphyseal fusion. *Proceedings of the National Academy of Sciences* 98(12): 6871–6876.
Worrall, H., Schweizer, R., Marks, E., Yuan, L., Lloyd, C. and Ramjan, R. (2018) The effectiveness of support groups: a literature review. *Faculty of Science, Medicine and Health — Papers: part A. 5441*. https://ro.uow.edu.au/cgi/viewcontent.cgi?article=6502&context=smhpapers (accessed January 2021).

FURTHER READING

ARTHRITIS AUSTRALIA

www.arthritisaustralia.com.au

This organisation works with patients and healthcare professionals to provide support and information for those living with all forms of arthritis, helping them to remain active. They fund high-quality research, educate healthcare professionals and provide information to those with arthritis and their carers.

AUSTRALIA AND NEW ZEALAND SARCOMA ASSOCIATION

https://sarcoma.org.au

The Australia and New Zealand Sarcoma Association (ANZSA) is the peak body for the sarcoma community. ANZSA aims to improve outcomes for sarcoma patients through research, education and awareness of sarcomas and related tumours. Sarcomas are rare cancers developing in the muscle, bone, nerves, cartilage, tendons, blood vessels, and the fatty and fibrous tissues.

OSTEOPOROSIS AUSTRALIA

www.osteoporosis.org.au

A national not-for-profit organisation responsible for providing osteoporosis information and services to the community and health professionals.

ACKNOWLEDGEMENTS

Photo: © Bunsinth-Nan-Pua / Shutterstock.com
Photo: © tommaso79 / Shutterstock.com
Photo: © fizkes / Shutterstock.com
Photo: © Rawpixel.com / Shutterstock.com
Photo: © Tetra Images, LLC / Alamy Stock Photo

CHAPTER 8

The circulatory system

TEST YOUR PRIOR KNOWLEDGE

- Compare and contrast arteries and veins.
- List the formed elements of the blood.
- List the functions of the blood cells.
- Discuss the life cycle of a red blood cell.
- List the functions of the lymphatic system.

LEARNING OUTCOMES

After reading this chapter you will be able to:

8.1 discuss the normal composition of blood

8.2 list the functions and explain the life cycle of the red blood cells, white blood cells and platelets

8.3 describe some of the differences between an artery and a vein

8.4 discuss the functions of the lymphatic circulation.

Body map

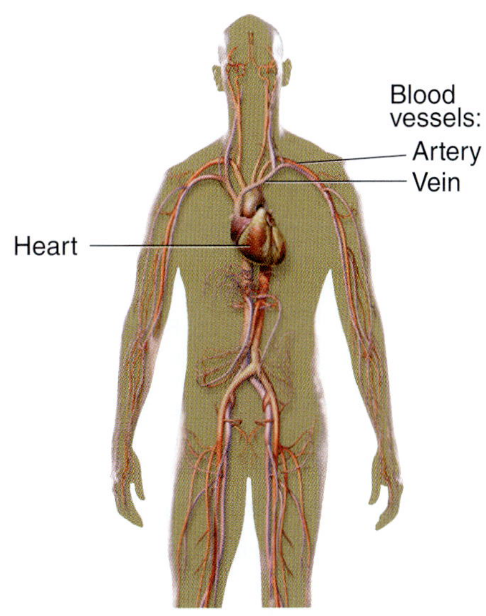

Introduction

The circulatory system is a complex system which deals with the distribution of nutrients, gases, **electrolytes** and hormones, as well as the removal of waste products of metabolism and other substances. The circulatory system includes the heart, the blood, the blood vessels and the lymphatic system. The blood vessels transport blood around the body.

Blood consists of formed elements within a fluid portion called plasma. The blood vessels form a network that allows blood to flow from the heart to all living cells and back to the heart. Blood has numerous functions including the transportation of nutrients, respiratory gases such as oxygen and carbon dioxide, metabolic wastes such as urea and uric acid, hormones, electrolytes and antibodies. As the blood is circulating throughout the body, cells are constantly exchanging nutrients, hormones, electrolytes, oxygen and other substances with it, as well as excreting unwanted wastes into the blood.

Blood is transported throughout the body by a network of blood vessels, some of which lead away from and some which return to the heart. The main types of blood vessels include arteries, arterioles, capillaries, venules and veins; each is designed to carry out a specific role(s). Another important part of the circulatory system is the lymphatic system, which drains a fluid called lymph. The lymphatic system consists of the lymph vessels, lymph nodes and lymph glands such as the spleen and the thymus gland.

This chapter will focus on the composition, structure and functions of various blood cells, the structure and functions of the blood vessels, factors affecting blood pressure and the structure and functions of the lymphatic system.

8.1 Components of blood

LEARNING OBJECTIVE 8.1 Discuss the normal composition of blood.

Blood consists of formed elements such as red blood cells (erythrocytes), leucocytes (white blood cells) and platelets (also called thrombocytes). Plasma, which is the fluid portion of blood, contains different types of proteins and other soluble molecules. When a blood sample is centrifuged to separate these components, the formed elements account for 45 per cent of the blood and plasma makes up 55 per cent of the total blood volume. Normally, more than 99 per cent of the formed elements are cells named for their red colour (red blood cells). White blood cells (pale in appearance) and platelets comprise less than 1 per cent of the formed elements. Between the plasma and erythrocytes lies the buffy coat, which consists of white blood cells and platelets (figure 8.1). The percentage of the formed elements constitutes the haematocrit or packed cell volume. Haematocrit is a blood test that measures the percentage of red blood cells in whole blood. The volume of blood is constant unless a person has physiological problems, such as haemorrhage.

FIGURE 8.1 Components of blood

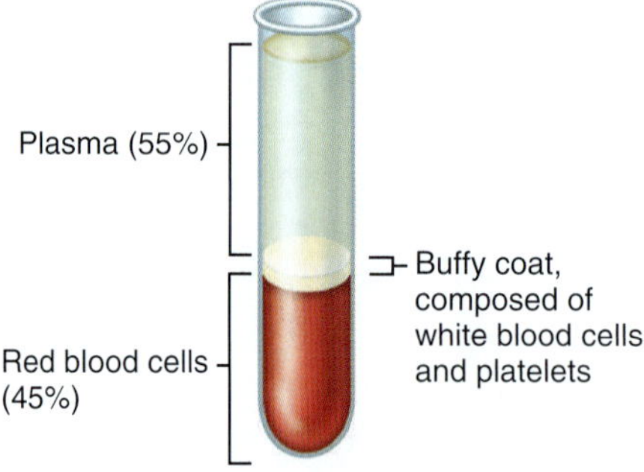

Source: Tortora and Derrickson (2009). Reproduced with permission of John Wiley & Sons.

Thus, blood is composed of plasma, a yellowish liquid containing nutrients, hormones, minerals and various cells, mainly red blood cells, white blood cells and platelets (figure 8.2). Both the formed elements and the plasma play an important role in homeostasis.

FIGURE 8.2 Cells of the blood

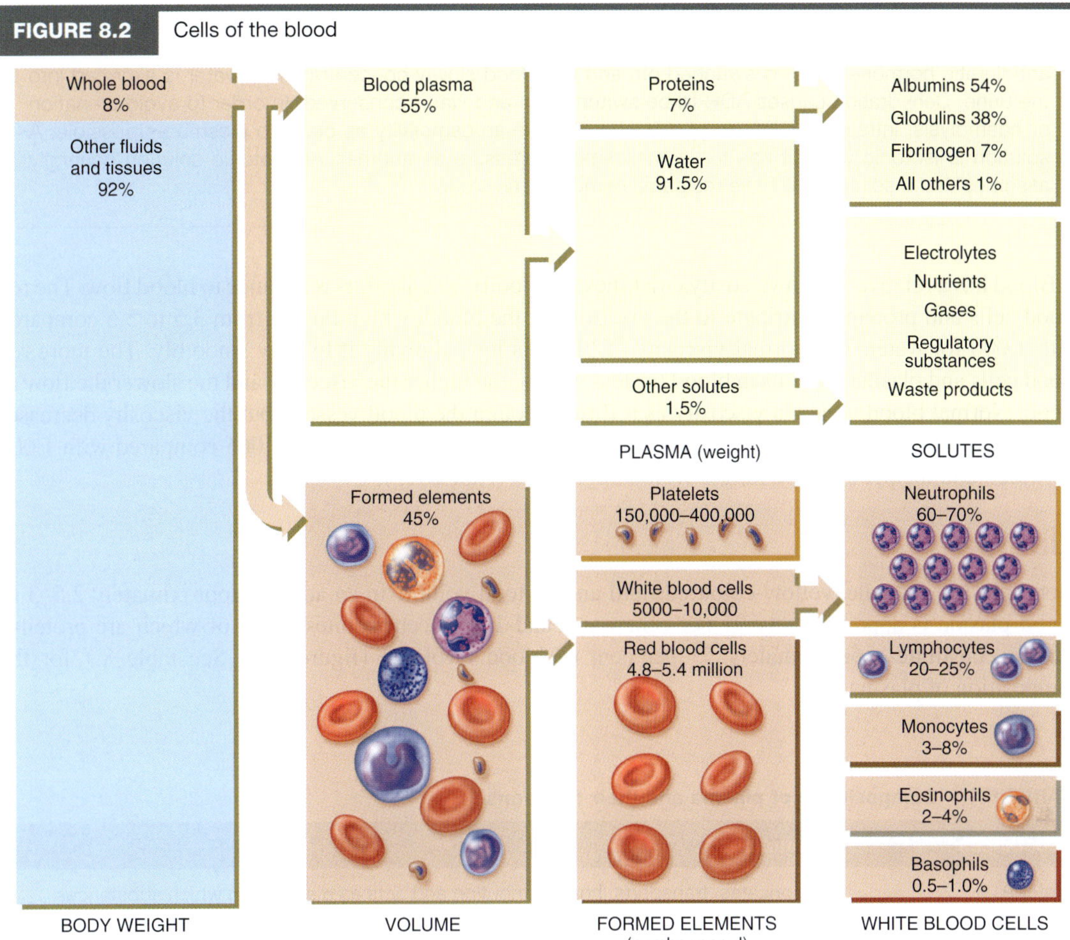

Source: Tortora and Derrickson (2009). Reproduced with permission of John Wiley & Sons.

Properties of blood

The average adult has a blood volume of approximately 5 L, which accounts for 7–9 per cent of the body's weight. Men have 5–6 L and women have 4–5 L. Blood is thicker, denser and flows much slower than water due to the red blood cells and large plasma proteins such as albumin and fibrinogen. Plasma proteins, including albumin, fibrinogen, prothrombin and the gamma globulins, constitute about 8 per cent of the blood plasma in the body. These proteins help maintain water balance (retaining fluid in the blood); as such, they affect **osmotic pressure**, increase blood viscosity and help maintain blood pressure. All the plasma proteins except the gamma globulins are synthesised in the liver.

HOMEOSTATIC IMBALANCE

Plasma osmolality

The normal osmolality of **extracellular** fluid is 285–295 mOsmol/kg. The osmolality of the blood is important for the cells to survive. Because osmolality affects the movement of fluids (with water moving from high to low areas to maintain homeostasis), changes in the osmolality of blood can lead to the unwanted movement of water. If blood osmolality is approximately 600 mOsmol (i.e. higher than normal, or **hypertonic**), the red blood cells could crenate (shrivel up) and die, as water leaves the cells to try and balance the osmolality; if, however, the osmolality is below 150 mOsmol (i.e. lower than normal, **hypotonic**), haemolysis (rupture) of the red blood cells could occur as water travels into the cell (like overinflating a balloon!). Massive haemolysis can be fatal, due to the ensuing lack of red blood cells. Plasma osmolality is tightly controlled by homeostatic mechanisms. Changes in plasma osmolality are detected by osmoreceptors in the circulatory system, directing specific regions of the brain (the hypothalamus). If the osmolality is too low (i.e. the blood is too dilute) the secretion of antidiuretic hormone (ADH) is switched off, and the blood slowly concentrates as water is excreted into the urine. Dehydration causes ADH to be switched on and water conserved. In order to avoid crenation or haemolysis, intravenous infusion fluids should have an osmolality as close to plasma as possible. A solution is isotonic when it has the same osmotic pressure as another. An isotonic solution generally assumes that a solution will have the same osmolality as blood.

Blood has a relatively high viscosity (stickiness of blood), which offers resistance to blood flow. The red blood cells and proteins contribute to the viscosity of the blood, which ranges from 3.5 to 5.5 compared with 1.000 for water. The normal viscosity of blood is low, allowing it to flow smoothly. The more red blood cells and plasma proteins in blood (or less water), the higher the viscosity and the slower the flow of blood. Normal blood varies in viscosity as it flows through the blood vessels, but the viscosity decreases as it reaches the capillaries. The specific gravity (density) of blood is 1.045–1.065 compared with 1.000 for water, and the pH of blood ranges from 7.35 to 7.45 (Nair 2013).

Plasma

Blood plasma is a pale, yellow-coloured fluid and its total volume in an adult is approximately 2.5–3 L. Blood plasma is approximately 91 per cent water and 10 per cent solutes, most of which are proteins. Plasma constitutes approximately 55 per cent of blood's volume (figure 8.2). See table 8.1 for the composition of plasma.

TABLE 8.1 Compositions of plasma and their functions

Substances	Functions
Water 91%	Lubricates, transports, heat distribution and acts as a solvent in which substances are dissolved
Plasma protein • albumin • globulin • prothrombin • fibrinogen	Responsible for maintaining osmotic pressure of blood (via colloid **osmosis**) and providing blood viscosity. These proteins carry out various specific functions, such as transporting hormones, fatty acids and calcium; providing protection from infections; transporting insoluble substances by allowing them to bind to protein molecules; and regulating pH of blood. An imbalance of plasma proteins can lead a patient to experience symptoms ranging from abnormally dilated blood vessels to a weakened immune system.
Electrolytes • sodium • potassium • calcium • bicarbonate • phosphate • chloride	Help maintain osmotic pressure, water distribution and cell functions
Nutrients • amino acids • fatty acids • glucose • glycerol • vitamins • minerals	Cell function growth and development
Gases	Cellular function and regulation of blood pH
Enzymes, hormones and vitamins	**Chemical reactions**, regulate growth and development and cofactors for enzymatic reaction

Waste products • urea • uric acid • creatinine • bilirubin • ammonia	Broken down and transported by blood to organs of excretion

Source: Adapted from Jenkins and Tortora (2013).

Water in plasma

Water constitutes approximately 91 per cent of plasma and is available to cells, tissues and extracellular fluid of the body to maintain homeostasis. It is considered the liquid portion of the blood. It is a solvent where chemical reactions between **intracellular** and extracellular reactions occur. Water contains solutes (dissolved within it); for example, see the list of electrolytes in table 8.1 whose concentrations change to meet body needs.

8.2 Functions of blood

LEARNING OBJECTIVE 8.2 List the functions and explain the life cycle of the red blood cells, white blood cells and platelets.

The functions of the blood are the following.

- *Transportation.* The blood is the means whereby all nourishment and respiratory gases are transported into and out of the cells.
- *Maintaining body temperature.* Blood helps to maintain the body temperature by distributing the heat produced by the chemical activity of the cells evenly, throughout the body.
- *Maintaining the acid–base balance.* Blood pH is maintained by the excretion or reabsorption of hydrogen ions and bicarbonate ions.
- *Regulation of fluid balance.* When the blood reaches the kidneys, excess fluid is excreted or reabsorbed to maintain fluid balance.
- *Removal of waste products.* The blood removes all waste products from the tissues and cells. These waste products are transported to the appropriate organs for excretion — lungs, kidneys, intestine, skin and so on.
- *Blood clotting.* By the mechanism of clotting, loss of blood cells and body fluids is prevented.
- *Defence action.* The blood aids in the defence of the body against the invasion of microorganisms and their toxins due to:
  - the phagocyte action of neutrophils and monocytes
  - the presence of antibodies and antitoxins.

CLINICAL CONSIDERATIONS

Intravenous fluid therapy

Intravenous (IV) fluid replacement is a common treatment used in hospitals and community settings to restore blood circulating volume, vital electrolytes and glucose.

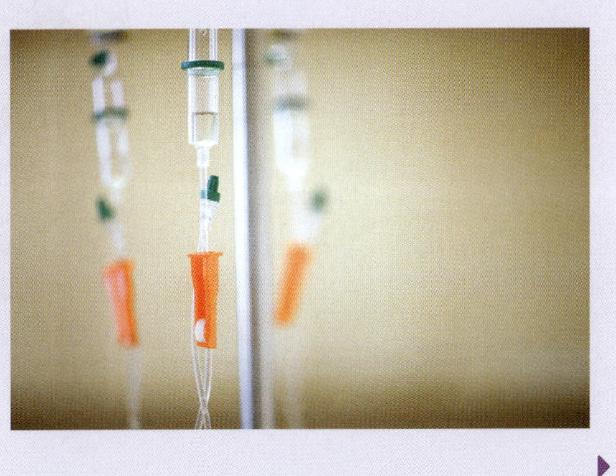

Acute fluid losses, which can occur from prolonged episodes of vomiting and diarrhoea, or dehydration in the very young or elderly populations, can lead to **hypovolaemia** (low blood volume) and is potentially fatal. Vital signs like low blood pressure and a high pulse and respirations are indicators of the body's attempt to compensate for intravascular fluid deficit. The severity of the fluid deficit is displayed through how much a vital sign deviates from the normal.

Another condition for which patients may require fluid replacement is sepsis, a life-threatening infection which causes circulatory collapse.

The aim of fluid replacement is to re-establish homeostatic fluid balance. The monitoring of patients during fluid therapy must be carefully managed.

Common conditions that require fluid replacement include:

- prolonged or severe vomiting
- prolonged or severe diarrhoea
- infection
- gastrointestinal (GI) suctioning
- heart failure
- septic shock
- respiratory failure
- haemorrhage
- cardiovascular collapse.

An accurate fluid balance chart must be maintained to track the intake and output of fluids in the body. Patients receiving IV fluids should also be observed for the normalisation of vital signs, a good indicator of how adequately volume is being replaced.

Note that IV fluids are replaced cautiously in patients with chronic heart failure (CHF). This is because supplemental IV fluids may cause additional stress to an already weak heart and lead to fluid overload (Pellicori et al. 2015). Patients with CHF may be on restricted IV fluid regimens and need to be weighed daily to observe for signs of fluid retention.

Formation of blood cells

Red blood cells and most white blood cells and platelets are produced in the bone marrow. The red blood and white blood cells and the platelets are the formed elements of blood (figure 8.3). The bone marrow is the soft fatty substance found in bone cavities. Within the bone marrow, all blood cells originate from a single type of unspecialised cell called a stem cell. When a stem cell divides, it first becomes an immature red blood cell, white blood cell or platelet-producing cell. The immature cell then divides, matures further and ultimately becomes a mature red blood cell, white blood cell or platelet (figure 8.1). Although this occurs mostly within the red bone marrow, some white blood cells develop in yellow bone marrow (see the chapter on the skeletal system and figure 17.1 in the chapter on the immune system).

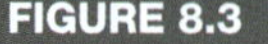

FIGURE 8.3 Formed elements of blood

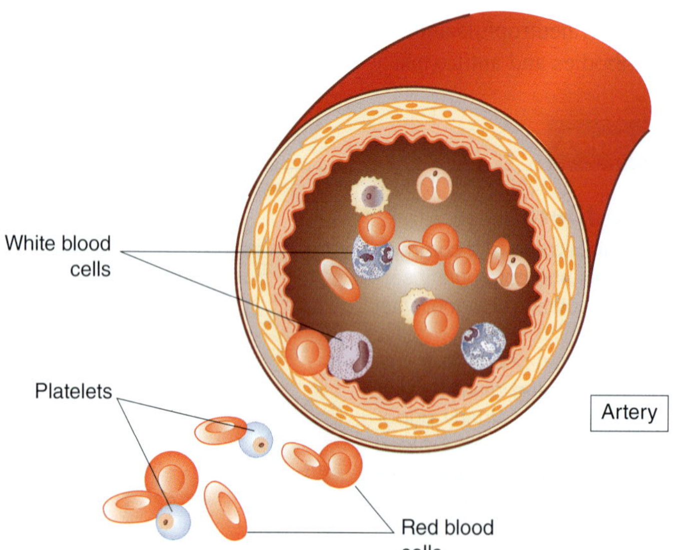

In order to produce blood cells, multipotent (also called pluripotent) stem cells divide into myeloid and lymphoid stem cells in the bone marrow. The myeloid stem cells further subdivide in the bone marrow to produce red blood cells, platelets (thrombocytes), basophils, eosinophils, neutrophils and monocytes (types of white blood cell). The lymphoid stem cells begin the development in the bone marrow as B- and T-lymphocytes. B-lymphocytes continue development in bone marrow, before migrating to other lymph organs such as the lymph nodes, spleen or tonsils. T-lymphocytes continue their development in the thymus, and may then migrate to other lymph tissues.

Red blood cells

Red blood cells (also known as erythrocytes) are the most abundant blood cells. They are biconcave discs (think of two dinner plates held back to back; see figure 8.4) and contain oxygen-carrying protein called haemoglobin. The biconcave shape is maintained by a network of proteins called spectrin. This network of protein allows the red blood cells to change shape as they are transported through the blood vessel. The **plasma membrane** of a red blood cell is strong and flexible. There are approximately 4 million to 5.5 million red blood cells in each cubic millimetre of blood. They are a pale buff colour that appears lighter in the centre. Young red blood cells contain a nucleus; however, the nucleus is absent in a mature red blood cell and without any **organelles** such as mitochondria, thus increasing the oxygen-carrying capacity of the red blood cell.

FIGURE 8.4 Red blood cells

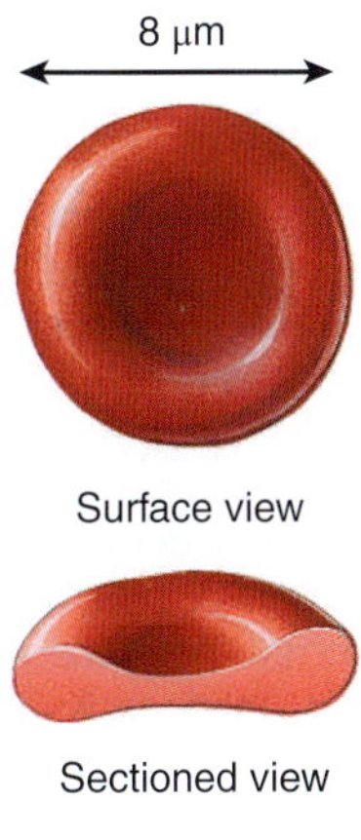

Source: Tortora and Derrickson (2009). Reproduced with permission of John Wiley & Sons.

The main function of haemoglobin in the red blood cell is to transport oxygen and carbon dioxide (approximately 20 per cent of carbon dioxide is carried in this way). As the blood flows through the capillaries in the tissues, carbon dioxide is picked up by the haemoglobin and oxygen is released. As the blood reaches the lungs, carbon dioxide is released and oxygen is picked up by the haemoglobin molecules. As red blood cells lack mitochondria to produce energy (**adenosine triphosphate**), they utilise anaerobic respiration to produce energy and do not use any of the oxygen they are transporting; movement of gases into and out of the red blood cell is via **passive transport**. Apart from transporting oxygen and carbon dioxide, the haemoglobin plays an important role in maintaining blood pressure and blood flow.

Haemoglobin

Haemoglobin is composed of a protein called globin bound to the iron-containing pigments called haem. Each globin molecule has four polypeptide chains consisting of two alpha and two beta chains (figure 8.5). Each haemoglobin molecule has four atoms of iron, and each atom of iron transports one molecule of oxygen; therefore, one molecule of haemoglobin transports four molecules of oxygen. There are approximately 250 million haemoglobin molecules in one red blood cell; therefore, one red blood cell transports 1 billion molecules of oxygen. At the capillary end the haemoglobin releases the oxygen molecule into the **interstitial** fluid, which is then transported into the cells.

FIGURE 8.5 Haemoglobin molecule

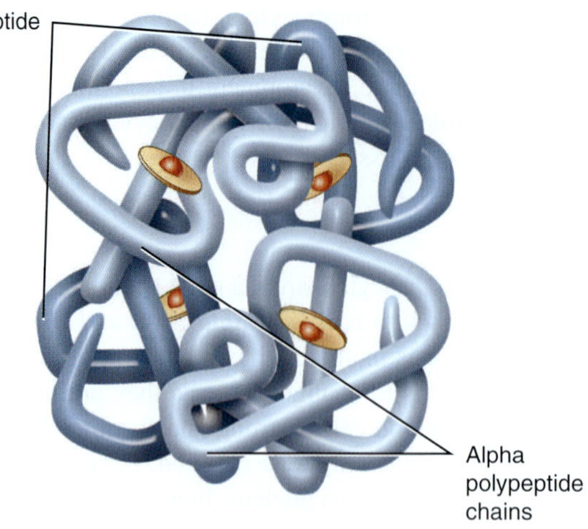

Source: Tortora and Derrickson (2009). Reproduced with permission of John Wiley & Sons.

MEDICINES MANAGEMENT

Iron deficiency anaemia

Anaemia occurs when the body does not have enough red, oxygen-carrying blood cells, which means the body's tissues and cells are not getting enough oxygen. It affects approximately 10 per cent of non-pregnant young women, and is estimated to be highly prevalent in Indigenous communities. Other at-risk groups include the very young and the very old, as well as those with restricted diets such as vegetarians and vegans.

Treatment for iron deficiency anaemia usually involves taking iron supplements and changing the diet to increase the iron levels, as well as treating the underlying cause. Iron supplements may be prescribed to restore the iron missing from the body; iron can also be restored via intravenous iron preparations. The most commonly prescribed supplement is ferrous sulphate which is taken as a tablet two or three times a day, often in tandem with appropriate dietary changes. Nurses need to be aware that patients receiving iron tablets may experience:

- abdominal pain
- constipation or diarrhoea
- heartburn
- feeling sick
- black stools (faeces).

Black stools may also result from an upper gastrointestinal bleed. If these symptoms persist, advise the patient to see their GP so that prompt action can be taken to alleviate the side effects.

See Baird-Gunning and Bromley (2016).

Formation of red blood cells

Erythroblasts undergo development in the red bone marrow to form red blood cells through a process known as erythropoiesis (figure 17.1). During maturation, red blood cells lose their nucleus and organelles and gain more haemoglobin molecules, thus increasing the amount of oxygen they transport. Mature red blood cells do not have a nucleus; their life span is approximately 120 days. It is estimated that approximately 2 million red blood cells are destroyed per second; however, an equal number are replaced each time to maintain the balance. The production of red blood cells is controlled by the hormone erythropoietin (EPO), which is produced by the kidney. Other essential components for the synthesis of red blood cells include:

- iron
- folic acid
- vitamin B_{12}.

CLINICALLY REASONED EPISODE OF CARE

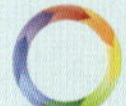

Thalassaemia

Consider the patient situation

Cristiana is a 5-year-old girl who has been brought into the general practice by her parents, Samara and Leo, as she has been unwell. She is seen by the practice nurse.

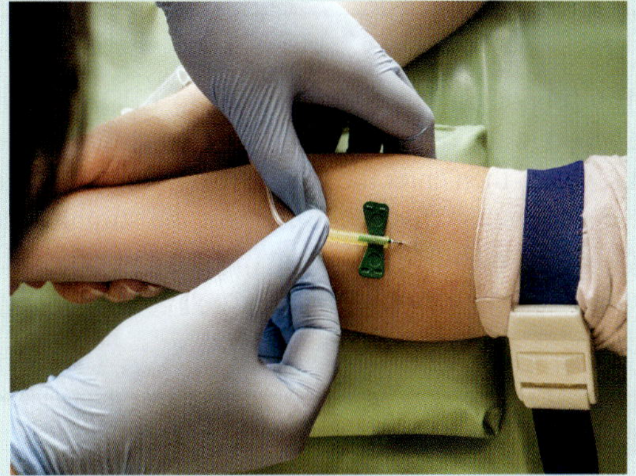

Collect cues and information

Samara notes that Cristiana appears to take longer to recover from common childhood illnesses and injuries. Samara is of Maltese descent. Cristiana has been sleeping more and is short of breath after activities; she is an otherwise healthy child who has hit all of the developmental milestones, although she has always been on the smaller end of the growth percentiles.

On arrival to the practice, Cristiana appears pale and has slightly yellow corneas. She is noted to be underweight for her age.

Process information

Thalassaemia is a genetically inherited anaemia caused by the abnormal formation of haemoglobin. People with thalassaemia produce either no or too little haemoglobin, which is used by red blood cells to carry oxygen around the body. Symptoms of thalassaemia include fatigue, weakness, paleness, slow growth, shortness of breath and skeletal deformities.

Thalassaemia is prevalent among Mediterranean cultures and ranges in severity. Due to the decreased oxygen-carrying haemoglobin, the body's ability to fight infection is impeded; thus people with thalassaemia are considered to be immunocompromised.

In its major form, people with the condition require regular blood transfusions and may have a limited life expectancy. Mild forms may not need treatment.

Cristiana's blood results report that she has a low haemoglobin count and small red blood cells. She is subsequently diagnosed with thalassaemia minor. Thalassaemia minor refers to people who have genetic changes in one copy of the HBB gene or in one copy in both HBA1 and HBA2 genes.

Establish goals

1. Refer to specialist nurse educator
2. Address nutritional needs
3. Commence treatment plan

Nursing actions

1. Refer to specialist nurse educator.
   Rationale:
   - Specialist nurse educators are well placed to provide targeted and detailed information about specific conditions.
   - Families should be educated so that they have a working knowledge of the condition, including treatment options and when and where to seek help.
2. Refer to dietician.
   Rationale:
   - People with thalassaemia can improve their condition through a healthy balanced diet that is low in fat and iron.
   - A dietician can work with families to assess their needs and create a diet plan which will encourage red blood cell production and energy.
3. Commence treatment for thalassaemia.
   Rationale:
   - Cristiana has been prescribed vitamin B supplements and folic acid. Vitamin B is important for cell health and red blood cell development; it improves energy levels and digestion and promotes nerve and muscle function. Folic acid is also essential for red blood cell development and growth.
   - Education on the timing and dosage of medication administration is essential to successful treatment regimes.

Evaluate outcomes

At her review three months later, Cristiana's blood tests show an improved haemoglobin count and Samara reports that Cristiana's energy levels have increased.

Reflect on new processes and learning

If a specialist nurse educator is not available, what learning and education resources are available for practice nurses to help educate patients and families?

Source: Based on the Clinical Reasoning Cycle, Levett-Jones (2013).

Erythropoietin, often abbreviated to EPO, is a hormone produced by the kidneys and transported by the blood to the bone marrow. In the bone marrow, erythropoietin stimulates the production of red blood cells, which then enter the bloodstream. The production and release of erythropoietin is through a negative feedback system (figure 8.6), where the stimulus (low oxygen levels, hypoxia) may result from factors such as low red blood cell count (e.g. anaemia, blood loss) or even impaired oxygen intake (e.g. respiratory problems, change in atmospheric oxygen levels).

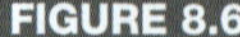

FIGURE 8.6 Negative feedback for erythropoiesis

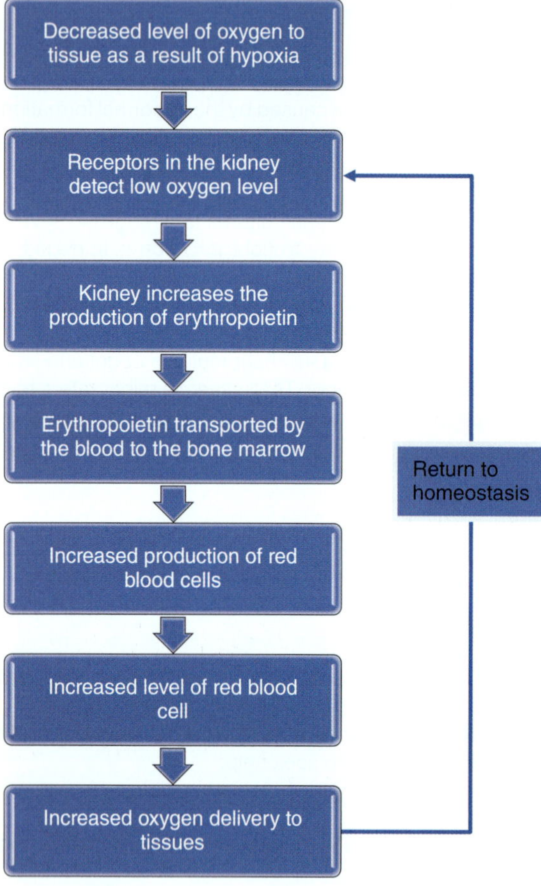

Life cycle of the red blood cell

Without a nucleus and other organelles, the red blood cell cannot synthesise new structures to replace the ones that are damaged, hence the limited life span. The breakdown (haemolysis) of the red blood cell is carried out by white blood cells called macrophages in the spleen, liver and the bone marrow (figure 8.7). The globin is broken down into individual amino acids which are then reused for protein synthesis. Iron is separated from haem and is stored in the muscles and the liver and reused in the bone marrow to manufacture new red blood cells. Haem is the portion of the haemoglobin that is converted to bilirubin and is transported by plasma albumin to the liver and eventually secreted in bile. In the large intestine, bacteria convert bilirubin into urobilinogen, some of which is reabsorbed into the bloodstream where it is converted into a yellow pigment called urobilin, which is excreted in urine, giving the urine a yellowish colour. The remainder of the urobilinogen is eliminated in faeces as a brown pigment called stercobilin. For this reason, pale-coloured stools can indicate issues with bile production/removal.

FIGURE 8.7 Destruction of the red blood cell

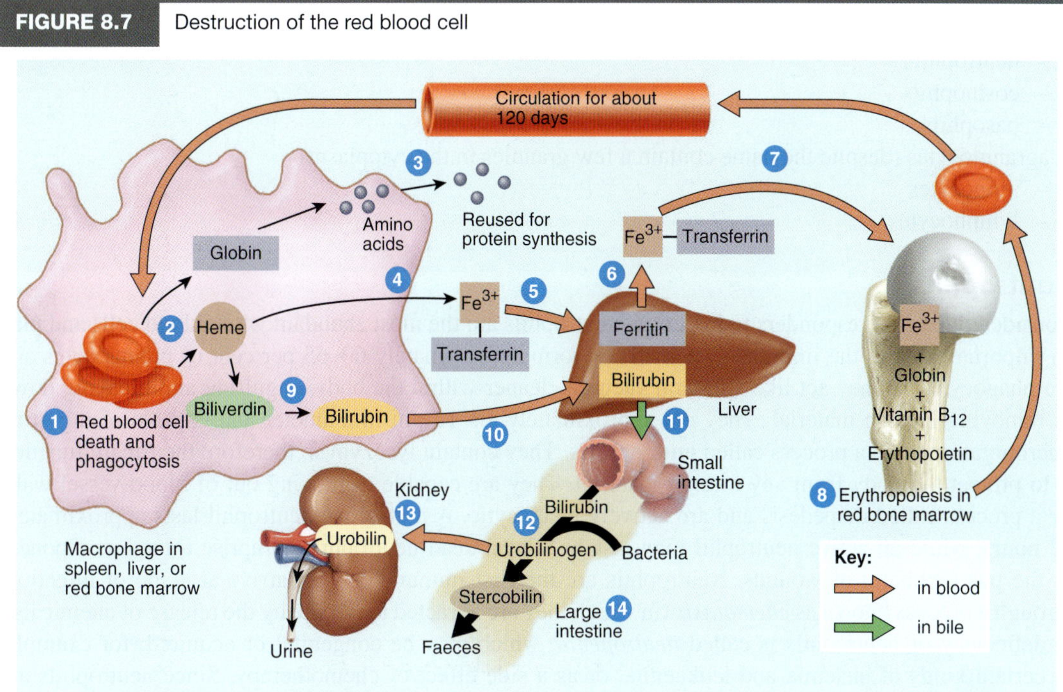

Source: Tortora and Derrickson (2009). Reproduced with permission of John Wiley & Sons.

Transport of respiratory gases

The major role of red blood cells is to transport oxygen from the lungs to the tissues. The oxygen in the alveoli (air sac) of the lungs combines with iron molecules in the haemoglobin of red blood cells to form oxyhaemoglobin. This is then transported by the blood to the tissues. As the oxygen level in the red blood cell increases it becomes bright red, and when the level of oxygen content drops the colour changes to dark bluish-red.

In addition to transporting oxygen from the lungs to the body tissues, red blood cells transport carbon dioxide from the tissues to the lungs. Carbon dioxide is transported in three ways:

- 10 per cent of the carbon dioxide is dissolved in the plasma
- 20 per cent of the carbon dioxide combines with haemoglobin of the red blood cell to form carbamino-haemoglobin
- 70 per cent of the carbon dioxide reacts with water to form carbonic acid, which is converted to bicarbonate and hydrogen ions:

$$CO_2 + H_2O \xleftrightarrow{\text{carbonic anhydrase}} \underset{\text{carbonic acid}}{H_2CO_3} \leftrightarrow \underset{\text{bicarbonate ion}}{HCO_3^-} + \underset{\text{hydrogen ion}}{H^+}$$

The reaction occurs primarily in red blood cells, which contain large amounts of carbonic anhydrase (an enzyme that facilitates the reaction). Once the bicarbonate ions are formed, they move out of the red blood cells into the plasma. At the lungs, this reaction can move in the opposite direction, forming water and carbon dioxide for removal (and maintaining blood pH levels).

White blood cells

White blood cells are also known as leucocytes. There are approximately 5000–10 000 white blood cells in every cubic millimetre of blood. The number may increase in infections to approximately 25 000 per cubic millimetre of blood, as the body attempts to fight the infection. An increase in white blood cells is called leucocytosis, and an abnormally low level of white blood cell is called leucopenia. Unlike red blood cells, white blood cells have nuclei and they are able to move out of blood vessel walls into the tissues. White blood cells are also able to produce a continuous supply of energy, unlike red blood cells. Finally, they are able to synthesise proteins, and thus their life span can be from a few days to years. There are two main types of white blood cells:

- granulocytes (contain granules in the **cytoplasm**)
  - neutrophils
  - eosinophils
  - basophils
- agranulocytes (despite the name contain a few granules in the cytoplasm)
  - monocytes
  - lymphocytes.

Neutrophils

Considered the first responders to infection, neutrophils are the most abundant white blood cells and play an important role in the immune system. They form approximately 60–65 per cent of granulocytes and are phagocytes — they act like a natural vacuum cleaner within the body, engulfing and breaking down or removing foreign material. They are approximately 10–12 μm in diameter and capable of ingesting microorganisms via a process called **endocytosis**. They contain lysozymes; therefore their main function is to protect the body from any foreign material. They are capable of moving out of blood vessel walls by a process called diapedesis and are actively phagocytic. A non-active neutrophil lasts approximately 12 hours, while an active neutrophil may last 1–2 days; dead neutrophils comprise a large component of the pus (exudate) of wounds. Neutrophils are the first immune cells to arrive at a site of infection, through a process known as *chemotaxis* (in which they are attracted to the site by the release of chemicals). A deficiency of neutrophils is called *neutropenia*, which may be congenital or acquired; for example, in certain kinds of anaemia and leukaemia, or as a side effect of chemotherapy. Since neutrophils are such an important part of the immune response, a lowered neutrophil count results in a compromised immune system.

The nuclei of the neutrophils are multi-lobed (figure 8.8). The number of neutrophils increases in:

- pregnancy
- infection
- leukaemia
- metabolic disorders such as acute gout
- inflammation
- myocardial infarction.

FIGURE 8.8 Neutrophil

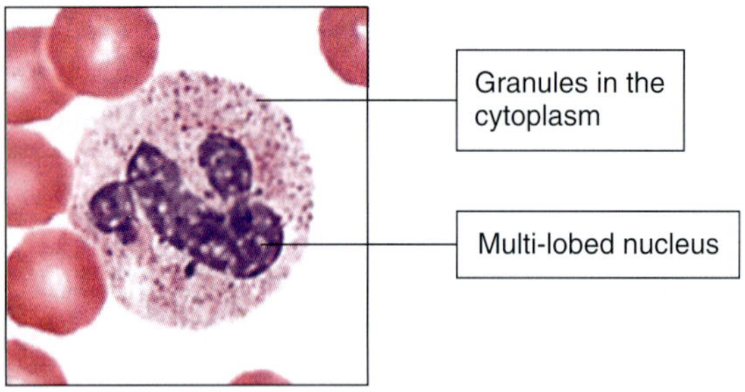

Source: Tortora and Derrickson (2009). Reproduced with permission of John Wiley & Sons.

Eosinophils

With the main job of killing parasites, eosinophils form approximately 2–4 per cent of granulocytes and have B-shaped nuclei (see figure 8.9). Like neutrophils, they too migrate from blood vessels and they are 10–12 μm in diameter. They are also phagocytes; however, they are not as active as neutrophils. They contain lysosomal enzymes and peroxidase in their granules, which are toxic to parasites, resulting in the destruction of the organism. Numbers increase in allergy (e.g. hay fever and asthma) and parasitic infection (e.g. tapeworm infection).

FIGURE 8.9 Eosinophil

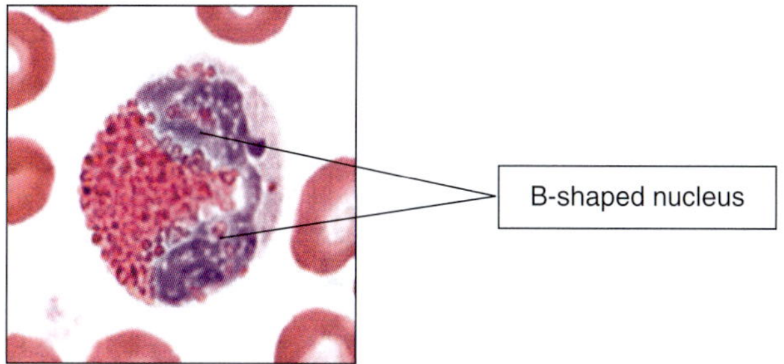

Source: Tortora and Derrickson (2009). Reproduced with permission of John Wiley & Sons.

Basophils

Basophils are the least abundant, accounting for approximately 1 per cent of granulocytes, and contain elongated lobed nuclei (figure 8.10). Basophils are 8–10 μm in diameter. In inflamed tissue they become mast cells and secrete granules containing heparin, histamine and other proteins that promote inflammation. They also secrete lipid mediators such as leukotrienes and several cytokines (via **exocytosis**). Basophils play an important role in providing immunity against parasites and also in the allergic response, as they have immunoglobulin E (IgE) on their surface and release chemical mediators that cause allergic symptoms when the IgE binds to its specific allergen.

FIGURE 8.10 Basophil

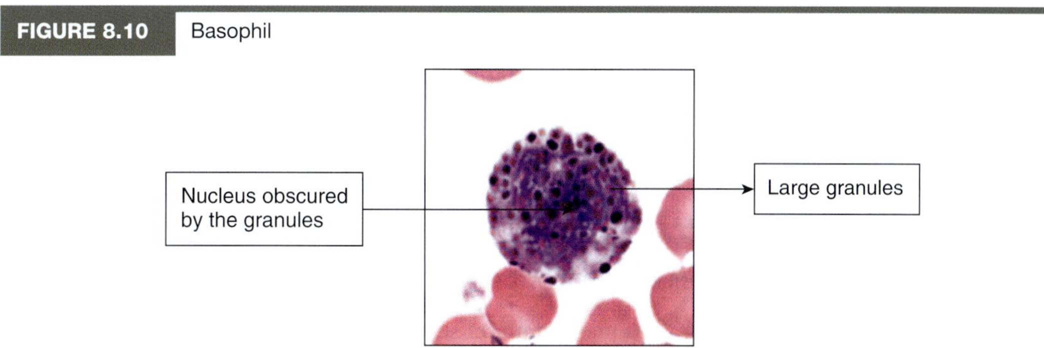

Monocytes

Working with neutrophils and lymphocytes to fight infection, monocytes account for 5 per cent of the agranulocytes and are circulating leucocytes (figure 8.11). Monocytes develop in the bone marrow and spread through the body in 1–3 days. They are approximately 12–20 μm in diameter. The nucleus of the monocyte is kidney- or horseshoe-shaped. These cells are known as monocytes in the blood, but can also migrate into body tissue where they develop into macrophages and engulf pathogens or foreign proteins to fight infection. Macrophages play a vital role in immunity and inflammation by destroying specific antigens (foreign body markers).

FIGURE 8.11 Monocytes

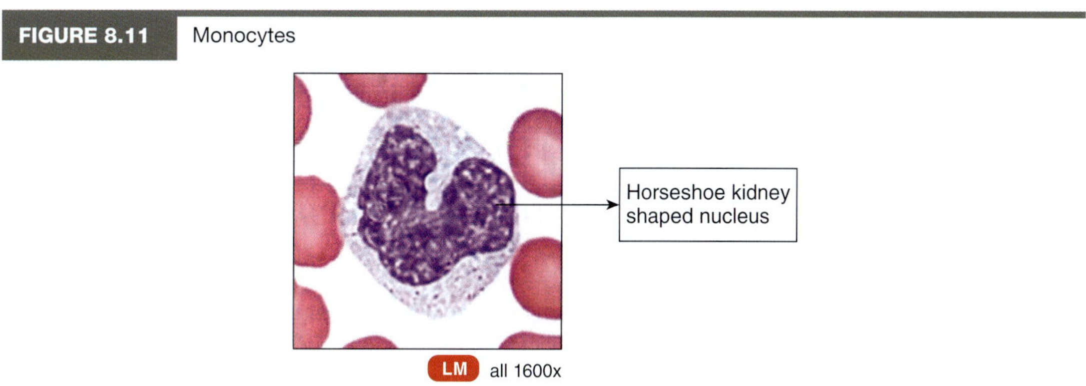

Source: Tortora and Derrickson (2009). Reproduced with permission of John Wiley & Sons.

Lymphocytes

Lymphocytes are the second-most abundant type of white blood cell and account for 25 per cent of the leucocytes. They are mostly found in the lymphatic tissue such as the lymph nodes and the spleen (figure 8.12). Small lymphocytes are approximately 6–9 µm in diameter, while the larger ones are 10–14 µm in diameter. They get their name from the lymph, the fluid that transports them. They can leave and re-enter the circulatory system, and their life span ranges from a few hours to years. The main difference between lymphocytes and other white blood cells is that lymphocytes are not phagocytes (they don't engulf foreign material). Two types of lymphocytes are identified, and they are T- and B-lymphocytes. T-lymphocytes originate from the thymus gland (hence the name), while B-lymphocytes originate in the bone marrow.

FIGURE 8.12 Lymphocyte

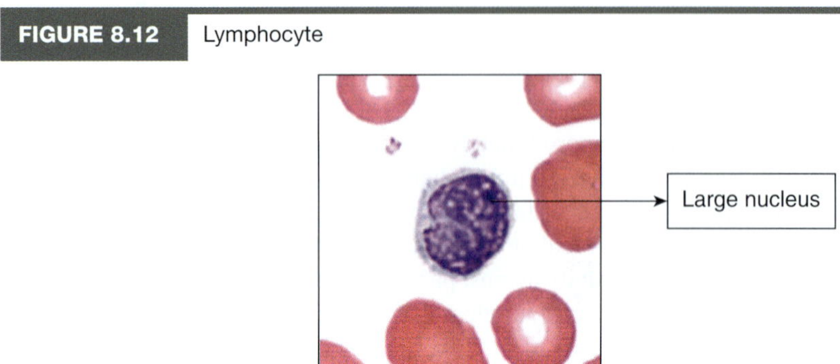

Source: Tortora and Derrickson (2009). Reproduced with permission of John Wiley & Sons.

T-lymphocytes mediate cellular immune response, which is part of the body's own defence, and can directly attack infected cells and tumours. The B-lymphocytes, on the other hand, become large plasma cells and produce antibodies that attach to foreign antigens — they patrol the blood plasma, acting like the alarm bells of the immune system when they recognise the antigens of foreign bodies such as viruses and bacteria.

Platelets

Platelets are small blood cells consisting of some cytoplasm surrounded by a plasma membrane and play a key role in the prevention of blood loss. They are produced in the bone marrow from megakaryocytes (bone marrow cells), and fragments of megakaryocytes break off to form platelets. They are approximately 2–4 µm in diameter but have no nucleus and the life span is approximately 5–9 days. Old and dead platelets are removed by macrophages in the spleen and the Kupffer cells in the liver. The surface of platelets contains proteins and glycoproteins that allow them to adhere to other proteins such as collagen in the connective tissues. Platelets play a vital role in blood loss by the formation of platelet plugs, which seal the holes in the blood vessels and release chemicals that aid blood clotting. If the platelet number is low, excessive bleeding can occur; however, if the number increases, blood clots (thrombosis) can form, leading to cerebrovascular accident, deep vein thrombosis, heart attack or pulmonary embolism.

Haemostasis

Haemostasis is a sequence of responses that stops bleeding and can prevent haemorrhage from smaller blood vessels. As such, haemostasis plays an important part in maintaining homeostasis (e.g. maintaining fluid balance, blood pressure, electrolyte levels), and it consists of three main processes:

- vasoconstriction
- platelet aggregation
- coagulation.

Vasoconstriction

- This constriction of blood vessels results from the contraction of the smooth muscle of the vessel wall, a reaction called vascular spasm.
- Constriction blocks small blood vessels, thus preventing blood flow through them, and limiting flow to the damaged site and reducing blood loss.

- The action of the sympathetic nervous system is to cause vasoconstriction, which restricts blood flow for several minutes or several hours.
- Platelets release thromboxanes, which belong to the lipid group eicosanoids. Thromboxanes are vasoconstrictors and potent hypertensive agents; they facilitate platelet aggregation.

Platelet aggregation

- Platelets adhere to the exposed collagen fibres of the connective tissue of the damaged blood vessels (due to a glycoprotein known as von Willebrand factor).
- Platelets release chemicals that make other platelets in the area stick (such as **adenosine diphosphate** and thromboxane), and they all clump together to form a platelet plug. Platelet plugs are very effective in preventing blood loss in small blood vessels, and with fibrin threads form tight plugs.

Coagulation

Blood coagulation is an important process to maintain homeostasis. If blood vessel damage is so extensive that platelet aggregation and vasoconstriction cannot stop the bleeding, the complicated process of coagulation (blood clotting) will begin to take place with the aid of clotting factors (table 8.2). Coagulation factors are a group of proteins essential for clotting; most of the clotting factors are synthesised in the liver, and some are obtained from our diet.

TABLE 8.2 **Blood clotting factors**

Factor	Common name
I	Fibrinogen
II	Prothrombin
V	Proaccelerin, labile factor
VII	Proconvertin
VIII	Antihaemophilic factor A
IX	Antihaemophilic factor B
X	Thrombokinase, Stuart–Prower factor
XI	Antihaemophilic factor C
XII	Hageman factor
XIII	Fibrin stabilising factor

Caused by blood reacting with the air/damaged cells and platelets, the simplified clotting process involves the following (see figure 8.13).

- Stage 1: Thromboplastinogenase is an enzyme released by the blood platelets and combines with antihaemophilic clotting factors to convert the plasma protein thromboplastinogen into thromboplastin.
- Stage 2: Thromboplastin combines with calcium ions to convert the inactive plasma protein prothrombin into thrombin (prothrombin is normally inactive in the blood so as not to continually clot).
- Stage 3: Thrombin acts as a catalyst to convert the soluble plasma protein fibrinogen into insoluble plasma protein fibrin. The subsequent mesh of fibrin threads traps blood cells to form a clot, plugging the cut/injury.

Once the clot is formed, the healing of the damaged blood vessel takes place, which restores the integrity of the blood vessel.

Two pathways are responsible for triggering a blood clot, known as intrinsic and extrinsic pathways. The extrinsic pathway is a rapid clotting system activated when the blood vessels are ruptured and tissue damage takes place and involves tissue factor (a clotting factor not normally circulating in the vessel). The intrinsic pathway is slower than the extrinsic pathway and is activated when the inner walls of the blood vessels are damaged (and involves only elements found within or intrinsic to the vascular system).

FIGURE 8.13 The stages of the simplified clotting process

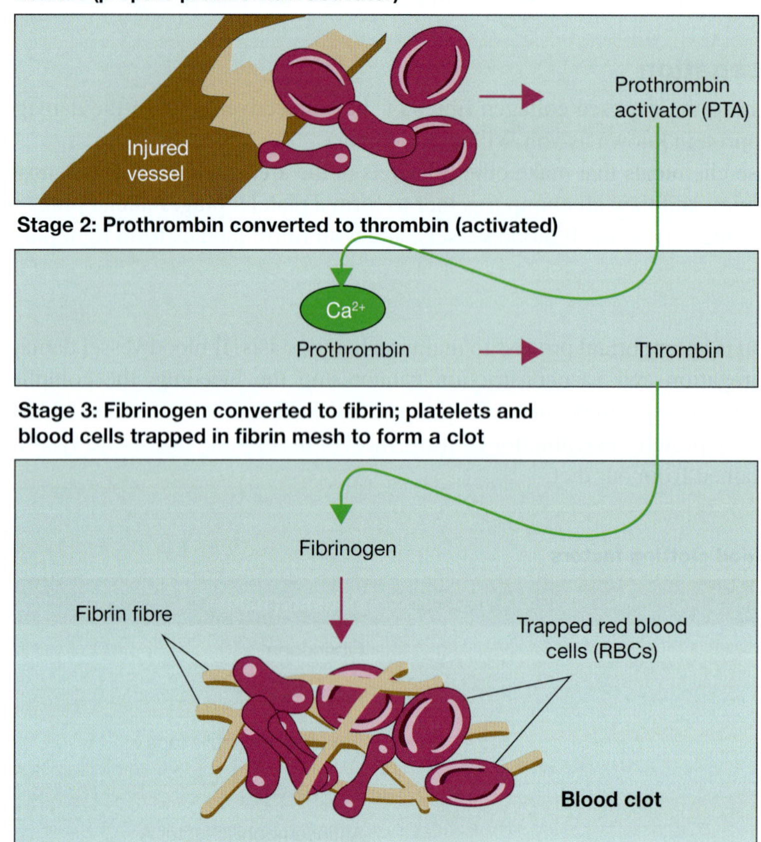

Source: Copyright © 2006, 2003 by Mosby, Inc. an affiliate of Elsevier Inc.

Although both pathways originate due to different damage (and involve different clotting factors), both have the end goal of creating a fibrin mesh to stabilise the platelet plug and prevent blood loss.

CLINICAL CONSIDERATIONS

Clotting disorders

Sometimes a blood clot forms within a blood vessel that has not been injured or cut. Some examples are listed below.

- A blood clot that forms within an artery supplying blood to the heart or brain is a common cause of heart attack and stroke. The platelets become sticky and clump next to patches of atheroma (accumulated fatty material) in blood vessels, activating the clotting mechanism.
- Sluggish blood flow can make the blood clot more readily than usual. This is a factor in deep vein thrombosis, which is a blood clot that sometimes forms in a leg vein, often due to poor venous return. There is an increased risk of such a clot during pregnancy or prolonged immobility (e.g. bed rest or even long-distance travel).
- Certain genetic conditions can make the blood clot more easily than usual.
- Certain medicines can affect the blood clotting mechanism, or increase the amount of some clotting factors, which may result in the blood clotting more readily.
- Liver disorders can sometimes cause clotting problems, as the liver makes some of the chemicals involved in preventing and dissolving clots.

There are a number of different blood tests which can identify clotting problems. The ones chosen depend on the circumstances and the suspected problem. Some of the tests are listed below.

- *Blood count*. Full blood count is a routine blood test that can count the number of red cells, white cells and platelets per millilitre of blood. It will detect a low level of platelets.

- *Bleeding time.* In this test, a tiny cut is made in the earlobe or forearm and the time taken for the bleeding to stop is measured. It is normally 3–8 minutes.
- *Blood clotting tests.* There are a number of tests that may be done. For example, the 'prothrombin time' and the 'activated partial thromboplastin time' are commonly done. These tests measure the time it takes for a blood clot to form after certain activating chemicals are added to the blood sample.
- *Platelet aggregation test.* This measures the rate at which, and the extent to which, platelets form clumps (aggregate) after a chemical is added that stimulates aggregation. It tests the function of the platelets.

See Knott (2017).

MEDICINES MANAGEMENT

Anticoagulants

Anticoagulant medicines reduce the ability of the blood to clot. This is necessary if the blood clots too much, as blood clots can block blood vessels and lead to conditions such as a stroke or a heart attack. The two most common anticoagulant medicines are:
- heparin
- warfarin.

Heparin and warfarin work slightly differently — heparin stops the activation of clotting factors, and so is faster acting, while warfarin blocks the production of further factors but not those that are currently in circulation, making it slower acting. Newer anticoagulants (such as rivaroxaban, dabigatran and apixaban) may be used as an alternative to warfarin for certain conditions; for example, warfarin is contraindicated during pregnancy because it can cross the placenta.

Some of the side effects for these medications include:
- passing blood in the urine or stool
- severe bruising
- excessive bleeding (haemorrhage)
- bleeding gums
- prolonged nose bleeds
- passing black faeces
- difficulty in breathing/chest pain
- in women, heavy or increased bleeding during a period, or any other bleeding from the vagina.

Patients taking anticoagulant medicines should be monitored closely to check that they are on the correct dose and not at risk of excessive bleeding (haemorrhage). The most common test for this is the international normalisation ratio.

See NPS Medicine Wise (2020).

CLINICALLY REASONED EPISODE OF CARE

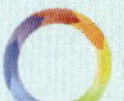

Haemophilia

Consider the patient situation

Jonathan is a 25-year-old male who, after a tackle during a rugby game, is taken to the emergency department with a heavy nosebleed. He is seen by the emergency nurse and he informs the nurse that he has haemophilia.

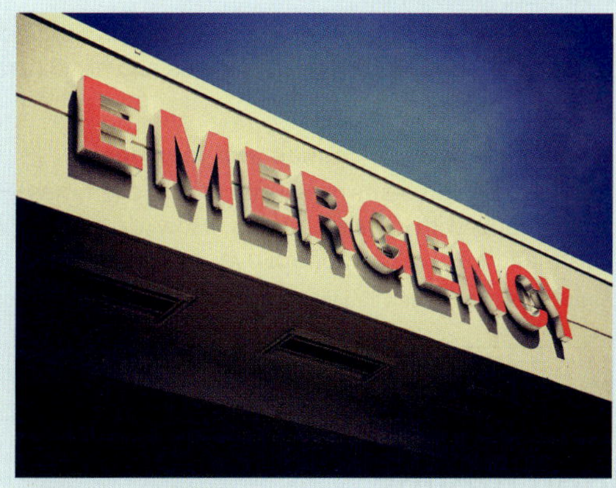

Collect cues and information

Jonathan is studying nursing and has a history of attention deficit disorder (ADD). He uses physical exercise (rugby) as a physical outlet for his pent-up energy.

His vital signs are recorded: temperature 37 °C; pulse 68 beats per minute; respiration 16 breaths per minute; and blood pressure 116/60 mmHg.

He informs the nurse that he was told to avoid contact sports but confesses that rugby is a good outlet for his ADD and that this strategy is important to him and for his studies. The nurse makes a note that

Jonathan's ADD has not impeded his capacity to understand the possible consequences of continuing to engage in a contact sport.

Process information

Haemophilia is a genetic condition which is characterised by the low level of clotting factors in the blood. Haemophilia A is classified as a deficiency in factor VIII, while haemophilia B is a deficit in factor IX. In Australia, around 2800 people live with haemophilia, of which the majority are male. This genetic condition is normally carried asymptomatically by women, but it is men who usually display the symptoms of the disorder. Due to the impaired clotting mechanisms, people with haemophilia bleed more easily, meaning that injuries could cause life-threatening haemorrhages.

Jonathan is also seen by the duty doctor, who carries out some blood tests. The results of the tests indicate that his activated partial thromboplastin time (APTT) is slightly delayed and his bleeding times are abnormal. APTT is a functional measure of the intrinsic and common pathways of the coagulation cascade. A normal APTT is between 30 and 40 seconds. Anything outside of this time represents an abnormal clotting time.

Treatment options for haemophilia are dependent on the type, blood results and clinical context. One option is desmopressin, which works by releasing factor VIII from stores in the body's tissues. It is used in people with mild and moderate haemophilia to increase a person's own factor VIII levels so that clotting can occur and stop bleeding.

Establish goals

1. Control bleeding via compression and pharmacological intervention
2. Monitor condition and efficacy of bleeding control
3. Education and information

Nursing actions

1. Control bleeding.
   Rationale:
   - Due to low clotting factors, people with haemophilia will continue to bleed. For a person with haemophilia, a bleeding event can represent a life-threatening situation.
   - Bleeding can be controlled via a nasal pack for compression, such as a Rapid Rhino®.
   - Pharmacological intervention, such as desmopressin, should also be administered as a priority in order to prevent further blood loss.
2. Monitor condition and the efficacy of the treatments implemented.
   Rationale:
   - Bleeding can lead to hypovolaemia, clinical deterioration, and in extreme cases death; therefore, monitoring blood loss and clinical vital signs at regular intervals is an important nursing action.
3. Educate Jonathan and his family.
   Rationale:
   - Nurses are well placed to work in a holistic framework and to consider the patient's psychosocial needs. For Jonathan, this will mean taking into consideration his study, ADD and haemophilia. Nurses can work with the patient to determine an outcome that is best for them.
   - Those with haemophilia should be aware that physical contact sports and activities are not recommended. Due to the risk of bleeding, these activities can present dangerous situations for the individual.
   - A referral to a specialist nurse educator may be appropriate to help educate Jonathan and his family.

Evaluate outcomes

As a result of the actions above, Jonathan is admitted for overnight observations and to assess the effect of the treatment. His bleeding resolves and his clinical observations remain stable. He is discharged home the next day.

Reflect on new processes and learning

Nursing often presents moral and ethical dilemmas. Reflect on the scenario above and Jonathan's decision to continue with contact sports. How do nurses work with individuals to ensure they have the right information as well as control over their daily activities?

Source: Based on the Clinical Reasoning Cycle, Levett-Jones (2013).

Blood groups

It is the red blood cells that define which blood group an individual belongs to. On the surface of the red cells there are markers called antigens, which are so small they cannot even be seen under a microscope.

Each person has different antigens (apart from identical twins) that are genetically inherited, and these antigens are the key to identifying blood types and must be matched in transfusions to avoid serious complications. The structure for defining blood groups is known as the ABO system. If an individual has blood group A, then they have A antigens covering their red cells. Group B has B antigens on their red blood cell, while group O has neither antigens and group AB has both antigens (Tortora & Derrickson 2011). In Australia, the most common blood groups are O and A, with AB being the rarest (Australian Red Cross Lifeblood 2021).

The ABO system also covers antibodies in the plasma that are the body's natural defence against foreign antigens. So, for example, blood group A has anti-B in their plasma (to recognise cells that are not 'self'), while B has anti-A. However, group AB has no antibodies and group O has both; a simple way to remember this is to think that each blood group needs to have both an A and a B somewhere, either as an antigen or an antibody (see figure 8.14). If these antibodies find the wrong red blood cells, they will attack them and destroy them (causing them to agglutinate, or clump together). That is why transfusing the wrong blood to a patient can be fatal. Table 8.3 shows that individuals with blood group O are able to donate to all blood types (as these cells have no antigens present), making them a universal donor. People with blood group AB have neither anti-A nor anti-B antibodies present in their blood plasma and so can receive all blood types.

FIGURE 8.14 ABO blood groups

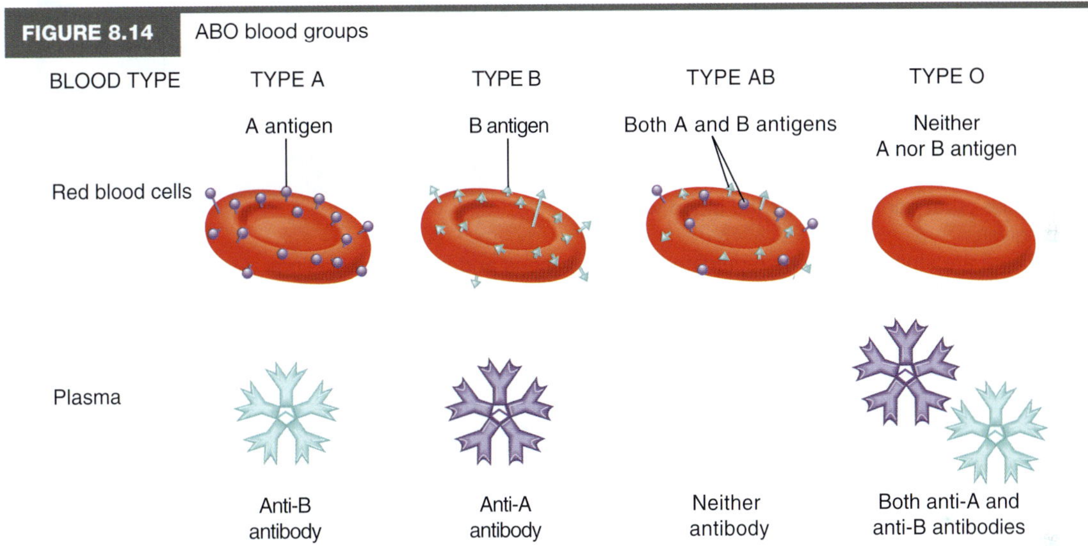

Source: Tortora and Derrickson (2009). Reproduced with permission of John Wiley & Sons.

TABLE 8.3 **Blood groups**

Blood type	Antigens	Antibodies	Can donate blood to	Can receive blood from
A	Antigen A	Anti-B	A, AB	A, O
B	Antigen B	Anti-A	B, AB	B, O
AB	Antigen A	None	AB	A, B, AB, O
	Antigen B			
O	None	Anti-A	A, B, AB, O	O
		Anti-B		

There is also another factor (factor D) to be considered — the rhesus factor (Rh) system, which makes a blood group 'positive' or 'negative'. Rh antigens can be present in each of the blood groups. Not everyone has the Rh antigen on the red blood cell; however, if a person has Rh antigen on their red blood cells then they are Rh positive and if they do not have the Rh antigen then they are Rh negative. A person with blood group A and Rh positive is known as A+, while if the Rh is negative they are A–. The same applies for B,

AB and O. In Australia, approximately 81 per cent of the population are rhesus positive; that is, they possess factor D on their red blood cells. The remaining 19 per cent of the population are rhesus negative as their red blood cells do not have factor D (Australian Red Cross Lifeblood 2021). It is important to consider the rhesus factor when cross-matching and transfusing blood to patients to avoid unnecessary complications such as agglutination (table 8.3). Rhesus positive blood should only be donated to Rh positive individuals, whereas Rh negative blood can be received by both positive and negative blood types; this makes the O– blood group the true universal donor, and for this reason it is kept on hand for emergency transfusions (when a person's blood group is not known).

SKILLS IN PRACTICE

Blood transfusion

Blood transfusion is the common term employed in medicine for the delivery of blood components directly (intravenously) into a person's circulation. Blood is usually administered through a plastic tube inserted into a vein in the arm. It can take between 30 minutes and 4 hours, depending on how much blood is needed.

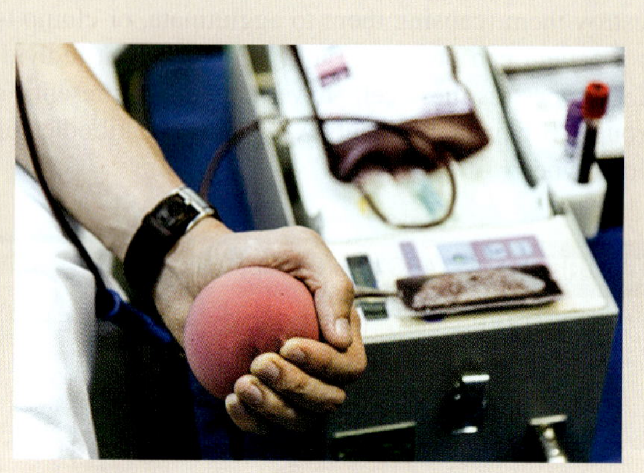

The components may be administered as a whole or individually. For example, a patient may need a replacement of red and white cells, as well as platelets and plasma, and receive a whole unit of blood. On the other hand, the patient may only require a platelet or plasma transfusion and the other components of the blood will not be given.

There are strict regulations regarding blood donations and blood transfusions. As well as ensuring it is safe for the potential donor to donate blood, the aim of these regulations is to minimise the risk of a person being given blood contaminated with a virus, such as hepatitis C, or receiving blood from a blood group that is unsuitable for them. For example, it is not possible for individuals who lived in the UK for over 6 months in the 1980s and early 1990s to give blood in Australia due to the risk of variant Creutzfeldt-Jakob disease (vCJD, sometimes known as 'mad cow disease').

Before the procedure, rigorous checks must be undertaken to ensure that the correct product and blood type is given to the correct patient. This includes careful confirmation of the patient's identity, their specific transfusion requirements, that the transfusion bag matches the details and blood typing on the patient's prescription and laboratory form, and that the product is in date and appears healthy and intact (Cowan & Davies 2018).

A patient receiving a blood transfusion will be placed under close observation during and after the procedure. Adverse reactions to a blood transfusion can be hazardous and potentially life-threatening.

Patients undertaking blood transfusions will have their vital signs, including respiration rate, pulse, blood pressure and temperature monitored carefully. Initial symptoms of a reaction may include shortness of breath and a fast pulse (Jones 2018). Any sign of a reaction requires that the transfusion is stopped immediately and that the patient is reviewed quickly by a doctor.

8.3 Blood vessels

LEARNING OBJECTIVE 8.3 Describe some of the differences between an artery and a vein.

Blood vessels are part of the circulatory system that transports blood throughout the body. There are three major types of blood vessels: the arteries, which carry the blood away from the heart; the capillaries, which enable the physical exchange of water, nutrients and chemicals between the blood and the interstitial fluid/tissues; and the veins, which carry blood from the capillaries back towards the heart (figure 8.15). All arteries, with the exception of the pulmonary and umbilical arteries, carry oxygenated blood, while most veins carry deoxygenated blood from the tissues back to the heart; exceptions are the pulmonary and umbilical veins, both of which carry oxygenated blood. The capillaries form the microcirculatory system, and it is at this point that nutrients, gases, water and electrolytes are exchanged between the blood and the interstitial fluid/tissue. Capillaries are tiny, extremely thin-walled vessels and act as a bridge between arteries and veins. The thin walls of the capillaries allow oxygen and nutrients to pass from the blood into tissue fluid and allow waste products to pass from tissue fluid into the blood.

FIGURE 8.15 Blood vessels

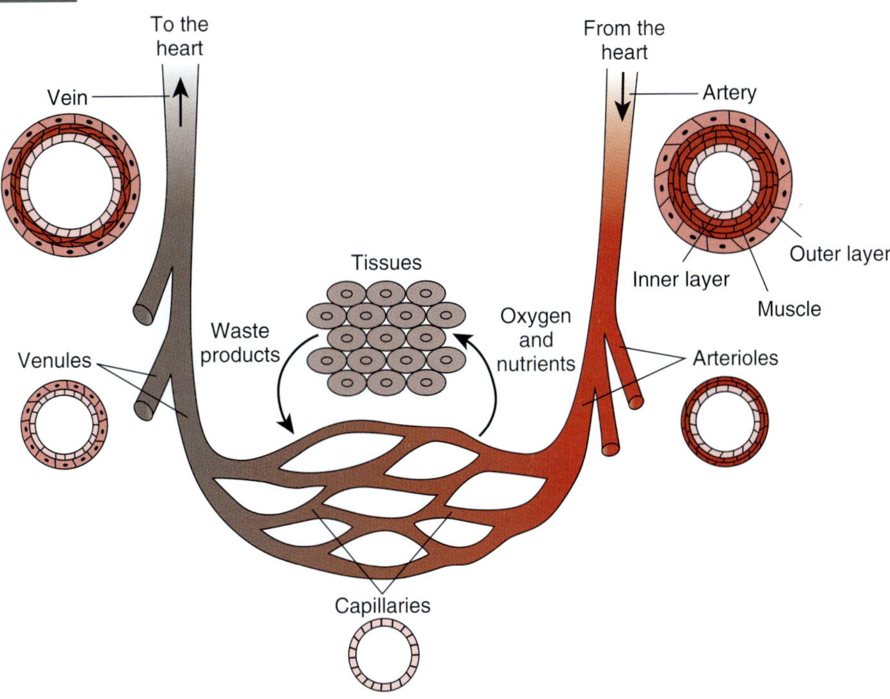

Structure and function of arteries and veins

For most of the blood vessels, the walls consist of three layers:

- the tunica interna
- the tunica media
- the tunica externa (adventia) (figure 8.16).

The *tunica interna* is the thin internal layer (only a few cells thick) of a vein and artery. It is sometimes referred to as the intima membrane. It is this layer that gives smoothness to the lining of the vessel, enhancing blood flow (and reducing blood pressure). It is lined by endothelial cells and elastic tissues; however, it varies in thickness between the blood vessels:

- arteries — most elastic tissue
- veins — very little tissue
- capillaries — no elastic layer.

The *tunica media* consists of elastic fibres and smooth muscle that allow for vasoconstriction, changing blood flow and pressure. The tunica media is supplied by the sympathetic branch of the autonomic nervous system. When stimulated, the walls contract, narrowing the lumen and increasing pressure within the blood vessel:

- arteries — varies by the size of the artery
- veins — thin layer
- capillaries — do not have tunica media.

The *tunica externa* (adventia) consists of collagen fibres and varies in thickness between the vessels. The collagen serves to anchor the blood vessel to nearby organs, giving it support and stability:

- arteries — relatively thick
- veins — relatively thick
- capillaries — very delicate.

Although the arteries and veins have similar layers, there are some clear differences between these two vessels. In particular, the thick elastic walls of arteries are important for withstanding higher blood pressures, while the valves in veins are essential in ensuring the return of blood to the heart (preventing backflow). For a summary, see table 8.4 and figure 8.17.

FIGURE 8.16 (a–e) Layers of a blood vessel

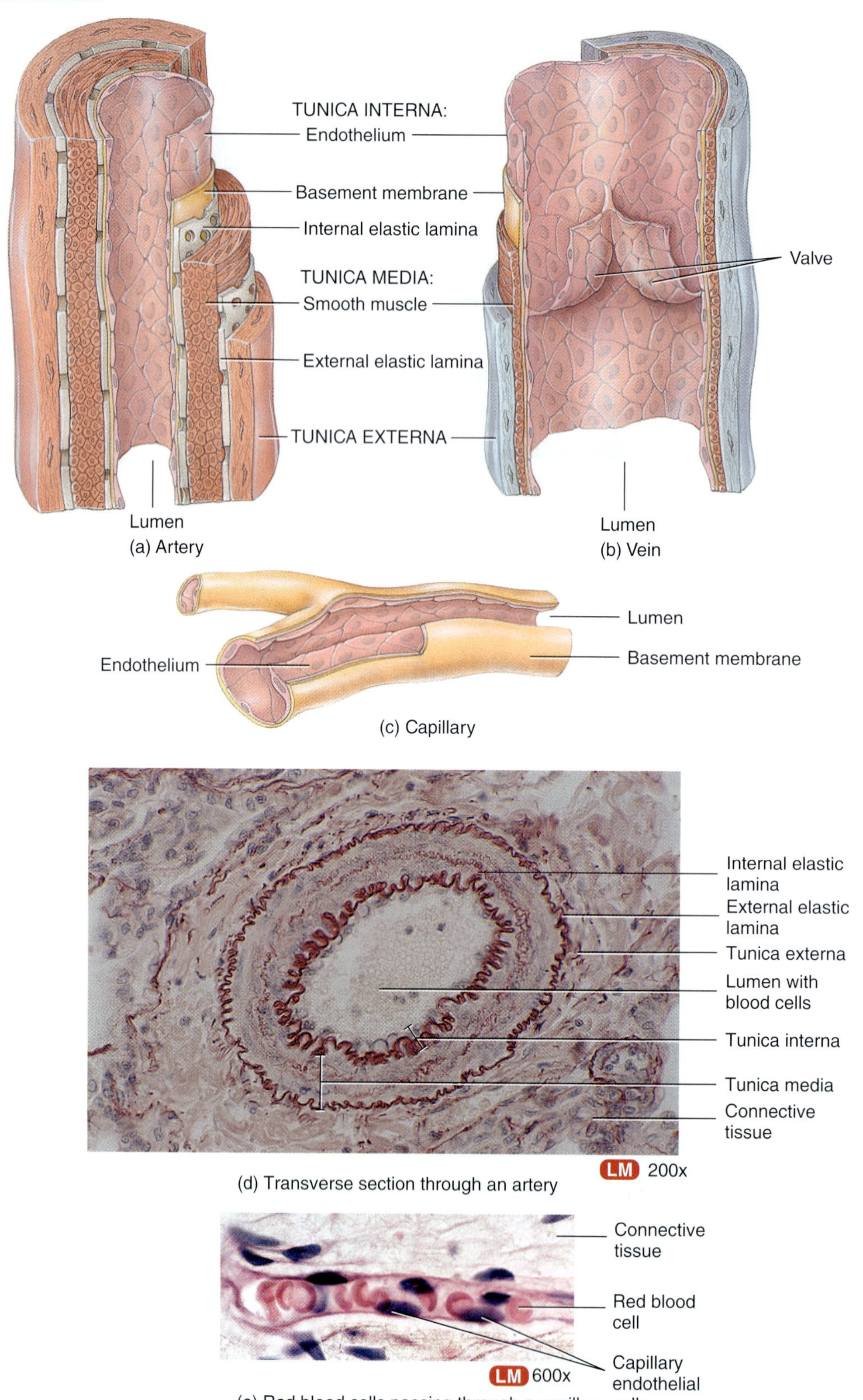

Source: Tortora and Derrickson (2009). Reproduced with permission of John Wiley & Sons.

TABLE 8.4 Differences between arteries and veins

Arteries	Veins
Transport blood away from the heart	Transport blood to the heart
Carry oxygenated blood, except the pulmonary and umbilical arteries	Carry deoxygenated blood, except the pulmonary and umbilical veins
Have a narrow lumen	Have a wider lumen
Have more elastic tissue	Have less elastic tissue
Do not have valves	Do have valves
Transport blood under high pressure	Transport blood under low pressure

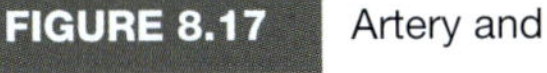
FIGURE 8.17 Artery and vein

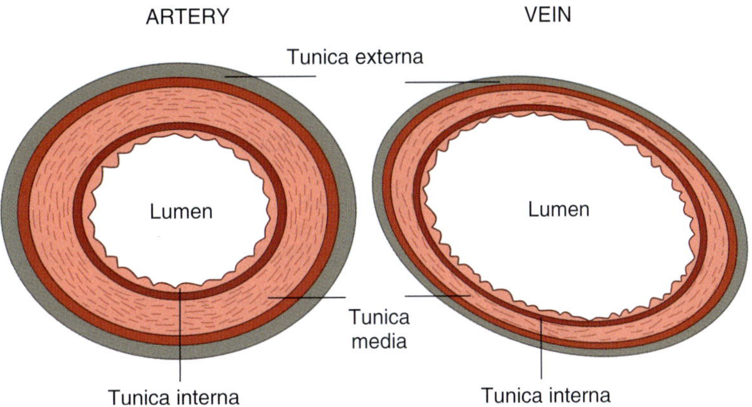

Capillaries

Capillaries are tiny blood vessels, approximately 5–20 μm in diameter. There are networks of capillaries (see figure 8.18) in most of the organs and tissues of the body. Capillary walls are only one cell thick, which allows exchange of material between the contents of the capillary and the surrounding interstitial fluid (and on to the tissue). The walls of capillaries are composed of a single layer of cells, the endothelium. This layer is so thin that molecules such as oxygen, water and lipids can pass through them by **diffusion** and enter the tissues. Waste products such as carbon dioxide and urea can diffuse back into the blood to be carried away for removal. Capillaries are so small that the red blood cells need to change shape in order to pass through them in single file.

SKILLS IN PRACTICE

Caring for a patient with an intravenous cannula

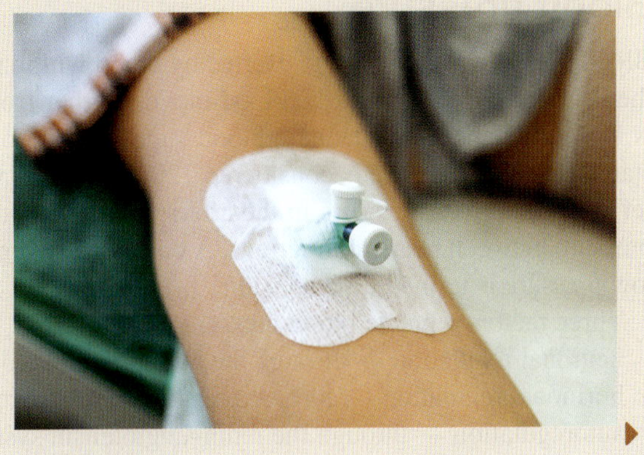

A cannula is a narrow tube which is inserted in a blood vessel or body cavity. It is a common procedure carried out in most healthcare facilities and the device may be kept in for a number of hours or days, depending on what it is needed for.

A peripheral intravenous cannula, also known as an intravenous catheter, is placed in a vein, usually in the lower arm. Its main purpose is to facilitate the administration of fluids or medications straight into the circulation; for example, administering fluids in a trauma case, or medications such as glucose to a hypoglycaemic patient, or pain relief. However, infections of the skin surrounding the device, or of the blood, can occur if it is not cared for properly.

Catheter-related bloodstream infections are a dangerous complication which can develop into sepsis, a life-threatening condition. Once the cannula is in place, it must be monitored carefully in order to prevent sepsis and other complications associated with an indwelling intravenous device. These include irritation of the site, **phlebitis** and blood or air **emboli** (Barton et al. 2017).

An assessment tool, such as the Visual Infusion Phlebitis score (Jackson 1999), is implemented to allow the catheter site to be monitored and maintained safely. The patient with an intravenous device is also advised to report symptoms such as pain, redness or swelling of the site so that any developing problems can be identified and treated quickly.

FIGURE 8.18 Capillary

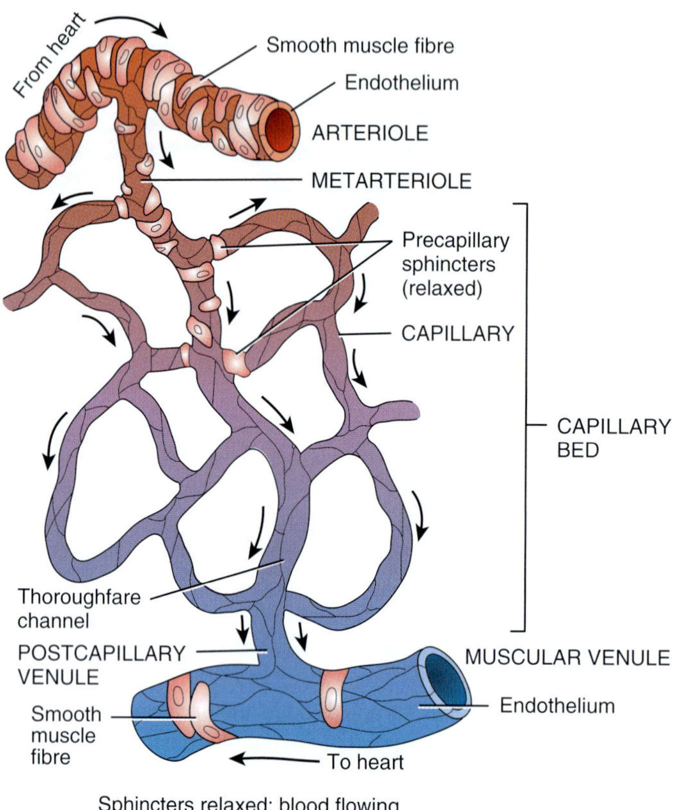

Source: Tortora and Derrickson (2009). Reproduced with permission of John Wiley & Sons.

Blood pressure

Blood pressure is the pressure exerted by blood within the blood vessel. The pressure is at its greatest near the heart and decreases as the blood moves further from the heart. Maintaining a healthy blood pressure is key to: 1) ensuring adequate blood supply to the organs; and 2) limiting strain on the heart. A gold standard blood pressure is considered 120/80 mmHg, where the first number (120, the systolic pressure) reflects the highest pressure in the arteries, and the latter number (80, the diastolic pressure) reflects the pressure between heart contractions. A consistently high blood pressure is termed 'hypertension', while a low pressure is termed 'hypotension'.

Three factors regulate blood pressure. They are:

- neuronal regulation — through the autonomic nervous system
- hormonal regulation — adrenaline, noradrenaline, renin and others
- autoregulation — through the renin–angiotensin system.

Physiological factors regulating blood pressure

There are several factors that affect blood pressure, including the following.

- *Cardiac output*. The volume of blood pumped out by the heart in 1 minute. Cardiac output is a function of heart rate and stroke volume. The heart rate is simply the number of heartbeats per minute. The stroke volume is the volume of blood, in millilitres, pumped out of the heart with each beat.
- *Circulating volume*. The volume of circulating blood perfusing tissues.
- *Peripheral resistance*. The resistance provided by the blood vessels.
- *Blood viscosity*. The measure of the resistance of blood flow. The resistance is provided by plasma proteins and other substances in the blood.
- *Hydrostatic pressure*. The pressure exerted by the blood on the vessel wall.

Control of arterial blood pressure

Blood pressure within the large systemic arteries must be maintained to ensure adequate blood flow to the tissues. This is maintained by the following.

- Baroreceptors situated in the arch of the aorta and the carotid sinus, which are sensitive to pressure changes within the blood vessel. When blood pressure increases, signals are sent to the cardio-regulatory centre (CRC) in the brainstem (medulla oblongata). The CRC increases the parasympathetic activity to the heart, reducing heart rate and inhibiting sympathetic activity to the blood vessels, causing vasodilatation. This reduces blood pressure. On the other hand, if the blood pressure falls, the CRC increases the sympathetic activity to the heart and the blood vessels, thus increasing heart rate and vasoconstriction, resulting in increased blood pressure.
- Chemoreceptors situated in carotid and aortic bodies help to regulate blood pressure by detecting changes in the levels of oxygen, carbon dioxide and hydrogen ions. Changes in the levels of carbon dioxide, oxygen and hydrogen ions can affect heart and respiration rates.
- Circulating hormones, such as antidiuretic and atrial natriuretic peptide hormones, help to regulate circulating blood volume, thus affecting blood pressure.
- The renin–angiotensin system helps to maintain blood pressure through its action on vasoconstriction.
- The hypothalamus responds to stimuli such as emotion, pain and anger and stimulates sympathetic nervous activity, affecting blood pressure.

CLINICAL CONSIDERATIONS

Hypertension: a national health priority

Blood pressure (BP) is a very common modifiable risk factor for adverse cardiovascular outcomes such as heart attack and stroke. Over 6 million Australians are reportedly hypertensive (broadly termed a BP ≥ 140/90 mmHg; see table 8.5) or taking BP-lowering medication. Hypertension is particularly common in low-income households and regional Australia, and a significant proportion of Aboriginal and Torres Strait Islander people are thought to experience untreated hypertension.

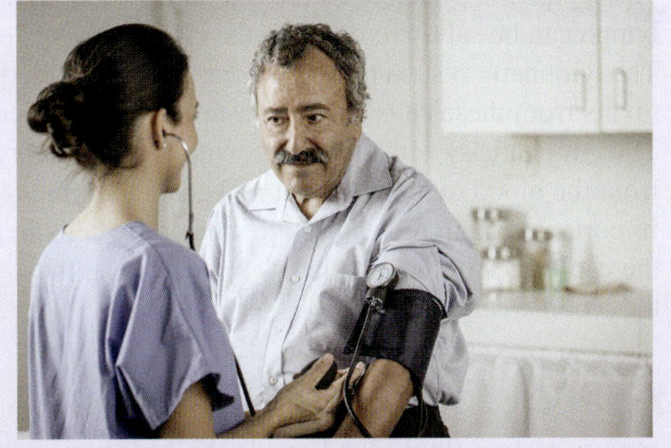

Controlling hypertension is a vital step in cardiovascular disease risk management; even small reductions in BP of 1–2 mmHg are known to reduce cardiovascular morbidity and mortality. The causes of hypertension are multifactorial, including but not limited to obesity, diabetes, older age, smoking, genetics, diet and physical inactivity. Treatment strategies encompass a combination of the following.

- *Lifestyle advice/changes*. These include not smoking, consuming a nutritious diet and participating in regular adequate exercise (recommended for all Australians, with or without hypertension).
- *Antihypertensive medication*. Many people will require medication to reduce/control their blood pressure. Medications such as ACE inhibitors, angiotensin receptor blockers (ARBs), calcium channel blockers and thiazide diuretics are common first-line antihypertensive drugs in patients with uncomplicated hypertension. However, a patient's comorbidities must be considered, as these could contraindicate the use of certain medications.

TABLE 8.5 **Classification of clinic blood pressure in adults**

Diagnostic category*	Systolic (mmHg)		Diastolic (mmHg)
Optimal	< 120	and	< 80
Normal	120–129	and/or	80–84
High–normal	130–139	and/or	85–89
Grade 1 (mild) hypertension	140–159	and/or	90–99
Grade 2 (moderate) hypertension	160–179	and/or	100–109
Grade 3 (severe) hypertension	≥ 180	and/or	≥ 110
Isolated systolic hypertension	> 140	and	< 90

*When a patient's systolic and diastolic blood pressure levels fall into different categories, the higher diagnostic category and recommended actions apply.

Source: National Heart Foundation of Australia (2016).

For more information, see Gabb et al. (2016).

8.4 Lymphatic system

LEARNING OBJECTIVE 8.4 Discuss the functions of the lymphatic circulation.

The lymphatic system (figure 8.19) is part of the circulatory system and it transports a clear fluid called lymph. The lymphatic system begins with very small, closed-end vessels called lymphatic capillaries (figure 8.20), which are in contact with the surrounding tissues and the interstitial fluid. The lymphatic system consists of:

- lymph
- lymph vessels
- lymph nodes
- lymphatic organs such as spleen and the thymus.

Functions of the lymphatic system involve the following.

- The lymphatic system aids the immune system in destroying pathogens and filtering waste so that the lymph can be safely returned to the circulatory system.
- The lymphatic system removes excess fluid, waste, debris, dead blood cells, pathogens, cancer cells and toxins from these cells and the tissue spaces between them.
- The lymphatic system also works with the circulatory system to deliver nutrients, oxygen and hormones from the blood to the cells that make up the tissues of the body.
- Important protein molecules are created by cells in the tissues. These molecules are too large to enter the capillaries of the circulatory system; thus, these protein molecules are transported by the lymph to the bloodstream.

Lymph

Lymph is a clear fluid found inside the lymphatic capillaries and has a similar composition to plasma. Lymph is the ultrafiltrate of the blood, which occurs at the capillary ends of the blood vessels. Blood pressure in the blood vessel forces fluid and other substances such as small protein (albumin) from the capillaries into the tissue space as interstitial fluid, which then enters the lymphatic capillaries as lymph. The body contains approximately 1–2 L of lymph, which forms about 1–3 per cent of body weight. Lymph transports plasma proteins, bacteria, fat from the small intestine and damaged tissues to the lymph nodes for destruction. The lymph contains lymphocytes and macrophages, giving it an important role in the immune system.

FIGURE 8.19 Lymphatic system

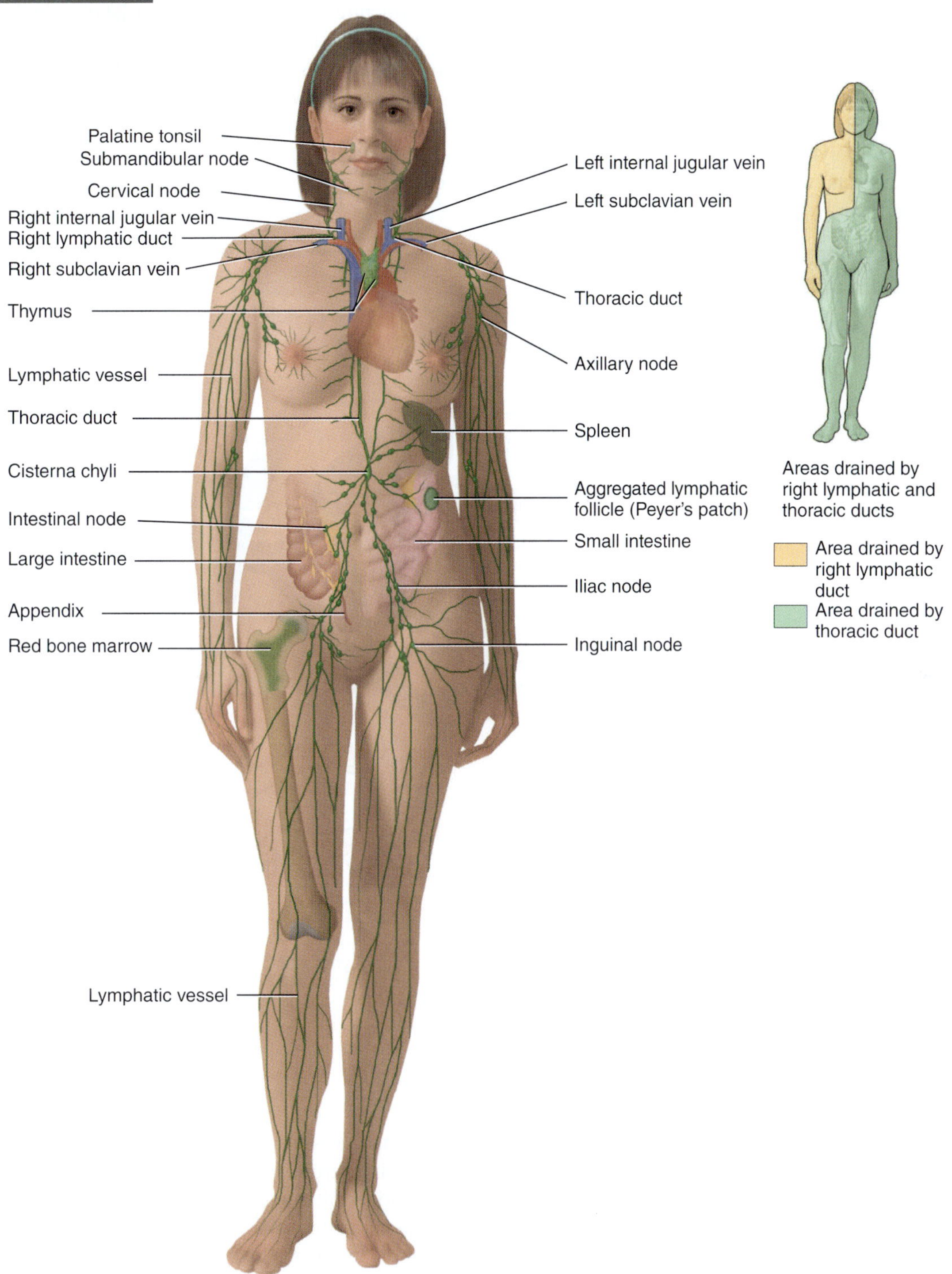

Anterior view of principal components of lymphatic system

Source: Tortora and Derrickson (2009). Reproduced with permission of John Wiley & Sons.

Lymph capillaries and large lymph vessels

Both the blood and the lymphatic capillaries have a similar structure, in that they both consist of a single-layered endothelial cell that allows movement of substances from the interstitial space into the lymphatic capillaries (figure 8.20). However, lymphatic capillaries are one-way vessels with a closed end (figure 8.21) in the interstitial space. Lymphatic vessels resemble veins in structure; however, the lymphatic vessels have thinner walls and more valves in them. The larger lymphatic vessels have numerous valves to prevent backflow of lymph. The lymphatic vessels combine to form two large ducts, the right lymphatic and thoracic ducts, which then empty into the subclavian veins (and on to the superior vena cava and then the heart).

FIGURE 8.20 Lymphatic capillaries

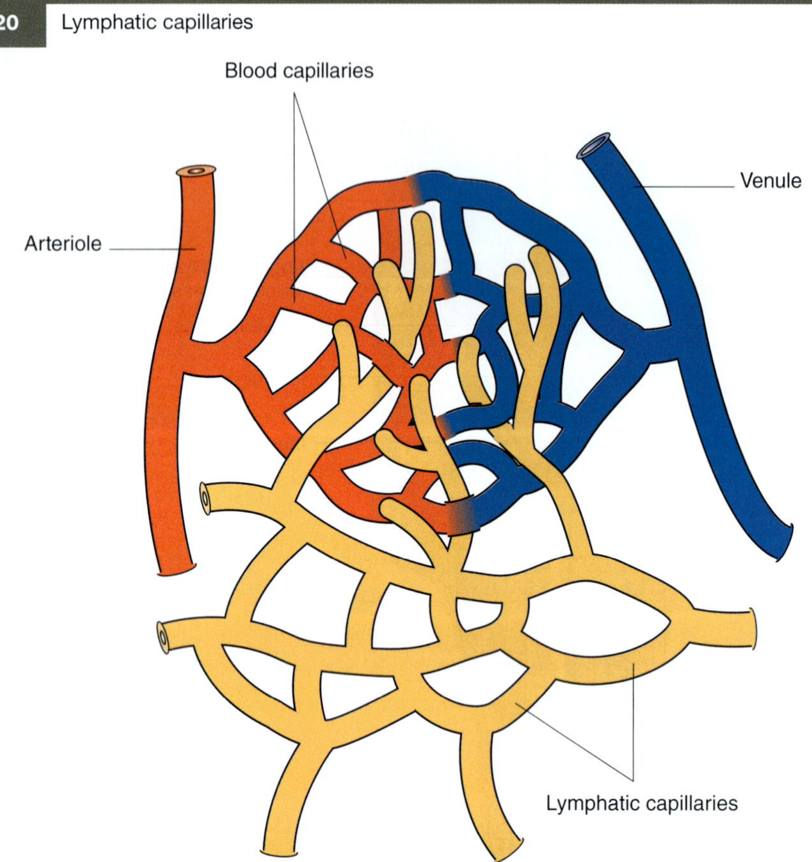

Lymph nodes

Lymph nodes are bean-shaped organs located along the lymphatic vessels. These nodes are found in the largest concentrations in the neck, armpit, thorax, abdomen and the groin; lesser concentrations are found behind the elbows and knees. The lymphocytes in the lymph nodes filter out harmful substances from the lymph and are sites for specific defences of the immune system; as such, lymph nodes play a key role in regulating harmful/foreign substances in the body. The lymph node is made up of an outer fibrous capsule that dips down into the node to form partitions (trabeculae), thus dividing the node into **compartments** (figure 8.22). Approximately four or five afferent vessels may enter a lymph node; however, only one or two efferent vessels will transport the lymph out of the node.

FIGURE 8.21 Lymphatic circulation

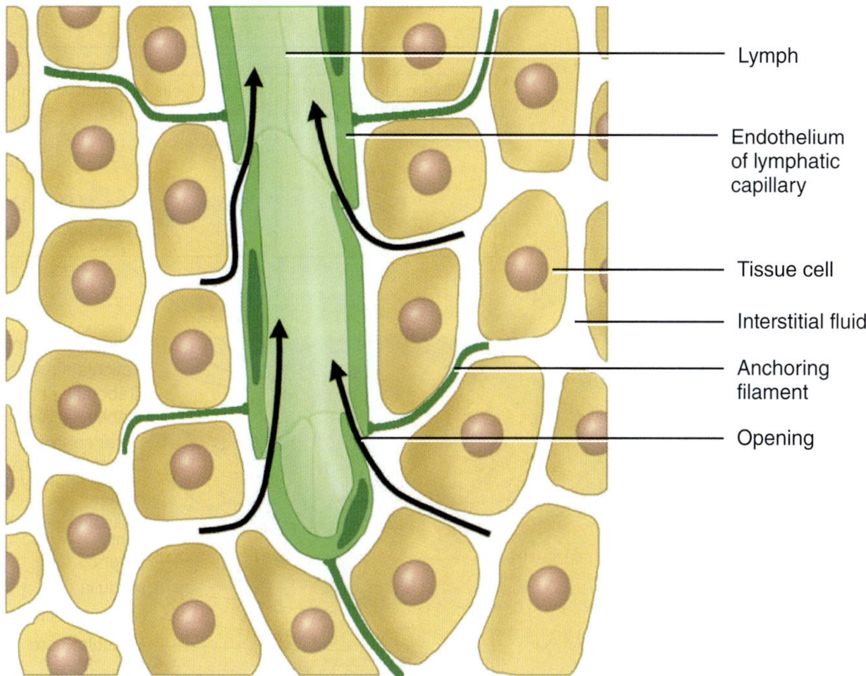

Details of a lymphatic capillary

Source: Tortora and Derrickson (2009). Reproduced with permission of John Wiley & Sons.

CLINICAL CONSIDERATIONS

Oedema

Oedema, previously known as dropsy, is the medical term for fluid retention in the body. The build-up of fluid causes affected tissue to become swollen. The swelling can occur in one particular part of the body — for example, as the result of an injury — or it can be more general.

The latter is usually the case with oedema that occurs as a result of certain health conditions, such as heart failure (an inability to pump blood effectively) or kidney failure (an inability to maintain fluid balance). Some of the possible symptoms include:

- skin discolouration
- areas of skin that temporarily hold the imprint of the finger when pressed (known as pitting oedema)
- aching, tender limbs
- stiff joints
- weight gain or weight loss
- raised blood pressure and pulse rate.

The treatment includes treating the underlying cause, including losing weight, exercise and diuretics to get rid of excess body water.

See Knott (2018).

FIGURE 8.22 A lymph node

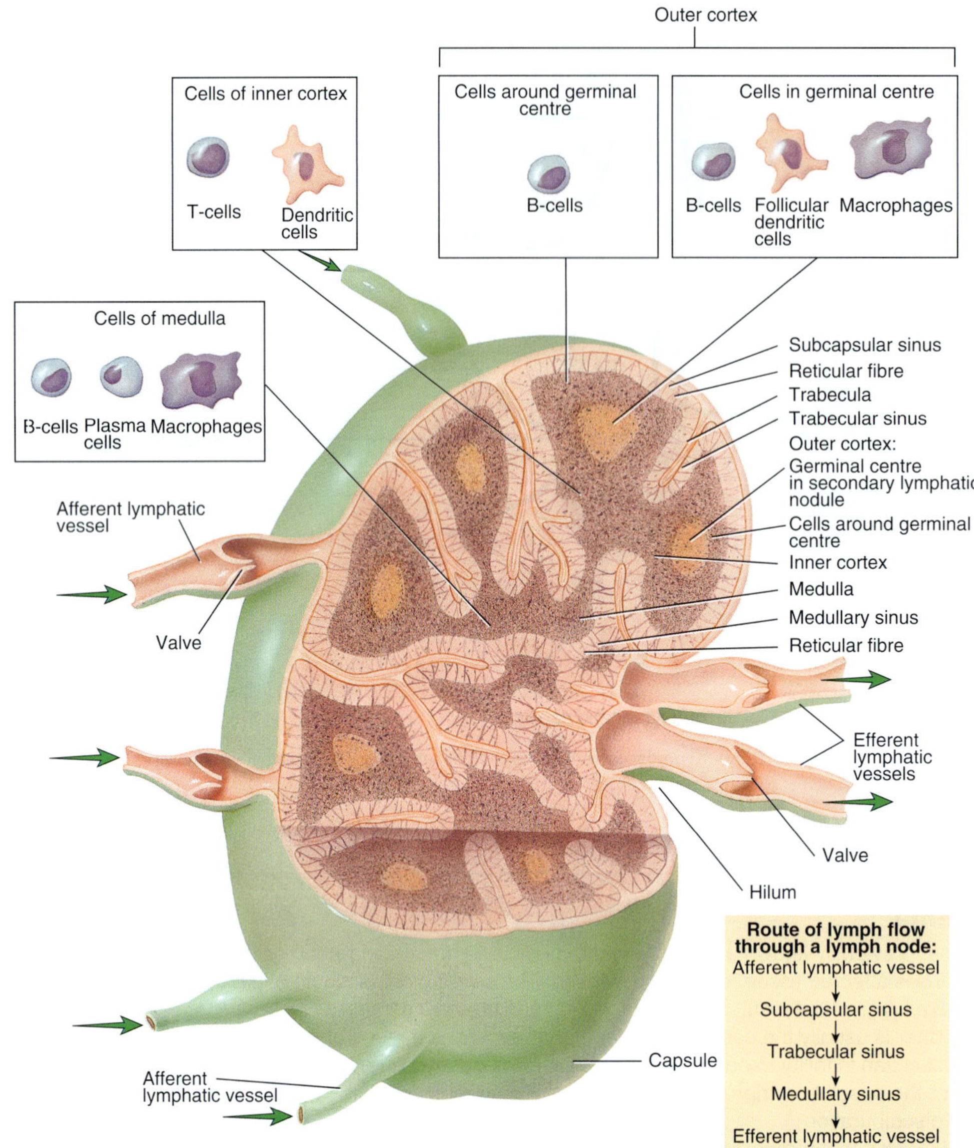

Source: Tortora and Derrickson (2009). Reproduced with permission of John Wiley & Sons.

MEDICINES MANAGEMENT

ABVD and chemotherapy treatments for Hodgkin lymphoma

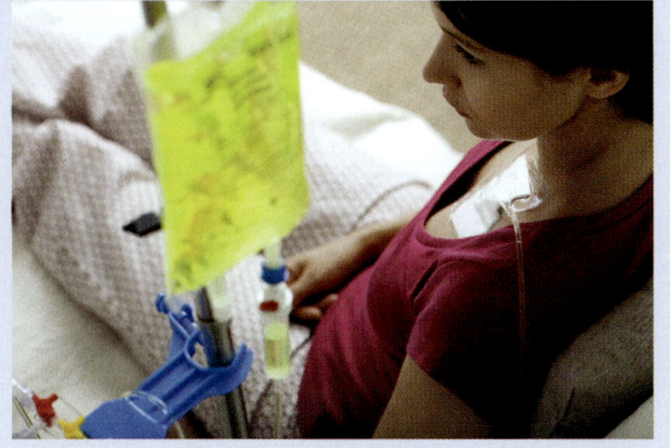

Hodgkin lymphoma is a blood cancer, and it develops in the lymph nodes of the lymphatic system. It is the most common form of blood cancer in teenagers and young adults. It appears as a solid tumour in the glands in the neck, chest, armpit or groin.

Chemotherapy for Hodgkin lymphoma uses combinations of different anticancer drugs rather than just one drug. This reduces the chances of the patient developing resistance to any one of the drugs. It also reduces the side effects, because lower doses of each individual drug are used. The drug combination most widely used for Hodgkin lymphoma is called ABVD (adriamycin, bleomycin, vinblastine and dacarbazine). This regimen is usually given in 4-week cycles by administering the drugs into the vein on days 1 and 15 of each cycle. Patients with late-stage Hodgkin lymphoma are given more cycles of treatment.

Side effects of chemotherapy include:

- nausea, which can be relieved using other medication
- hair loss
- low white blood cell count (neutropenia) and compromised immunity.

Specific side effects of ABVD include:

- heart problems caused by adriamycin
- fever or rash caused by bleomycin
- lung condition called fibrosis caused by bleomycin
- ulcers or blisters caused by vinblastine
- headaches, fatigue or diarrhoea caused by dacarbazine.

For more information, see the Australian Council Research Foundation (n.d.) and the Cancer Institute NSW (2020).

Lymphatic organs

Spleen

The two main organs of the lymphatic system are the spleen and the thymus gland. The spleen is the largest lymphoid organ and is approximately 12 cm in length, 7 cm wide and 2.5 cm thick. It weighs about 200 g and is purplish in colour. The main functions of the spleen are:

- filtering the blood — the destruction of old red blood cells and the remnants of manufacturing phagocytic lymphocytes and monocytes
- storage of blood — approximately 350 mL at any one time.

The structure of the spleen is similar to the lymph node. The spleen is surrounded by a capsule of connective tissue and, like the lymph nodes, it is divided into compartments by trabeculae. The two main functional sections of the spleen are the red and the white pulp. It is in contact with the stomach, the left kidney and the diaphragm. The blood supply to the spleen derives from the splenic artery, and the splenic vein transports the blood out of the spleen.

The thymus gland

The thymus gland is a ductless, pinkish-grey mass of lymphoid tissue located in the thorax. At birth it is about 5 cm in length, 4 cm in breadth and about 6 mm in thickness. The organ enlarges during childhood and atrophies (deteriorates) at puberty. The thymus gland consists of two lobes joined by connective tissue, and each lobe is covered by an outer cortex and an inner portion called the medulla. Each lobe is divided into lobules by trabeculae, and each lobule has an outer cortex and inner medulla. Acting like a T-lymphocyte school, the cortex contains many immature lymphocytes which migrate from the bone marrow to the thymus gland to become specialised T-lymphocytes (T-cells). Mature T-cells then migrate to the medulla and it is from the medulla that the mature T-cells enter the general circulation, where they are transported by the blood to the spleen and the lymph nodes.

SUMMARY

The circulatory system is a very efficient and complex system. It ensures that all the cells and tissues of the body receive all they need, including oxygen, nutrients and electrolytes to ensure that all systems are functioning efficiently. The blood transports many substances, such as red blood cells, white blood cells, hormones and electrolytes essential for cellular function. It also plays a major role in the body's defence against bacteria and other organisms through the action of the white blood cells. The blood also transports waste products of metabolism; for example, urea, carbon dioxide and uric acid.

Blood that is pumped out of the left ventricle of the heart is transported by a network of vessels called arteries and the blood is returned to the heart by the veins. There are three types of blood vessels: arteries, veins and capillaries. Arteries carry blood away from the heart, while the veins transport blood to the heart. The blood vessels of the circulatory system are a closed system, in that blood does not leave or leak out of the blood vessels unless they are damaged. It is at the capillary end that nutrients and other products essential for cellular function leave the blood vessels. White blood cells may also leave the blood vessels at the capillary end; however, red blood cells are contained within the circulatory system.

The lymphatic system is also known as the secondary circulation. It transports fluid called lymph, which is an ultrafiltrate of the blood. It plays an important part in the immune system. The fluid lymph is transported by the lymphatic system from all parts of the body and returned to the circulatory system via the right lymphatic and thoracic ducts, which then empty into the subclavian veins.

KEY TERMS

adenosine diphosphate The end product that results when adenosine triphosphate loses one of its phosphate groups located at the end of the molecule.

adenosine triphosphate A compound that is necessary for cellular energy.

chemical reactions Reactions that involve molecules, in which they are formed, changed or broken down.

compartments Spaces.

cytoplasm Fluid found inside the cell.

diffusion The most common form of passive transport of materials; it is the means by which gases, liquids and solutes disperse randomly and occupy any space available so that there is an equal distribution.

electrolytes Substances that dissociate in water to form ions.

emboli A mass that travels through the bloodstream, with the potential to clog up a blood vessel.

endocytosis Processes by which cells ingest foodstuffs and infectious microorganisms.

exocytosis The system of transporting material out of cells.

extracellular Space found outside the cell.

hypertonic Solution that has a large amount of solutes dissolved in it.

hypotonic Solution that has a low concentration of solutes.

hypovolaemia Decreased volume of circulating blood.

interstitial Space between cells.

intracellular Space inside the cell.

organelles Structural and functional parts of a cell.

osmosis Movement of water through a selectively permeable membrane so that concentrations of substances in water are the same on either side of the membrane.

osmotic pressure The pressure that must be exerted on a solution.

passive transport The process by which substances move on their own down a concentration gradient without utilising cellular energy.

phlebitis Inflammation of a vein.

plasma membrane Outer layer of the cell.

FIND OUT MORE

1 Explain why blood is called connective tissue.
2 Within the classification of white blood cells there are some grouped under the term granulocytes. List these white blood cells and their functions.
3 What is acute myeloid leukaemia?
4 List the checks you would make to ensure that the patient is receiving the correct blood transfusion.
5 Describe the forces that move fluid across capillary walls.
6 Describe the physiological factors affecting blood pressure.
7 Explain the term 'essential hypertension'.
8 Describe the flow of lymphatic fluid through the lymphatic system.
9 In our body there are MALT tissues. Explain the term MALT and its function.
10 How does the structure of a lymph node aid lymphocytes and macrophages in their protective function?

CONDITIONS

Below is a list of conditions that are associated with the circulatory system. Take some time and write notes about each of the conditions. You may make the notes taken from textbooks or other resources (e.g. people you work with in a clinical area) or you may make the notes as a result of people you have cared for. If you are making notes about people you have cared for, you must ensure that you adhere to the rules of confidentiality.

Atherosclerosis
Thrombocyte disorders
Aplastic anaemia
Deep vein thrombosis
Peripheral vascular disease
Non-Hodgkin's lymphoma

REFERENCES

Australian Council Research Foundation (n.d.) Hodgkin lymphoma. www.acrf.com.au/support-cancer-research/types-of-cancer/hodgkin-lymphoma (accessed February 2021).

Australian Red Cross Lifeblood (2021) About blood types. www.donateblood.com.au/learn/about-blood (accessed 15 January 2021).

Baird-Gunning, J. and Bromley J. (2016) Correcting iron deficiency. *Australian Prescriber* 39: 193–199.

Barton, A., Ventura, R. and Vavrick, B. (2017) Peripheral intravenous cannulation: protecting patients and nurses. *British Journal of Nursing* 26(8): 28–33.

Cancer Institute NSW (2020) Patient information — Hodgkin lymphoma: ABVD (doxorubicin, bleomycin, vinblastine, dacarbazine) early stage. www.eviq.org.au/haematology-and-bmt/lymphoma/hodgkin-lymphoma/57-early-stage-abvd-doxorubicin-bleomycin-vinblas/patient-information#side-effects (accessed February 2021).
Cowan, K. and Davies, A. (2018) How to undertake a blood component transfusion. *Nursing Standard* 33(5): 79–82.
Gabb, G.M., Mangoni, A.A., Anderson, C.S., Cowley, D., Dowden, J.S., Golledge, J., ... and Arnolda, L. (2016). Guideline for the diagnosis and management of hypertension in adults — 2016. *Medical Journal of Australia* 205(2): 85–89.
Jackson, A. (1999) Infection control: a battle in vein infusion phlebitis. *Nursing Times* 94(4): 68–71.
Jenkins, G. and Tortora, G.J. (2013) *Anatomy and Physiology: From Science to Life, vol. 2*, 3rd edn. Hoboken, NJ: John Wiley & Sons, Inc.
Jones, A. (2018) Safe transfusion of blood components. *Nursing Standard* 32(25): 50–63.
Knott, L. (2017) Blood clotting tests. www.patient.co.uk/health/blood-clotting-tests (accessed 10 December 2018).
Knott, L. (2018) Oedema (swelling). https://patient.info/signs-symptoms/oedema-swelling (accessed 15 January 2021).
Levett-Jones, T. (2013) *Clinical Reasoning: Learning to Think Like a Nurse*. Pearson Australia.
Nair, M. (2013) The blood and associated disorders. In Nair, M. and Peate, I. (eds), *Fundamentals of Applied Pathophysiology: An Essential Guide for Nursing and Healthcare Students*, 2nd edn. Chichester: John Wiley & Sons, Ltd.
National Heart Foundation of Australia (2016) Guideline for the diagnosis and management of hypertension in adults. www.heartfoundation.org.au/getmedia/c83511ab-835a-4fcf-96f5-88d770582ddc/PRO-167_Hypertension-guideline-2016_WEB.pdf (accessed February 2021).
NPS Medicine Wise (2020) Anticoagulant medicines and how to take them. www.nps.org.au/consumers/warfarin-apixaban-eliquis-dabigatran-pradaxa-and-rivaroxaban-xarelto-anticoagulants-and-how-to-take-them (accessed 14 January 2021).
Pellicori, P., Kaur, K. and Clark, A.L. (2015) Fluid management in patients with chronic heart failure. *Cardiac Failure Review* 1(2): 90–95.
Tortora, G.J. and Derrickson, B.H. (2009) *Principles of Anatomy and Physiology*, 12th edn. Hoboken, NJ: John Wiley & Sons, Inc.
Tortora, G.J. and Derrickson, B.H. (2011) *Principles of Anatomy and Physiology*, 13th edn. Hoboken, NJ: John Wiley & Sons, Inc.

FURTHER READING

ANAEMIA — IRON DEFICIENCY

Baird-Gunning, J. and Bromley J. (2016) Correcting iron deficiency. *Australian Prescriber* 39: 193–199.

In this article you will find the background of and recommendations in the treatment and management of iron deficiency anaemia.

BLOOD CLOTTING DISORDERS

https://patient.info/doctor/bleeding-disorders

This link provides information on the investigation and diagnosis, treatment and management of clotting disorders.

NON-HODGKIN LYMPHOMA — RITUXIMAB

www.lymphoma.org.au/about-lymphoma/treatments/immunotherapy/antibody-therapy/monoclonal-antibodies

Learn about Lymphoma Australia's guidance on the use of rituximab (MabThera) to treat aggressive non-Hodgkin lymphoma.

ACKNOWLEDGEMENTS

Photo: © Anna Jurkovska / Shutterstock.com
Photo: © vasara / Shutterstock.com
Photo: © Annette Shaff / Shutterstock.com
Photo: © coldsnowstorm / Getty Images
Photo: © Patryk Kosmider / Shutterstock.com
Photo: © Amble Design / Shutterstock.com
Photo: © Image Point Fr / Shutterstock.com
Figure 8.13: © 2006, 2003 by Mosby Inc. an affiliate of Elsevier Inc.
Table 8.5: © National Heart Foundation of Australia. Guideline for the diagnosis and management of hypertension in adults, 2016.

CHAPTER 9

The cardiac system

TEST YOUR PRIOR KNOWLEDGE

- Name the chambers of the heart.
- Describe blood flow through the heart.
- Name one of the valves in the heart.
- Describe the position of the heart in the body.
- Describe the factors that affect heart rate.

LEARNING OUTCOMES

After reading this chapter you will be able to:

9.1 describe the structure of the heart

9.2 describe the cardiac action potential and nervous system controls

9.3 list the arteries and veins that supply blood to the heart muscle

9.4 describe the electrical excitation of the heart

9.5 discuss the cardiac cycle.

Body map

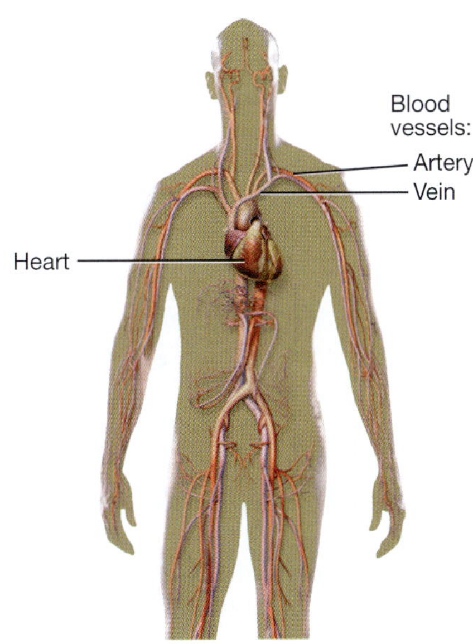

Introduction

The heart is a muscular organ containing four chambers. Its main function is to pump blood around the circulatory system, including the **pulmonary circulation** that passes through the lungs and the **systemic circulation** that supplies the rest of the body. In the average day the heart beats about 100 000 times and never rests. It must continue its cycle of contraction and relaxation in order to provide a continuous blood supply to the tissues and ensure the delivery of nutrients and oxygen and the removal of waste products. The purpose of this chapter is to review the structure and function of the heart, including:

- the size and location of the heart
- the overall structure of the heart
- the heart muscle and the cells of the heart
- the blood supply to the heart muscle
- the flow of blood through the heart
- the electrical pathways of the heart
- the **cardiac cycle**
- factors affecting **cardiac output**.

9.1 Size and location of the heart

LEARNING OBJECTIVE 9.1 Describe the structure of the heart.

The heart weighs 250–390 g in men and 200–275 g in women and is a little larger than the owner's closed fist, being approximately 12 cm long and 9 cm wide (Jenkins & Tortora 2013). It is located in the thoracic cavity (chest) in the mediastinum (between the lungs), behind and to the left of the sternum (breastbone) (see figure 9.1).

FIGURE 9.1 Location of the heart

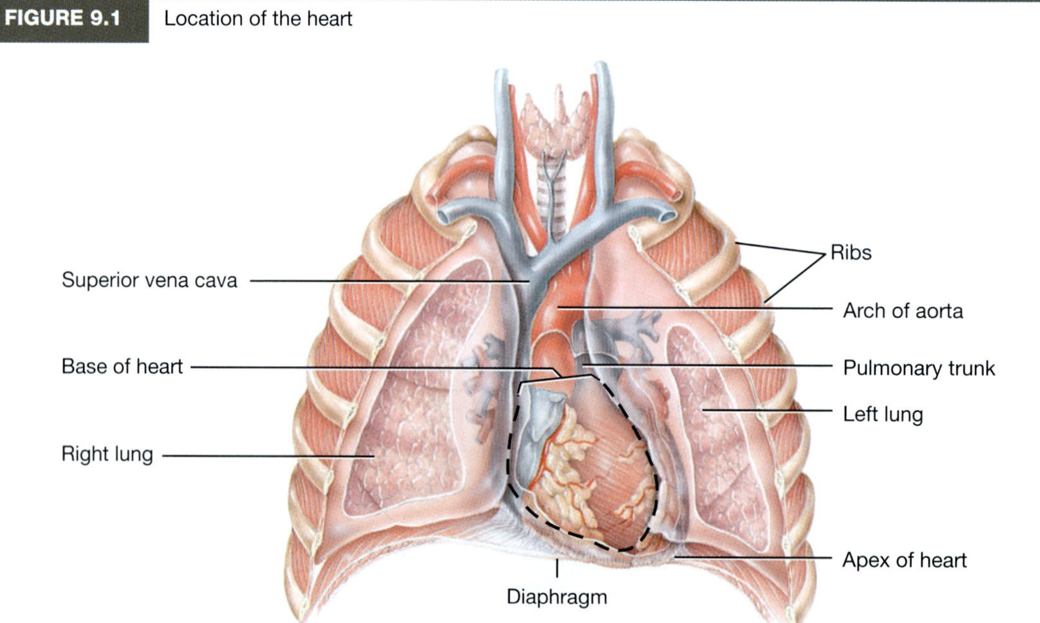

Source: Tortora and Derrickson (2009). Reproduced with permission of John Wiley & Sons.

As can be seen, the apex of the heart (the pointed end) is below the base of the heart and lies on the diaphragm. The base of the heart is itself made up of two of the chambers of the heart known as the **atria** (atrium is the singular of atria).

The structures of the heart

Heart wall

Pericardium

The heart is surrounded by a membrane called the **pericardium** (peri = around). This is often referred to as a single sac surrounding the heart but is in fact made up of two sacs (the **fibrous pericardium** and the **serous pericardium**) that are closely connected to each other (see figure 9.2). These two sacs have very different structures (Jenkins & Tortora 2013).

- *The fibrous pericardium.* This is a tough, inelastic layer made up of dense, irregular connective tissue. The role of this layer is to prevent the overstretching of the heart. It also protects the heart and anchors it in place.
- *The serous pericardium.* This is a thinner, more delicate layer that forms a double layer around the heart, comprising:
  - the **parietal pericardium**, which is the outer layer fused to the fibrous pericardium
  - the **visceral pericardium** (otherwise known as the epicardium), which adheres tightly to the surface of the heart.

FIGURE 9.2 Heart wall

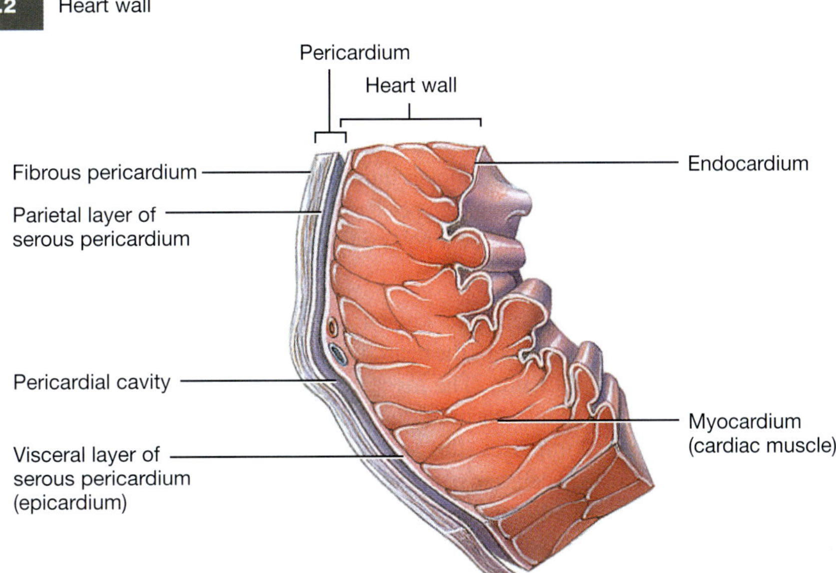

Source: Tortora and Derrickson (2009). Reproduced with permission of John Wiley & Sons.

HOMEOSTATIC IMBALANCE

Pericarditis

Pericarditis is a common condition which usually presents as severe, progressive chest pain that can radiate to the arms and neck, complicating differential diagnosis given the symptomatic overlap with myocardial ischaemia. It has multiple potential causes including trauma, myocardial infarction, vasculitis, connective tissues disease, some cancers or infection. Despite advances in diagnostic techniques, most cases remain idiopathic. Fortunately, most cases are benign and self-limiting, with treatment in the form of non-steroidal anti-inflammatory drugs (NSAIDs) such as ibuprofen and indometacin to relieve fever and manage pain. Occasionally, pericarditis can be accompanied by pericardial effusion or the build-up of fluid in the pericardial cavity. If this build-up is slow, the pericardium can stretch to accommodate even large fluid volumes without compromising filling of the heart. However, if the accumulation is rapid, intrapericardial pressure will increase, limiting the ability of the heart to fill (cardiac tamponade), and is potentially fatal if untreated (figure 9.3).

FIGURE 9.3 (Top) Inflamed parietal pericardium in inflamed effusive constrictive pericarditis; and (bottom) the same patient following pericardiectomy

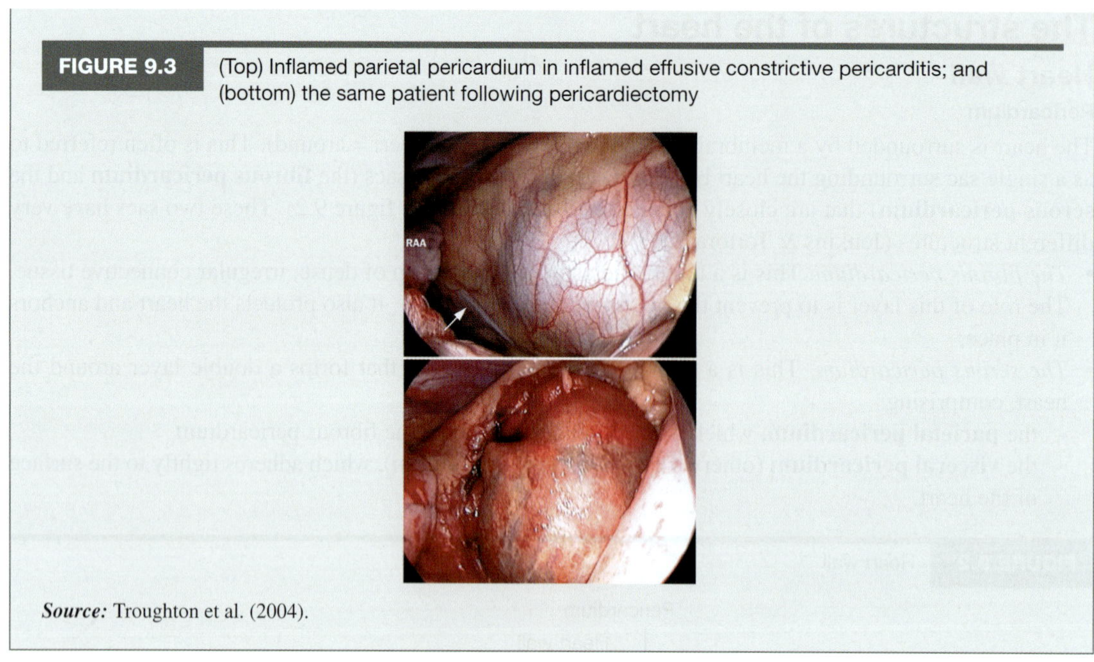

Source: Troughton et al. (2004).

Between the parietal and visceral pericardium is a thin film of fluid (**pericardial fluid**) that reduces the friction between the membranes as the heart moves during its cycle of contraction and relaxation. The space containing the pericardial fluid is known as the pericardial cavity; however, it must be noted that this 'space' is so small it is normally considered to be a potential space.

Myocardium

Underlying the pericardium is the heart muscle known as the **myocardium** (myo = muscle). The myocardium makes up the majority of the bulk of the heart. It is a type of muscle only found within the heart and is specialised in its structure and function. The myocardium can be divided into two categories: the majority is specialised to perform mechanical work (contraction); the remainder is specialised to the task of initiating and conducting electrical impulses (this second type of cardiac muscle cell will be reviewed later in the chapter). The cardiac muscle cells (**myocytes**) are held together in interlacing bundles of fibres that are arranged in spiral or circular bundles. Compared with skeletal muscle fibres, cardiac muscle fibres are shorter in length and have branches (see figure 9.4). The ends of the cardiac myocytes are attached to the adjacent cells in an end-to-end fashion. At this point there is a thickening of the **sarcolemma** (plasma membrane) known as intercalated discs. These discs contain two types of junction.

- **Desmosomes** hold the cells together so that the fibres do not pull apart.
- **Gap junctions** allow the rapid passage of **action potentials** (electrical current) between cells.

FIGURE 9.4 Cardiac muscle cells (cardiac myocytes)

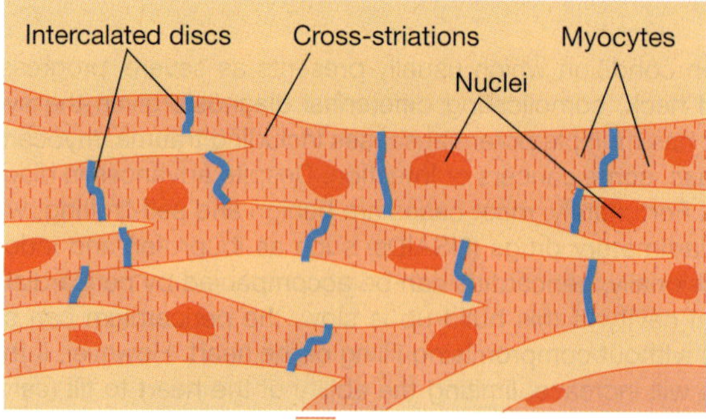

Compared with skeletal muscle cells, the cardiac myocyte contains one nucleus (or occasionally two nuclei) and the mitochondria are larger and more numerous, making cardiac muscle cells less prone to fatigue. However, cardiac muscle requires a large supply of oxygen and is less able to cope with reductions in the amount of available oxygen.

The cardiac muscle cells are divided into two discrete networks separated by a fibrous layer, the atria and the **ventricles**, and these two networks contract as separate units. Thus, the atria contract separately from the ventricles (see later). Within each myocyte are long contractile bundles of myofibrils. Myofibrils are in turn made up of smaller units known as sarcomeres. Contraction of the cardiac muscle is by the shortening of its sarcomeres.

CLINICALLY REASONED EPISODE OF CARE

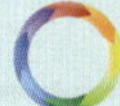

Hypertropic cardiomyopathy

Consider the patient situation

Stephen is a 14-year-old boy who is reporting increasing shortness of breath when playing sports at school. His mother has hypertrophic cardiomyopathy. Stephen is referred for an echocardiogram.

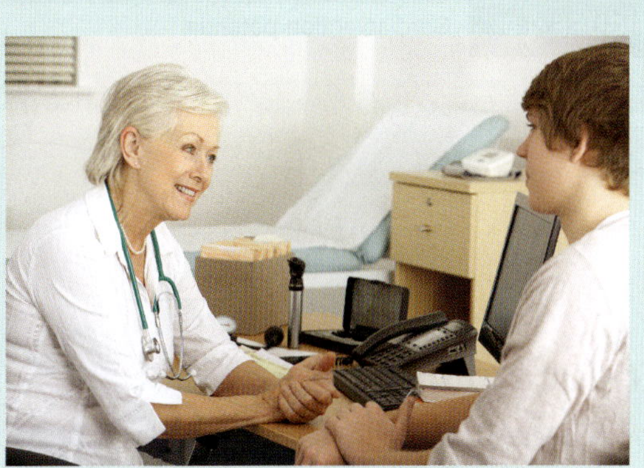

Collect cues and information

The echocardiogram shows development of hypertrophy of the ventricular **septum** (the wall between the ventricles), which is causing some obstruction of blood flow into the **aorta**.

Stephen reports no problems in everyday life, but when exercising the reduction in blood flow out of the heart leads to a reduction of blood flow to the tissues and the shortness of breath he has been experiencing when playing sports.

Stephen has further testing including 24-hour ECG monitoring, which shows no evidence of cardiac arrhythmias, and an echocardiography while exercising (stress echo).

Process information

Hypertrophic cardiomyopathy (HCM) is the most common inherited cardiac condition (about 1:500 live births), and for many, it causes no symptoms. HCM is a condition that leads to the muscles of the heart (the myocardium) becoming thickened and stiff.

In cases like Stephen's, the thickening of the muscles of the septum between the ventricles can lead to the obstruction of blood flow out of the heart into the aorta — this is known as hypertrophic obstructive cardiomyopathy (HOCM). HCM nearly always affects the left ventricle, but occasionally it will affect the right ventricle as well.

Nursing actions

1. Provide reassurance, support and education for Stephen and his mother prior to and during the procedures.
   Rationale:
   - Quality patient education and support reduces patient anxiety.
2. Provide education around prescribed beta blockers.
   Rationale:
   - Commonly used medications are beta blockers and calcium channel blockers. If there is evidence of arrhythmias (disturbance of the heart rhythm) then anti-arrhythmic medications (such as amiodarone) will be prescribed. In severe cases an implantable cardioverter-defibrillator (ICD) will be implanted into the patient's chest. Severe cases of HCM may require surgical reduction of the heart muscle thickness, or in very severe cases heart transplant.
   - Patient education supports concordance with recommended therapies which will promote good outcomes for the person.
3. Provide education around lifestyle changes.
   Rationale:
   - Recommendations include minimising alcohol, stopping smoking, reducing salt intake, maintaining a healthy weight and reducing caffeine intake. While patients with HCM can (and should) exercise, the levels of exercise recommended differ from patient to patient and should be discussed with a doctor before a new exercise regimen is started.
   - Making lifestyle adjustments will help to reduce the impact of HCM on the life of the person.

Evaluate outcomes

Stephen will have regular medical reviews to check progression of the condition so that therapeutic management can be adjusted.

For more information on HCM (and other cardiomyopathies) see the Cardiomyopathy Association of Australia, www.cmaa.org.au.

Source: Based on the Clinical Reasoning Cycle, Levett-Jones (2013).

9.2 The cardiac action potential

LEARNING OBJECTIVE 9.2 Describe the cardiac action potential and nervous system controls.

Unlike the normal skeletal muscle, in response to a single action potential a cardiac muscle fibre develops a prolonged contraction that is approximately 10–15 times longer in duration than a skeletal muscle contraction due to a plateau phase. Cardiac muscle fibres also have a longer refractory period, and thus a new contraction cannot be initiated until muscle relaxation is well advanced. Thus, a sustained contraction (**tetany**) cannot occur in cardiac muscle (figure 9.5).

FIGURE 9.5 Cardiac action potential

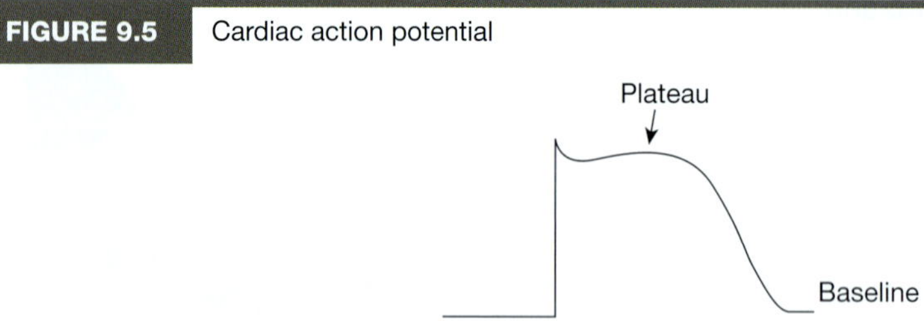

Endocardium

The **endocardium** (endo = within) is a layer of smooth simple **epithelium** lining the inside of the heart muscle (see figure 9.2) and the heart valves. It is connected seamlessly with the lining of the large blood vessels that are connected to the heart.

The heart chambers

The heart is divided into four chambers (see figure 9.6): the atria (entry halls or chambers) and the ventricles (little bellies). Even though the heart is referred to as a pump, it is better to think of it as two pumps.

- The right heart pump receives deoxygenated blood (blood that has given up some of its oxygen to the cells) from the tissues and pumps it out into the pulmonary circulation (the lungs).
- The left heart pump receives oxygenated blood from the pulmonary circulation and pumps it out to the rest of the body (the systemic circulation).

FIGURE 9.6 The chambers of the heart

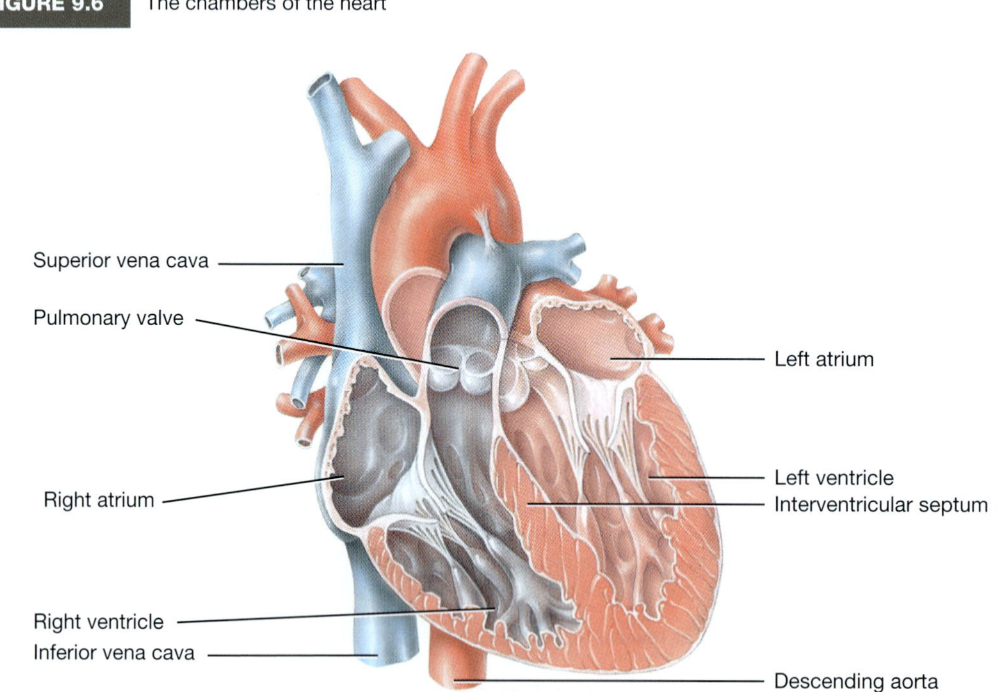

Source: Tortora and Derrickson (2009). Reproduced with permission of John Wiley & Sons.

Atria

The atria are the smaller chambers of the heart and lie superior to (above) the ventricles. There are two atria.

- The right atrium receives blood from three veins: the **superior vena cava**, the **inferior vena cava** and the **coronary sinus**. The superior vena cava drains blood from the upper parts of the body, the inferior vena cava drains blood from the lower parts of the body and the coronary sinus drains blood from the circulation of the heart itself.
- The left atrium forms most of the base of the heart and receives blood from the lungs through four **pulmonary veins**.

Between the atria is a thin dividing wall, the **interatrial septum** (inter = between, septum = dividing wall).

The thickness of a chamber's wall varies according to the work the chamber has to perform. As the atria are only pumping blood into the ventricles they have much thinner walls than the ventricles, which have to pump blood around the pulmonary and systemic circulation.

Between the atria and the ventricles are two valves (the **atrioventricular (AV) valves**).

- The **tricuspid valve** is made up of three cusps (leaflets) and lies between the right atrium and the right ventricle.
- The **bicuspid (mitral) valve** is made up of two cusps and lies between the left atrium and the left ventricle.

The purpose of the AV valves is to prevent the backward flow of blood from the ventricles into the atria during ventricular contraction.

Ventricles

There are two ventricles: the right ventricle and the left ventricle. Each ventricle pumps the same amount of blood per beat (**stroke volume**) but they have very different pressures.

- The right ventricle receives blood from the right atrium and pumps this blood out into the pulmonary circulation (the lungs). As the pressure in the pulmonary circulation is quite low the right ventricle has a thinner wall than the left ventricle.
- The left ventricle receives blood from the left atrium and pumps this blood out into the systemic circulation (the rest of the body) via the aorta. As the left ventricle has to pump against a higher pressure and over a greater distance it has a much thicker (more muscular) wall.

Between the ventricles is a dividing wall, the **interventricular septum**. Thus, with the septum between the atria and the septum between the ventricles there is no mixing of blood between the two sides.

At the outlet of each ventricle is a valve. Both of these valves are made up of three semilunar (half-moon-shaped) cusps (leaflets).

- The **pulmonary valve** lies between the right ventricle and the pulmonary arteries and prevents the backward flow of blood into the right ventricle from the pulmonary arteries during ventricular relaxation.
- The **aortic valve** lies between the left ventricle and the aorta (the main artery leading to the systemic circulation) and prevents the backward flow of blood into the left ventricle from the systemic circulation during ventricular relaxation.

CLINICAL CONSIDERATIONS

Rheumatic heart disease: a national health priority

Improving the health and wellbeing of Aboriginal and Torres Strait Islander communities remains one of Australia's national priority areas due to the disparities between these communities and other Australians, particularly in terms of both burden of disease and decreased overall life expectancy. One significant area of concern is the high rates of both acute rheumatic fever and rheumatic heat disease. Rheumatic heart disease is a potentially life-threatening complication of acute rheumatic fever (caused by group A streptococcus) and is a major cause of valvopathies in the Indigenous population. During rheumatic fever, the valves of the heart (and other structures) become inflamed due to immune cross-reactions between anti-streptococcal antibodies and the endothelial tissues of the heart. This cross-reaction leads to inflammation and scarring that results in valve incompetence (figure 9.7) (Marijon et al. 2012).

Globally, rates of rheumatic heart disease have declined profoundly in the last century but have remained at disproportionately high rates in the Aboriginal community, particularly in the Northern Territory. Between 2013 and 2017, there were 1900 people in Australia diagnosed with rheumatic heart disease. Of those diagnosed, approximately 93 per cent were of Aboriginal descent, largely due to issues of domestic overcrowding and low levels of functioning hygiene equipment (such as bathing facilities and laundry equipment) in affected communities as a result of both socioeconomic disparities and the remote nature of the communities in the Northern Territory (AIHW 2020a; Davey 2021). Another feature of remote communities is decreased access to timely healthcare, therapies and support services, which also contributes to poorer health outcomes.

FIGURE 9.7 A rheumatic **mitral valve** showing the damage typical of rheumatic heart disease

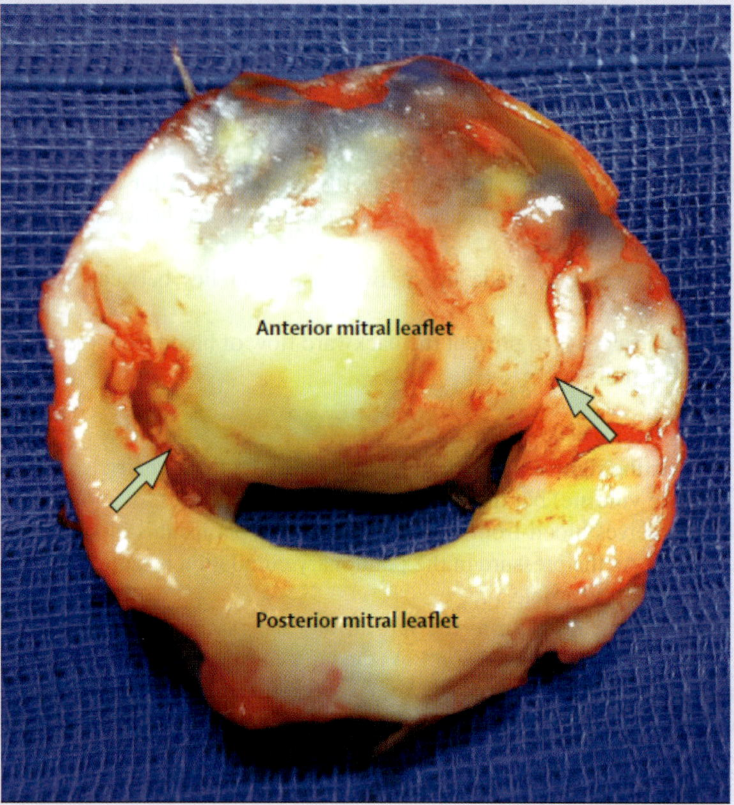

Source: Marijon et al. (2012).

CLINICALLY REASONED EPISODE OF CARE

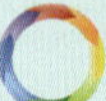

Heart defect

Consider the patient situation

Daisy is a 43-year-old woman with Down syndrome (trisomy 21) living in residential care. She has been reporting increasing shortness of breath on exertion and regular chest pain. Daisy has difficulty describing her symptoms and this has led to her reports often being ignored.

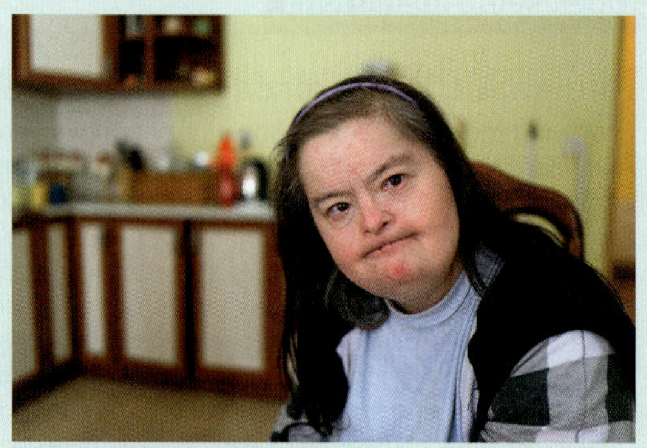

Collect cues and information

Daisy's shortness of breath seems suspicious to the clinician, and so Daisy's heart and lungs are auscultated. Though her lungs are clear, the clinician hears a murmur when listening to Daisy's heart sounds. Daisy is referred to a cardiologist.

The cardiologist refers Daisy for an electrocardiogram and an echocardiogram. The echocardiogram shows mild regurgitation of the aortic valve with a normal heart size.

Process information

Any of the four valves of the heart can become disordered in their functioning. There are two main processes that can affect the valves (Clare 2007).

1. *Valvular incompetence (regurgitation)*. The valve becomes unable to close properly and thus there is backward flow of blood into the heart chamber behind the valve. Incompetence is most common in the mitral and aortic valves; it is very rare in both the tricuspid and pulmonary valves. Common causes of incompetence include age-related degeneration of the valve, infection of the valve and coronary artery disease.
2. *Valve stenosis*. The valve becomes stiff and the leaflets of the valve may fuse together, thus narrowing the opening that blood can pass through. Stenosis is rare in the pulmonary valve and is usually only found in the tricuspid valve in conjunction with aortic and/or mitral valve stenosis. Common causes of stenosis are rheumatic fever and age-related changes in the case of aortic valve stenosis.

Congenital heart defects are common in people with Down syndrome (Pfitzer et al. 2018). As screening programs improve, the rates of diagnosed congenital heart disease in those with Down syndrome are likely to increase. However, undiagnosed congenital heart disease remains common in the adult Down syndrome population (Vis et al. 2010).

People with valve disease may require valve replacement surgery.

Nursing actions

1. Provide support for Daisy at all medical appointments to ensure that she feels heard, her health complaints are recognised and she understands all therapeutic interventions.
   Rationale:
   - All people have a right to healthcare in Australia, and Australia is a signatory to the Convention on the Rights of Persons with Disabilities, which recognises that persons with disabilities have the right to the enjoyment of the highest attainable standard of health without discrimination. See the United Nations Department of Economic and Social Affairs (2016).
2. Provide education and multidisciplinary referrals for Daisy on lifestyle decisions which will help to minimise risks of obesity.
   Rationale:
   - People with Down syndrome are at higher risk of obesity than the general population. The multidisciplinary approach will involve others who support Daisy and will include education, diet plans and regular health checks.
   - Obesity predisposes patients to diabetes and coronary heart disease and exacerbates any congenital heart problems already present.

Evaluate outcomes

Daisy can articulate her understanding of her health issues, the therapeutic interventions and the lifestyle decisions that will help to slow progress of her condition and minimise its impact on her life.

Source: Based on the Clinical Reasoning Cycle, Levett-Jones (2013).

SKILLS IN PRACTICE

Auscultation of heart sounds

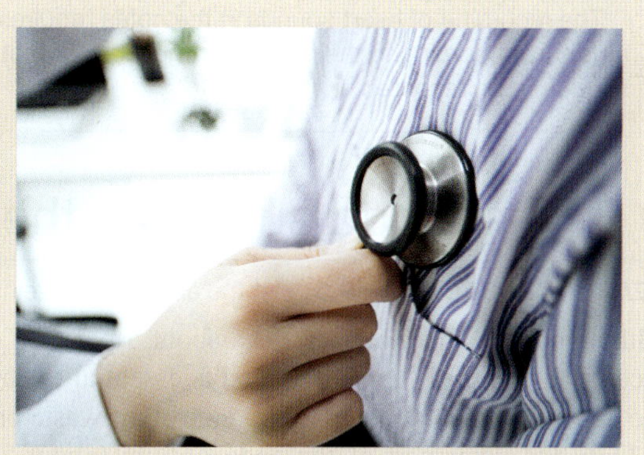

The auscultation of heart sounds requires a stethoscope and good hearing (amplified stethoscopes are available for nurses with hearing impairments). A normal heart will have two sounds: 'lub' (known as S1), which is the closing of the atrioventricular valves, and 'dub' (S2), which is caused by the closing of the **semilunar valves** (between atrium and ventricle). Other sounds that may be heard (adventitious sounds) include the following.

- *Murmurs*. These are caused by turbulent blood flow. The most common murmurs are related to heart valve disease.
- *Rubs*. A rub will almost always be a pericardial friction rub that is almost diagnostic of pericarditis (inflammation of the pericardium).

- *Clicks*. Clicks are difficult to hear; the aid of modern imaging technology has helped with the appreciation of these sounds. These sounds occur at the maximal opening of flexibly stenotic aortic or pulmonary valves in combination with pulmonary artery or aortic dilation.

Listening to heart sounds requires the placement of the stethoscope in four positions that correspond to different parts of the heart (see figure 9.8)

FIGURE 9.8 Auscultation sites for heart sounds

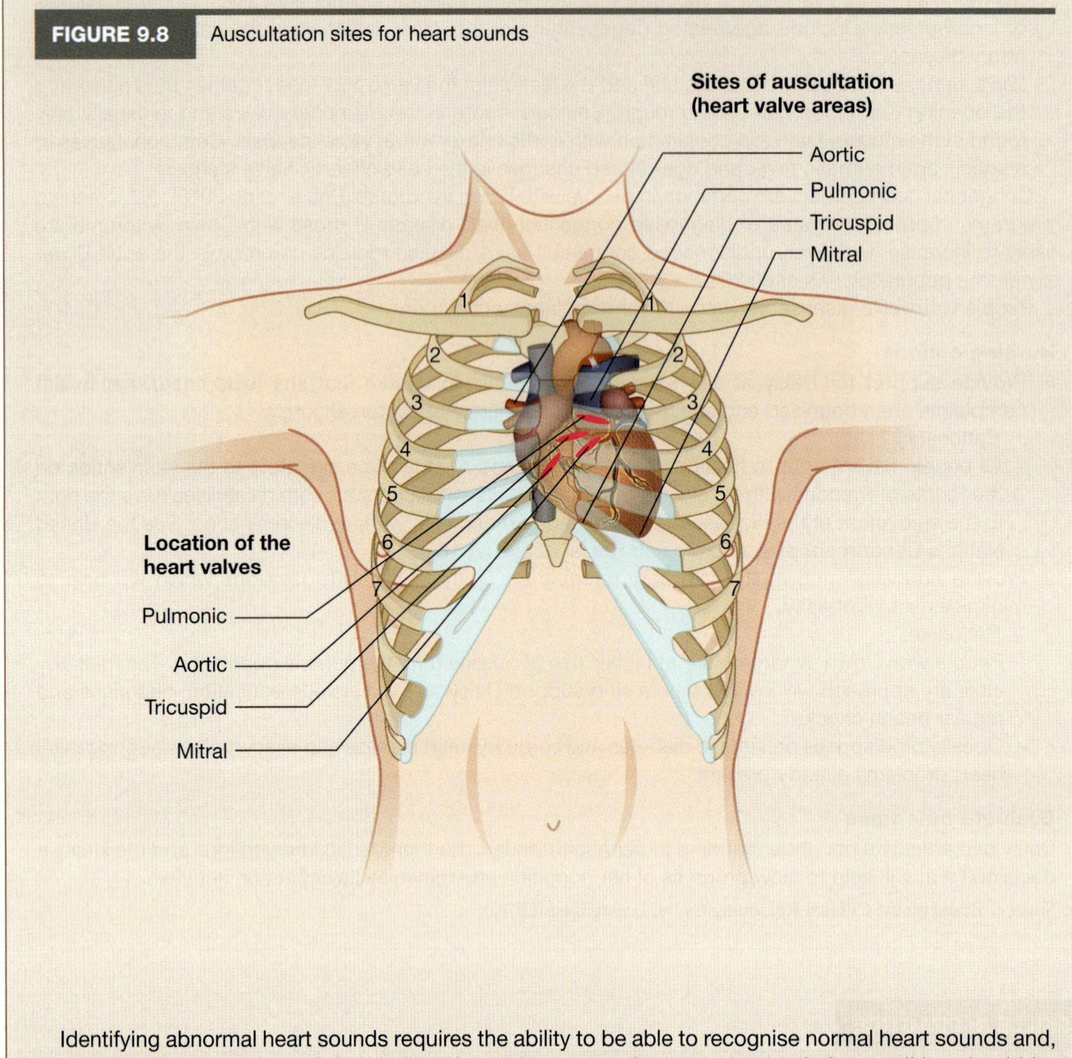

Identifying abnormal heart sounds requires the ability to be able to recognise normal heart sounds and, as such, until a nurse is proficient in listening to heart sounds, any suspected abnormalities should be reported to medical staff.

The recording of heart sounds in the notes requires the use of specific notation and the ability to grade murmurs according to their intensity and is a skill that can be learned after the nurse is able to identify the sounds to be recorded.

9.3 The blood supply to the heart

LEARNING OBJECTIVE 9.3 List the arteries and veins that supply blood to the heart muscle.

Although small, the heart receives about 5 per cent of the body's blood supply. Ensuring that the heart receives a plentiful supply of blood is essential to ensuring a constant supply of oxygen and nutrients to the myocardium and the efficient removal of waste products.

Only the inner part of the endocardium (about 2 mm in thickness) is supplied with blood directly from the inside of the heart chambers. The rest of the heart is supplied by the **coronary arteries**. The coronary arteries come directly off the aorta just after the aortic valve. They continuously divide into smaller branches, forming a web of blood vessels to supply the heart muscle. Figure 9.9 shows the main coronary arteries.

FIGURE 9.9 Coronary arteries

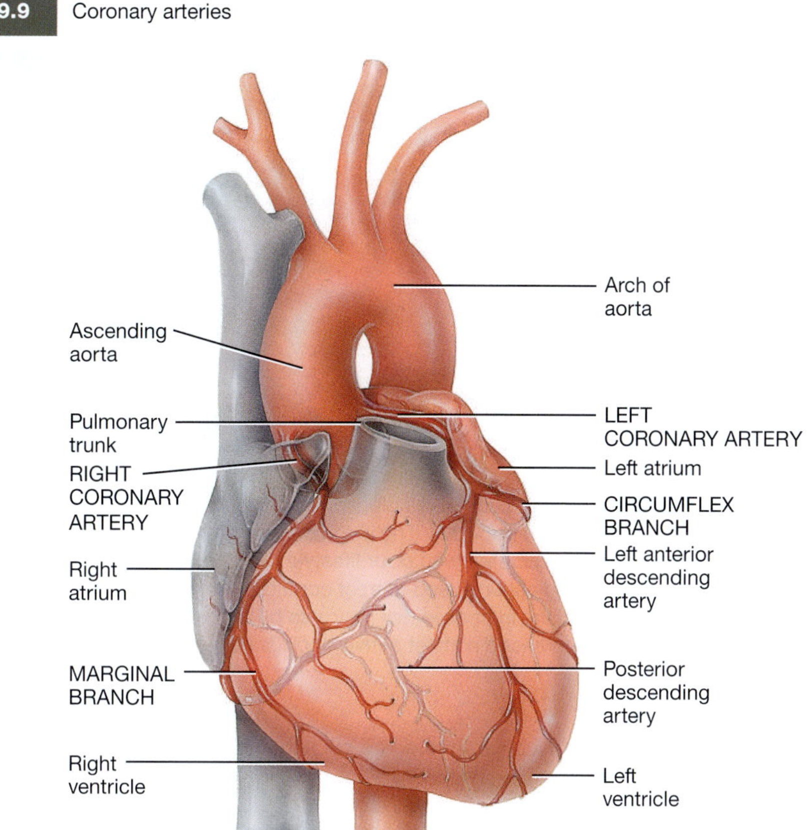

Source: Tortora and Derrickson (2009). Reproduced with permission of John Wiley & Sons.

Each artery (and its branches) supplies different areas of the heart muscle; table 9.1 gives a summary of the main arteries, their branches and the areas of the heart they supply. It is important to note that table 9.1 gives the anatomy as it pertains to most people, but there are normal variations in this pattern of blood supply in as much as 30 per cent of the population. These variations have no significance in the normal, healthy person but can be important in the treatment of cardiac patients.

TABLE 9.1 **Names of the coronary arteries, their major branches and the areas of the heart they supply**

Artery	Area of the heart supplied	Major branches
Left anterior descending (LAD)	Front and side of the left ventricle, apex of the heart	Diagonals Septals
Circumflex artery	Back and side of the left ventricle	Oblique marginal
Right coronary artery (RCA)	Right ventricle, base of the heart and interventricular septum	Posterior descending artery

As the coronary arteries are compressed during each heart beat, blood does not flow through the coronary arteries at this time. Thus, blood flow to the myocardium occurs during the relaxation phase; this is the opposite of every other part of the body.

CLINICALLY REASONED EPISODE OF CARE

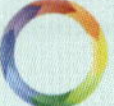

Chest pain and mental illness

Consider the patient situation

George is a 45-year-old Indigenous Australian who has been complaining of recurrent chest pain for the last few weeks. His GP has referred him to the local hospital for investigation. Given George's test results and his risk factors for coronary artery disease, the cardiologist decides that George should undergo an angiogram (cardiac catheter).

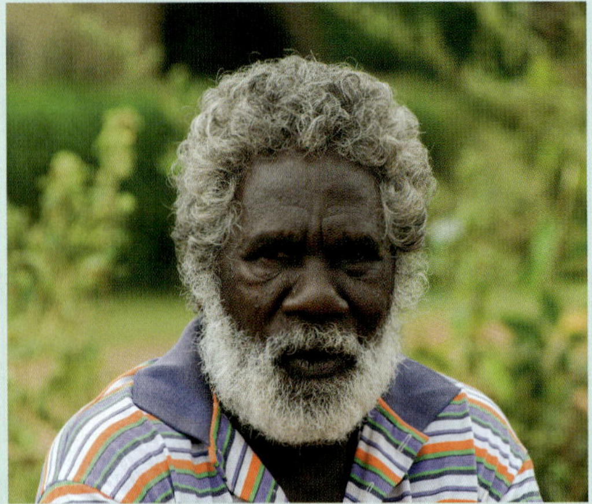

Collect cues and information

Health history: George was diagnosed with schizophrenia at the age of 21. After trying other antipsychotics over several years, he has now been taking clozapine (a second generation or atypical antipsychotic) for15 years.

Process information

The side effects of clozapine include weight gain, raised blood sugar, hypertension and raised cholesterol levels. George is a known smoker and has a poor diet. The increased risk of heart disease in patients with mental ill health has traditionally been associated with poor lifestyle choices (smoking, a lack of exercise and poor diet) and the side effects of medications used to treat conditions. In recent years there has been a growing evidence base to suggest that the increased risk may also be a direct result of the mental illness itself. Proposed mechanisms include increased platelet activity, cortisol levels and inflammatory markers (De Hert 2018).

Nursing actions

1. Provide reassurance, support and education for George prior to and during the procedure. Support George to provide informed consent.
   Rationale:
   - The procedure is carried out under local anaesthetic and complications are rare, and usually minor.
   - Quality patient education reduces anxiety and ensures informed consent (Australian Commission on Safety and Quality in Health Care 2020).
2. Assist with the procedure as required.
   Rationale:
   - Cardiac catheterisation is the insertion of a catheter through a large artery (normally in the groin or the arm) to the heart where X-ray dye (contrast) can be injected into the coronary arteries in order to obtain an image of any narrowing of the lumen that may be reducing blood flow to the cardiac muscle (figure 9.10).
   - This diagnostic procedure can determine what intervention may be required to support myocardial tissue perfusion.
3. Provide post-procedure care by:
   - monitoring left femoral access site for bleeding and swelling, left limb peripheral perfusion, and vital signs
   - maintaining flat bed rest and then sitting up at 30° until cleared by doctor for mobilisation
   - monitoring pressure dressing on wound
   - encouraging oral fluids to assist with excretion of radio-opaque dye used for procedure.

   Rationale:
   - Cardiac catheterisation uses a large artery for access. Puncturing an artery carries risk of bleeding and formation of a haematoma (clot). The clot can obstruct **arterial** flow, resulting in compromised perfusion of the limb. A pressure dressing and restriction of mobility can reduce this risk.
   - Cardiac catheterisation can trigger dysrhythmias, and vital signs can detect changes to patient status.
   - Contrast dyes cause increased fluid loss in urine (osmotic diuresis) and encouraging oral fluids will replace fluid lost from the body.
4. Provide health promotion education.
   Rationale:
   - This should focus on modifying cardiovascular risk factors — weight loss, smoking cessation and exercise. Follow up discussion with written materials and offer resources such as those found at the Heart Foundation (2021) and St Vincent's Hospital Heart Health (n.d.).

- Health promotion delivered at the point the patient is attending for diagnosis or investigation is known as opportunistic health promotion. Although there is little George can do about the physiological effects of his mental illness and some of the side effects of the antipsychotic medication, healthcare professionals should encourage and support him with any lifestyle modification which he may be open to.

FIGURE 9.10 Cardiac catheterisation

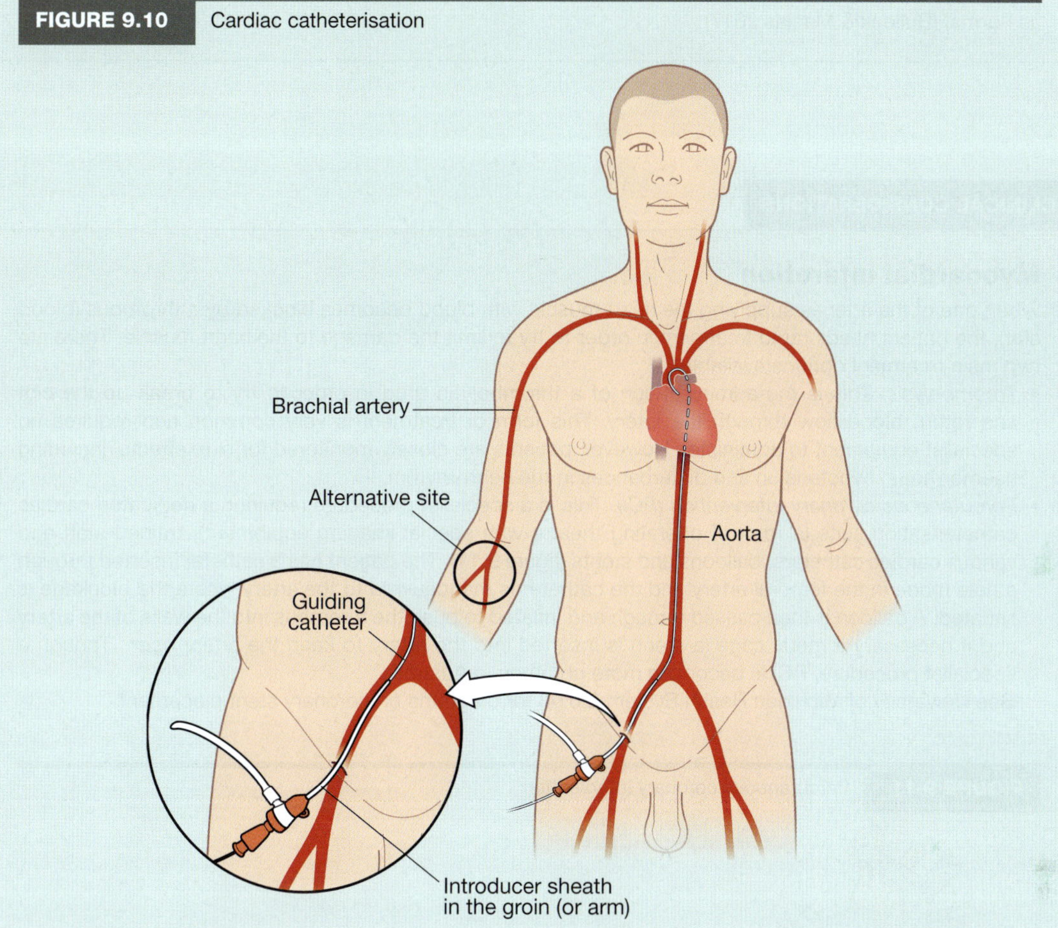

Evaluate outcomes

George recovers from his procedure with no complications. He reports changes to his lifestyle which will reduce his risk of heart disease.

Source: Based on the Clinical Reasoning Cycle, Levett-Jones (2013).

MEDICINES MANAGEMENT

Cardiac medication

Following his angiogram, George is informed that he has narrowing in some of his coronary arteries and the pain he is experiencing is angina due to an imbalance between the heart muscles' need for oxygen and the ability of blood to flow through the narrowed arteries. The cardiologist prescribes George a drug called diltiazem to help stop the pain from affecting his day-to-day life.

Diltiazem is one of a class of drugs known as calcium channel blockers. In angina they work by reducing the force of contraction of the heart by reducing the influx of calcium into the myocytes. This reduction in the force of contraction reduces the work of the heart, and therefore the need for oxygen.

Calcium channel blockers are also commonly used in the treatment of hypertension.

The side effects of calcium channel blockers include swollen ankles, ankle or foot pain, constipation, skin rashes, a flushed face, headaches, dizziness or tiredness (Bullock & Manias 2017). Both diltiazem and clozapine are known to increase the risk of low blood pressure (hypotension); thus it is recommended that George reports any episodes of dizziness to his GP and his blood pressure is monitored regularly (BNF 2019).

While diltiazem is not known to be affected, many of the calcium channel blockers are affected by grapefruit, and thus patients are generally advised not to drink grapefruit juice or eat grapefruit when taking calcium channel blockers. Other citrus fruits do not seem to have the same effect and can be eaten as normal (Bullock & Manias 2017).

CLINICAL CONSIDERATIONS

Myocardial infarction

When one of the arteries supplying the heart muscle with blood becomes blocked by a thrombus (blood clot), the patient needs rapid treatment in order to try to limit the damage to the heart muscle. There are two main treatment options available.

- *Thrombolysis.* This is the administration of a thrombolytic drug in order to try to break up the clot and return blood flow through the artery. This form of treatment is very common and requires no specialist equipment to administer. However, patients are closely monitored for side effects, including haemorrhage, hypotension and disturbances in the heart rhythm.
- *Percutaneous coronary intervention (PCI).* This is a specialist procedure requiring a dedicated cardiac catheterisation suite (a form of operating theatre with special imaging equipment), trained staff and various cardiac catheters, balloons and stents (figure 9.11). The patient has a catheter inserted through a hole made in the femoral artery and the catheter is manoeuvred to the artery where the blockage is situated. A balloon is then passed through and inflated to push the thrombus into the walls of the artery and if necessary a metal cage (a stent) is inserted into the artery to keep the artery open. Though a specialist procedure, PCI is becoming more common in Australia.

See University of Michigan Health System (2014) for diagrams on coronary stent placement.

FIGURE 9.11 Percutaneous coronary intervention

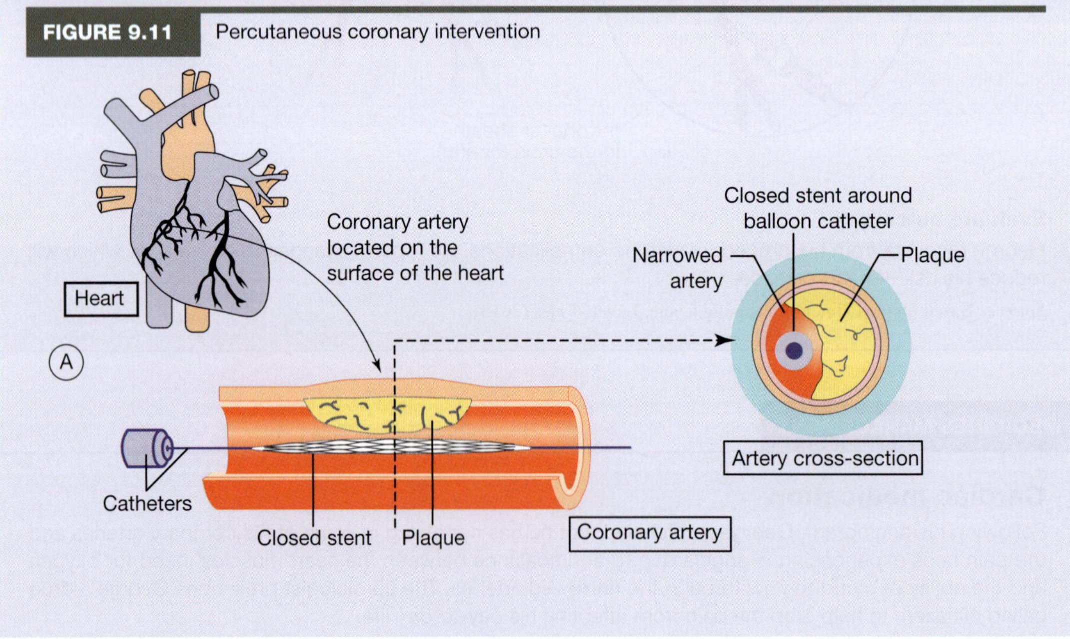

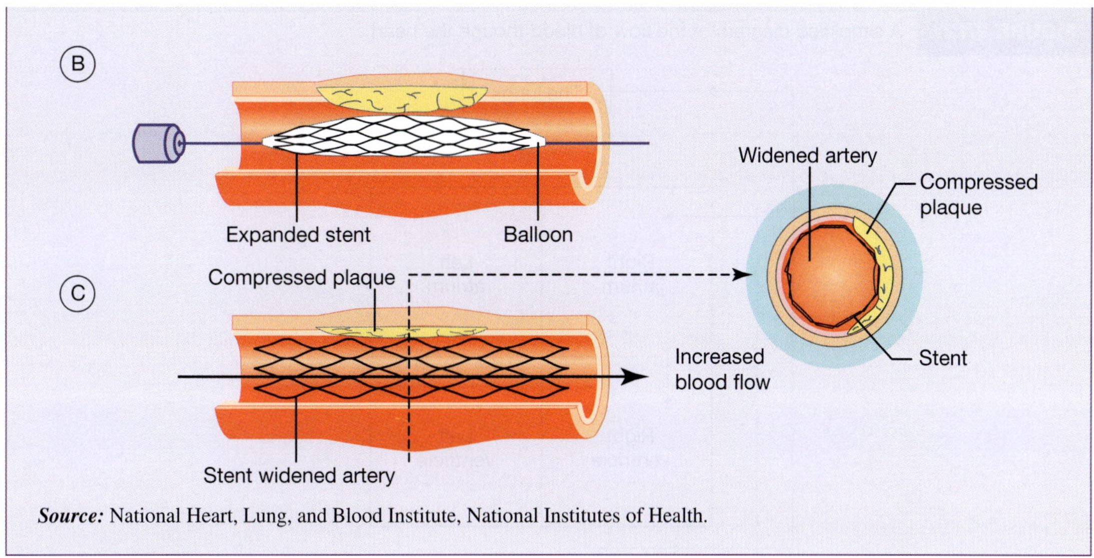

Source: National Heart, Lung, and Blood Institute, National Institutes of Health.

CLINICAL CONSIDERATIONS

Premature myocardial infarction: a national health priority

Myocardial infarction (subsequent to ischaemic heart disease) is the leading cause of death both in Australia and globally. In Australia 11.6 per cent of deaths in the wider community and 11.5 per cent in Aboriginal and Torres Strait Islander communities are attributable to myocardial infarction (Davey 2021). While these rates are similar, the mean age of onset is considerably lower in Indigenous communities (~50 years) when compared with the rest of the community (~80 years).

The underlying causes of this trend represent a number of Australia's national health priorities such as diabetes, dyslipidaemia, chronic kidney disease and hypertension, which all contribute to atherosclerosis, plaque calcification, and ultimately coronary artery disease (Davey 2021). Another significant factor is higher rates of tobacco use in Indigenous communities, with 43 per cent of adults using tobacco products compared with 11.6 per cent of Australian adults overall (AIHW 2020b). Limited access to appropriate nutrition and cardiac rehabilitation services combined with low referral rates to these services further complicate the treatment of myocardial infarction and contribute to premature death in remote communities (Field et al. 2018).

Blood flow through the heart

As noted earlier in the chapter, though the heart is a single organ it is best to think of it as two pumps, the right and the left heart pumps. Each pump is made up of two chambers (atrium and ventricle) and their associated valves.

- The right heart pump receives blood from the systemic circulation (the body) and pumps it through the pulmonary circulation (the lungs).
- The left heart pump receives blood from the pulmonary circulation and pumps it out around the systemic circulation.

Figure 9.12 gives a simplified explanation of the flow of blood through the heart. In this diagram, deoxygenated blood is in blue and oxygenated blood is in red. It is important to note that 'deoxygenated blood' does not refer to blood that has no oxygen in it but to blood that has given up some of its oxygen to the tissues. Typically, deoxygenated blood contains 75 per cent of the oxygen that oxygenated blood carries.

So, as can be seen, deoxygenated blood returns from the body to the right atrium and then into the right ventricle, from where it is pumped out to the lungs. In the lungs the waste gases are exchanged for oxygen and the oxygenated blood flows into the left atrium and into the left ventricle. From the left ventricle the blood is then pumped into the circulation of the body.

FIGURE 9.12 A simplified diagram of the flow of blood though the heart

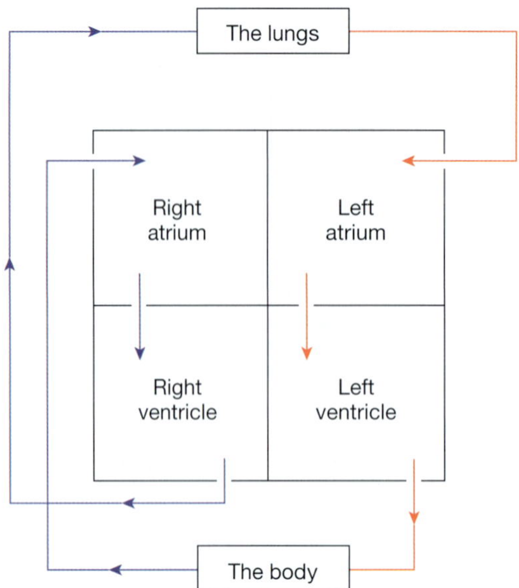

A more detailed and anatomical view can be seen in figure 9.13. Blood enters the right atrium via the superior vena cava and inferior vena cava and leaves the right ventricle via the pulmonary arteries. Note that even though it is deoxygenated blood leaving the right ventricle it is the vessels that the blood is carried in that make it arterial or **venous**. Thus:

- blood entering the atria is carried in veins and is therefore **venous blood**
- blood leaving the ventricles is carried in arteries and is **arterial blood**.

FIGURE 9.13 Anatomical view of the blood flow through the heart

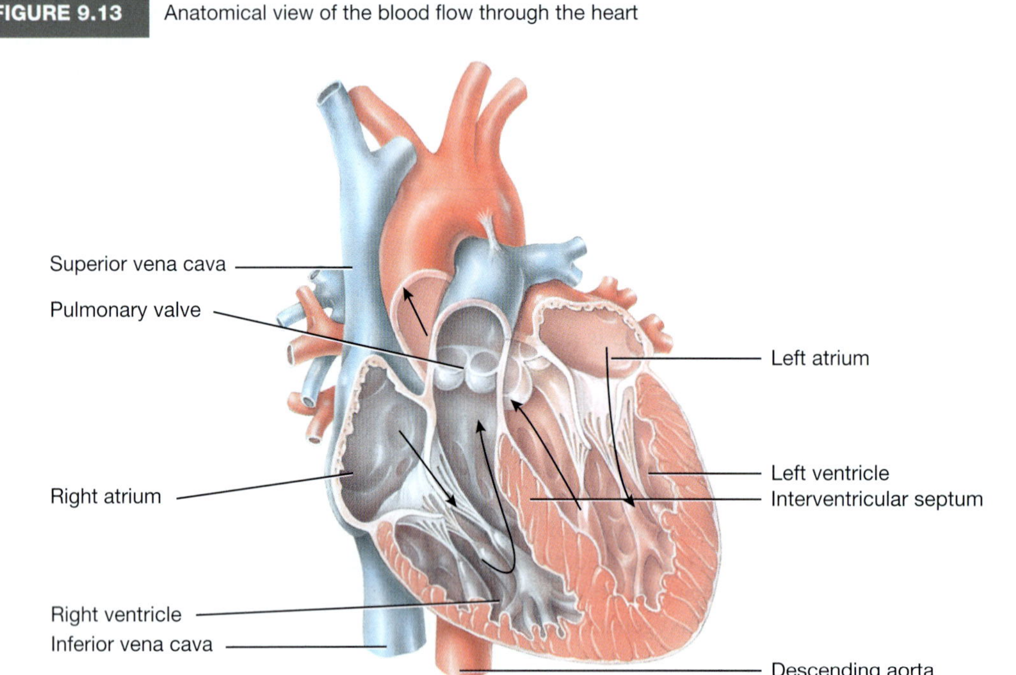

Source: Tortora and Derrickson (2009). Reproduced with permission of John Wiley & Sons.

Blood is transported through the pulmonary circulation and returned to the left atrium through the pulmonary veins; it is then pumped out by the left ventricle into the aorta.

9.4 The electrical pathways of the heart

LEARNING OBJECTIVE 9.4 Describe the electrical excitation of the heart.

Within the heart there is a specialised network of electrical pathways dedicated to ensuring the rapid transmission of electrical impulses. This ensures that the myocardium is excited rapidly in response to an initiating impulse so that the chambers contract and relax in the right order and the different pairs of chambers (atria and ventricles) contract at the same time. So, for instance, the left and right ventricles will contract simultaneously in response to an impulse (but after the atria). Also, the way in which the conduction system is organised means that the ventricles contract in a specific way to ensure they eject blood effectively. For example, if you wanted to empty out a tube of toothpaste you would squeeze from the base to ensure maximum effect. Likewise, the ventricles contract in such a way as to push blood towards and through the semilunar valves.

The cardiac muscles have a specialised property not seen in any other part of the body. All cells within the myocardium have the ability to create their own action potential without external excitation from another cell or a **hormone**. This is known as **automaticity** (or auto-rhythmicity). The problem with this is that, uncontrolled, the cells would all act independently and the heart would not beat effectively as there would be no coordination of the electrical activity and the subsequent muscle contractions. This is overcome by specialised cells in the conduction system. These cells create and distribute an electrical current that leads to a controlled and effective heart contraction. An overview of the anatomy of the conduction system can be seen in figure 9.14.

FIGURE 9.14 Conduction system of the heart

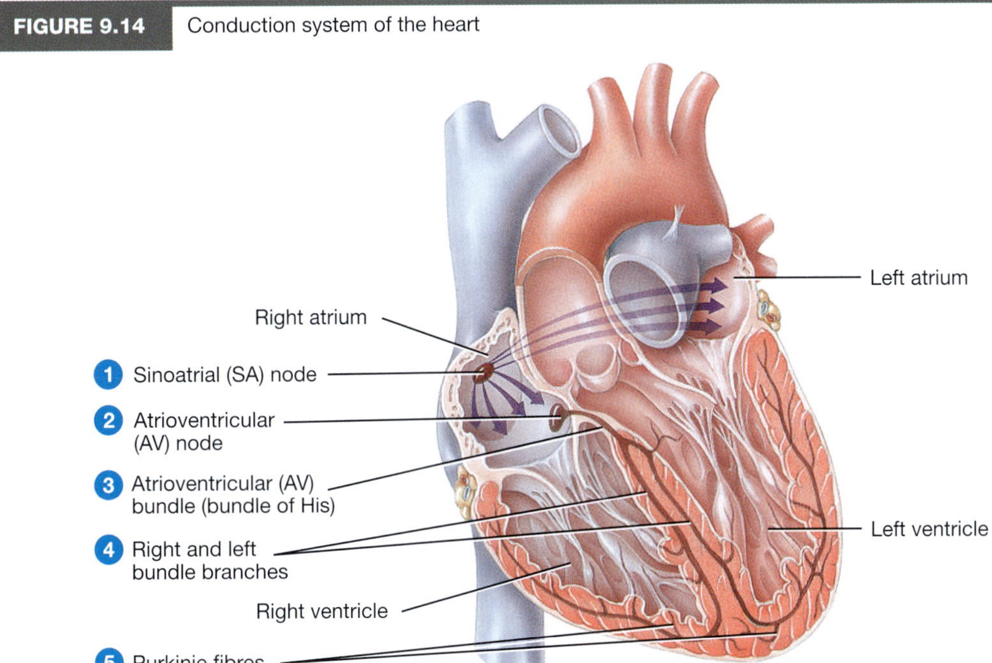

Source: Tortora and Derrickson (2009). Reproduced with permission of John Wiley & Sons.

Normal electrical excitation/distribution begins in the **sinoatrial (SA) node**, which is located in the right atrium, and is rapidly transmitted across the atria by fast pathways. This ensures that the right and left atria are excited together and beat as one unit. The impulse is transmitted to the **atrioventricular (AV) node**, where further transmission is delayed for approximately 0.1 s (Martini et al. 2014). This ensures that the atria have completely contracted before ventricular contraction is initiated. It should be noted that the atria and the ventricles are electrically isolated from each other by a band of non-conducting fibrous tissue, and thus the only electrical connection between the two is the **bundle of His** (**atrioventricular (AV) bundle**) (figure 9.15).

Once the impulse has been 'held' in the AV node it is then transmitted down the bundle of His (AV bundle) to the fast pathways of the two bundle branches (one bundle branch per ventricle). The bundles then divide into the smaller and smaller branches of the **Purkinje fibres system**, which transmits the impulses to the muscles of the ventricles.

FIGURE 9.15 Normal electrical conduction

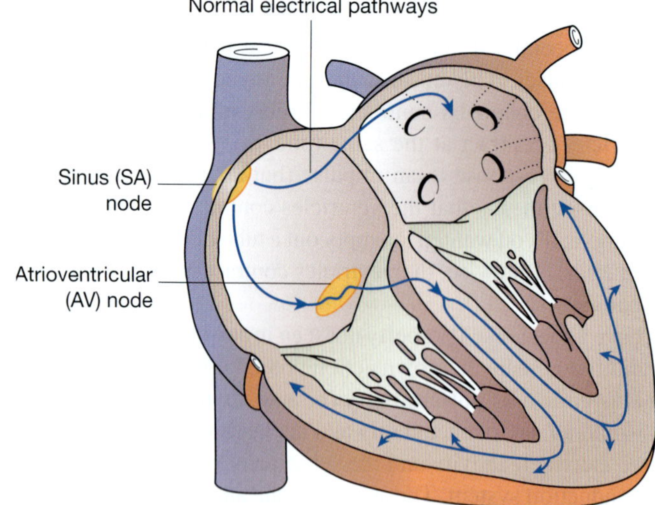

Source: Tortora and Derrickson (2009). Reproduced with permission of John Wiley & Sons.

MEDICINES MANAGEMENT

Digoxin

Pauline is a 72-year-old woman admitted to the coronary care unit with a heart rate of 35 and a blood pressure of 90/40 mmHg. She is feeling very unwell and is restless, confused and agitated. The ECG recording of her heart shows signs of digoxin toxicity and on questioning Pauline's daughter it appears Pauline had been prescribed digoxin a few months ago.

Digoxin is a cardiac glycoside used in the treatment of heart failure and arrhythmias of the atria. Once a very popular drug, its use has reduced, but it is still prescribed. Digoxin slows and strengthens the heart beat (decreasing heart rate and increasing force of contraction). Owing to these effects, an excess of digoxin in the blood can lead to a slow heart rate, which can cause dizziness. In the elderly, excretion of digoxin is reduced and thus digoxin levels can rise above the therapeutic threshold even on normal doses.

The signs of digoxin toxicity include nausea, vomiting, confusion, delirium and headache. It can also lead to very high levels of blood potassium. In life-threatening cases, the digoxin can be counteracted by the use of digoxin-specific antibodies (digibind) infused into the blood. Otherwise, supportive treatment and monitoring may be instituted and the digoxin withheld.

When administering digoxin, the nurse is required to take the pulse of the patient; if it is below 60 beats per minute, the drug should be withheld and medical advice sought. The actions the nurse has taken must also be documented (Bullock & Manias 2017).

CLINICAL CONSIDERATIONS

Nodal cells

Otherwise known as pacemaker cells, these are specialised cells that not only create electrical impulses but also create them at regular intervals.

Nodal cells are divided into two groups.

1. The SA node is located in the right atrium, which generates electrical impulses at approximately 70–80 impulses per minute.
2. The AV node is located just above the point where the atria and ventricles meet. This node generates impulses at 40–60 impulses per minute.

The difference in the rate of impulse creation is important in the normal functioning of the heart as every time an impulse is transmitted down the electrical system it 'resets' the cells 'lower down'. Hence, the SA node is the normal pacemaker of the heart as it creates impulses faster than the AV node.

Thus, like a military command structure, the SA node could be seen to be a general who commands the captain (AV node), but if the general no longer issues commands then the captain will take over command.

Even with the 'command structure' created by the nodal cells the conduction system of the heart can slow considerably and the patient can become very unwell. For instance, if the AV node no longer transmits impulses into the bundle of His, the cells in the lower parts of the conduction system can produce action potentials of their own, but this will be at a very slow rate (between 20 and 35 impulses per minute). In order to rectify this problem the patient would need to have a permanent pacemaker fitted (figure 9.16).

FIGURE 9.16 Pacemaker

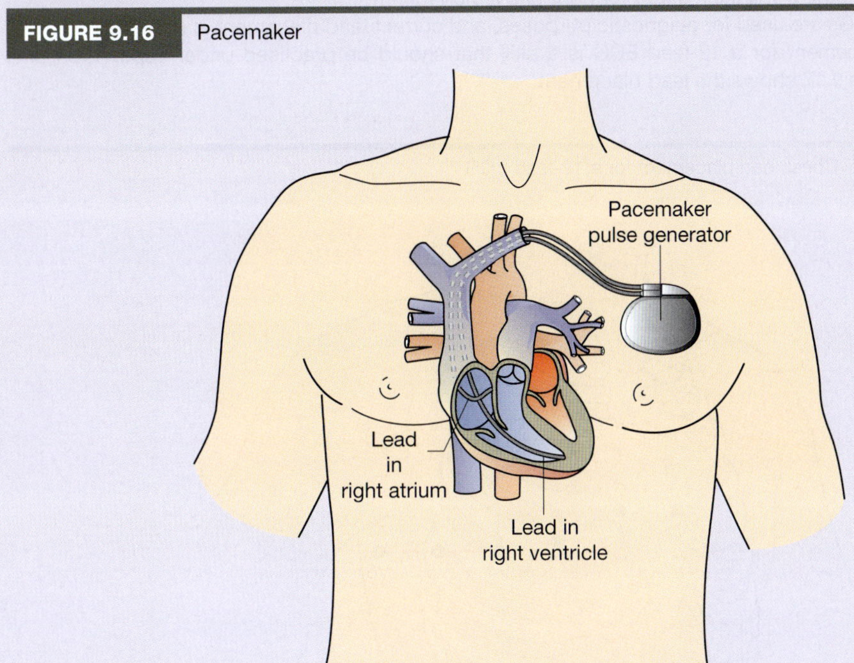

The 'generator' (battery and circuitry) is contained in a small box that is buried beneath the skin of the chest wall. Wires lead from the generator through a vein into the patient's heart. Depending on the type of pacemaker fitted, there may be one or two wires. So, for instance, in the case of a failed AV node the pacemaker would have two wires: one in the right atrium and one in the right ventricle. The pacemaker would sense the atrial action potential and then (after a short delay to mimic the action of the AV node) the ventricle would receive an electrical impulse, causing it to contract. Thus, the pacemaker acts as a replacement AV node (O'Grady 2007).

SKILLS IN PRACTICE

ECG

On admission to the coronary care unit, Pauline required a 12-lead ECG and cardiac monitoring. While they both record the electrical activity of the heart, 3-lead monitoring and a 12-lead ECG have different purposes.

Three-lead cardiac monitoring is used for the continuous monitoring of the heart rhythm in patients thought to be at risk of a heart rhythm disturbance. The lead placement is as follows.

Red lead	Right arm
Yellow lead	Left arm
Green lead	Left leg
Or	
Black lead	Right leg

It should be noted that the leads of a monitoring system are normally attached to the relevant shoulder for the arm leads and the lower chest for the leg leads, thus leaving the patient freedom of movement and leaving the chest clear for resuscitation (if required).

For a 12-lead ECG, the limb leads are placed as noted above but at the wrists and ankles; the chest leads are then attached. Many nurses use mnemonics to remember limb lead placement such as: '**R**ide **Y**our **G**reen **B**ike'; others will think of *red for right* and *lemon for left*.

Twelve-lead ECGs are used for diagnostic purposes, and correct lead placement is essential.

Chest lead placement for a 12-lead ECG is a skill that should be practised under supervision until competent. Figure 9.17 shows the lead placement.

FIGURE 9.17 Chest lead placement for a 12-lead ECG

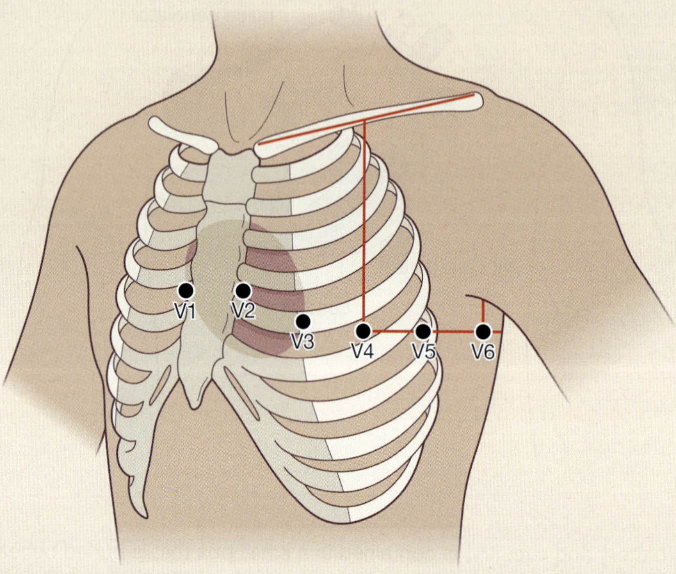

- V1: fourth intercostal space, right sternal border
- V2: fourth intercostal space, left sternal border
- V3: midway between V2 and V4
- V4: fifth intercostal space, left midclavicular line
- V5: level with V4, left anterior axillary line
- V6: level with V4, left mid axillary line.

In female patients, electrodes are never placed on top of the breast unless you cannot gain access to the normal position. If you do have to move onto the breast, document this on the recording.

9.5 The cardiac cycle

LEARNING OBJECTIVE 9.5 Discuss the cardiac cycle.

The cardiac cycle is the name given to the mechanical activity of the heart and is best understood by looking at the pressure changes in the heart chambers and the aorta and relating these to the mechanical activity of the heart and its chambers.

HOMEOSTATIC IMBALANCE

Atrial fibrillation

Atrial fibrillation (AF) is a common form of cardiac arrhythmia that occurs where sinus rhythm is disrupted by rapid and irregular ectopic **depolarisation** of the atria (figure 9.18). This causes the atria to 'quiver' rather than contract in an effective and coordinated manner, leading to inadequate filling of the heart. AF is important in the context of both cardiovascular disease and Australia's health priorities as the risk of AF is increased in the presence of congestive heart failure, pericarditis, coronary heart disease and hypertension, and is itself a major contributor to both mortality and morbidity in these diseases. Under normal circumstances the heart will beat at a rate of approximately 60 beats per minute at rest; this can increase to between 180 and 200 beats per minute during exercise to meet the metabolic needs of the body. In contrast, the atrial cells are responding to between 400 and 600 stimuli per minute during AF. It is commonly treated with drugs, such as amiodarone and dronedarone, that block Na^+, K^+ and Ca^{++} channels, beta blockers and direct current cardioversion to restore sinus rhythm.

FIGURE 9.18 ECG of normal versus atrial fibrillation

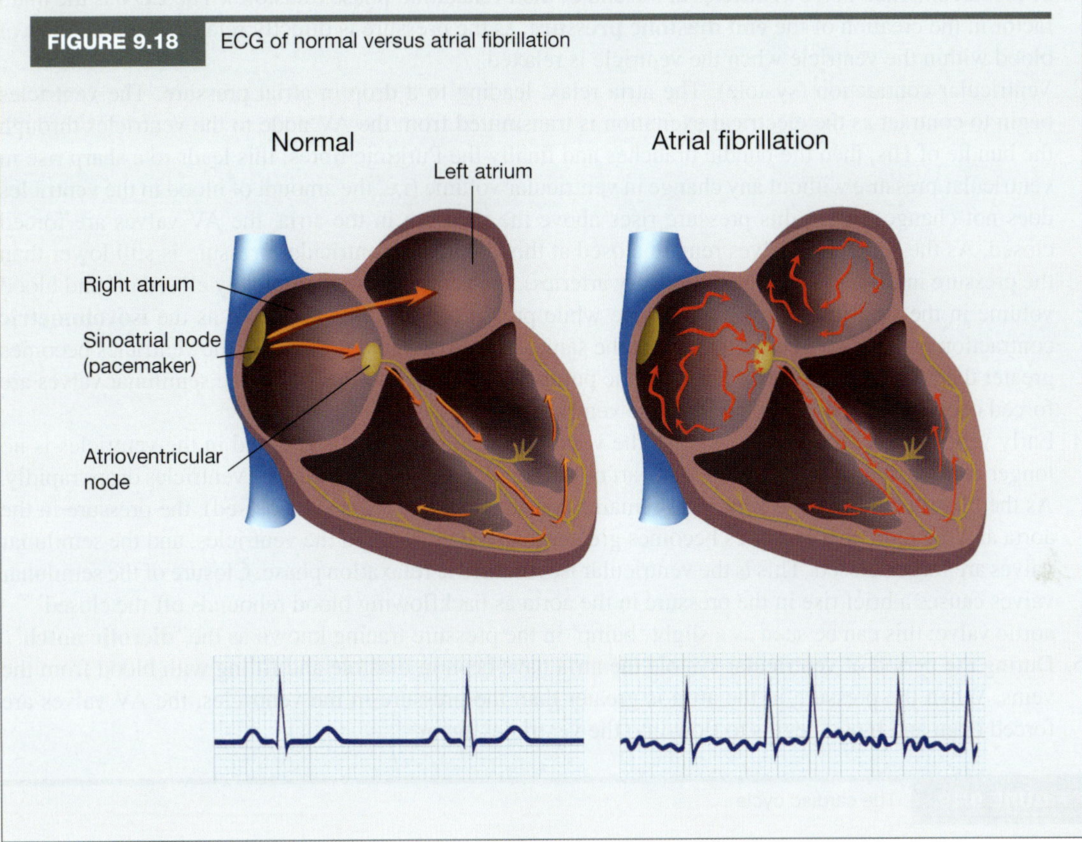

Systole and diastole

These are two terms that require definition as they are unique in anatomy and physiology to the functioning of the heart.

- **Systole**: the contraction of a heart chamber (atrium or ventricle).
- **Diastole**: the relaxation of a heart chamber (atrium or ventricle).

The cardiac cycle can be seen in figure 9.19. Note, the diagram refers to the pressures in the left side of the heart (atrium and ventricle); the cardiac cycle is the same on the right side but the pressures are lower. The cardiac cycle can be broken down into a series of steps that are detailed below. The flow of blood in the heart and the circulatory system is always from a point of higher pressure to a point of lower pressure.

The cardiac cycle is usually divided into five phases.

1. A period of ventricular filling in mid to late relaxation (ventricular diastole). Pressure in the ventricle is low. Blood that is returning to the heart through the vena cava is flowing passively through the atria and the open AV valves into the ventricle. The pressure in the atria is higher than that in the ventricles and this forces the bicuspid and tricuspid valves open. As the pressure in the ventricles rises due to the increased amount of blood in the ventricles, the leaflets of the AV valves begin to drift upwards to their closed positions. The semilunar valves (the aortic and the pulmonary valves) are closed; the pressure in the aorta and the pulmonary arteries is greater than that in the ventricles, thus forcing these valves shut. About 70 per cent of ventricular filling happens during this phase.

2. Late in this phase the atria begin to contract (atrial systole) in response to excitation by an action potential from the SA node; this compresses the blood in the atria, leading to a slight rise in the pressure in the atria. This rise in pressure leads to a greater flow of blood into the ventricles from the atria. The ventricles remain in diastole as the electrical excitation that led to atrial contraction is delayed in the AV node. By the end of this point in time the ventricles are in the last part of their relaxation phase and contain the largest amount of blood they will contain during the cardiac cycle. This is known as the **end diastolic volume** (EDV) and is about 130 mL of blood (Jenkins & Tortora 2013); that is, the volume of blood contained in the ventricles at the end of their relaxation phase (diastole). The EDV is the main factor in the creation of the **end diastolic pressure**, as the pressure is directly related to the amount of blood within the ventricle when the ventricle is relaxed.
3. Ventricular contraction (systole). The atria relax, leading to a drop in atrial pressure. The ventricles begin to contract as the electrical excitation is transmitted from the AV node to the ventricles through the bundle of His, then the bundle branches and finally the Purkinje fibres; this leads to a sharp rise in ventricular pressure without any change in ventricular volume (i.e. the amount of blood in the ventricles does not change). Once this pressure rises above the pressure in the atria, the AV valves are forced closed. As the semilunar valves remain closed at this point (the ventricular pressure is still lower than the pressure in the aorta and the pulmonary arteries), the ventricles are completely closed off and blood volume in the ventricles remains the same while pressure rises. This is known as the **isovolumetric** contraction phase ('iso' means remaining the same). Eventually, the pressure in the ventricles becomes greater than the pressure in the aorta and the pulmonary arteries. At this point, the semilunar valves are forced open and blood is ejected from the ventricles.
4. Early ventricular diastole (relaxation). The ventricles begin to relax. The blood in the ventricles is no longer compressed by the action of the heart muscle, and the pressure within the ventricles drops rapidly. As the blood volume in the ventricles remains constant (the AV valves are closed), the pressure in the aorta and the pulmonary arteries becomes greater than the pressure in the ventricles, and the semilunar valves are forced closed. This is the ventricular isovolumetric relaxation phase. Closure of the semilunar valves causes a brief rise in the pressure in the aorta as backflowing blood rebounds off the closed aortic valve; this can be seen as a slight 'bump' in the pressure tracing known as the '**dicrotic notch**'.
5. During the period of ventricular systole the atria have been in diastole and filling with blood from the veins. When the pressure in the atria is greater than the pressure in the ventricles, the AV valves are forced open and blood begins to flow into the ventricles again.

FIGURE 9.19 The cardiac cycle

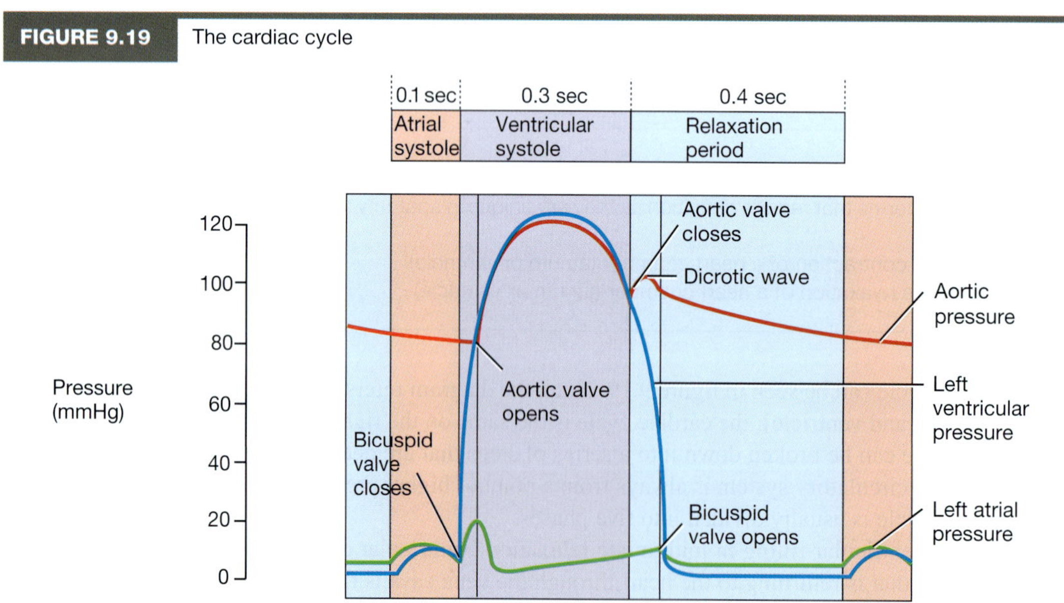

Source: Tortora and Derrickson (2009). Reproduced with permission of John Wiley & Sons.

CLINICAL CONSIDERATIONS

Electrocardiogram and the cardiac cycle

Though the cardiac cycle refers to the mechanical action of the heart, the electrical activity that stimulates this mechanical action can be seen by the use of an ECG, an electrical tracing produced by attaching electrodes to the patient's skin and generated by an ECG machine. However, it is possible for the electrical tracing to be present without mechanical activity in certain types of cardiac arrest.

The normal ECG of one cycle of the heart is shown in figure 9.20.

FIGURE 9.20 Normal ECG of one cycle of the heart

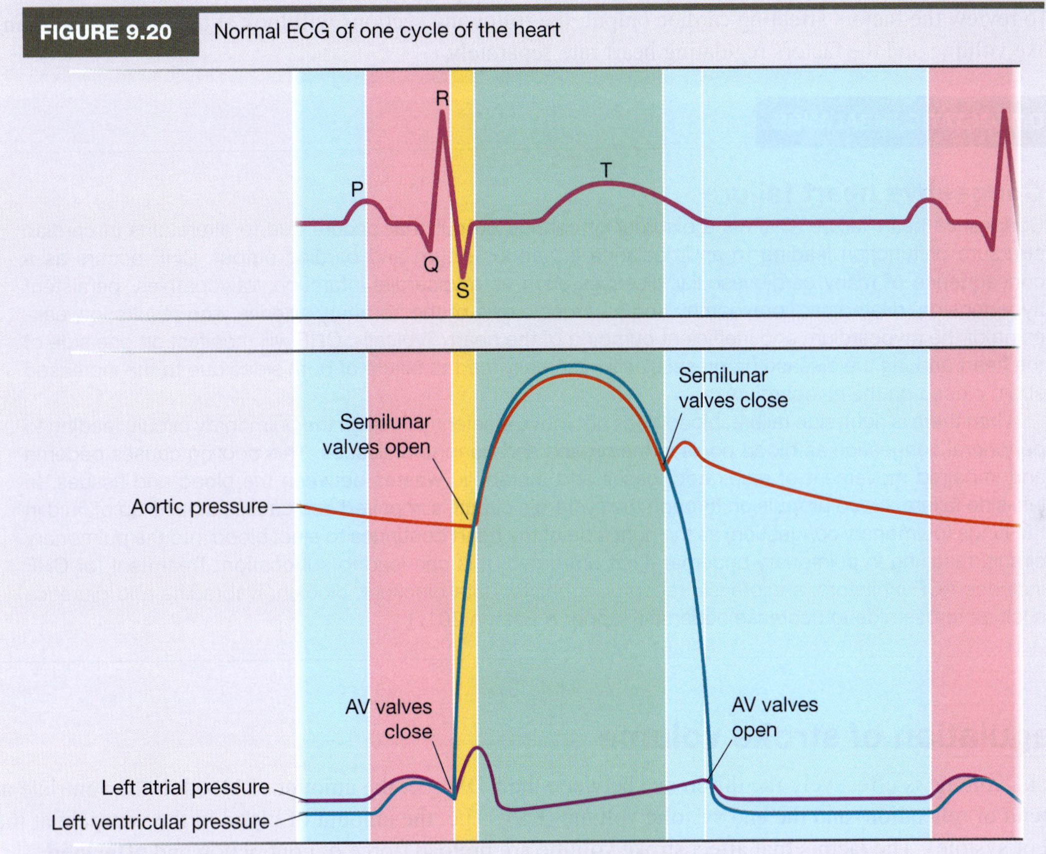

Source: Adapted from Jenkins and Tortora (2013). Reproduced with permission of John Wiley & Sons.

The changes from the baseline on the ECG are labelled by letters of the alphabet:

- P — atrial depolarisation; corresponds to atrial contraction
- QRS — ventricular depolarisation; corresponds approximately to ventricular contraction (though this happens just after the peak of the R wave)
- T — ventricular **repolarisation**; corresponds to the relaxation phase of the ventricle; atrial repolarisation cannot be seen as it is hidden by the greater electrical activity of ventricular depolarisation.

Despite this appearing to be a long process, if we assume a heart rate of 75 beats per minute then the average cardiac cycle would take approximately 0.8 s. The atria are in systole for 0.1 s and then in diastole for 0.7 s, while the ventricles are in systole for 0.3 s and diastole for 0.5 s. As heart rate increases, the cardiac cycle becomes shorter due to the shortening of the diastolic phase; the systolic phase remains the same. As already noted, the heart muscle is supplied with blood during the diastolic (relaxation) phase, as blood cannot flow in the coronary arteries when the heart is contracting; thus, as heart rate increases, blood flow in the coronary arteries (and blood supply to the heart muscle) is reduced.

Factors affecting cardiac output

This section gives an overview of the factors affecting the cardiac output. 'Cardiac output' is a term relating to the amount of blood the heart pumps out in 1 minute and is defined by

$$\text{Cardiac output (CO)} = \text{Stroke volume (SV)} \times \text{Heart rate (HR)}$$

Thus, the amount of blood the heart pumps out in a minute is made up of the amount of blood ejected from the ventricle in one beat (SV) times the heart rate (HR) in beats per minute. This gives a total volume. Thus, if we said that SV is 70 mL and the heart rate is 75, then cardiac output is $70 \times 75 = 5250$ mL (or 5.25 L) per minute.

To review the factors affecting cardiac output, the following sections will look at the factors regulating stroke volume and the factors regulating heart rate separately.

HOMEOSTATIC IMBALANCE

Congestive heart failure

Congestive heart failure (CHF) is a disorder of cardiac output that occurs due to alterations in cardiac structure or function leading to an imbalance in venous return and cardiac output. CHF occurs as a consequence of many cardiovascular diseases such as myocardial infarction, valvopathies, persistent hypertension, dilated cardiomyopathy and atherosclerosis of the coronary arteries, and results in weakening of the myocardium and inefficient pumping of the heart. Typically, CHF will manifest on one side of the heart and, as the disease progresses, will eventually lead to failure of both sides due to the increased strain placed on the myocardium.

When there is right-side failure, blood does not move efficiently through the pulmonary circuit, leading to peripheral congestion as blood pools in the organs and peripheral tissues. This pooling causes oedema and impaired movement of respiratory gases and metabolic wastes between the blood and tissues. In left-side failure, blood propulsion through the systemic circuit is impaired and causes a build-up of fluid in the lungs (pulmonary congestion) as the right side of the heart continues to eject blood into the pulmonary circuit, resulting in pulmonary oedema. If left untreated, this can lead to suffocation. Treatment for CHF includes ACE inhibitors, angiotensin receptor agonists, beta blockers, digoxin, ivabradine and diuretics such as furosemide to decrease oedema (Hopper & Easton 2017).

Regulation of stroke volume

Stroke volume is effectively the difference between the EDV (i.e. the amount of blood in the ventricle at the end of relaxation) and the end systolic volume (ESV) (i.e. the amount of blood in the ventricle at the end of systole). The factors that affect stroke volume are preload, force of contraction and **afterload**.

Preload

The force the cardiac muscle fibres contract with during systole is affected by the amount of stretch they are subjected to (the greater the stretch, the greater the force). This is known as the Frank–Starling law.

The stretch of the cardiac muscle is directly related to the amount of blood in the ventricle at the end of diastole (EDV), which is, in turn, dependent on the volume of blood returned to the heart via the veins (venous return). Thus, venous return is related to the force of contraction of the ventricles. Anything that affects the speed or volume of venous return affects EDV, and therefore force of contraction, such as the following.

- A slower heart rate allows for more time for blood to fill the ventricle, increasing the volume of blood in the ventricle at the end of diastole.
- Exercise increases venous return, as the increase in heart rate increases the pressure in the veins and the speed of venous return and the effect of skeletal muscle activity squeezes the veins 'pushing' blood back to the heart (skeletal muscle pumps). Conversely, standing still means that venous return is reduced. Thus, the guardsmen who have to stand still outside Buckingham Palace are taught to discretely contract and relax their feet to aid venous return and prevent fainting.
- Hormonal and nervous influences. The release of adrenaline or the excitation of the sympathetic nervous system leads to the contraction of the veins and the 'squeezing' of blood back to the heart.
- Very fast heart rates reduce the diastolic filling time, and thus there is less time for the ventricle to receive blood before systole starts.

- Certain heart arrhythmias stop the atria contracting effectively, and thus atrial systole is no longer effective at 'pushing' the last bit of blood into the ventricles.
- A reduced blood volume (for instance, due to a haemorrhage) reduces venous return.

Force of contraction

Though EDV is a major component of the force of contraction (because of the Frank–Starling law), force of contraction can also be affected by other factors. The contractility of the heart can be affected by several factors.

- Hormones, such as adrenaline, glucagon and thyroxine, all increase the force of contraction.
- Sympathetic nervous system activity increases the force of contraction through the action of noradrenaline.
- Contractility can be reduced by acidaemia (excess hydrogen **ions** in the blood) and high potassium levels in the blood.

Afterload

Afterload refers to the pressure in the arteries leading from the ventricles (aorta or pulmonary arteries) that the ventricle must overcome in order to eject blood. In the normal adult the pressure is 80 mmHg in the aorta and 8 mmHg in the pulmonary arteries. This difference in the pressure to be overcome is reflected in the relative thickness of the ventricular walls, with the left ventricular wall being thicker (more muscular) than the right (see previous discussion on the structure of the heart).

In the average adult, aortic and pulmonary pressure is not an important factor in determining afterload as it is constant, but changes in anatomy and/or physiology, such as hypertension or aortic valve disease, can increase afterload. Increased afterload increases the amount of blood left in the ventricle after each systole, and thus also has an effect in increasing the preload (by increasing ventricular ESV and therefore pressure).

MEDICINES MANAGEMENT

Hypercholesterolemia (high cholesterol levels)

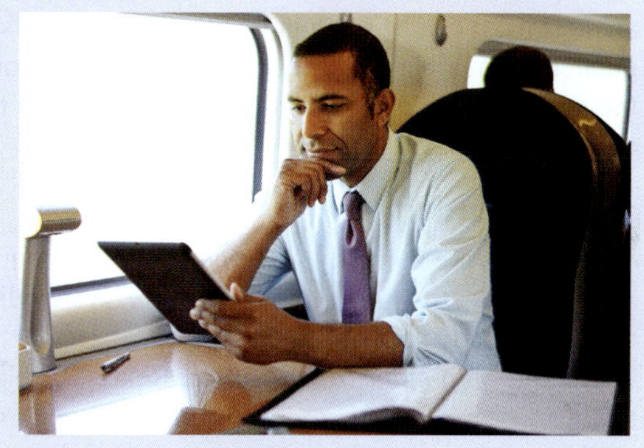

Dave is a 45-year-old office worker who has recently returned to work after a myocardial infarction (MI). The rehabilitation nurse has given Dave a lot of information on healthy eating and exercise, but she notes his blood cholesterol test result is significantly higher than is advisable for someone who has had an MI. The nurse consults with the medical team and Dave is prescribed 80 mg atorvastatin once a day.

Atorvastatin is a cholesterol-lowering medication that lowers the amount of cholesterol produced in the body. It is commonly used in patients who have had an MI and have high cholesterol as it has been shown to reduce the chance of another MI. The patient is still required to maintain a healthy diet as atorvastatin will not treat the dietary intake of cholesterol and fat by the patient.

The nurse advises Dave to take the atorvastatin at night as one of the more common side effects is muscle pain and the patient is less likely to notice this when asleep. Dave is also advised not to eat grapefruit or drink grapefruit juice while taking atorvastatin as it can interact (Bullock & Manias 2017).

Regulation of heart rate

Heart rate is controlled by two main mechanisms:

- autonomic nervous system activity
- hormone activity.

Resting heart rate is also affected by factors such as age, gender, temperature and physical fitness (Jenkins & Tortora 2013).

Autonomic nervous system activity

When activated by a stimulus, such as exercise or stress, the sympathetic nerve fibres release the neurotransmitter noradrenaline at their axon terminals. This leads to the excitation of the SA node and an increase in its production of action potentials, thus increasing in heart rate.

Alternatively, when the parasympathetic nervous system is stimulated, this results in the release of acetylcholine at the parasympathetic cardiac nerve endings, which has the effect of reducing the rate of action potential generation in the SA node, thus reducing heart rate.

Both the sympathetic and parasympathetic nervous systems are active at all times, but the parasympathetic nervous system is normally the dominant influence. This can be seen if the vagus nerve (cranial nerve X) is cut — for instance, in heart transplant patients. In these situations the SA node will normally produce action potentials at a rate of 100 a minute and therefore the heart rate increases to 100 beats per minute. The removal of the influence of the parasympathetic nervous system (by the disconnection of the vagus nerve) removes the heart rate reduction effect of this system.

Baroreceptors and the cardiovascular centre

Baroreceptors are specialised mechanical receptors located in the carotid sinus and the aortic arch. They are sensitive to the amount of stretch placed on these blood vessels and have a direct connection (via the autonomic nervous system) to the **cardiovascular centre** in the **medulla oblongata**.

The cardiovascular centre of the medulla oblongata is the main control centre for autonomic nervous activity affecting the heart. As can be seen in figure 9.21, the cardiovascular centre is made up of two sub-centres.

- The **cardioinhibitory centre** directly controls parasympathetic outflow to the heart (especially the SA node); thus, increased outflow from this centre has the effect of reducing heart rate.
- The **vasomotor centre** is further divided into the pressor area and the depressor area. The pressor area has a relatively constant outflow of action potentials to the heart via the sympathetic nervous system. This has a direct effect on both heart rate and the force of ventricular contraction (and therefore stroke volume) as well as effects on the vasculature, which subsequently will affect heart function by changing preload and afterload. Outflow from the pressor area is moderated by nerves transmitting impulses from the depressor area that have a directly inhibiting effect on the transmission of impulses from the pressor area. Thus, it can be thought that the nerve impulses of the depressor area act like a 'collar' or tap: the greater the number of impulses from the depressor area, the tighter the collar or tap is made, reducing the number of impulses from the pressor area to the heart, and thus the effect on heart rate and force of contraction.

Hormone activity

Two hormones are normally associated with the control of heart rate.

- *Adrenaline — from the adrenal medulla.* Adrenaline has the same effect as noradrenaline released by the sympathetic nervous system.
- *Thyroxine — from the thyroid gland.* Released in large quantities, thyroxine has the effect of increasing the heart rate.

FIGURE 9.21 Baroreceptor reflex

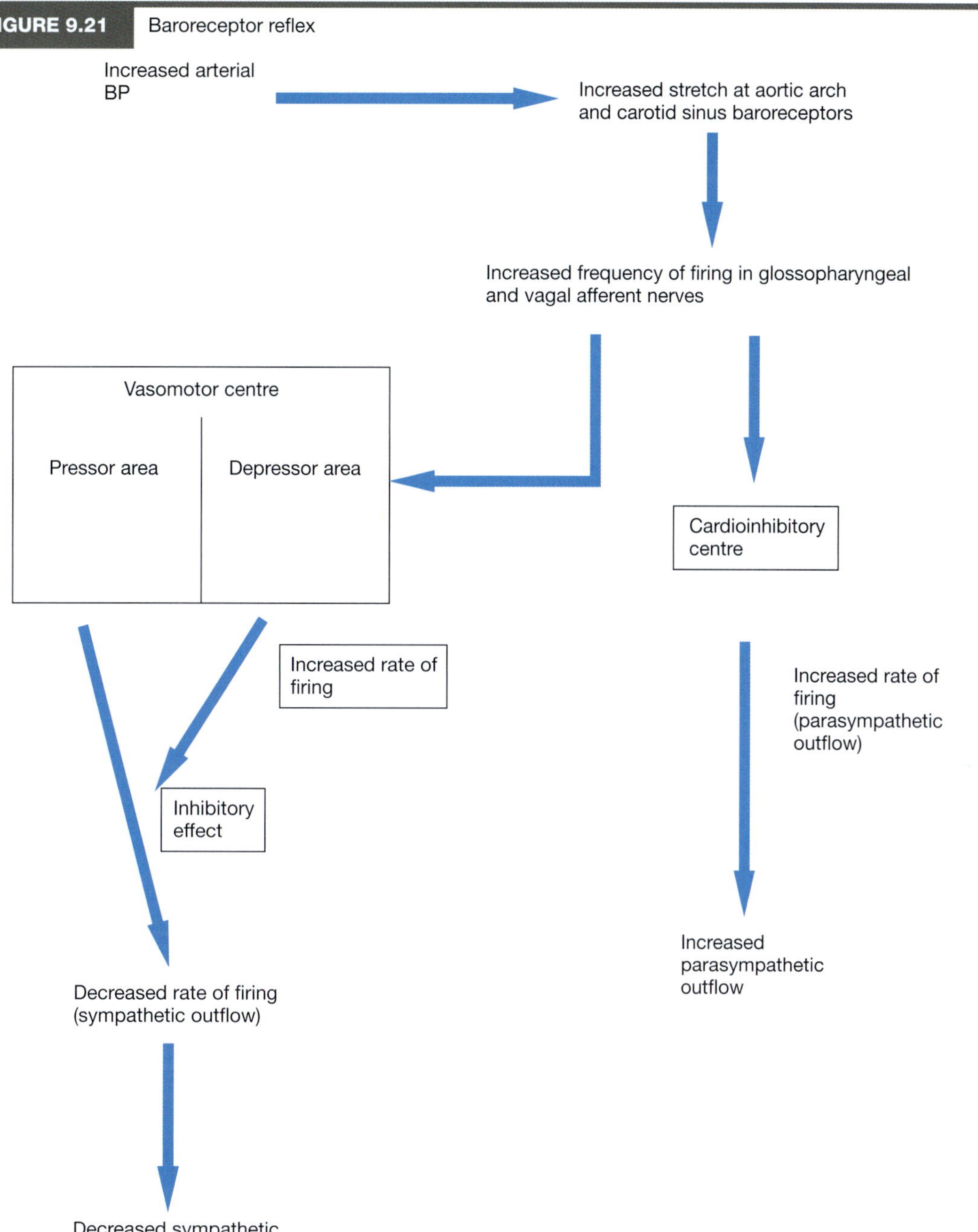

SUMMARY

The heart is a single organ situated in the thoracic cavity between the lungs. Though a single organ, the heart is effectively two separate pumps made up of four chambers.

- The right heart pump, comprising the right atrium and right ventricle, pumps blood through the pulmonary circulation.
- The left heart pump, comprising the left atrium and the left ventricle, pumps blood through the systemic circulation.

Surrounding the heart is a double protective sac called the pericardium. Underlying the pericardium is the heart muscle (myocardium), which is a specialised type of muscle that is branched in its structure and is laid down in spiral bundles to make up the walls of the various heart chambers.

Control of the heart muscle is achieved by the use of a specialised series of nerve cells that make up the conduction system of the heart, including:

- the SA node, the pacemaker of the heart
- the AV node, an area of the heart's conduction system that controls the delivery of the action potential to the ventricles
- Purkinje fibres, conductive fibres that aid rapid distribution of the action potential throughout the ventricles.

Blood flow through the heart is based on changes of pressure in the cardiac cycle. These pressure changes also lead to the opening and closing of the cardiac valves, thus further controlling blood flow.

Regulation of the heart's activity is based on the actions of:

- hormones, especially adrenaline
- autonomic nervous system activity; for instance via the cardiovascular centres.

KEY TERMS

action potentials Momentary change in the electrical status of a cell wall.

afterload The 'load' that the heart has to pump against, mostly created by the blood pressure in the aorta and pulmonary arteries.

aorta Main artery leading from the left ventricle.

aortic valve Semilunar valve that lies between the left ventricle and the aorta.

arterial Pertaining to the arteries.

arterial blood Blood carried in the arteries.

atria Upper chambers of the heart (singular = atrium).

atrioventricular (AV) bundle Otherwise known as the AV bundle. Bundle of conductive nerve fibres that transmit action potentials from the AV node to the ventricular conduction system. Otherwise known as the bundle of His.

atrioventricular (AV) node Otherwise known as the AV node. Specialised area of cardiac cells located just above the point where the right atrium and right ventricle meet.

atrioventricular (AV) valves Collective name for the two valves that lie between the atria and the ventricles (bicuspid and tricuspid).

automaticity The ability of certain cells to generate their own action potential without an external stimulus.

baroreceptors Specialised mechanical receptors located in the aortic arch and the carotid sinus.

bicuspid (mitral) valve The AV valve that lies between the left atrium and the left ventricle. Also known as the mitral valve.

bundle of His See atrioventricular bundle.

cardiac action potential Specialised action potential of the heart muscle cells; it is of longer duration than normal cellular action potentials.

cardiac cycle The sequence of events that occurs when the heart beats.

cardiac output The amount of blood pumped out by a ventricle in millilitres per minute.

cardioinhibitory centre Part of the cardiovascular centre; when stimulated, the major effect is to slow down the heart rate.

cardiovascular centre Located in the medulla oblongata, this centre controls most of the nervous activity that affects the heart.

coronary arteries Arteries that supply the myocardium with oxygenated blood.
coronary sinus Collection of veins that come together to form a single large vessel that returns blood from the myocardium to the right atrium.
depolarisation Change in the electrical potential of a cell membrane to a more positive charge.
desmosomes A specialised cell structure whose function is to hold cells together.
diastole The relaxation of a heart chamber (atrium or ventricle).
dicrotic notch A small bump in the pressure tracing of the arteries created by a backflow of blood after the closure of the aortic valve.
end diastolic pressure The pressure created by the blood in a named chamber (usually the left ventricle) at the end of diastole.
end diastolic volume The volume of blood in a named chamber (usually the left ventricle) at the end of diastole.
endocardium Innermost layer that lines the chambers of the heart and also lines the cardiac valves.
epithelium Layer of body tissue that lines the inside of cavities and the surface of many structures.
fibrous pericardium The outer, tough layer of the pericardium that provides protection to the heart, prevents overstretching of the heart and helps to anchor the heart in place.
gap junctions A specialised connection between cell membranes that allows the passage of ions and molecules.
hormone Chemical substance that is released into the blood by the endocrine system and has a physiological control over the function of cells or organs other than those that created it.
inferior vena cava Large vein that returns blood to the right atrium from the lower parts of the body.
interatrial septum Dividing wall between the atria.
interventricular septum Dividing wall between the ventricles.
ions Electrically charged atoms or molecules.
isovolumetric No change in volume (amount).
medulla oblongata The lower half of the brainstem.
mitral valve See bicuspid valve.
myocardium Muscle layer of the heart.
myocytes Cardiac muscle cell.
nodal cells Otherwise known as pacemaker cells, these are specialised cells that not only create electrical impulses but create them at regular intervals. The two main groupings of these cells are located in the SA node and the AV node.
pericardial fluid A thin film of fluid that reduces the friction between the pericardial membranes as the heart moves during its cycle of contraction and relaxation.
pericardium Double-layered sac that surrounds the heart.
parietal pericardium The outer layer of the serous pericardium; it is fused to the fibrous pericardium.
pulmonary circulation Circulatory system of the lungs.
pulmonary valve Semilunar valve that lies between the right ventricle and the pulmonary circulation.
pulmonary veins Veins of the pulmonary circulation that return blood from the lungs to the left atrium.
Purkinje fibres (system) Specialised conductive fibres that rapidly transport action potentials through the ventricle walls.
repolarisation Return of the electrical potential of a cell membrane to a negative resting state.
sarcolemma Cell membrane of a muscle cell.
semilunar valves The valves that lie between the ventricles and the pulmonary or systemic circulation (aortic valve and pulmonary valve).
septum A dividing wall.
serous pericardium Inner (double) layer of the pericardium comprised of the parietal and visceral pericardial layers.
sinoatrial (SA) node Otherwise known as the SA node. Specialised area of cardiac cells located in the upper part of the right atrium. Usually referred to as the pacemaker of the heart.
stroke volume The amount of blood ejected by a ventricle in one beat.
superior vena cava The large vein that returns blood to the right atrium from the upper part of the body.
systemic circulation The circulatory system of the body (excluding the lungs).
systole The contraction of a heart chamber (atrium or ventricle).
tetany Sustained involuntary contraction of a muscle.
tricuspid valve The AV valve that lies between the right atrium and ventricle.

vasomotor centre Part of the cardiovascular centre; has effects on heart rate and the force of contraction of the heart.

venous Pertaining to the veins.

venous blood Blood carried in the veins.

ventricles The large lower chambers of the heart.

visceral pericardium The inner layer of the serous pericardium (otherwise known as the epicardium); adheres tightly to the surface of the heart.

CONDITIONS

The following is a list of conditions that are associated with the cardiac system. Take some time and write notes about each of the conditions. You may make the notes taken from textbooks or other resources (e.g. people you work with in a clinical area), or you may make the notes as a result of people you have cared for. If you are making notes about people you have cared for, you must ensure that you adhere to the rules of confidentiality.

Heart failure
Myocardial infarction
Aortic stenosis
Mitral regurgitation
Pericarditis

REFERENCES

Australian Commission on Safety and Quality in Health Care (2020) Informed consent — Fact sheet for clinicians. www.safetyandquality.gov.au/publications-and-resources/resource-library/informed-consent-fact-sheet-clinicians (accessed February 2021).

Australian Institute of Health and Welfare (2020a) Health risk factors among Indigenous Australians. www.aihw.gov.au/reports/australias-health/health-risk-factors-among-indigenous-australians (accessed 31 January 2021).

Australian Institute of Health and Welfare (2020b) Tobacco smoking. www.aihw.gov.au/reports/australias-health/tobacco-smoking (accessed 31 January 2021).

British National Formulary (2019) Interactions — Clozapine. https://bnf.nice.org.uk/interaction/clozapine-2.html (accessed 5 June 2019).

Bullock, S. and Manias, E. (2017) *Fundamentals of Pharmacology*, 8th edn. Sydney: Pearson Australia.

Clare, C. (2007) Valve disorders. In Hatchett, R. and Thompson, D.R. (eds), *Cardiac Nursing: A Comprehensive Guide*. London: Churchill Livingstone Elsevier; pp. 357–382.

Davey, R.X. (2021) Health disparities among Australia's remote-dwelling Aboriginal people: a report from 2020. *JALM* 126: 125–141.

De Hert, M., Detraux, J. and Vancampfort, D. (2018) The intriguing relationship between coronary heart disease and mental disorders. *Dialogues in Clinical Neuroscience* 20(1): 31–40.

Heart Foundation (2021) I am interested in heart health. www.heartfoundation.org.au (accessed February 2021).

Hopper, I. and Easton, K. (2017) Chronic heart failure. *Australian Prescriber* 40: 128–136.

Field, P.E., Franklin, R.C., Barker, R.N., Ring, I. and Leggat, P.A. (2018) Cardiac rehabilitation services for people in rural and remote areas: an integrative literature review. *Rural and Remote Health* 18: 4738.

Jenkins, G.W. and Tortora, G.J. (2013) *Anatomy and Physiology: From Science to Life*, 3rd edn. Hoboken, NJ: John Wiley & Sons, Inc.

Levett-Jones, T. (2013). *Clinical Reasoning: Learning to Think Like a Nurse*. Pearson Australia.
Marijon, E., Mirabel, M., Celermajer, D.S. and Jouven, X. (2012) Rheumatic heart disease. *Lancet* 379: 953–964.
Martini, F.H., Nath, J.L. and Bartholemew, E.F. (2014) *Fundamentals of Anatomy and Physiology*, 10th edn. San Francisco, CA: Pearson Benjamin Cummings.
O'Grady, E. (2007) *A Nurse's Guide to Caring for Cardiac Intervention Patients*. Chichester: John Wiley & Sons, Ltd.
Pfitzer, C., Helm, P.C., Rosenthal, L.M., Berger, F., Bauer, U.M.M. and Schmitt, K.R. (2018) Dynamics in prevalence of Down Syndrome in children with congenital heart disease. *European Journal of Pediatrics* 177(1): 107–115.
Prystowsky, E.N., Padanilam, B.J. and Fogel, R.I. (2015) Treatment of atrial fibrillation. *JAMA* 314(3): 278–288.
St Vincent's Hospital Heart Health (n.d.) Heart health. www.svhhearthealth.com.au/aboriginal-heart-health (accessed February 2021).
Tortora, G.J. and Derrickson, B.H. (2009) *Principles of Anatomy and Physiology*, 12th edn. Hoboken, NJ: John Wiley & Sons, Inc.
Troughton, R.W., Asher, C.R. and Klein, A.L. (2004) Pericarditis. *Lancet* 363(9410): 717–727.
United Nations Department of Economic and Social Affairs (2016) Convention on the Rights of Persons with Disabilities (CRPD). www.un.org/development/desa/disabilities/convention-on-the-rights-of-persons-with-disabilities.html (accessed February 2021).
University of Michigan Health System (2014) Coronary angioplasty and stenting. www.med.umich.edu/cardiac-surgery/patient/adult/adultcandt/coronary_angioplasty.shtml (accessed 5 June 2019).
Vis, J.C., de Bruin-Bon, R.H., Bouma, B.J., Huisman, S.A., Imschoot, L., van den Brink, K. and Mulder, B.J. (2010) Congenital heart defects are under-recognised in adult patients with Down's syndrome. *Heart* 96: 1480–1484.

FURTHER READING

AUSTRALIAN HEART FOUNDATION

www.heartfoundation.org.au

The Australian Heart Foundation is Australia's largest charity for heart disease. The website has many useful resources for patients and professionals.

ARRHYTHMIA ALLIANCE

www.heartrhythmalliance.org/aa/au

Arrhythmia Alliance (A-A) – Australia is a health promotion charity working to improve the diagnosis, treatment and quality of life for all those affected by arrhythmias.

RESUSCITATION COUNCIL (AUSTRALIA)

https://resus.org.au

The Australian Resuscitation Council is a voluntary coordinating body which represents all major groups involved in the teaching and practice of resuscitation.

ACKNOWLEDGEMENTS

Photo: © Monkey Business Images / Shutterstock.com
Photo: © muroPhotographer / Shutterstock.com
Photo: © kokouu / Getty Images
Photo: © LittlePanda29 / Shutterstock.com
Photo: © Monkey Business Images / Shutterstock.com
Figure 9.3: © Troughton, R.W., Asher, C.R. and Klein, A.L. (2004) Pericarditis. *Lancet* 363(9410): 717–727. doi:10.1016/s0140-6736(04)15648-1
Figure 9.7: © Marijon, E., Mirabel, M., Celermajer, D.S. and Jouven, X. (2012) Rheumatic heart disease. *Lancet* 379(9819): 953–964. doi:10.1016/s0140-6736(11)61171-9
Figure 9.18: © Aila Medical Media / Shutterstock.com

CHAPTER 10

The digestive system

TEST YOUR PRIOR KNOWLEDGE

- What is the main function of the digestive system?
- List the structures that form the digestive system.
- List the hormones and enzymes involved in the digestive system.
- Name the main food groups.
- Differentiate between macronutrients and micronutrients.

LEARNING OUTCOMES

After reading this chapter you will be able to:

10.1 identify the organs of the digestive system and describe the functions of each of these organs, as well as the overall function of the digestive system

10.2 describe the structure and function of the accessory organs of the digestive system

10.3 explain the action of the enzymes and hormones associated with the digestion of proteins, carbohydrates and fats, and how the products of digestion are utilised within the body

10.4 list the common vitamins and minerals and the problems associated with a deficit or excess.

Body map

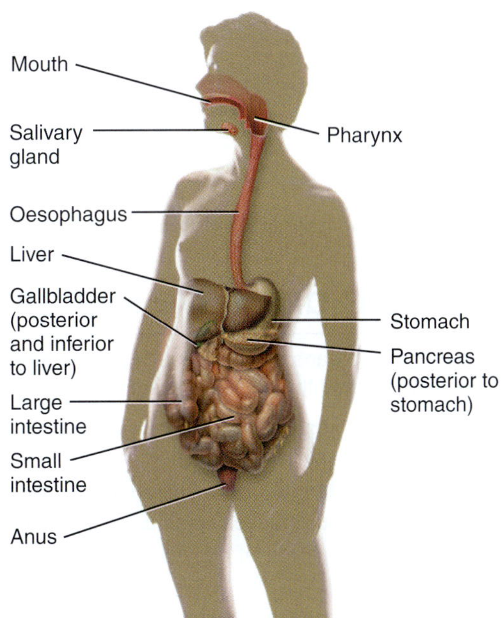

Introduction

The digestive system is also known as the gastrointestinal system or the alimentary canal. This vast system is approximately 10 m long. It travels the length of the body from the mouth through the thoracic, abdominal and pelvic cavities, where it ends at the **anus** (see figure 10.1). The digestive system has one major function: to convert food from the diet into a form that can be utilised by the cells of the body in order to carry out their specific functions. This chapter discusses the structure and function of the digestive system and explains how dietary **nutrients** are broken down and used by the body for cell **metabolism** and for growth and repair.

FIGURE 10.1 The digestive system

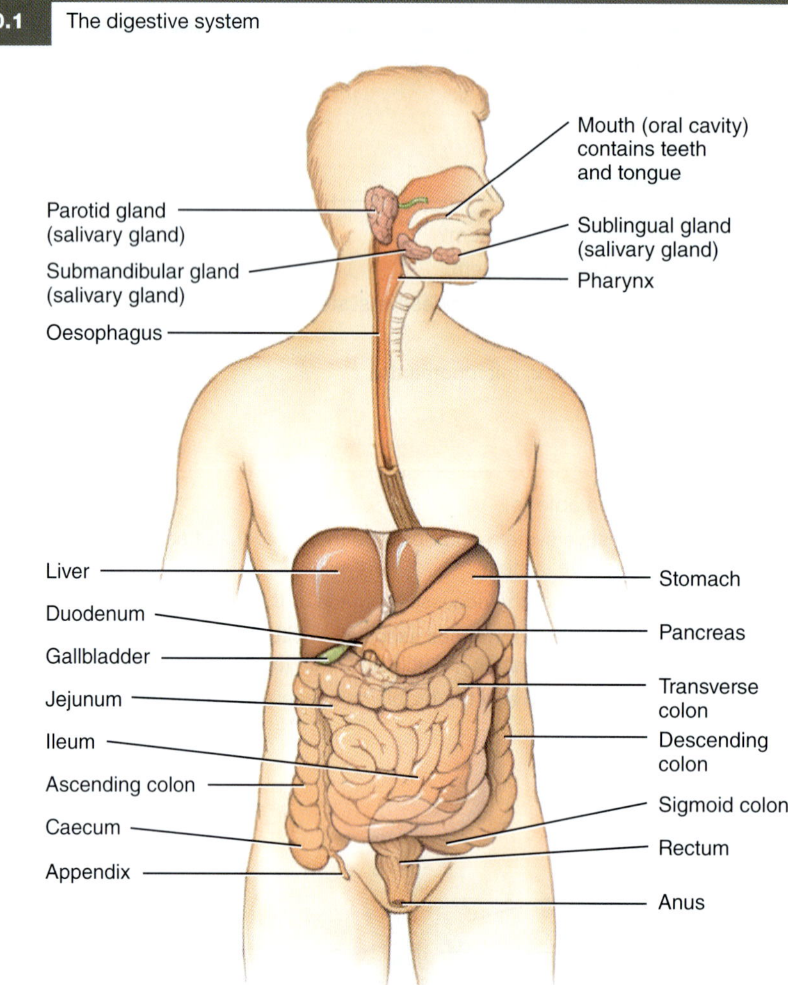

Source: Tortora and Derrickson (2009). Reproduced with permission of John Wiley & Sons.

10.1 The activity of the digestive system

LEARNING OBJECTIVE 10.1 Identify the organs of the digestive system and describe the functions of each of these organs, as well as the overall function of the digestive system.

The activity of the digestive system can be categorised into five processes:

- **ingestion** — taking food into the digestive system
- **propulsion** — moving the food along the length of the digestive system
- **digestion** — breaking down food; this can be achieved *mechanically* as food is chewed or moved through the digestive system, or *chemically* by the action of *enzymes* mixed with the food as it moves through the digestive system
- **absorption** — the products of digestion exit the digestive system and enter the blood or lymph capillaries for distribution to where they are required
- elimination — the waste products of digestion are excreted from the body as **faeces**.

The organisation of the digestive system

The digestive system consists of the main digestive system structures and the accessory organs. The main digestive system structures include the mouth, **pharynx**, **oesophagus**, **stomach**, small intestine and large intestine. Accessory organs also contribute to the function of the digestive system. The accessory organs are the salivary glands, the **liver**, the gall bladder and the pancreas.

The digestive system organs

The mouth (oral cavity)

Food enters the mouth or **oral cavity**, and this is where the process of digestion begins. The oral cavity consists of several structures (see figure 10.2). Food enters the oral cavity in a process called ingestion. The food mixes with saliva.

FIGURE 10.2 The oral cavity

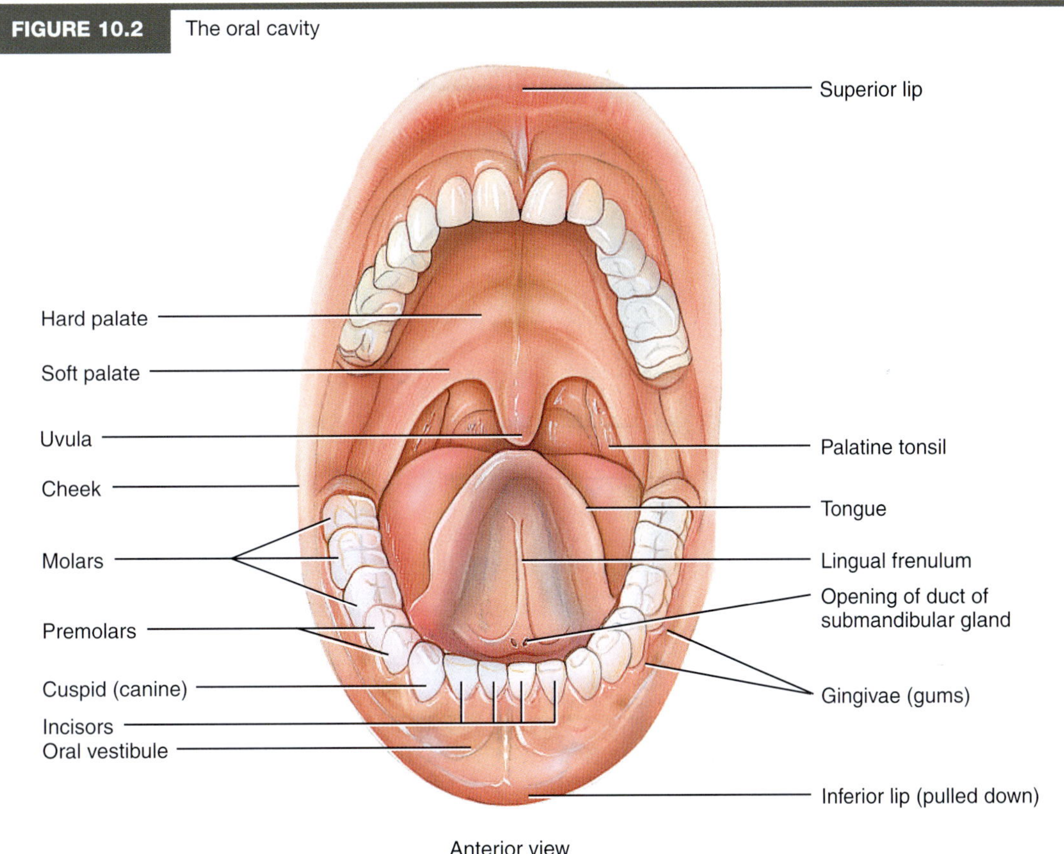

Source: Tortora and Derrickson (2009). Reproduced with permission of John Wiley & Sons.

The lips and cheeks are formed of muscle and connective tissue. This allows the lips and cheeks to move food mixed with saliva around the mouth and begin mechanical digestion. The teeth contribute to mechanical digestion by grinding and tearing food. This process of chewing and mixing food with saliva is called **mastication**. The oral cavity can be exposed to very hot and very cold food as well as rough food particles. It is lined with mucus-secreting, stratified squamous epithelial cells. This layer provides some protection against abrasion, the effects of heat and continuous wear and tear.

The lips and cheeks are also involved in speech and facial expression.

Tongue

The tongue is a large, voluntary muscular structure that occupies much of the oral cavity. It is attached posteriorly to the **hyoid bone** and inferiorly by the lingual **frenulum** (see figure 10.2).

The superior surface of the tongue is covered in stratified squamous epithelium for protection against wear and tear. This surface also contains many little projections called **papillae**. The papillae (or tastebuds) contain the nerve endings responsible for the sense of taste (Tortora & Derrickson 2012). The tastebuds contribute to our enjoyment of food. As well as taste, other functions of the tongue include swallowing (**deglutition**), holding and moving food around the oral cavity and speech.

Palate

The **palate** forms the roof of the mouth and consists of two parts: the hard palate and the soft palate. The hard palate is located anteriorly and is bony. The soft palate lies posteriorly and consists of skeletal muscle and connective tissue (see figure 10.2). The palate plays a part in swallowing. The palatine tonsils lie laterally and are lymphoid tissue. The **uvula** is a fold of tissue that hangs down from the centre of the soft palate.

Pharynx

The pharynx consists of three parts: the oropharynx, the nasopharynx and the **laryngopharynx**. The nasopharynx is considered a structure of the respiratory system. The **oropharynx** and the laryngopharynx are passages for both food and respiratory gases (see figure 10.3). The **epiglottis** is responsible for closing the entrance to the larynx during swallowing, and this essential action prevents food from entering the larynx and obstructing the respiratory passages.

FIGURE 10.3 (a, b) Swallowing

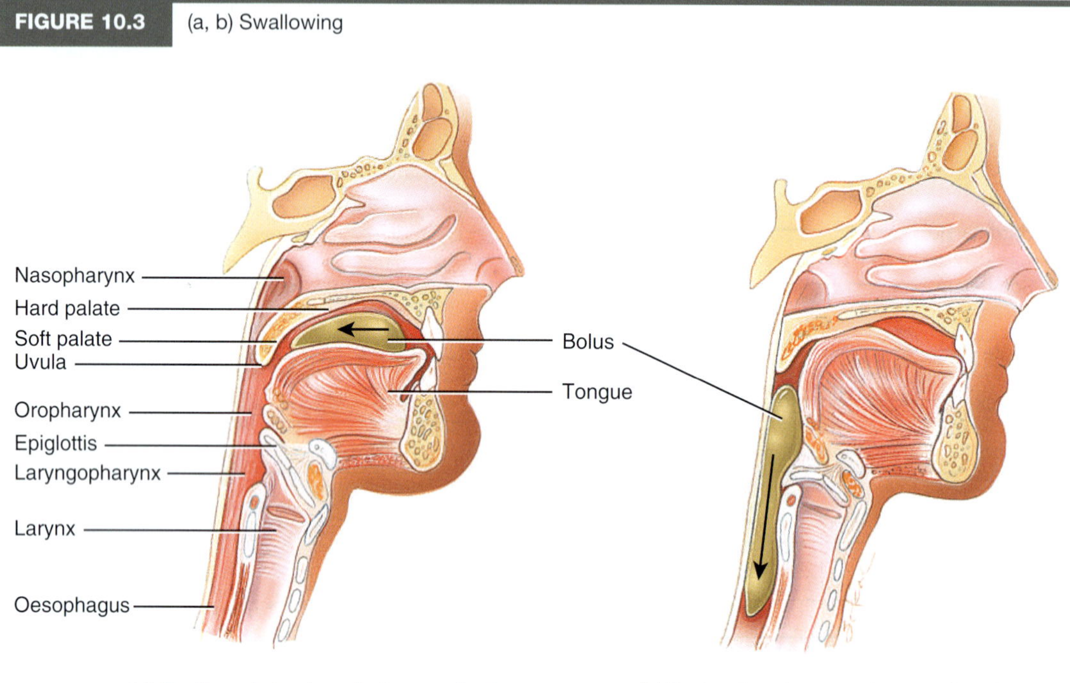

(a) Position of structures before swallowing (b) During the pharyngeal stage of swallowing

Source: Tortora and Derrickson (2009). Reproduced with permission of John Wiley & Sons.

Swallowing (deglutition)

Once ingested food has been adequately chewed and formed into a bolus, it is ready to be swallowed. Swallowing (deglutition) occurs in three phases.

1. *The **voluntary phase**.* During this phase the action of the voluntary muscles serving the oral cavity manipulates the food bolus into the oropharynx. The tongue is pressed against the palate and this prevents the food from moving forward again.
2. *The **pharyngeal phase**.* During this phase a reflex action is initiated in response to the sensation of the food bolus in the oropharynx. This reflex is coordinated by the swallowing centre in the medulla oblongata, and the motor response is contraction of the muscles of the pharynx. The soft palate elevates, closing off the nasopharynx and preventing the food bolus from using this route. The larynx moves up and moves forward, allowing the epiglottis to cover the entrance to the larynx so the food bolus cannot move into the respiratory passages.
3. *The oesophageal phase.* The food bolus moves from the pharynx into the oesophagus. Waves of oesophageal muscle contractions move the food bolus down the length of the oesophagus and into the stomach. This wave of muscle contraction is known as **peristalsis** (see figure 10.4).

FIGURE 10.4 Peristalsis in the oesophagus

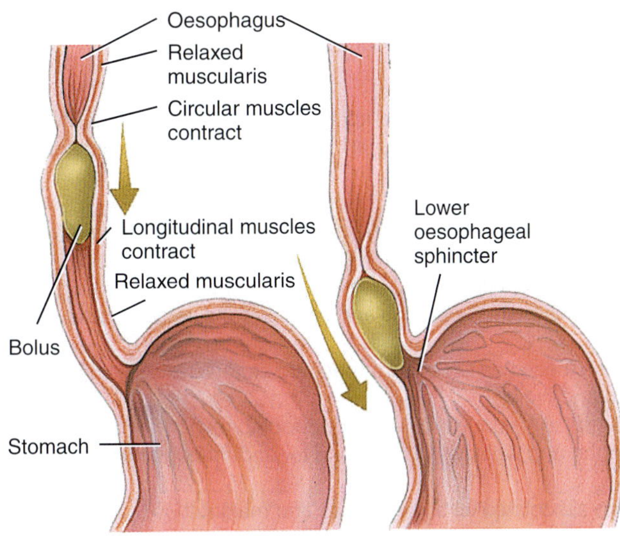

Anterior view of frontal sections of peristalsis in oesophagus

Source: Tortora and Derrickson (2009). Reproduced with permission of John Wiley & Sons.

CLINICALLY REASONED EPISODE OF CARE

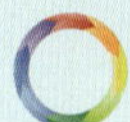

Dysphagia

Consider the patient situation

Asif is a 34-year-old man with a moderate learning disability. He lives in a community care home which is staffed by nursing and care staff.

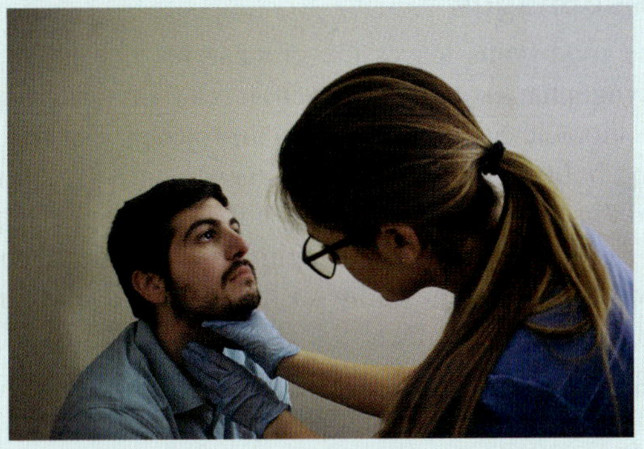

Collect cues and information

Asif has recently had two upper respiratory tract infections and has been coughing frequently at mealtimes. The care staff at the community home care centre report that he has been losing weight.

The care staff are concerned about Asif's changing condition and have sent him to the doctor for investigation. His symptoms include eating and drinking difficulties.

Process information

Dysphagia is a medical term used to describe swallowing difficulties. Dysphagia can occur at any of the four stages of swallowing. Signs and symptoms of dysphagia include choking while eating and drinking, feeling that food gets stuck in the throat, and/or difficulties controlling and swallowing liquids. These symptoms can lead to aspiration, where ingested food and fluids make their way into the airway and lungs.

People with a disability are more likely to develop dysphagia. The health risks to people with learning disabilities include chest infections, asphyxia, chronic lung conditions, obstructive sleep apnoea and hypoxemia when eating. Dysphagia increases the risk of dehydration, malnutrition and the frequency of upper respiratory tract infections, aspiration pneumonia and choking.

Asif is experiencing several of these symptoms. Asif is not on any medications that may affect his dysphagia and therefore medications are eliminated as a source.

Identify problems/issues

1. Eating and drinking difficulties leading to malnutrition and weight loss
2. Frequent chest infections secondary to dysphagia

Nursing actions

1. Refer to GP and speech and language therapist for a comprehensive assessment of swallow, mouth and tongue movements, breathing assessment and possible video fluoroscopy.
   Rationale:
   - A speech and language assessment is an essential element of caring for someone with dysphagia.
   - The speech pathologist comprehensively assesses the mouth and swallowing and is able to make a diagnosis of dysphagia. The assessment leads to a diagnosis and management plan for Asif.
2. Implement actions from the speech review including supervision while eating, sitting Asif upright during mealtimes, cutting food into small portions and checking oral hygiene after eating.
   Rationale:
   - Implementing these measures will ensure that care staff are giving Asif the best chance of avoiding aspiration of food and fluid.
   - These care measures will reduce the risk of developing respiratory tract infections and pneumonia.
3. Implement a food chart and weekly weigh to monitor and manage how much Asif is eating.
   Rationale:
   - Dysphagia is often associated with weight loss and malnutrition.
   - This measure allows staff to monitor Asif's nutritional needs and his weight.

Evaluate outcomes

As a result of the nursing actions implemented within the community care team, Asif is back to his normal weight one month later and has had no further upper respiratory tract infections.

Reflect on new processes and learning

Reflect on the role of community nursing. How can community nurses, who care for people in their homes, drive positive outcomes for people with learning disabilities?

Source: Based on the Clinical Reasoning Cycle, Levett-Jones (2013).

Oesophagus

The food bolus leaves the oropharynx and enters the oesophagus. The oesophagus extends from the laryngopharynx to the stomach. It is a thick-walled structure, measuring about 25 cm in length, and lies in the thoracic cavity, posterior to the trachea. The function of the oesophagus is to transport substances (the food bolus) from the mouth to the stomach. Thick mucus is secreted by the **mucosa** of the oesophagus, and this aids the passage of the food bolus and also protects the oesophagus from abrasion.

The **upper oesophageal sphincter** regulates the movement of substances into the oesophagus, and the **lower oesophageal sphincter** (also known as the cardiac sphincter) regulates the movement of substances from the oesophagus to the stomach. The muscle layer of the oesophagus differs from the rest of the digestive tract, as the superior portion consists of skeletal (voluntary) muscle and the inferior portion consists of smooth (involuntary) muscle. Breathing and swallowing cannot occur at the same time (Nair & Peate 2018).

MEDICINES MANAGEMENT

Omeprazole

Omeprazole is a medicine used to treat a number of digestive system conditions, including dyspepsia, acid reflux, oesophagitis and peptic ulcer disease. It belongs to a group of medicines known as proton pump inhibitors (Galbraith et al. 2007). **Hydrochloric acid** produced in the stomach can escape into the oesophagus or the **duodenum** of the small intestine and irritate the delicate epithelium in these areas. Omeprazole works on the **parietal cells** in the stomach, inhibiting the production of hydrochloric acid.

Omeprazole is usually prescribed as 20–40 mg once daily.

The common side effects for patients taking omeprazole are:

- vomiting
- diarrhoea
- constipation

- pain (stomach)
- headaches
- increased flatulence
- nausea.

GESA (2011) has produced guidance on the investigation and management of dyspepsia.

The structure of the digestive system

There are four layers of tissue or tunicas that exist throughout the length of the digestive tract from oesophagus to anus (see figure 10.5).

FIGURE 10.5 Structure of the digestive tract

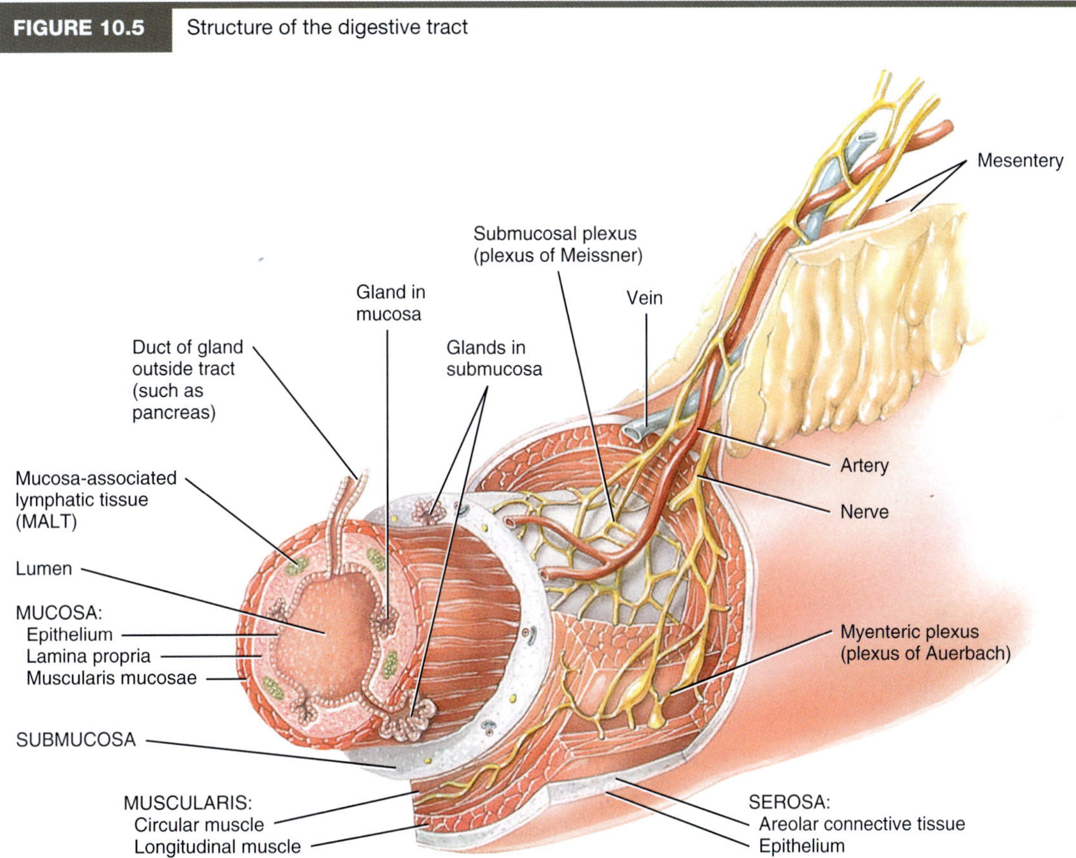

Source: Tortora and Derrickson (2009). Reproduced with permission of John Wiley & Sons.

The mucosa is the innermost layer. The products of digestion are in contact with this layer as they pass through the digestive tract. The mucosa consists of three layers. The mucosal epithelium (mucous membrane) is involved in the secretion of mucus and other digestive system secretions such as saliva or gastric juice. This layer helps to protect the digestive system from the continuous wear and tear it endures; in the small intestine this layer is involved in absorption of the products of digestion. The next layer is the **lamina propria**, which consists of loose connective tissue that has a role in supporting the blood vessels and lymphatic tissue of the mucosa. The outermost layer is called the **muscularis mucosa** and consists of a thin smooth muscle layer that helps to form the gastric pits or the **microvilli** of the digestive system.

The **submucosa** is a thick layer of connective tissue. It contains blood and lymphatic vessels and some small glands. It also contains **Meissner's plexus** — nerves that stimulate the intestinal glands to secrete their products.

The muscularis consists of an inner layer of circular smooth muscle and an outer layer of longitudinal smooth muscle. The stomach has three layers of smooth muscle, and the upper oesophagus has skeletal muscle. Blood and lymph vessels and the **myenteric plexus** (a network of sympathetic and parasympathetic nerves) are located between the two layers of smooth muscle. The wave-like contraction and relaxation of this muscle layer are responsible for moving food along the digestive tract — a process known as peristalsis (see figure 10.5). Peristalsis helps to churn and mechanically digest food.

The outer layer of the digestive tract is the **serosa** (adventitia). The largest area of serosa is found in the abdominal and pelvic cavities and is known as the **peritoneum**. The peritoneum is a closed sac. The **visceral peritoneum** covers the organs of the abdominal and pelvic cavity, and the parietal peritoneum lines the abdominal wall. A small amount of serous fluid lies between the two layers. The peritoneum has a good blood supply and contains many lymph nodes and lymphatic vessels. It acts as a barrier, protecting the structures it encloses, and can act to isolate areas of infection to prevent damage to neighbouring structures.

Stomach

The stomach lies in the abdominal cavity. It lies between the oesophagus superiorly and the duodenum of the small intestine inferiorly. It is divided into regions (see figure 10.6).

FIGURE 10.6 The stomach

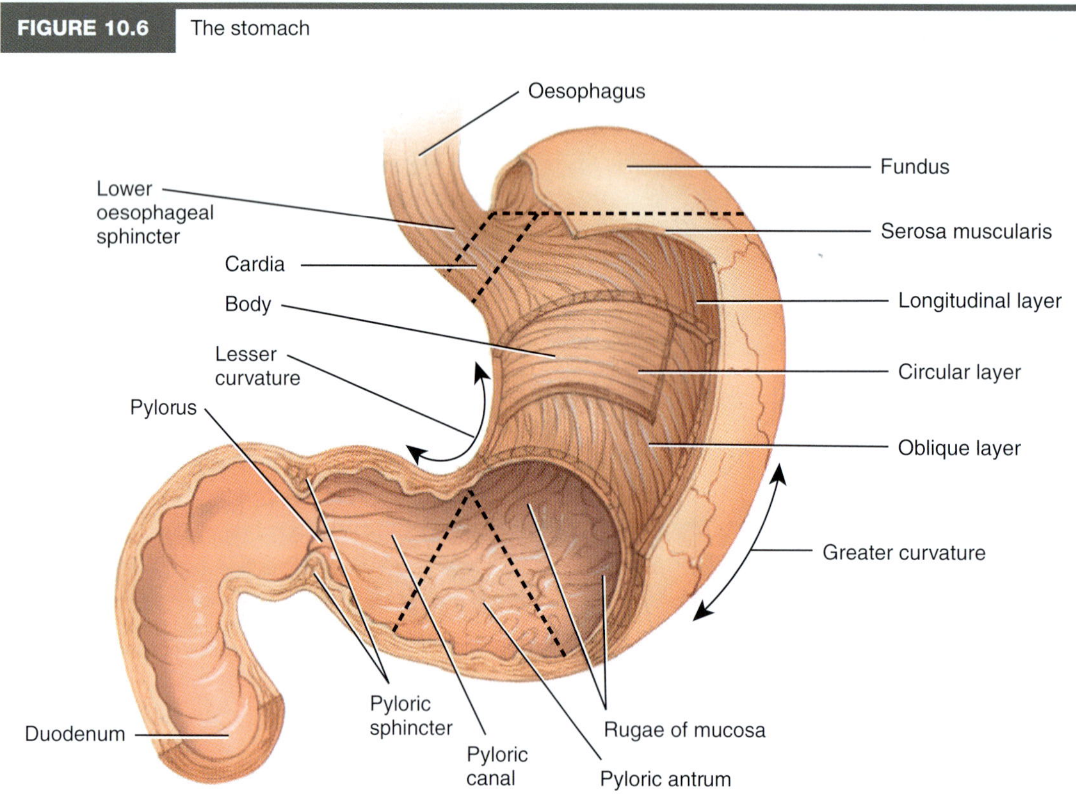

Source: Tortora and Derrickson (2009). Reproduced with permission of John Wiley & Sons.

The entrance to the stomach from the oesophagus is via the lower oesophageal sphincter or cardiac sphincter. This leads to a small area within the stomach called the **cardiac region** or cardia. The **fundus** is the dome-shaped region in the superior part of the stomach. The **body region** occupies the space between the lesser and greater curvature of the stomach, and the **pyloric region** narrows into the **pyloric canal**. The **pyloric sphincter** controls the exit of chyme from the stomach into the small intestine. **Chyme** is the name given to the food bolus as it leaves the stomach.

The stomach is supplied with arterial blood from a branch of the celiac artery, and venous blood leaves the stomach via the hepatic vein. The vagus nerve innervates the stomach with parasympathetic fibres that stimulate gastric motility and the secretion of gastric juice. Sympathetic fibres from the celiac plexus reduce gastric activity.

The stomach has the same four layers of tissue as the digestive tract, but with some differences. The muscularis contains three layers of smooth muscle instead of two. It has longitudinal, circular and oblique muscle fibres. The extra muscle layer facilitates the churning, mixing and mechanical digestion of food that occurs within the stomach, as well as supporting the onward journey of the food by peristalsis.

The mucosa within the stomach is also different from the rest of the digestive tract. When the stomach is empty, the mucosal epithelia falls into long folds known as **rugae**. The rugae fill out when the stomach is full. A very full stomach can contain approximately 4 L, while an empty stomach contains only about 50 mL. The shape and size of the stomach vary from person to person and depending on the quantity of food stored within it.

The mucosa contains many gastric glands that secrete many different substances (see figure 10.7).

- **Surface mucous cells** produce thick bicarbonate-coated mucus. This thick layer of mucus protects the stomach mucosal epithelia from corrosion by acidic gastric juice. When these cells become damaged, they are quickly shed and replaced.
- **Mucous neck cells** also secrete mucus — this mucus is different from surface cell mucus.
- Parietal cells produce hydrochloric acid and **intrinsic factor**. Intrinsic factor is necessary for the absorption of **vitamin** B_{12}. This vitamin is essential for the production of mature erythrocytes. Hydrochloric acid creates the acidic environment of the stomach (pH 1–3) and begins denaturing dietary **protein** in preparation for the action of **pepsin**.
- **Chief cells** produce **pepsinogen**, which is converted to pepsin in the presence of hydrochloric acid. Pepsin is necessary for the breakdown of protein into smaller peptide chains.
- Enteroendocrine cells, such as G cells, produce a variety of hormones, including gastrin. These hormones help regulate gastric motility.

This concoction of secretions plus water and mineral salts is more commonly called gastric juice. About 2 L of gastric juice is produced daily.

FIGURE 10.7 Gastric glands and cells

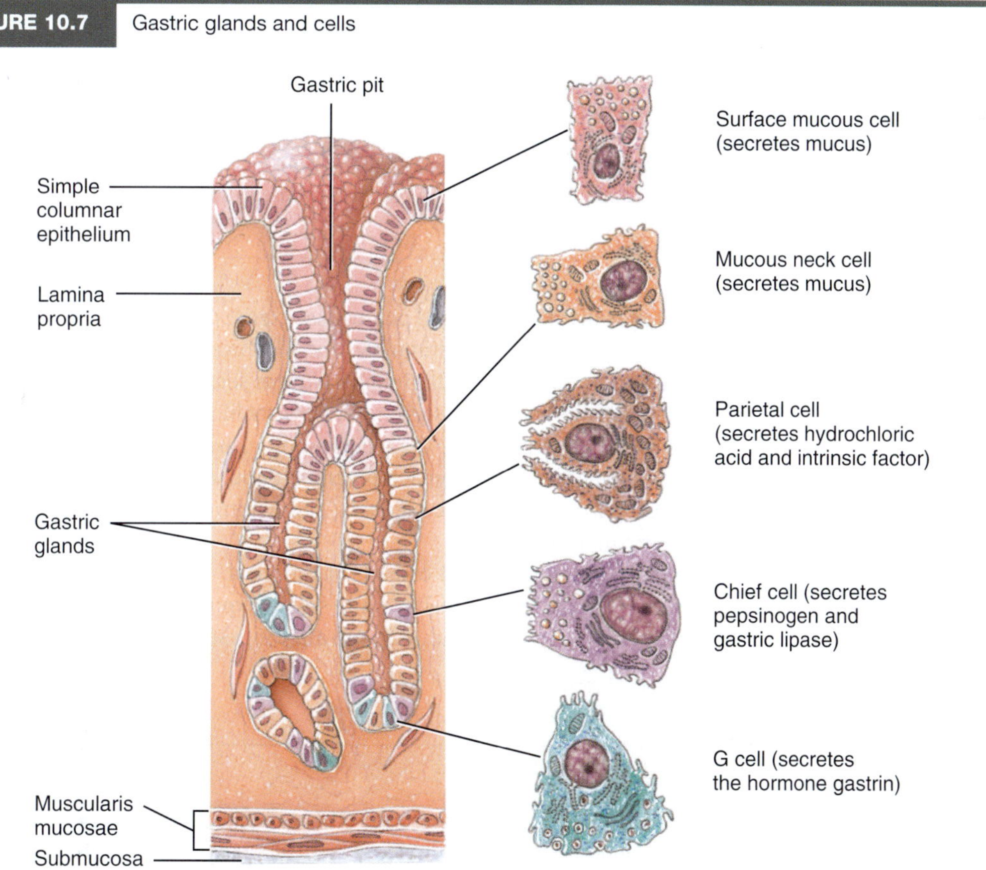

Source: Tortora and Derrickson (2009). Reproduced with permission of John Wiley & Sons.

CLINICAL CONSIDERATIONS

Enteral feeding

Enteral feeding is the ingestion of food via the digestive tract.

Food is mainly ingested via the oral cavity but there are times when this route is not possible; for example, during critical illness, when consciousness is affected or when swallowing is affected. Other methods of providing enteral nutrition include via the following.

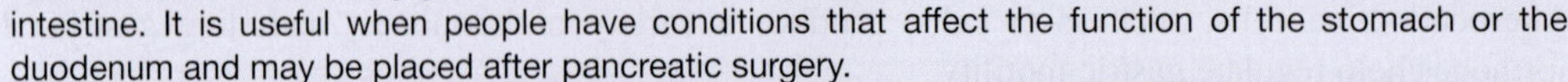

- *Nasogastric tube*. This is a thin tube inserted via the nose, down the oesophagus and into the stomach.
- *Nasojejunal tube*. This is a tube inserted as per the nasogastric tube. However, it passes the stomach and enters the **jejunum** of the small intestine. It is useful when people have conditions that affect the function of the stomach or the duodenum and may be placed after pancreatic surgery.
- *Percutaneous endoscopic gastrostomy (PEG) tube*. This tube is placed where longer-term enteral feeding is required. The tube is inserted via the abdominal wall into the stomach. This procedure requires the appropriate healthcare practitioner to use endoscopy to place the tube in the correct position. Sedation is administered for this procedure.
- *Percutaneous endoscopic jejunostomy (PEJ) tube*. This tube is placed in the same way as a PEG tube; however, it bypasses the stomach and is placed beyond the duodenum in the jejunum. PEJ may be chosen over PEG if the patient has a condition affecting the stomach.

Enteral tubes are often required in clinical practice. They can be placed for short-term use — for example, for aspirating the gastric contents — or more longer term for enteral nutrition including the administration of medicines.

The healthcare worker must ensure that they understand the care required for each tube including the risks associated with misplacement, the tube blocking and pressure where the tubes are in contact with the skin.

Regulation of gastric juice secretion is divided into three phases (see figure 10.8).

1. *The cephalic phase*. The sight, taste or smell of food stimulates the secretion of gastric juice.
2. *The gastric phase*. When food enters the stomach, the hormone gastrin is secreted into the bloodstream, and this stimulates the secretion of gastric juice. The secretion of hydrochloric acid reduces the pH of the stomach contents, and when the pH drops below 2 the secretion of gastrin is inhibited.
3. *The intestinal phase*. As the acidic contents of the stomach enter the duodenum of the small intestine, the hormones **secretin** and **cholecystokinin** (CCK) are secreted. These hormones also act to reduce the secretion of gastric juice and gastric motility.

The rate of gastric emptying depends on the size and content of the meal. A large meal takes longer than a small meal. Liquids quickly pass through the stomach, while solids require longer to be thoroughly mixed with gastric juice. Most meals will have left the stomach 4 h after ingestion.

HOMEOSTATIC IMBALANCE

Diabetic gastroparesis

Diabetic gastroparesis refers to delayed gastric emptying (GE) and decreased gastric motility due to hyperglycaemia, inflammation of enteric neuromuscular tissues and autonomic neuropathy. Diabetic gastroparesis is relatively common and occurs in roughly 50 per cent of patients with poor glycaemic control. Symptoms vary from being very mild to severe, and include bloating, vomiting, nausea, weight loss, premature satiety and upper abdominal pain (Bharucha et al. 2019).

Additionally, diabetic gastroparesis can have significant effects on quality of life, with impacts similar to those experienced by sufferers of rheumatoid arthritis and inflammatory bowel disease. Treatment usually involves changes to dietary composition but can progress to prokinetic medications, supplemental nutrition or electrical gastric stimulation (Bharucha et al. 2019).

FIGURE 10.8 Phases of gastric juice secretion

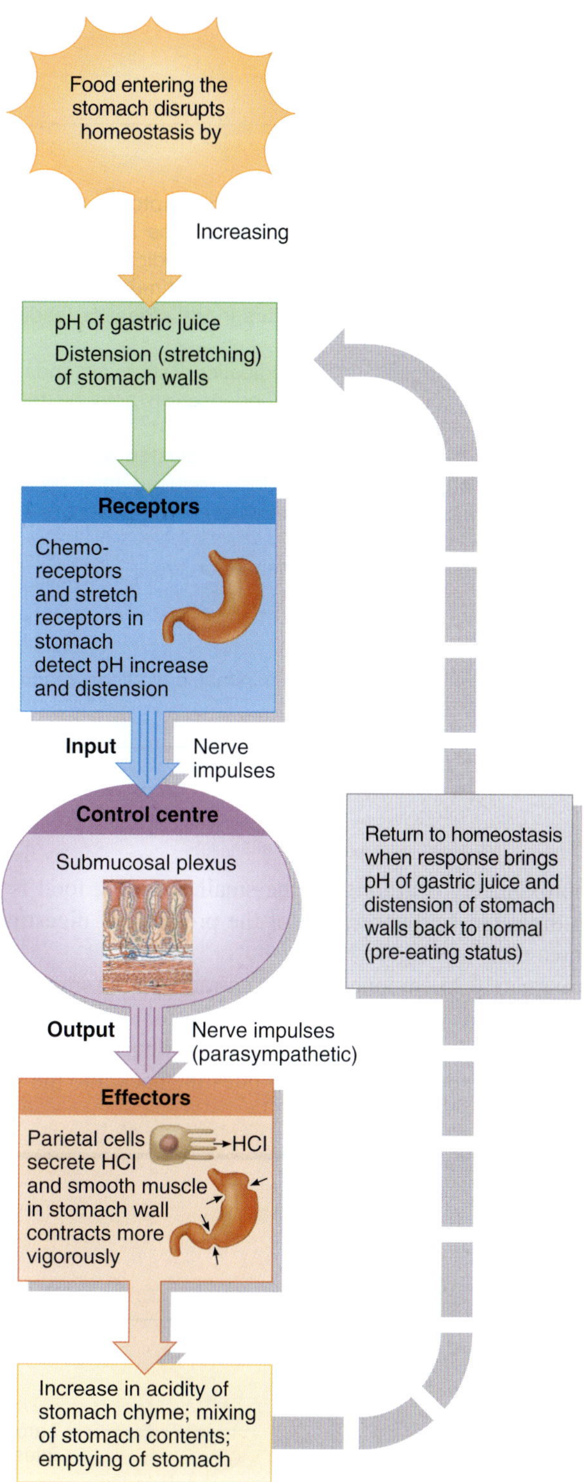

Source: Tortora and Derrickson (2009). Reproduced with permission of John Wiley & Sons.

The functions of the stomach are:

- to act as a storage site for food
- production of mucus to protect the stomach
- mechanical digestion, by the churning action facilitated by an additional layer of smooth muscle
- mixing food with hydrochloric acid to help eradicate pathogens and denature proteins in preparation for the action of pepsin

- production of chyme
- production of intrinsic factor.

MEDICINES MANAGEMENT

Ondansetron

Nausea and vomiting are the most common digestive system symptoms. Vomiting (emesis) occurs when the emetic or vomiting centre in the brain is activated. It can be activated as a result of irritation in the stomach. The irritation may be due to bacteria, or often medication. Some medications cross the blood–brain barrier and stimulate the vomiting centre. When stimulated, the abdominal muscles and diaphragm are activated and a reverse peristalsis occurs in the stomach, leading to the ejection of the stomach contents.

This unpleasant reaction can be treated with medications such as ondansetron, which belongs to a group of medications known as antiemetics. Ondansetron acts by blocking serotonin, which promotes vomiting.

The usual adult dose is 8 mg twice daily. This can be adjusted according to need. Ondansetron is often prescribed during chemotherapy, and the dose required may be increased if this is prescribed. Ondansetron may also be prescribed intravenously if the patient is too nauseous to tolerate oral medication.

The most common side effects associated with ondansetron are:

- constipation
- headaches
- flushing.

The side effects associated with this medication are minimal, and allergy reactions are sometimes seen when given intravenously (Galbraith et al. 2007).

Small intestine

The small intestine is approximately 6 m long. In the small intestine, food is further broken down by mechanical and chemical digestion, and absorption of the products of digestion takes place. The small intestine is divided into three parts (see figure 10.9).

1. The duodenum is approximately 25 cm long. It is the entrance to the small intestine.
2. The jejunum measures 2.5 m and is the middle part of the small intestine.
3. The **ileum** measures 3.5 m. It meets the large intestine at the **ileocaecal valve**. This valve prevents the backflow of the products of digestion from the large intestine back into the small intestine.

FIGURE 10.9 The small intestine

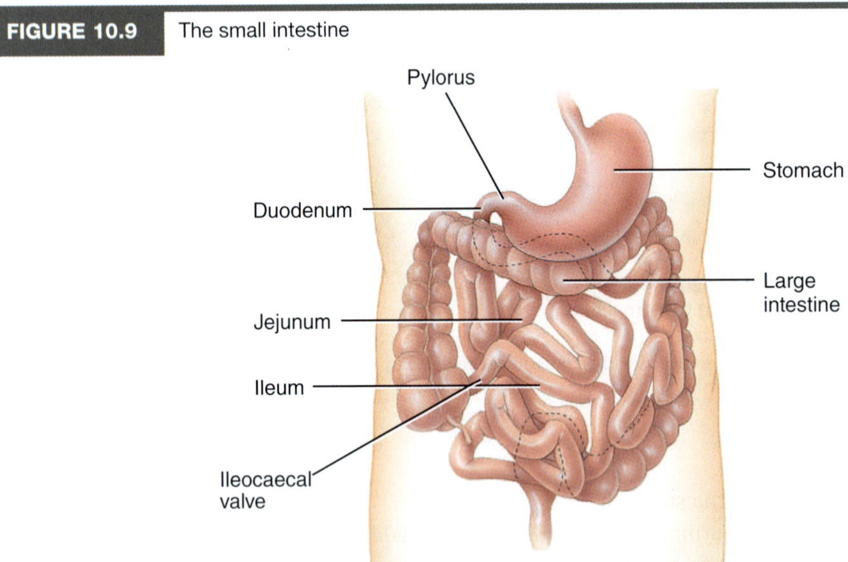

Source: Tortora and Derrickson (2009). Reproduced with permission of John Wiley & Sons.

The small intestine is innervated with both parasympathetic and sympathetic nerves. It receives its arterial blood supply from the **superior mesenteric artery** and nutrient-rich venous blood drains into the **superior mesenteric vein** and eventually into the **hepatic portal vein** towards the liver.

There are four types of cell present in the mucosa of the small intestine (see figure 10.10).

- The absorptive cell produces digestive enzymes and absorbs digested foods.
- **Goblet cells** secrete mucus to protect the intestine from abrasion and from the acidic chyme entering the small intestine.
- Enteroendocrine cells produce regulatory hormones such as secretin and CCK. These hormones are secreted into the bloodstream and act on their target organs to release pancreatic juice and **bile**.
- **Paneth cells** produce lysozyme, which protects the small intestine from pathogens that have survived the acid conditions of the stomach. **Peyer's patches** (lymphatic tissue of the small intestine) also protect the small intestine.

FIGURE 10.10 The cells within the villi of the small intestine

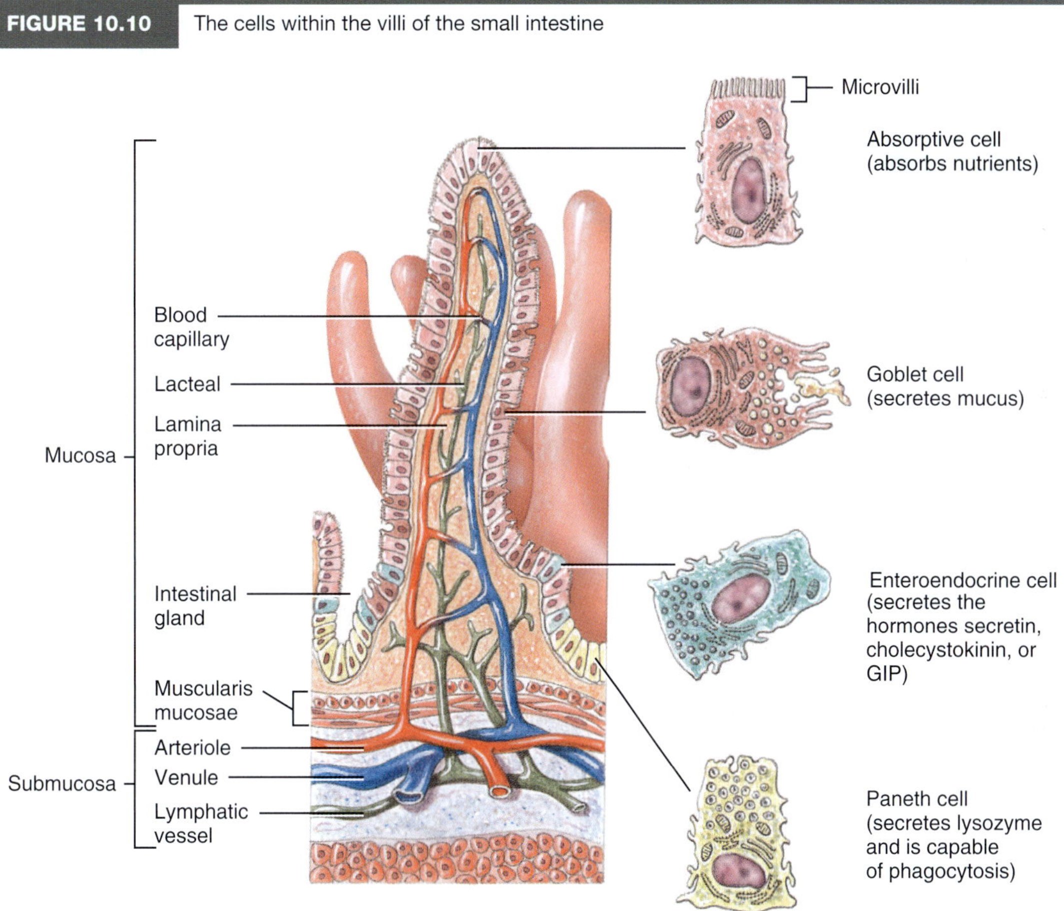

Source: Tortora and Derrickson (2009). Reproduced with permission of John Wiley & Sons.

Partially digested food enters the small intestine and spends 3–6 h moving through its 6 m length. The smooth muscle activity within the small intestine continues the process of mechanical digestion. There are two types of mechanical digestion in the small intestine: segmental contractions, which help to mix the various enzymes in the small intestine with the contents of the chyme; and peristalsis, which propels the food down the length of the small intestine as well as facilitating mixing.

Chemical digestion completes the breakdown of the carbohydrates, **fats** and proteins. Pancreatic juice from the pancreas, bile from the gall bladder and intestinal juice contribute to this.

Function of the small intestine

- Production of mucus to protect the duodenum from the effects of the acidic chyme.
- Secretion of intestinal juice and pancreatic juice from the pancreas increase the pH of the chyme to facilitate the action of the enzymes.

- Bile enters the small intestine to emulsify fat so that it can be further broken down by the action of lipase.
- Many enzymes are secreted to complete the chemical digestion of carbohydrates, proteins and fats.
- Mechanical digestion is by peristalsis and **segmentation** and slows down to allow adequate mixing and maximum absorption.
- The small intestine is structurally designed with a large surface area for maximum absorption of the products of digestion.
- The small intestine is where the majority of nutrients, electrolytes and water are absorbed.

The large intestine

The contents of the large intestine move slowly through it by a process called segmentation. This allows time to complete digestion and absorption. Entry to the large intestine is controlled by the ileocaecal sphincter. The sphincter opens in response to the increased activity of the stomach and the action of the hormone gastrin and prevents the backflow of food residue into the ileum (see figure 10.11).

FIGURE 10.11 The large intestine

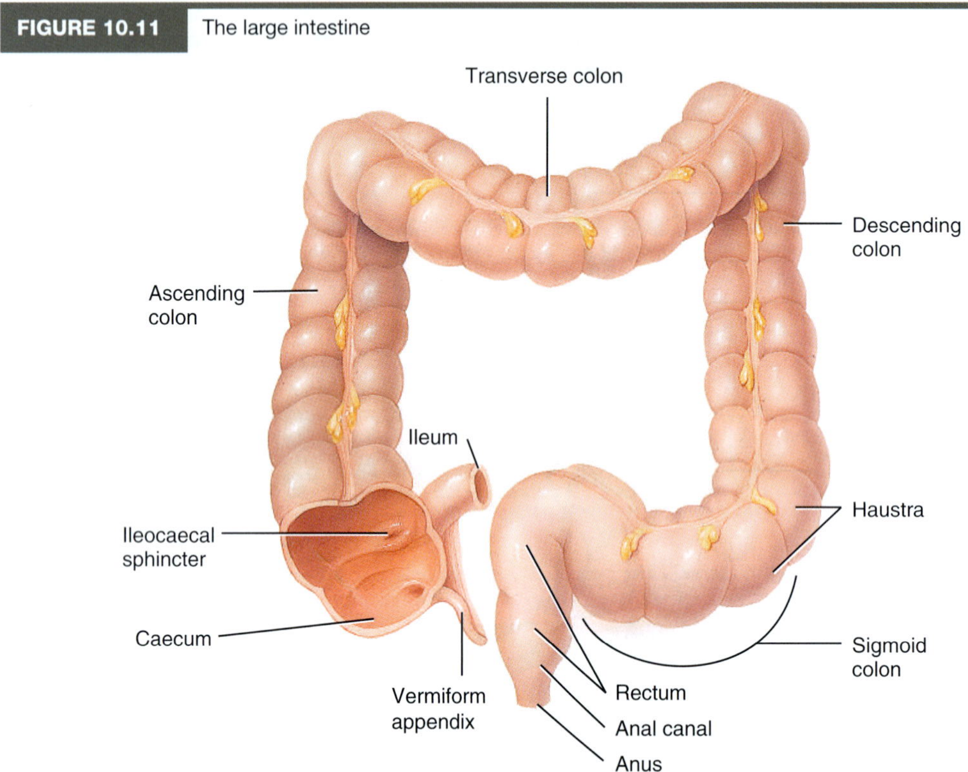

Source: Tortora and Derrickson (2009). Reproduced with permission of John Wiley & Sons.

The large intestine measures 1.5 m in length and 7 cm in diameter. It is continuous with the small intestine from the ileocaecal valve and ends at the anus.

Food residue enters the **caecum** and moves up the ascending colon along the transverse colon, down the descending colon and out of the body via the **rectum**, anal canal and anus. The caecum is a descending, sac-like opening into the large intestine. The **vermiform appendix** is a narrow, tube-like structure that leaves the caecum but is closed at its distal end. It is composed of lymphoid tissue and has a role in immunity. Two sphincter muscles control exit from the anus. The internal anal sphincter is smooth muscle and is under the control of the parasympathetic nervous system, whereas the external anal sphincter is composed of skeletal muscle and is under voluntary control.

CLINICAL CONSIDERATIONS

Appendicitis

The narrow lumen of the appendix does not allow much room for inflammation. If it becomes blocked by faecoliths (hard faecal material) or becomes twisted and kinked, this results in inflammation of the appendix. The swelling associated with this can lead to ulceration of the mucosal lining. This presents initially as central abdominal pain that eventually localises at the region of the appendix. Appendicitis can subside, but it can result in abscess formation and even rupture.

The large intestine mucosa contains large numbers of goblet cells that secrete mucus to ease the passage of faeces and protect the walls of the large intestine. The simple columnar epithelium changes to stratified squamous epithelium at the anal canal. Anal sinuses secrete mucus in response to faecal compression. This protects the anal canal from the abrasion associated with defecation.

The longitudinal muscle layer of the large intestine is formed into bands called the **taeniae coli**. These give the large intestine its gathered appearance. The sac created by this gathering is called a **haustrum**.

The food residue from the ileum is fluid when it enters the caecum and contains few nutrients. While the small intestine is responsible for some of the absorption of water, the primary function of the large intestine is to absorb water and turn the food residue into semi-solid faeces. The large intestine also absorbs some vitamins, minerals, electrolytes and drugs. Food residue usually takes 24–48 h to pass through the large intestine; 500 mL of food residue enters the large intestine daily and approximately 150 mL leaves as faeces.

As faeces enters the rectum, the stretching of the walls of the rectum initiates the defecation reflex. Acquired, voluntary control of the defecation reflex occurs between the ages of 2 and 3 years. The external anal sphincter is under voluntary control, and, if it is appropriate to do so, defecation can occur. Contraction of the abdominal muscles and diaphragm (the Valsalva manoeuvre) increases intra-abdominal pressure and assists in the process of defecation. If it is not appropriate to defecate, it can be postponed, as it is under voluntary control. After a few minutes the urge to defecate will subside and will only be felt again when the next mass movement (prolonged peristaltic contractions unique to the large intestine) through the large intestine occurs.

Faeces is a brown, semi-solid material. It contains fibre, **stercobilin** (from the breakdown of bilirubin), water, fatty acids, shed epithelial cells and microbes. Stercobilin gives faeces its brown colour. An excess of water in faeces results in diarrhoea. This occurs when food residue passes too quickly through the large intestine, so that the absorption of water cannot occur. Conversely, constipation occurs if food residue spends too long in the large intestine.

MEDICINES MANAGEMENT

Lactulose

Lactulose belongs to a group of medications called laxatives or aperients. It is used to treat constipation. Constipation occurs as a result of insufficient fluid intake or dehydration, a lack of exercise or immobility, during pregnancy or due to a lack of dietary fibre.

People who experience constipation should try to increase their mobility and fluid intake. They should examine their diet to see whether additional fibre can be taken to increase faecal water retention (faecal bulking). Lactulose may also be prescribed.

The usual adult dose for lactulose is 15 mL three times a day. Lactulose acts in the large intestine and can take 48 h to have an effect. Increasing fluid intake to 2 L will also help.

Lactulose is an osmotic laxative (Galbraith et al. 2007) and leads to a change in the osmotic pressure in the bowel, and therefore more water is available in the intestine. This leads to the stool having more water content, making it pass through the intestine easier.

The side effects of taking lactulose include:

- nausea
- diarrhoea
- flatulence
- abdominal discomfort.

Selby and Corte (2010) have produced a clinical knowledge summary on constipation.

10.2 Accessory organs of the digestive system

LEARNING OBJECTIVE 10.2 Describe the structure and function of the accessory organs of the digestive system.

Teeth

Temporary teeth are also known as deciduous teeth or milk teeth. Temporary teeth begin to appear at about 6 months old. There are 20 temporary teeth, and these are replaced by permanent teeth from about the age of 6 years (Nair & Peate 2018). There are 32 permanent teeth. Sixteen are located in the maxilla arch (upper) and 16 are located in the mandible (lower) (see figure 10.12).

FIGURE 10.12 (a, b) Teeth

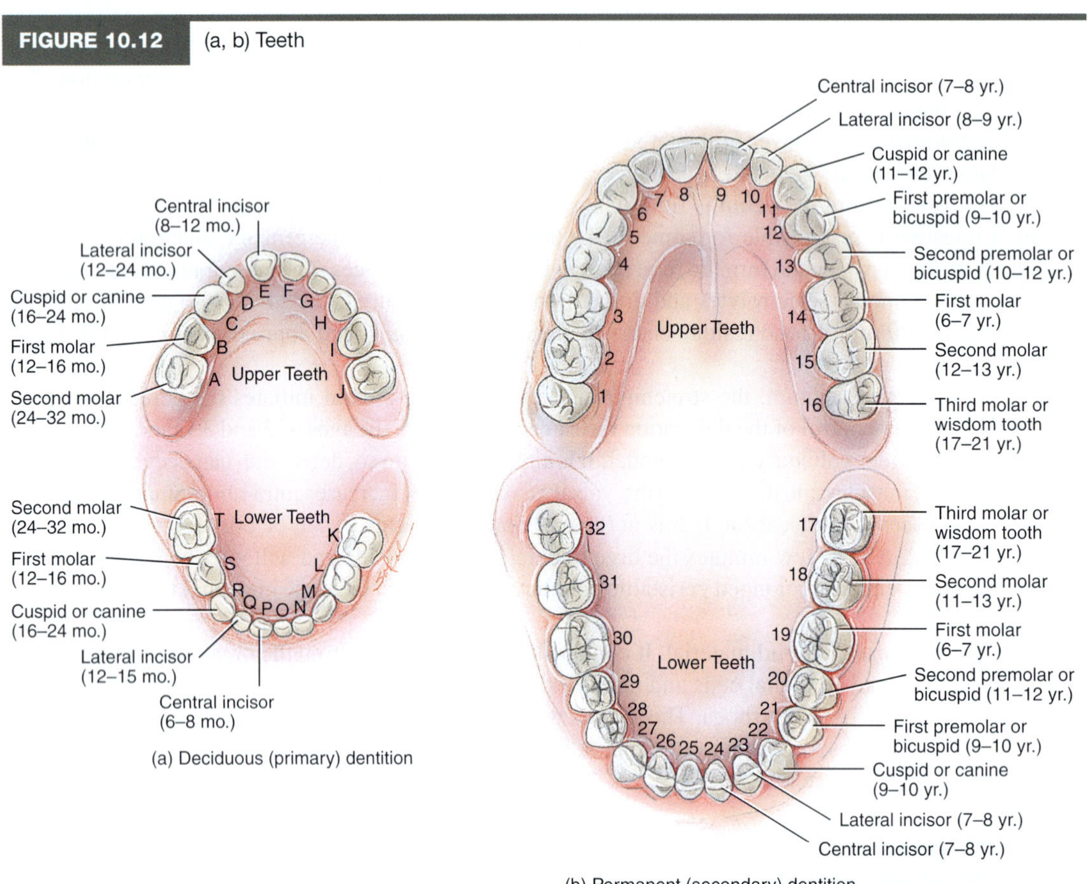

Source: Tortora and Derrickson (2009). Reproduced with permission of John Wiley & Sons.

Canines and **incisors** are cutting and tearing teeth. **Premolars** and **molars** are used for the grinding and chewing of food. Despite their different functions and shape, the structure of each tooth is the same. The visible part of the tooth is called the crown. The crown sits above the gum or gingiva. The centre of the tooth is called the **pulp cavity**. Blood and lymph vessels as well as nerves enter and leave the tooth here. The tooth receives nutrients and sensations via the pulp. Surrounding this is a calcified matrix, not unlike bone, called the dentine. Surrounding the dentine is a very hard, protective material called **enamel**. The neck of the tooth is where the crown meets the root. The teeth are anchored in a socket with a bone-like material called cementum, and the function of the teeth is to chew (masticate) food.

Salivary glands

There are three pairs of salivary glands (see figure 10.13). The **parotid glands** are the largest and they are located anterior to the ears. Saliva from the parotid glands enters the oral cavity close to the level of the second upper molar tooth. The **submandibular glands** are located below the jaw on each side of the face. Saliva from these glands enters the oral cavity from beside the lingual frenulum of the tongue. The **sublingual glands** are the smallest. They are located in the floor of the mouth.

FIGURE 10.13 Salivary glands

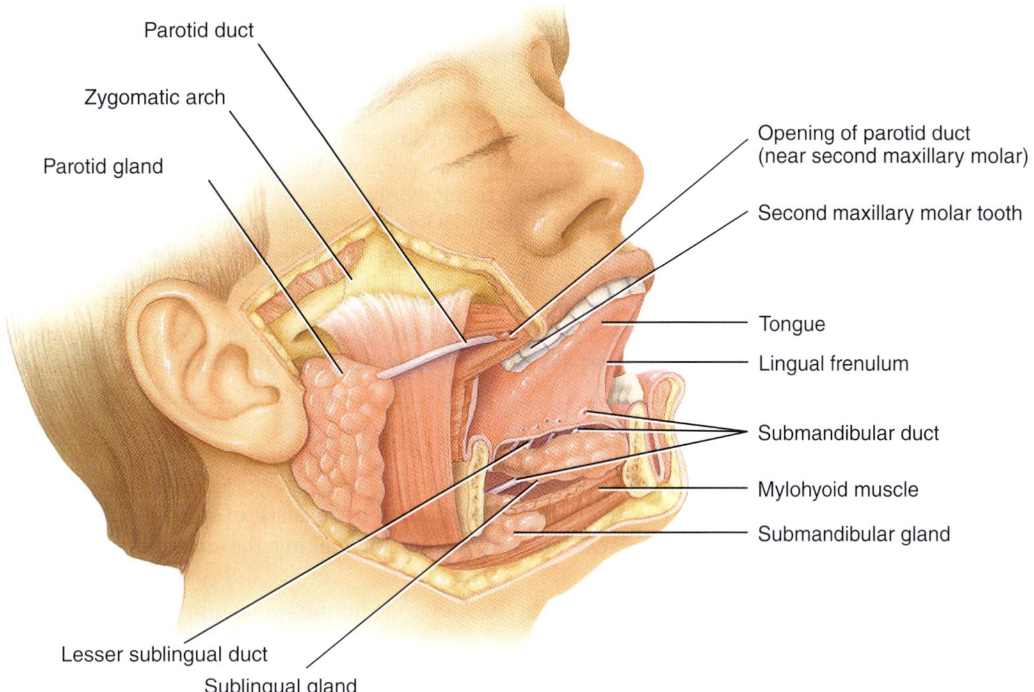

Although saliva is continuously secreted in order to keep the oral cavity moist, the activity of the **parasympathetic fibres** that innervate the salivary glands will lead to an increased production of saliva in response to the sight, smell or taste of food. The action of sympathetic fibres leads to a decreased secretion of saliva.

In health, approximately 1–1.5 L of saliva is secreted daily. Saliva consists of:

- water
- **salivary amylase**
- mucus
- **mineral salts**
- **lysozyme**
- immunoglobulins
- blood clotting factors.

Saliva has several important functions.

- Salivary amylase is a digestive enzyme responsible for beginning the breakdown of **carbohydrate** molecules from complex polysaccharides to the disaccharide maltase.
- The fluid nature of saliva helps to moisten and lubricate food that enters the mouth. This makes it easier to hold the food in the mouth and also assists in forming the food into a bolus in preparation for swallowing.
- The continuous secretion of saliva is cleansing and helps to maintain moisture in the oral cavity. A lack of moisture can lead to oral mucosal infections and formation of mouth ulcers.
- The oral cavity is an entry route for pathogens from the external environment. Lysozyme, a constituent of saliva, has an antibacterial action. Immunoglobulin and clotting factors also contribute to the prevention of infection.
- Taste is only possible when food substances are moist. Saliva is required to moisten food.

SKILLS IN PRACTICE

Mouth care

Patients who are ill can also be dehydrated and therefore their production of saliva is reduced. This can lead to an increased risk of oral infections, as wear and tear within the oral cavity increases. Reduced amounts of saliva leads to less washing away of pathogens to the acid environment of the stomach where they may be destroyed. The oral cavity provides a route for pathogens to enter the respiratory tract, and therefore good oral hygiene practices may help prevent respiratory infections, particularly in patients who are vulnerable due to acute illness, cancer treatments or immobility.

When patients are ill, a sufficient dietary intake is essential for tissue repair and healing; however, a lack of saliva will lead to the food not tasting as it should. The food will not easily form into the required bolus size for ease of swallowing. This may put the patient off eating and drinking and may lead to the patient losing their appetite and potentially delay healing.

Ill health can lead to neglect of hygiene standards for individuals. Mouth care is easy for patients to ignore when they are feeling poorly. However, it is an essential consideration for nursing.

The pancreas

The pancreas is composed of exocrine and endocrine tissue. It consists of a head, body and tail (see figure 10.14). The cells of the pancreas are responsible for making the endocrine and exocrine products.

- The islet cells of the islets of Langerhans produce the endocrine hormones insulin and glucagon. These hormones control carbohydrate metabolism.
- The **acini glands** of the exocrine pancreas produce 1.2–1.5 L of pancreatic juice daily. Pancreatic juice travels from the pancreas via the **pancreatic duct** into the duodenum at the **hepatopancreatic ampulla**.
- The cells of the pancreatic ducts secrete bicarbonate ions, which gives pancreatic juice its high pH (pH 8). This helps to neutralise acidic chyme from the stomach, thus protecting the small intestine from damage by the acidity. Additionally, the actions of **amylase** and lipase are most effective at the higher pH (pH 6–8).

FIGURE 10.14 The liver, gall bladder and pancreas

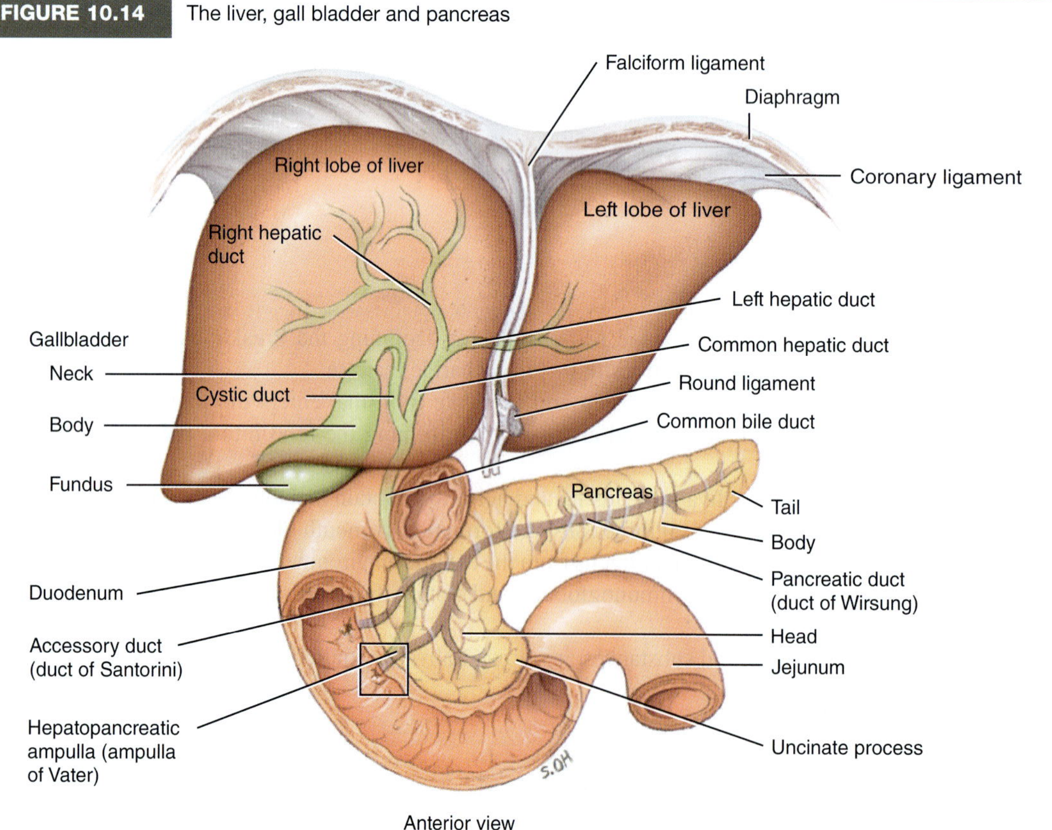

Source: Tortora and Derrickson (2009). Reproduced with permission of John Wiley & Sons.

Pancreatic juice consists of:

- water
- mineral salts
- pancreatic amylase, which completes the digestion of carbohydrates
- lipase, used in the digestion of fat
- trypsinogen, chymotrypsinogen and procarboxypeptidase, which are released in an inactive form to protect the digestive system structures from the protein-digesting enzymes that they become — once they enter the duodenum they are activated by enterokinase from intestinal juice and become trypsin, chymotrypsin and carboxypeptidase respectively and are then used in the digestion of protein.

Two hormones regulate the secretion of pancreatic juice. Secretin, produced in response to the presence of hydrochloric acid in the duodenum, promotes the secretion of bicarbonate ions. CCK, secreted in response to the intake of protein and fat, promotes the secretion of the enzymes present in pancreatic juice. Parasympathetic vagus nerve stimulation also promotes the release of pancreatic juice.

In summary, the exocrine function of the pancreas is to secrete pancreatic juice into the duodenum. The actions of pancreatic juice lead to the further breakdown of carbohydrate, fat and protein.

MEDICINES MANAGEMENT

Creon

Creon is a medication prescribed for patients who have cystic fibrosis or pancreatic insufficiency. It contains the following enzymes:

- amylase — for the breakdown of carbohydrate
- lipase — for the breakdown of fats
- proteases — for the breakdown of protein.

Pancreatic insufficiency can occur as a result of pancreatic cancer, pancreatic surgery and acute or chronic pancreatitis. In cystic fibrosis the ducts that transport the pancreatic enzymes become obstructed with the increased mucus production associated with this disease pathway.

The dosage of creon required will depend on the diet of the patient. If the symptoms of loose stool and weight loss persist, then the dose of creon may be increased. Creon is usually taken for life. Side effects associated with creon include:

- abdominal distension
- nausea
- vomiting
- diarrhoea
- constipation.

The tablets are enteric coated to protect them from inactivation in the stomach (Galbraith et al. 2007).

Turner (2015) has produced a clinical knowledge summary on managing chronic pancreatitis.

CLINICALLY REASONED EPISODE OF CARE

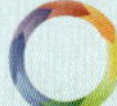

Crohn's disease

Consider the patient situation

Zoe is 10 years old. She complains constantly to her mum that she is tired and does not want to go to school. Her teachers have reported lethargy and an inability to join in with the other children for any length of time.

Zoe attends the dentist for her routine 6-monthly check-up and the dentist reports mouth ulcers. Zoe's mum is concerned as all of the symptoms, including a failure to gain weight and develop, are starting to mount up.

Zoe visits the GP with her mum.

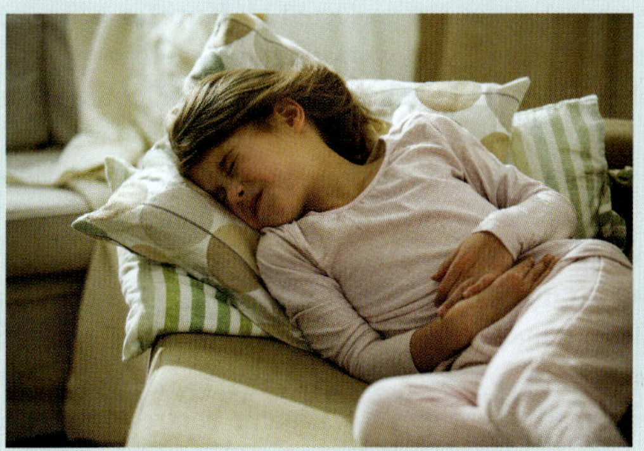

Collect cues and information

Zoe provides a stool sample and while there is no evidence of blood, it is sent off for analysis. Zoe's stool sample does reveal blood in the stool and her blood tests show anaemia.

Zoe is referred to a consultant and she discusses her symptoms which include:

- diarrhoea
- crampy tummy pain
- mouth ulcers
- tiredness
- weight loss.

Following additional tests, including an MRI scan, the consultant diagnoses Crohn's disease.

Process information

Crohn's disease is an inflammatory bowel disease. While the symptoms of Crohn's disease can occur at any time, they often begin in childhood. The causes of Crohn's disease are unknown but are thought to be linked to a number of things including the immune system, genetic makeup, abnormal gut flora and the after-effects of a viral illness.

The inflammation in Crohn's disease may occur anywhere in the digestive tract. It may be patchy and cover small areas, or it may extend further and deeper into the tissue. It is a chronic condition.

Nursing actions

1. Provide reassurance, support and education for Zoe and her mother during and after consultations.
   Rationale:
   - Quality patient education and support reduces patient anxiety.
2. Provide education around the prescribed anti-inflammatory medications.
   Rationale:
   - Patient education supports concordance with recommended therapies which will promote good outcomes for the person.
3. Provide referrals to other healthcare professionals such as dieticians, and recommend patient support groups for people with inflammatory bowel disease; see www.crohnsandcolitis.com.au.
   Rationale:
   - People living with chronic health conditions benefit both emotionally and psychologically by establishing a support network.

Evaluate outcomes

Zoe and her mother articulate an appropriate level of understanding of Zoe's condition and therapeutic interventions.

Source: Based on the Clinical Reasoning Cycle, Levett-Jones (2013).

The liver and production of bile

The liver is the body's largest gland. It weighs between 1 and 2 kg. It lies under the diaphragm partly protected by the ribs. The liver occupies most of the right **hypochondriac region** and extends through part of the epigastric region into the left hypochondriac region. The right lobe is the largest of the four liver lobes. On the posterior surface of the liver there is an entry and exit to the organ called the **portal fissure**. Blood, lymph vessels, nerves and **bile ducts** enter and leave the liver through the portal fissure.

The liver is composed of tiny hexagonal-shaped lobules that contain **hepatocytes** (see figure 10.15). The hepatocytes are protected by **Kupffer cells** (hepatic macrophages). The Kupffer cells deal with any foreign particles and worn-out blood cells.

Each corner of the hexagonal-shaped lobule has a **portal triad**. A branch of the hepatic artery, a branch of hepatic portal vein and a bile duct are present here. The hepatic artery supplies the hepatocytes with oxygenated arterial blood. The hepatic portal vein delivers nutrient-rich deoxygenated blood from the digestive tract to the hepatocytes. The hepatocytes' function is to filter, detoxify and process the nutrients from the digestive tract. Nutrients can be used for energy, stored or used to make new molecules. The **liver sinusoids** are large, leaky capillaries that drain the blood from the hepatic artery and hepatic portal vein into the central vein. This processed blood is then drained into the hepatic vein and on to the inferior vena cava.

As the blood flows towards the centre of the triad to exit at the central vein, the bile produced by the hepatocyte as a metabolic by-product moves in the opposite direction towards the bile canaliculi and on to the bile ducts. Bile then leaves the liver via the common hepatic duct towards the duodenum of the small intestine.

FIGURE 10.15 Liver lobule

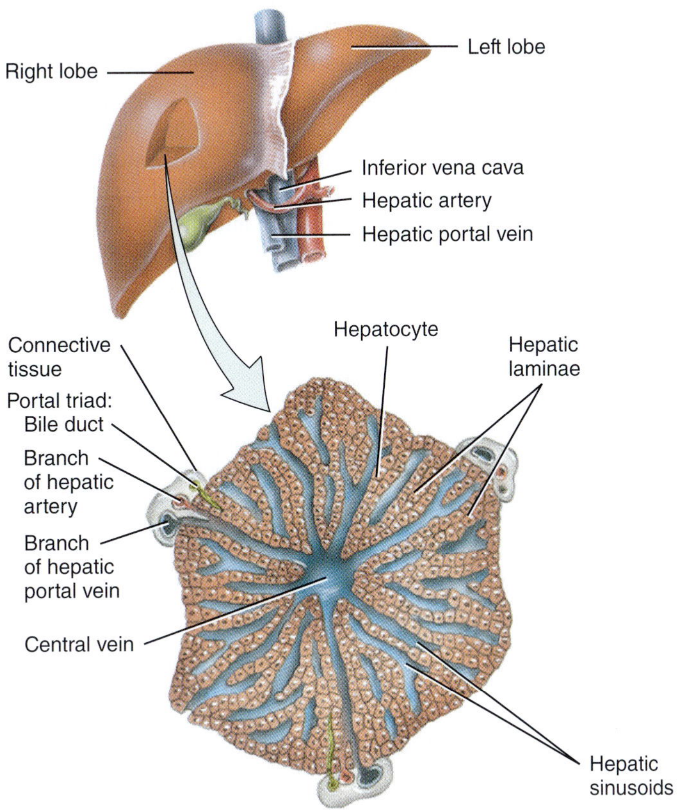

Overview of histological components of liver

Source: Tortora and Derrickson (2009). Reproduced with permission of John Wiley & Sons.

The liver produces and secretes up to 1 L of yellow/green alkaline bile per day. Bile is composed of:

- bile salts, such as bilirubin from the breakdown of haemoglobin
- cholesterol
- fat-soluble hormones
- fat
- mineral salts
- mucus.

The function of bile is to emulsify fats, giving the fat-digesting enzyme lipase a larger surface area to work on.

Bile is stored and concentrated in the gall bladder.

The functions of the liver

Apart from the production of bile and the metabolism of carbohydrate, fat and protein (discussed further on in this chapter), the liver has many additional functions:

- detoxification of drugs — the liver deals with medication, alcohol, ingested toxins and the toxins produced by the action of microbes
- recycling of erythrocytes
- deactivation of many hormones, including the sex hormones, thyroxine, insulin, glucagon, cortisol and aldosterone
- production of clotting proteins
- storage of vitamins, minerals and glycogen
- synthesis of vitamin A
- heat production.

The gall bladder

The gall bladder is a small, green, muscular sac that lies posterior to the liver. It functions as a reservoir for bile. It also concentrates bile by absorbing water. The mucosa of the gall bladder, like the rugae of the stomach, contains folds that allow the gall bladder to stretch in order to accommodate varying volumes of bile. When the smooth muscle walls of the gall bladder contract, bile is expelled into the cystic duct and down into the common bile duct before entering the duodenum via the hepatopancreatic ampulla.

The stimulus for gall bladder contraction is the hormone CCK. This enteroendocrine hormone, secreted from the small intestine into the blood, is produced in response to the presence of fatty chyme in the duodenum. CCK stimulates the secretion of pancreatic juice and the relaxation of the **hepatopancreatic sphincter**. When the sphincter is relaxed, both bile and pancreatic juice can enter the duodenum.

HOMEOSTATIC IMBALANCE

Cholelithiasis

Cholelithiasis, or gallstones, occurs when cholesterol or bile pigments solidify or crystallise within the gall bladder. These gallstones can then lodge in the bile ducts, causing inflammation and the impairment or blockage of bile flow into the duodenum.

Cholelithiasis is a very common condition and can range from being completely asymptomatic to causing symptoms such as nausea, jaundice, abdominal pain and vomiting. Treatment options range from dietary changes to surgical removal of the gallstones or complete removal of the gall bladder (cholecystectomy) (Health Direct 2020).

10.3 Digestive hormones

LEARNING OBJECTIVE 10.3 Explain the action of the enzymes and hormones associated with the digestion of proteins, carbohydrates and fats, and how the products of digestion are utilised within the body.

Many hormones are responsible for the activity of the digestive system. A summary of their role is contained in table 10.1.

TABLE 10.1 **Summary of the role of the digestive system hormones**

Hormone	Origin	Target	Action	Stimulus
Gastrin	Stomach	Stomach	Increases gastric gland secretion of hydrochloric acid Gastric emptying	Presence of protein in the stomach
Secretin	Duodenum	Stomach	Inhibits gastric gland secretion Inhibits gastric motility	Acidic and fatty chyme in the duodenum
		Pancreas	Increases pancreatic juice secretion Promotes cholecys-tokinin action	
		Liver	Increases bile secretion	
Cholecystokinin	Duodenum	Pancreas	Increases pancreatic juice secretion	Chyme in the duodenum
		Gall bladder	Stimulates contraction	
		Hepatopancreatic sphincter	Relaxes — entry to duodenum opens	

Chemical digestion

Within the small intestine, any carbohydrates that have not been broken down by the action of salivary amylase will be broken down by pancreatic amylase.

Bile will emulsify fat and fatty acids, making it easier for **lipase** (also from the pancreatic juice) to break the fats into fatty acids and glycerol. Proteins are denatured by hydrochloric acid in the stomach. In the small intestine they are further acted upon by the enzymes trypsin, chymotrypsin and carboxypeptidase. The end product of protein digestion are tripeptidases, dipeptidases and amino acids.

The small intestine produce 1–2 L of intestinal juice daily. It is secreted from the cells of the **intestinal crypts** (crypts of Lieberkühn) (located between the **villi**) in response to either acidic chyme irritating the intestinal mucosa or distension from the presence of chyme in the small intestine. Intestinal juice is slightly alkaline (pH 7.4–8.4) and watery. Intestinal juice and pancreatic juice from the pancreas mix with the acidic chyme as it enters the duodenum and increase the pH, thus preventing the corrosive action of chyme on the mucosa of the duodenum. Intestinal juice contains mucus, which helps protect the intestinal mucosa, mineral salts and enterokinase.

The primary function of the small intestine is absorption of water and nutrients, and it has several anatomical adaptations to facilitate this.

- Permanent circular folds, called **plicae circulars**, within the mucosa and submucosa slow down the movement of the products of digestion, allowing time for absorption of nutrients to occur.
- On the surface of the mucosa are tiny, finger-like projections called villi. At the centre of the villi is a capillary bed and a **lacteal** (lymph capillary). This allows nutrients to be absorbed directly into the blood or the lymph.
- On the surface of the villi are cytoplasmic extensions called microvilli. The presence of the microvilli greatly increases the surface area available for absorption. The appearance of the microvilli resembles the surface of a brush; hence it is called the brush border. The brush border produces some enzymes used to further break down carbohydrates such as lactase, maltase, dextrinase and sucrase. It also produces enzymes to further break down proteins: aminopeptidase, carboxypeptidase and dipeptidase.

The absorption of nutrients occurs by diffusion or active transport. Some nutrients will be absorbed into the blood capillary and some will be absorbed into the lacteal.

10.4 Nutrition, chemical digestion and metabolism

LEARNING OBJECTIVE 10.4 List the common vitamins and minerals and the problems associated with a deficit or excess.

This chapter has hitherto concentrated on how the digestive tract deals with food ingested in order to break it down into its constituent parts for use by the cells of the body. This section will consider nutrition and the role of a balanced diet in health.

An adequate intake of nutrients is essential for health. Nutrition also has an important role in social and psychological wellbeing. If managed inappropriately, nutrition can lead to many physical and psychological illnesses. Therefore, it is important to have an understanding of the role of nutrients within the body in order to understand how a lack or excess of nutrients will lead to ill health.

The remainder of this chapter will identify the **macronutrients** and **micronutrients** and the food groups that provide the source of macronutrients and micronutrients. It will examine what the nutrients are broken down into and how the body uses these constituent parts.

Nutrients

A nutrient is a substance that is ingested and processed by the gastrointestinal system. It is digested and absorbed and can be used by the body to produce energy or become the building block for a new molecule or to participate in essential chemical reactions. Nutrients are required for body growth, repair and maintenance of cell function. Not all of the food ingested can be classed as nutrients. Some indigestible plant fibres are not nutrients (dietary fibre/resistant starches) but are required for healthy functioning of the digestive system and the gut microbiome.

Balanced diet

The body has the ability to break down some nutrients in order to create new molecules, but this ability is finite and there remains a group of essential nutrients that the body cannot make but are required to be ingested in the diet for homeostasis to be maintained. A balanced diet is therefore essential for health (NHMRC 2013). The daily recommended portions of food groups required for a balanced diet are often shown in a food pyramid (see figure 10.16). Lack of a balanced diet can lead to malnourishment, and overindulgence can lead to obesity.

FIGURE 10.16 The food pyramid

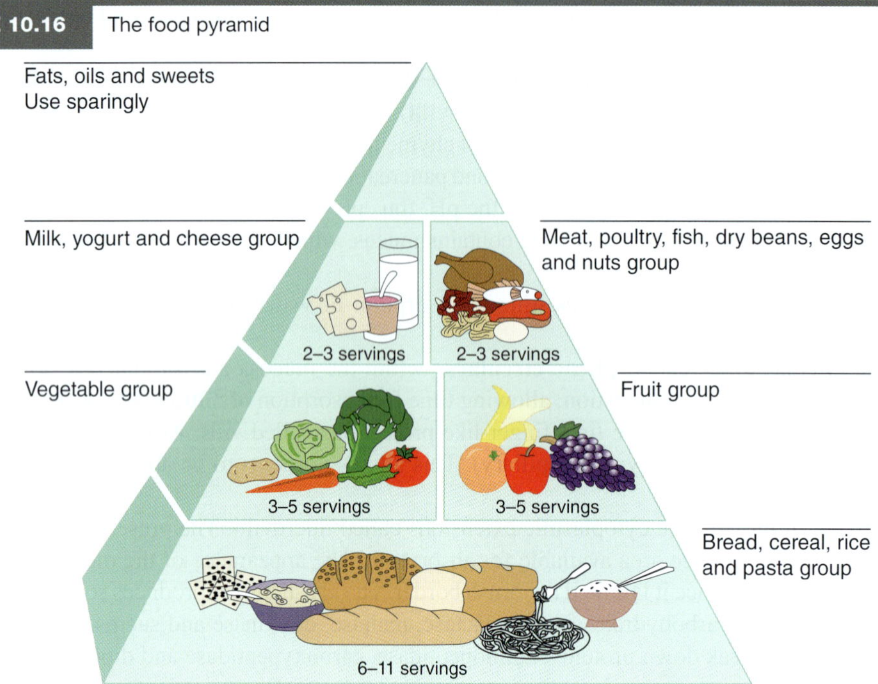

Source: Tortora and Derrickson (2009). Reproduced with permission of John Wiley & Sons.

CLINICAL CONSIDERATIONS

Bariatric surgery

Bariatric surgery is used as a last resort to treat those who are severely obese. The procedure works by reducing the intake or the absorption of calories and is used to treat people with potentially life-threatening obesity if other treatments (e.g. lifestyle changes) have not worked. Indications include the following.

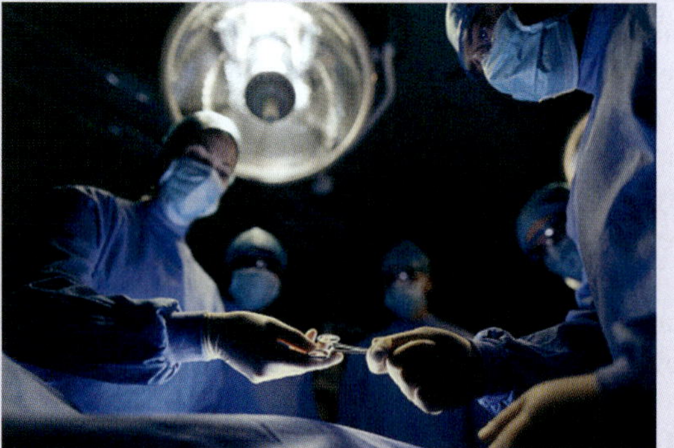

- The person has a body mass index (BMI) greater than 40, or the person has a BMI of 35 or above and another serious health condition that may be improved if weight is lost (e.g. type 2 diabetes or hypertension).
- Other non-surgical methods have failed to maintain weight loss for at least 6 months.
- The person commits to long-term follow-up.

Weight loss surgery can help to significantly and quickly reduce excess body fat for those who meet the criteria. Bariatric surgery has to be undertaken in a specialist centre with long-term follow-up of patients. National guidelines are available concerning bariatric surgery. Contraindications include those who are unfit for surgery and those people with an uncontrolled alcohol or drug dependency.

Dietary nutrients begin life as large food molecules. They enter the digestive tract and are broken down into smaller molecules. This process is called **catabolism**. Digestive enzymes facilitate the breakdown of foods by a process called **hydrolysis**. Hydrolysis is the addition of water to break down the chemical bonds of the food molecules. Each of the three different types of food is broken down (lysed) by different enzymes.

Nutrient groups

Carbohydrates, proteins and lipids (fats) are known as the major nutrients or macronutrients. They are required in quite large quantities. Vitamins and minerals are required in much smaller quantities, but they are also crucial for the maintenance of health — they are also known as the micronutrients. There are therefore six classes of nutrients:

- water
- carbohydrates
- lipids (fats)
- proteins
- vitamins
- minerals.

Water

Water is essential for the action of many digestive system functions. It is required to produce the many different juices of the digestive system. As the enzymes act on the different food molecules within the diet, water is added as chemical bonds are broken. This process is known as hydrolysis (Cohen & Hull 2018).

Carbohydrates

Monosaccharides, disaccharides and polysaccharides are all carbohydrates. The dietary source of carbohydrates is plants. However, the milk sugar lactose is a form of carbohydrate found in cow and human milk. Carbohydrates are found in many foods, such as bread, pasta, cereal, biscuits, vegetables and fruit.

Carbohydrates consist of carbon, hydrogen and oxygen. They can be complex, such as the polysaccharides starch and glycogen, or simple, such as the disaccharides sucrose (table sugar) and lactose (milk sugar) and the monosaccharides glucose, fructose and galactose.

Digestion of carbohydrates supplies the body with fructose, galactose and glucose. The liver converts fructose and galactose to glucose as glucose is the molecule used by the body's cells.

Digested carbohydrates are absorbed into the blood via the villi of the small intestine. They enter the hepatic portal circulation and are transported to the liver for processing. The liver is a highly metabolic organ that requires a plentiful supply of glucose to carry out its metabolic activity.

Glucose is used by the cells to produce adenosine triphosphate (ATP). Glucose plus oxygen makes ATP, carbon dioxide and water. The process of breaking down glucose is called **glycolysis**.

Insufficient carbohydrate intake will lead to an inability to meet the cells' energy demands. If this happens, the body will break down amino acids and lipids to create new glucose, a process called **gluconeogenesis**.

Excess glucose is converted to glycogen and stored in the liver and skeletal muscle. It can also be converted to fat and stored.

Fats

Dietary sources of fat include butter, eggs, cheese, milk, oily fish and the fatty part of meat. These contain saturated fat, which is mainly saturated fatty acids and glycerol. Vegetable oils and margarine are sources of unsaturated fats. The body can also create fat from excess carbohydrates and proteins.

Fat also contains carbon, hydrogen and oxygen, but in a different combination from carbohydrates.

When fat enters the small intestine it mixes and is emulsified by bile. The action of pancreatic lipase completes the digestion of fat and it is broken down into monoglycerides, glycerol and fatty acids. The monoglycerides and some of the fatty acids enter the lacteals of the villi and are transported via the lymph to the thoracic duct and then into the circulation, where they eventually reach the liver. Glycerol and the remaining fatty acids are absorbed more directly into the capillary blood and reach the liver via the hepatic portal vein.

The liver uses some of the fatty acids and glycerol to produce energy and heat. In fact, hepatocytes and skeletal muscle use triglycerides as their major energy source. Excessive triglycerides can also be stored as lipid inclusions in adipose tissue, and this can also be used as an energy source when glucose is not available to body cells.

Dietary fats make food seem tender and lead to increased feelings of satisfaction with food during eating. They are necessary for the absorption of fat-soluble vitamins. Adipose tissue protects, cushions and insulates vital organs in the body. Phospholipids are required to form the myelin sheath and cell membranes. Cholesterol is obtained from egg yolk and dairy produce but is also synthesised in the body to form steroid hormones and bile salts.

Excess fat in the diet can lead to obesity and cardiovascular disease. A lack of fat in the diet can lead to weight loss, poor growth and skin lesions.

Proteins

Dietary sources of protein include meat, eggs and milk. Beans and peas (legumes), nuts, cereals and leafy green vegetables are also sources of amino acids.

Protein digestion begins in the stomach and is completed in the small intestine. Proteins are broken down into amino acids. They are absorbed via the villi of the small intestine, where they reach the capillaries and enter the hepatic portal circulation to the liver or pass into the general circulation.

Proteins are used by the body for many purposes. They are used to form muscle, collagen and elastin, necessary for body structure and tissue repair. The hormones insulin and growth hormone are required for this. Amino acids are also used to form hormones and enzymes within the body. To produce a protein, all of the amino acids required to form that protein must be available within the cell in order for it to be made. This is called the all or nothing rule. Protein can also be used as a source of energy for the body. The amino acids are broken down mainly at the liver, where the nitrogenous part of the amino acid is removed and converted first to ammonia and then to urea. Urea is excreted as a waste product in urine. The remainder of the amino acid is used to produce energy. Protein cannot be stored by the body. Any excess amino acids are converted to carbohydrate or fat to be stored in adipose tissue.

Too much protein in the diet can lead to obesity. A lack of dietary protein can lead to muscle/tissue wasting and weight loss. A lack of plasma proteins can lead to oedema.

Vitamins

Vitamins are organic molecules that are required in small amounts for healthy metabolism. Essential vitamins cannot be manufactured by the body and must come from the diet, highlighting again the importance of a balanced diet. Some vitamins can be manufactured. Vitamin K is synthesised by intestinal bacteria; the skin makes vitamin D; and vitamin A is made from beta-carotene, found for example in carrots.

Many vitamins act as *coenzymes* (Seeley et al. 2008). These vitamins combine with enzymes to make them functional. For example, the formation of clotting proteins requires the presence of vitamin K.

Vitamins are either fat soluble or water soluble. The fat-soluble vitamins combine with lipids from the diet and are absorbed in this way. Apart from vitamin K, the fat-soluble vitamins can be stored in the body; therefore, there can be problems associated with toxicity when these vitamins accumulate.

The water-soluble vitamins are absorbed with water along the digestive tract. They cannot be stored, and any excess ingested will be excreted in urine. A summary of vitamins and their functions is given in table 10.2.

Minerals

Small quantities of inorganic compounds called minerals are required by the body for many purposes. For example, calcium gives structure and strength to tissues, and sodium forms ions essential for maintaining osmotic balance. They also form approximately 5 per cent of the body weight (Nair & Peate 2018).

There are minerals that are required in moderate amounts, such as calcium and magnesium, and many others known where trace amounts are required, such as cobalt and copper. A summary of some of the minerals and their function is given in table 10.3.

TABLE 10.2 Vitamins summary

Vitamin	Source	Function	Deficiency
		Fat soluble	
A, retinol	Manufactured from beta-carotene. Egg yolk, cream, fish oil, cheese, liver	Skin, mucosa integrity; bone and tooth development during growth; photoreceptor pigment synthesis in the retina, normal reproduction, antioxidant	Night blindness; dry skin and hair; loss of skin integrity; increased infection, particularly respiratory, gastrointestinal and urinary
D	Manufactured by the skin. Cheese, eggs, fish oil, liver	Regulates calcium and phosphate metabolism	Rickets in children, osteomalacia in adults
E	Egg yolk, wheat germ, whole cereals, milk and butter	Antioxidant	In severe deficiency, ataxia and visual disturbances, decreased life span of red blood cells
K	Synthesised by bacteria in the large intestine. Liver, fish, fruit and leafy green vegetables	Formation of clotting proteins at the liver	Prolonged clotting times, bruising, bleeding
		Water soluble	
B_1, thiamine	Egg yolk, liver, nuts, meat, legumes cereal germ	Coenzyme required for carbohydrate metabolism	Beriberi — muscle wasting, stunted growth polyneuritis and infection. Vision disturbances, confusion, unsteadiness, memory loss, fatigue, tachycardia, heart enlargement
B_2, riboflavin	Milk, green vegetables, yeast, cheese, fish roe, liver	Coenzyme required for carbohydrate and protein metabolism	Skin-cracking, particularly around the corners of the mouth, blurred vision, corneal ulcers, intestinal mucosa lesions
Folic acid	Liver, kidney, yeast, fresh leafy vegetables, eggs, whole grains	Coenzyme essential for DNA synthesis, red blood cell formation	Anaemia, spina bifida in newborn, increased risk of heart attack and stroke
Niacin, nicotinic acid	Liver, cheese, yeast, eggs, cereals, nuts, fish	Coenzyme involved in glycolysis, fat breakdown — assists with breakdown and inhibits cholesterol production	Pellagra — skin reddening to light, anorexia, nausea and dysphagia, delirium and dementia
B_6, pyridoxine	Meat, liver, fish, grains, bananas, yeast	Coenzyme involved in amino acid metabolism	Increased risk of heart disease, eye and mouth lesions. In children, nervous irritability, convulsions, abdominal pain and vomiting
B_{12} cyanocobal-amin	Meat, fish, liver, eggs, milk	Coenzyme in all cells, involved in DNA synthesis. Formation and maintenance of myelin around nerves	Pernicious anaemia, peripheral neuropathy
B_5 pan-tothenic acid	Meat, grains, legumes, yeast, egg yolk	Coenzyme associated with amino acid metabolism and formation of steroids	Non-specific symptoms
Biotin	Egg yolk, liver, legumes, tomatoes	Coenzyme in carbohydrate metabolism	Pallor, anorexia, nausea, fatigue
C, ascorbic acid	Fruit, particularly citrus fruit, vegetables	Antioxidant, enhances iron absorption and use, maturation of red blood cells	Poor wound healing, joint pain, anaemia, scurvy

TABLE 10.3 Minerals summary

Mineral	Source	Function	Deficiency (D)/excess (E)
Calcium	Milk, egg yolk, shellfish, cheese, green vegetables	Bones and teeth, cell membrane permeability, nerve impulse transmission, muscle contraction, heart rhythm, blood clotting	D: osteomalacia, osteoporosis, muscle tetany. In children — rickets and retarded growth E: lethargy and confusion, kidney stones
Chloride	Table salt	Works with sodium to maintain osmotic pressure of extracellular fluid	D: alkalosis, muscle cramps E: vomiting
Magnesium	Nuts, milk, legumes, cereal	Constituent of coenzymes. Muscle and nerve irritability	D: neuromuscular problems, irregular heartbeat E: diarrhoea
Sodium	Table salt	Extracellular cation. Works with chloride to maintain osmotic pressure of extracellular fluid. Muscle contraction, nerve impulse transmission, electrolyte balance	D: rare — nausea E: hypertension, oedema
Potassium	Fruit and vegetables and many foods	Intracellular cation. Muscle contraction, nerve impulse transmission electrolyte balance	D: Rare — muscle weakness, nausea, tachycardia E: cardiac abnormalities, muscular weakness
Iron	Liver, kidney, beef, green vegetables	Constituent of haemoglobin	D: anaemia E: haemochromatosis, liver damage
Iodine	Saltwater fish, vegetables	Constituent of thyroid hormones	D: hypothyroidism E: thyroid hormone synthesis depressed

CLINICAL CONSIDERATIONS

Obesity

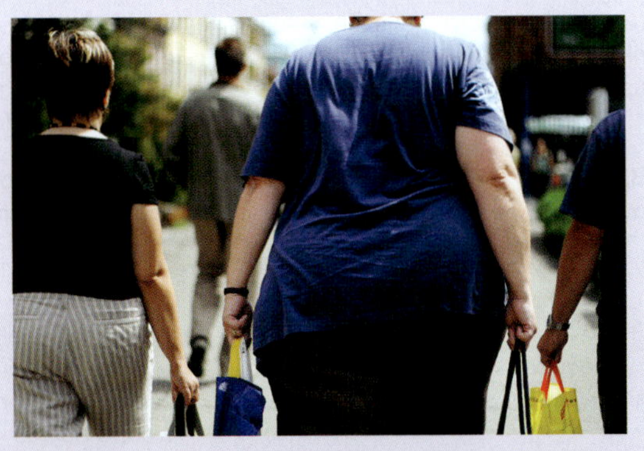

Obesity is increasing globally. Obesity occurs when dietary calorie intake is greater than what is required to maintain basic bodily functions and activity (repair, energy generation, etc.); this is referred to as positive energy balance. Increased globalisation has led to widespread access to affordable, calorie-dense foods which, when combined with decreasing rates of physical activity, leads to persistent positive energy balance and appears to be the main cause for this global increase in body weight. However, changes in gut microbiota and several other factors associated with increased urbanisation (decreased sleep duration, noise/light pollution, etc.) have also been implicated, particularly the gut microbiome which has been implicated in both obesity and a number of other disorders (Ng et al. 2014; Malik et al. 2013).

Obesity has increased markedly over the past 30 years, with approximately 39 per cent of the world's adult population being categorised as overweight and a further 13 per cent described as obese (body mass index (BMI) > 25 kg/m^2) in 2016 (WHO 2018). The costs associated with treating obesity and its associated comorbidities (such as type 2 diabetes and metabolic syndrome) haveincreased pressure on medical systems worldwide and led to an increase in the incidence of comorbidities such as coronary heart disease, metabolic syndrome and type 2 diabetes mellitus. Additionally, obesity predisposes people to indigestion, gallstones, hernias, cardiovascular disease, some cancers, varicose veins, osteoarthritis and depression. For these reasons, obesity is one of Australia's national health priorities.

Currently, 36 per cent of Australian adults are considered overweight. A further 31 per cent are classified as obese, which is a higher rate than that seen in the international data. A further consideration in Australia is the higher rates of obesity in lower socio-economic and remote communities, given the reduced access to healthcare and nutritious food in these communities (AIHW 2020). More alarming are the rates of obesity in Aboriginal and Torres Strait Islander communities, where 76.8 per cent of adults are classified as either overweight or obese. Given the links between obesity and type 2 diabetes mellitus and cardiovascular disease, there is a desperate need to improve education and treatment of obesity in affected communities.

SUMMARY

Digestion and nutrition play a vital role in the maintenance of health. The digestive tract processes ingest nutrients by breaking them down chemically and mechanically. Accessory structures (such as the pancreas, liver and gall bladder) have an essential role in providing the digestive tract with bile and pancreatic juices to facilitate the digestion of the macronutrients (proteins, carbohydrates and fats). The small intestine provides a large surface area for the absorption of nutrients, and the liver processes the products of digestion that are absorbed in the small intestine. The large intestine plays an excretory role, ridding the body of the waste products from digestion and absorbing any remaining water back into the body.

The maintenance of homeostasis is achieved through the ingestion of a balanced diet, containing a variety of elements from each of the food groups.

Without these activities, normal cell functioning would be at risk and this would lead to poor health. Digestive health contributes all aspects of physical, psychological and social wellbeing.

KEY TERMS

absorption Process whereby the products of digestion move into the blood or lymph fluid.
acini glands Produce pancreatic juice.
amylase Carbohydrate-digesting enzyme.
anus End of the digestive tract.
bile Fluid produced by the liver and required for the digestion of fat.
bile ducts Tubes that carry bile from the liver.
body region Largest region of the stomach.
caecum Beginning of the large intestine.
canines Type of tooth.
carbohydrate One of the major food groups.
cardiac region Region of the stomach closest to the oesophagus.
catabolism Process of breaking down substances into simpler substances.
chief cells Pepsinogen-producing cells.
cholecystokinin Digestive system hormone.
chyme Creamy, semi-fluid mass of partially digested food mixed with gastric secretions.
deglutition Swallowing.
digestion The chemical and mechanical breakdown of food for absorption.
duodenum First part of the small intestine.
enamel Covering of the tooth.
epiglottis Cartilage that covers the larynx during swallowing.
faeces Brown, semi-solid digestive system waste.
fats One of the major food groups.
frenulum Fold between the lip and gum.
fundus Anatomical base region of the stomach.
gluconeogenesis The creation of glucose from non-carbohydrate molecules.
glycolysis The anaerobic breakdown of glucose to form pyruvic acid.
goblet cells Mucus-producing cells.
haustrum Sac-like section of the large intestine.
hepatic portal vein Vein that delivers dissolved nutrients to the liver.
hepatocytes Liver cells.
hepatopancreatic ampulla The site where the bile duct and pancreatic duct meet.
hepatopancreatic sphincter Muscular valve that controls the entrance of pancreatic juice and bile to the duodenum.
hydrochloric acid Acid produced by the parietal cells of the stomach.
hydrolysis Addition of water to break down food molecules.
hyoid bone Bone that acts as the base of the tongue.
hypochondriac region Upper lateral divisions of the abdominopelvic cavity.
ileocaecal valve Site where the small and large intestine meet.
ileum The end part of the small intestine.

incisors Type of tooth.
ingestion The process of taking food into the body via the mouth.
intestinal crypts Also known as the crypts of Lieberkühn — glands found in the villi of the small intestine.
intrinsic factor Substance required for the absorption of vitamin B_{12}.
jejunum The middle part of the small intestine between the duodenum and the ileum.
Kupffer cells Hepatic macrophage.
lacteal Lymphatic capillary of the small intestine.
lamina propria Loose connective tissue layer of the digestive tract.
laryngopharynx Where the larynx and pharynx meet.
lipase Fat-digesting enzyme.
liver Accessory organ located in the abdominal cavity that has many metabolic and regulatory functions.
liver sinusoids Liver capillaries.
lower oesophageal sphincter Valve between the oesophagus and stomach.
lysozyme Bactericidal enzyme.
macronutrients Food consumed in large quantities.
mastication Chewing.
Meissner's plexus Nerves of the small intestine.
metabolism Sum total of the chemical reactions occurring in the body.
micronutrients Nutrients required in small quantities.
microvilli Cytoplasmic extensions of the villi.
minerals salts Inorganic compounds.
molars Type of tooth.
mucosa Layer of the digestive tract.
mucous neck cells Mucous-secreting cells of the stomach.
muscularis mucosa Muscular layer of the digestive tract.
myenteric plexus Digestive tract innervation.
nutrients Products obtained from the digestion of food and used by the body.
oesophagus Muscular tube from laryngopharynx to stomach.
oral cavity The first part of the digestive system.
oropharynx Part of the pharynx closest to the oral cavity.
palate Roof of the mouth.
pancreatic duct Duct that links the pancreas and common bile duct.
Paneth cell Cell that produces lysozyme.
papillae Small mucosal projections.
parasympathetic fibres Autonomic nervous system nerve fibres.
parietal cells Hydrochloric acid-producing cell of the stomach.
parotid glands Salivary glands located close to the ears.
pepsin Enzyme required for the breakdown of protein.
pepsinogen Enzyme precursor of pepsin.
peristalsis Wave-like contractions that move food through the digestive tract.
peritoneum Serous membrane that lines the abdominal cavity.
Peyer's patches Lymphatic tissue of the small intestine.
pharyngeal phase Second phase of swallowing.
pharynx Tube between the mouth and the oesophagus.
plicae circulars Permanent circular folds in the small intestine.
portal fissure Area where blood vessels and nerves enter and leave the liver.
portal triad Corner of liver lobule.
premolars Type of tooth located between the canine and molar teeth.
propulsion The process of moving the food along the length of the digestive system.
protein Substance that contains carbon, hydrogen, oxygen and nitrogen.
pulp cavity Centre of the tooth.
pyloric canal Area where the stomach opens into the small intestine.
pyloric region Area of the stomach that occurs where the stomach meets the small intestine.
pyloric sphincter Valve that controls food movement from the stomach to the small intestine.
rectum Final portion of the large intestine.
rugae Folds or ridges found in the digestive tract.

salivary amylase Carbohydrate-digesting enzyme found in saliva.
secretin Hormone that regulates secretion of pancreatic juice.
segmentation Movement of chyme in the small intestine.
serosa Outer layer of the digestive tract.
stercobilin Waste product of bilirubin breakdown.
stomach Reservoir for food involved in both chemical and mechanical digestion.
sublingual glands Salivary gland located on the floor of the mouth.
submandibular glands Salivary glands located below the jaw bilaterally.
submucosa Thick connective tissue layer of the digestive tract.
superior mesenteric artery Vessel that supplies the small intestine with arterial blood.
superior mesenteric vein Blood vessel that drains venous blood from the small intestine.
surface mucous cells Mucus-secreting cells of the stomach.
taeniae coli Muscle bands in the large intestine.
upper oesophageal sphincter Controls the movement of food into the oesophagus from the oropharynx.
uvula Small piece of tissue that protrudes from the soft palate.
vermiform appendix Blind-ended tube connected to the caecum and composed of lymphatic tissue.
villi Tiny, finger-like projections found on the surface of the mucosa of the small intestine.
visceral peritoneum The innermost part of the peritoneum that is in contact with the abdominal organs.
vitamin An essential organic compound required in small amounts.
voluntary phase The first phase of swallowing.

ACTIVITIES

TRUE OR FALSE

1. The large intestine is colonised with bacteria.
2. The first section of small intestine is called the jejunum.
3. Pancreatic juice reaches the duodenum through the cystic duct.
4. The function of bile is to emulsify fats.
5. There are 20 milk teeth.
6. The enzyme that acts on carbohydrate is lipase.
7. The sense of taste is improved when food is not dry.
8. The oesophagus contains only smooth muscle.
9. Intrinsic factor is produced by enteroendocrine cells.
10. The secretion of gastric juice is increased during the intestinal phase.

FIND OUT MORE

1. What is gingivitis and what advice would you give to help prevent this condition?
2. Oral candidiasis (oral thrush) affects many hospital inpatients. Can you suggest why this might be and discuss the treatment available?
3. What is the role of the nurse in caring for a patient with dysphagia?
4. Discuss the conditions that may lead to a patient requiring an ileostomy.
5. Differentiate between colostomy and ileostomy.
6. A 28-year-old woman has had a colostomy formed. She asks you how the colostomy would be affected should she become pregnant. How would you advise this patient?
7. Discuss how the digestive system would respond to starvation.
8. Investigate the services available to patients who have irritable bowel syndrome to help them manage everyday life.
9. A range of medications is available to minimise or eliminate digestive system conditions associated with the acid environment of the stomach. Research these medications and consider when they may be used.
10. Constipation is a very common digestive system condition. What is the role of the nurse in relation to prevention of constipation?

TEST YOUR LEARNING

1. Where does bile and pancreatic juice enter the duodenum?
2. Which teeth are used for grinding of food?
3. What is the exocrine pancreatic product essential for?
4. What are carbohydrates broken down into?
5. List the enzymes involved in the breakdown of protein.

CONDITIONS

The following is a list of conditions that are associated with the digestive system. Take some time and write notes about each of the conditions. You may make the notes taken from textbooks or other resources (e.g. people you work with in a clinical area), or you may make the notes as a result of people you have cared for. If you are making notes about people you have cared for, you must ensure that you adhere to the rules of confidentiality.

Peptic ulcer
Peritonitis
Ulcerative colitis
Paralytic ileus
Obesity
Malnutrition

REFERENCES

Australian Institute of Health and Welfare (2020) Overweight and obesity: an interactive insight. www.aihw.gov.au/reports/overweight-obesity/overweight-and-obesity-an-interactive-insight/contents/what-is-overweight-and-obesity (accessed 2 February 2021).

Bharucha, A.E., Kudva, Y.C. and Prichard, D.O. (2019) Diabetic gastroparesis. *Endocrine Reviews* 40: 1318–1352.

Cohen, B.J. and Hull, K.L. (2018) *Memmlers's The Human Body in Health and Disease*, 14th edn. Philadelphia, PA: Wolters Kluwer.

Galbraith, A., Bullock, S., Manias, E., Hunt, B. and Richards, A. (2007) *Fundamentals of Pharmacology: An Applied Approach for Nursing and Health*, 2nd edn. Abingdon: Routledge.

GESA (2011) *Gastro-oesophageal Reflux Disease in Adults Clinical Update*, 5th edn. Gastroenterological Society of Australia and Gastroenterological Nurses College of Australia. www.gesa.org.au/public/13/files/Education%20%26%20Resources/Clinical%20Practice%20Resources/GORD/Reflux_Disease.pdf (accessed 22 December 2020).

Health Direct (2020) Gallstones. www.healthdirect.gov.au/gallstones (accessed 20 February 2020).

Levett-Jones, T. (2013). *Clinical Reasoning: Learning to Think Like a Nurse*. Pearson Australia.

Malik, V.S., Willett, W.C. and Hu, F.B. (2013) Global obesity: trends, risk factors and policy implications. *Nature Reviews Endocrinology* 9(1): 13–27.

Nair, M. and Peate, I. (2018) *Fundamentals of Applied Pathophysiology. An Essential Guide for Nursing and Healthcare Students*, 3rd edn. Chichester: John Wiley & Sons, Ltd.

National Health and Medical Research Council (2013) *Eat for health: Australian dietary guidelines.* Canberra, Australia: NHMRC.
Ng, M., Fleming, T., Robinson, M., Thomson, B. et al. (2014) Global, regional, and national prevalence of overweight and obesity in children and adults during 1980–2013: a systematic analysis for the Global Burden of Disease Study 2013. *Lancet*. 384(9945): 766–781.
Seeley, R.R., Stephens, T.D. and Tate, P. (2008) *Anatomy and Physiology*, 8th edn. New York: McGraw-Hill.
Selby, W. and Corte, C. (2010) Managing constipation in adults. *Australian Prescriber* 33: 116–119.
Tortora, G.J. and Derrickson, B.H. (2009) *Principles of Anatomy and Physiology*, 12th edn. Hoboken, NJ: John Wiley & Sons, Inc.
Tortora, G.J. and Derrickson, B.H. (2012) *Essentials of Anatomy and Physiology*, 9th edn. New York: John Wiley & Sons, Inc.
Turner, R. (2015) Chronic pancreatitis: negotiating the complexities of diagnosis and management. *AFP Abdomen*. 44: 718–722.
World Health Organization (2018) *Obesity and Overweight Fact Sheet*. Geneva, Switzerland: WHO.

FURTHER READING

CROHN'S & COLITIS AUSTRALIA

www.crohnsandcolitis.com.au

Crohn's & Colitis Australia is the national peak patient body representing the 75 000 Australians diagnosed with Crohn's disease or ulcerative colitis.

www.gesa.org.au/public/13/files/Education%20%26%20Resources/Patient%20Resources/IBD/IBD%20-%20Crohns%20Colitis%203rd%20Ed.pdf

Clinical guidelines on Crohn's disease: management in adults, children and young people.

AUSTRALIAN COUNCIL OF STOMA ASSOCIATIONS

https://australianstoma.com.au/

The Australian Council of Stoma Associations Inc. (ACSA) is the national body representing 21 ostomy associations and, through the membership of these associations, approximately 46 000 persons living with an ostomy throughout Australia.

ACKNOWLEDGEMENTS

Photo: © Brookie Cookie / Shutterstock.com
Photo: © sfam_photo / Shutterstock.com
Photo: © Aleksandra Suzi / Shutterstock.com
Photo: © Shannon Fagan / Getty Images
Photo: © Jakub Cejpek / Shutterstock.com

CHAPTER 11

The renal system

TEST YOUR PRIOR KNOWLEDGE

- Name the functions of the kidneys.
- List the organs of the renal system.
- Describe the components of a nephron.
- List the composition of urine.
- Describe the structure and function of the bladder.

LEARNING OUTCOMES

After reading this chapter you will be able to:

11.1 describe the functions of the kidney
11.2 describe the external and internal structures of the kidney
11.3 describe the microscopic structures of the kidney
11.4 explain glomerular filtration
11.5 list the chemical compositions of urine.

Body map

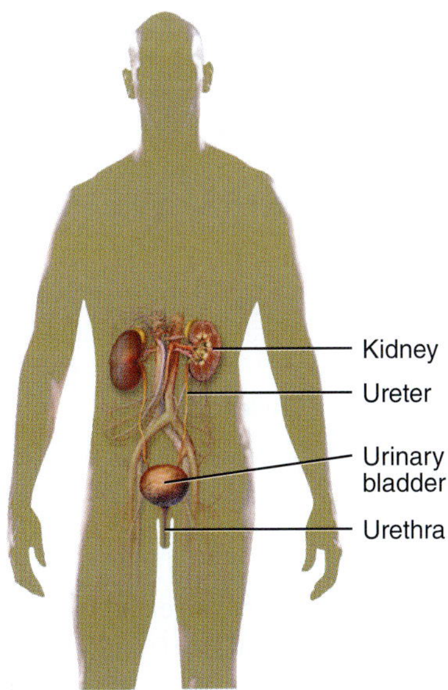

Introduction

The **kidneys** play an important role in maintaining homeostasis. They remove waste products through the production and **excretion** of urine and regulate fluid balance in the body. As part of their function, the kidneys filter essential substances from the blood, such as sodium and potassium, and selectively reabsorb substances essential to maintain homeostasis. Any substances not essential are excreted in the urine. The formation of urine is achieved through the processes of **filtration**, selective reabsorption and excretion. The kidneys also have an endocrine function, secreting hormones such as **renin** and **erythropoietin**. This chapter will discuss the structure and functions of the renal system. It will also include some common disorders and their related nursing management and treatment.

11.1 Functions of the kidney

LEARNING OBJECTIVE 11.1 Describe the functions of the kidney.

The renal system, also known as the urinary system, consists of:

- kidneys, which filter the blood to produce urine
- **ureters**, which convey urine to the bladder
- urinary bladder, a storage organ for urine until it is eliminated
- **urethra**, which conveys urine to the exterior.

See figure 11.1 for the organs of the renal system.

FIGURE 11.1 Organs of the renal system

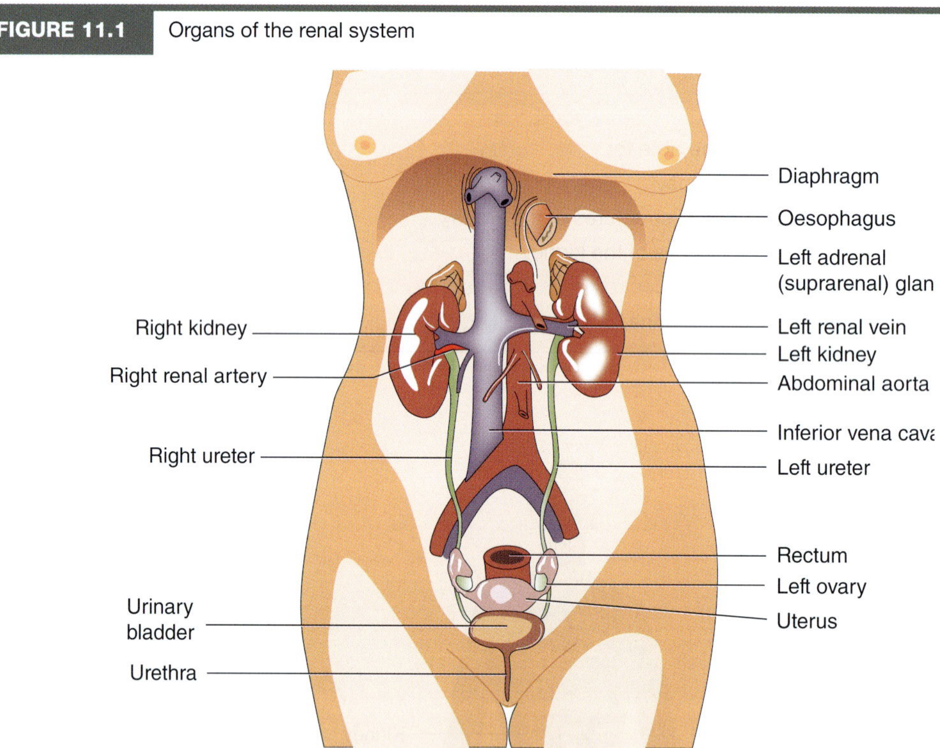

Source: Tortora and Derrickson (2009). Reproduced with permission of John Wiley & Sons.

The organs of the renal system ensure that a stable internal environment is maintained for the survival of cells and tissues in the body — homeostasis.

The kidneys maintain fluid balance, electrolyte balance and the acid–base balance of the blood.

- The kidneys remove waste products and excess water (fluid) collected by, and carried in, the blood as it flows through the body. Approximately 190 L of blood enter the kidneys every day via the **renal arteries**. Millions of tiny filters, called **glomeruli**, inside the kidneys separate waste products and water from the blood. Most of these unwanted substances come from what we eat and drink. The kidneys automatically remove the right amount of salt and other minerals from the blood to leave just the quantities the body needs.

- By removing just the right amount of excess fluid, healthy kidneys maintain what is called the body's fluid balance. In women, fluid content stays at about 55 per cent of total weight. In men, it stays at about 60 per cent of total weight. The kidneys maintain these proportions by balancing the amount of fluid that leaves the body against the amount entering the body. When a large volume of fluid is drunk, healthy kidneys remove the excess fluid and produce a lot of urine. On the other hand, if fluid intake is low, the kidneys retain fluid and the patient does not pass much urine. Fluid also leaves the body through sweat, breath and faeces. If the weather is hot and we lose a lot of fluid by sweating, then the kidneys will not produce much urine.
- Kidneys synthesise hormones such as renin and angiotensin. These hormones regulate how much sodium (salt) and fluid the body keeps, and how well the blood vessels can expand and contract. This, in turn, helps control blood pressure.
- Kidneys produce a hormone known as erythropoietin, which is carried in the blood to the bone marrow where it stimulates the production of red blood cells. These cells carry oxygen throughout the body. Without enough healthy red blood cells, anaemia develops, a condition that causes weakness, cold, tiredness and shortness of breath.
- Healthy kidneys keep bones strong by producing the hormone calcitriol. Calcitriol maintains the right levels of calcium and phosphate in the blood and bones. Calcium and phosphate balance are important to keep bones healthy. When the kidneys fail they may not produce enough calcitriol. This leads to abnormal levels of phosphate, calcium and vitamin D, causing renal bone disease. For a summary of the functions of the kidney, see table 11.1.

TABLE 11.1 Summary of the functions of the kidneys

Summary of the functions of the kidneys
Regulation of electrolytes — help to regulate ions such as sodium, potassium, calcium, chloride and phosphate ions
Regulation of blood pH — excrete hydrogen ions into the urine and conserve bicarbonate ions, thus helping to regulate pH of blood
Regulation of blood volume — by conserving or eliminating water in the urine
Secretes renin (regulates blood pressure) and erythropoietin (production of red blood cells)
Production of calcitriol for the regulation of calcium level
Aids in regulation of blood glucose level by gluconeogenesis
Detoxification of free radicals and drugs
Excretion of waste products, such as urea, uric acid and creatinine

11.2 Kidneys: external and internal structures

LEARNING OBJECTIVE 11.2 Describe the external and internal structures of the kidney.

External structures

There are two kidneys, one on each side of the spinal column. They are approximately 11 cm long, 5–6 cm wide and 3–4 cm thick. They are said to be bean-shaped organs, where the outer border is convex; the inner border is known as the **hilum** (also known as hilus), and it is here that the renal arteries, **renal veins**, nerves and the ureters enter and leave the kidneys. The renal artery carries blood to the kidneys; and once the blood is filtered, the renal vein takes the blood away. The right kidney is in contact with the liver's large right lobe, and hence the right kidney is approximately 2–4 cm lower than the left kidney.

Covering and supporting the kidneys are three layers:

- renal fascia
- adipose tissue
- renal capsule.

The renal fascia is the outer layer and consists of a thin layer of connective tissue that anchors the kidneys to the abdominal wall and the surrounding tissues. The middle layer is called the adipose tissue and surrounds the capsule. It cushions the kidneys from trauma. The inner layer is called the renal capsule. It consists of a layer of smooth connective tissue that is continuous with the outer layer of the ureter.

The renal capsule protects the kidneys from trauma and maintains their shape. See figure 11.2 for the external layers.

FIGURE 11.2 External layers of the kidney

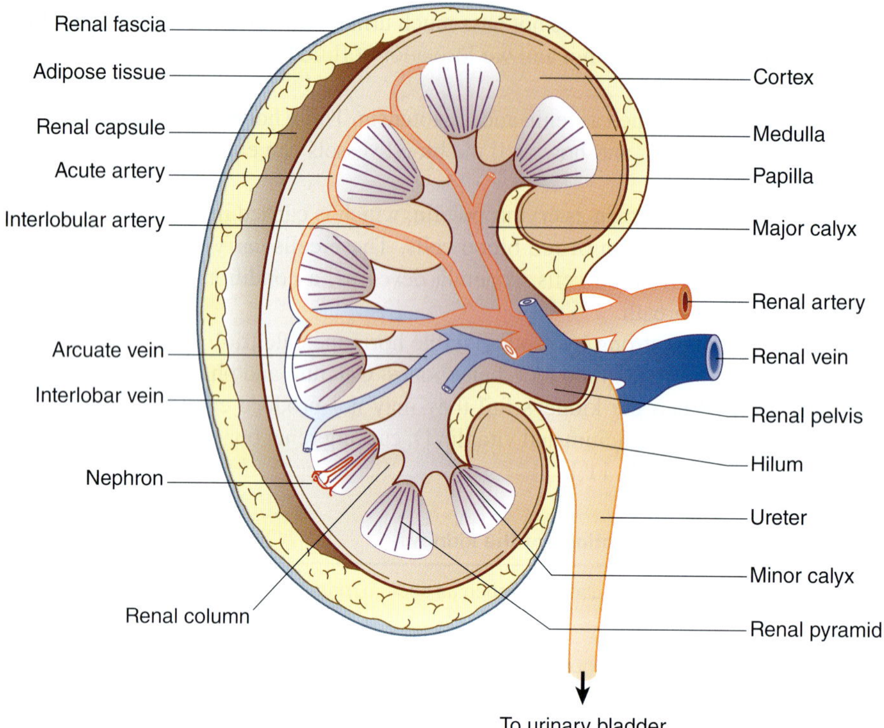

Blood supply of the kidney

The role of the kidney is to filter at least 20–25 per cent of blood during the resting cardiac output. Approximately 1200 mL of blood flows through the kidney each minute. Each kidney receives its blood supply directly from the aorta via the renal artery, which is divided into **anterior** and **posterior** renal arteries. There are several arteries that deliver blood to the kidneys. They are the:

- renal artery — arises from the abdominal aorta at the level of first lumbar vertebra
- segmental artery — branch of the renal artery
- interlobar artery — branch of the segmental artery
- arcuate artery — renal columns leading to the corticomedullary junction
- interlobular arteries — divisions of the arcuate arteries.

CLINICAL CONSIDERATIONS

Acute kidney injury

When the kidneys suddenly stop working this is known as acute kidney injury (AKI). It occurs for many reasons with the most common reason being a reduction in fluid volume or pressure. This can be caused by a reduction in blood volume from loss of blood or fluid or from a reduction in pressure caused by sepsis or reduced cardiac output. The incidence of AKI is increasing globally. In Australia, AKI accounts for significant morbidity and mortality and is a significant contributor to hospitalisation and death rates of Indigenous Australians (AIHW 2015).

There are two ways to determine if the kidneys are working effectively. The first is with blood tests to measure changes in creatinine and the other is to measure urine output.

Clinical assessment of hydration status can be difficult to determine. However, some signs and symptoms can help you to decide if a patient has had too little or too much fluid.

- A visual inspection of the skin and mucus membranes: consider temperature, colour and dryness of the skin, lips and mouth (should be moist and pink).

- Assessment of peripheral circulation can be undertaken by measuring the capillary refill time (CRT): apply enough pressure to the fingernail bed to cause blanching (up to 5 seconds). Measure the time until the skin returns to normal. This should be less than 2 seconds in a well-hydrated person.
- Assessment of skin turgor (elasticity): pinch a small section of skin between thumb and index finger over the anterior chest, abdomen or forearm. Skin is slowly released and should return to normal quickly. Decreased skin turgor can indicate dehydration.
- A useful indicator of reduced blood volume is the body's compensatory mechanisms. A raised MEWS (modified early warning score) including reduced blood pressure, raised heart rate and breathing rate can all be a sign.
- A variation in lying and standing blood pressure (a drop in standing blood pressure indicates fluid volume deficit).
- Visible signs of oedema usually found in the peripheries (pitting oedema) or occasionally the lungs (frothy sputum).

SKILLS IN PRACTICE

Undertaking a fluid balance

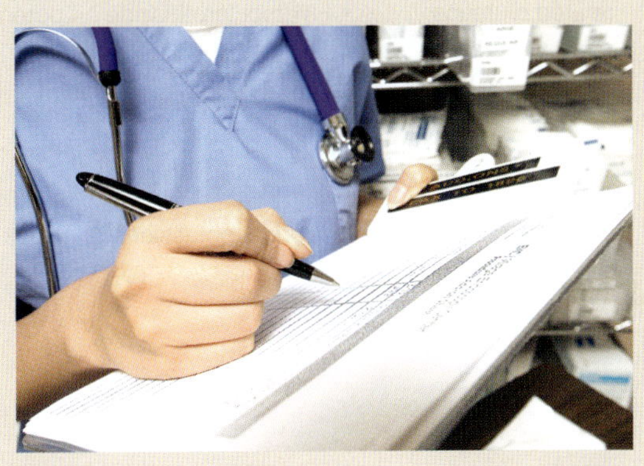

A fluid balance chart is designed to identify fluid intake and fluid output to determine what the balance of fluid is. An accurate fluid balance chart is essential for managing an unwell patient and it can be a key sign in identifying when the kidneys are not working correctly. When calculating fluid balance, it is important to consider all types of fluid that will influence hydration status. Any drinks, soups, gravy and custard need to be accounted for. As well as accurately documenting input, output needs to be accounted for. This includes all urine, any drains, vomiting and diarrhoea. Other considerations include fluid loss that cannot be measured. This is known as insensible loss; when the environment is hot or when a person has an elevated temperature or a high respiratory rate, more fluid will be lost.

To accurately measure fluid intake, make sure you are aware of the volumes contained in cups, mugs, soup bowls and so on so that the correct volume can be recorded. Ask the patient to keep a note, if appropriate, of what they have drunk and when. Measure all urine output, by asking the patient to use a urinal or a measuring device that can be placed in the toilet, or weighing pads to determine the fluid volume. Fluid balance is a team effort and requires teamwork.

Daily fluid balance total and daily weights can supplement any clinical assessment regarding fluid status and can be a useful indicator when determining how to manage a patient.

1 kg increase in weight = 1 litre of fluid.

Any short-term elevation in weight could indicate that the patient is retaining fluid.

MEDICINES MANAGEMENT

Blood pressure management

High blood pressure (hypertension) is a common comorbidity and is regularly managed using blood pressure medication and lifestyle changes. Elevated blood pressure can have a direct effect on the heart and vascular system meaning that patients are at increased risk of coronary heart disease and stroke.

There are many different types of blood pressure medications (antihypertensives) and patients may be on combinations of medications in order to achieve the desired effect.

Angiotensin-converting enzyme inhibitors, such as captopril, ramipril and lisinopril, are known as ACE inhibitors. They work by interrupting the renin angiotensin cycle instigated by the juxtaglomerular cells located near the glomerulus of the nephron. Angiotensin II has powerful vasoconstriction properties which cause a rise in blood pressure. ACE inhibitors work by stopping the conversion of angiotensin I to angiotensin II. While on this medication, patients must drink plenty of fluids and avoid dehydration.

Other antihypertensive medications include the following groups: thiazides and related diuretics, sartans (angiotensin II antagonists and angiotensin receptor antagonists), calcium channel blockers and beta-blockers (see table 11.2) (Australian Medicines Handbook 2020).

TABLE 11.2 Antihypertensives

Antihypertensive group	Examples of antihypertensive	Mode of action	Nursing and paramedic considerations/actions
ACE inhibitors	Captopril Eanalapril Fosinopril Perindopril Quinapril Ramipril Trandolapril	Angiotensin-converting enzyme inhibitors	May cause orthostatic hypotension, headache, cough, fatigue, nausea; patient may feel dizzy on standing when taking this class of drugs; patient should get up gradually from sitting or lying to standing; sit or lie down if feeling dizzy. Patients do not take potassium supplements while on this medication unless otherwise advised.
Thiazides and related diuretics	Thiazide: • Hydrochlorothiazide Thiazide related: • Chlortalidone • Indapamide	Moderately potent diuretics	May cause orthostatic hypotension, headaches, weakness, muscle cramps, polyuria, electrolyte disturbances; patient may feel dizzy on standing when taking this class of drugs; patient should get up gradually from sitting or lying to standing; sit or lie down if feeling dizzy.
Other diuretics	Amiloride (potassium sparing)	Weak diuretic	May cause orthostatic hypotension, weakness, headache, nausea, vomiting, constipation, muscle cramps; patient may feel dizzy on standing when taking this class of drugs; patient should get up gradually from sitting or lying to standing; sit or lie down if feeling dizzy. Patients do not take potassium supplements while on this medication unless otherwise advised.
Sartans	Candesartan Eprosartan Irbesartan Losartan Olmesartan Telmisartan Valsartan	Angiotensin II antagonists and angiotensin receptor antagonists (ARA) or blockers (ARB)	May cause orthostatic hypotension and headache; patient may feel dizzy on standing when taking this class of drugs; patient should get up gradually from sitting or lying to standing; sit or lie down if feeling dizzy. Patients do not take potassium supplements while on this medication unless otherwise advised.
Calcium channel blockers	Dihydropyridines: • Amlodipine • Clevidipine • Felodipine • Lercanidipine • Nifedipine • Nimodipine Non-dihydropyridines: • Diltiazem • Verapamil	Block inward current of calcium into cells in vascular smooth muscle, myocardium and cardiac conducting system via L type calcium channels.	Patient may experience nausea, headache, dizziness, flushing, hypotension and peripheral oedema.

Beta-blockers	Atenolol Bisoprolol Carvedilol Esmolol Labetalol Metoprolol Nebivolol Pindolol Propanolol Sotalol	Blocks beta receptors in heart, peripheral vasculature, bronchi, kidney, brain, liver, pancreas and uterus.	Contraindicated in bradycardia (45–50 bpm); may cause bradycardia and orthostatic hypotension; patient may experience nausea, diarrhoea, dyspnoea, cold extremities, fatigue, dizziness, altered vision; patient should get up gradually from sitting or lying to standing; sit or lie down if feeling dizzy.

Source: Adapted from Australian Medicines Handbook (2020).

CLINICALLY REASONED EPISODE OF CARE

Diarrhoea and vomiting

Consider the patient situation

Jamie is a 47-year-old male with Down syndrome. Jamie lives with high blood pressure, type 2 diabetes and chronic back pain. He has presented to the emergency department feeling weak secondary to diarrhoea and vomiting.

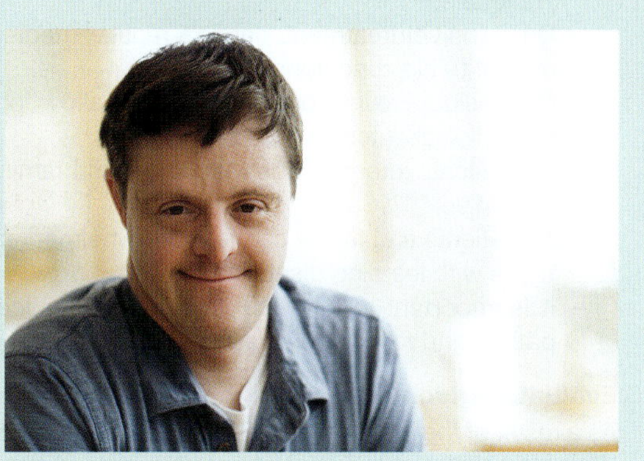

Collect cues and information

Jamie has had diarrhoea and been vomiting for three days. He is alert and orientated in the emergency department; however, the nurse observes that he has dry lips and skin. He is hypotensive at 105/65 mmHg and complains that he feels dizzy. Jamie does not recall the last time that he passed urine. Blood results confirm that Jamie has an acute kidney injury (AKI).

Process information

AKI, previously known as acute renal failure, encompasses a wide spectrum of injury to the kidneys, not just kidney failure. An AKI can occur for several reasons — one being acute dehydration secondary to diarrhoea and vomiting. Diarrhoea and vomiting can lead to decreased circulating blood volume and therefore reduced blood flow to the kidneys. AKI is seen in 13 to 18 per cent of all people admitted to hospital, with older adults being particularly affected.

Jamie is demonstrating clinical signs of dehydration, including dry cracked lips and a low blood pressure. This, in conjunction with Jamie's comorbidities and medications, has led to the AKI. An AKI is diagnosed from serum creatinine levels of > 0.3 mg/dL within 48 hours and decreased urine output.

Jamie has now been admitted to the ward under the care of the nursing staff.

Establish goals

1. Intravenous therapy/fluid rehydration
2. Fluid balance monitoring
3. Evaluate interventions and monitor blood pressure
4. Review of medications, in particular antihypertensives
5. Communication with Jamie and his carer and family

Nursing actions

1. Commence intravenous fluid therapy 0.9% sodium chloride.

   Rationale:
   - The commencement of intravenous therapy will be guided by test results and will be ordered by the medical team.
   - Intravenous therapy will replace volume lost through diarrhoea and vomiting.
   - Fluid therapy will replace electrolytes lost through diarrhoea and vomiting.

2. Conduct strict fluid balance monitoring.

   Rationale:
   - Fluid overload in AKI is associated with poor outcomes and thus fluid input and output should be monitored closely.
   - A fluid balance chart and strict monitoring of urine output will allow nurses and medical staff to assess the efficacy of the intervention.
   - Jamie has presented with oliguria (urine output less than 0.5 mL/kg/hour), therefore this should be closely monitored for improvement.
3. Perform urine dipstick testing.

   Rationale:
   - The assessment of AKI should include a urine dipstick for blood, protein, leucocytes, nitrites and glucose in all people as soon as AKI is suspected or detected.
   - These results may contribute to treatment and management goals.
4. Evaluate interventions and monitor blood pressure.

   Rationale:
   - To avoid further injury, AKI requires ongoing assessment and evaluation of intervention efficacy.
   - Evaluation should include observations, including blood pressure, urine input and output, and symptoms of dizziness.
5. Organise medication review, particularly antihypertensives.

   Rationale:
   - During initial treatment, Jamie's regular medication, including his antihypertensives, may be detrimental to his conditions.
   - Organising a review of medication will allow for the adjustment of regular medications to ensure the best clinical outcomes for Jamie.
6. Communicate interventions with Jamie and family.

   Rationale:
   - All patients and family can feel overwhelmed and anxious while being treated in hospital, especially those with learning disabilities.
   - It is important to take the time to communicate interventions and procedures to ensure that the patient and family are aware of what is happening and why.

Evaluate outcomes

As a result of the interventions above, Jamie recovers in hospital after three days and is discharged home. His blood tests and clinical observations have improved, and he is no longer experiencing diarrhoea, vomiting or dizziness.

Reflect on new processes and learning

Reflect on the role of the nurse. How do nurses assess the efficacy of their interventions in a case such as Jamie's?

Source: Based on the Clinical Reasoning Cycle, Levett-Jones (2013).

Internal structures

There are three distinct regions inside the kidney:

- **renal cortex**
- **renal medulla**
- **renal pelvis**.

The renal cortex is the outermost part of the kidney. In adults, it forms a continuous, smooth outer portion of the kidney with a number of projections (renal columns) that extend down between the pyramids. The renal column is the medullary extension of the renal cortex. The renal cortex is reddish in colour and has a granular appearance, which is due to the capillaries and the structures of the **nephron**. The medulla is lighter in colour and has an abundance of blood vessels and tubules of the nephrons (see figure 11.3). The medulla consists of approximately 8–12 **renal pyramids** (see figure 11.3). The renal pyramids, also called malpighian pyramids, are cone-shaped sections of the kidneys. The wider portion of the cone faces the renal cortex, while the narrow end points internally, and this section is called the renal papilla. Urine formed by the nephrons flows into cup-like structures, called **calyces**, via papillary ducts. Each kidney contains approximately 8–18 minor calyces and two or three major calyces. The minor calyces receive urine from the renal papilla, which conveys the urine to the major calyces. The major calyces unite to form the renal pelvis, which then conveys urine to the bladder (see figure 11.4). The renal pelvis forms the expanded upper portion of the ureter, which is funnel-shaped and it is the region where two or three calyces converge.

FIGURE 11.3 (a, b) Internal structures showing blood vessels

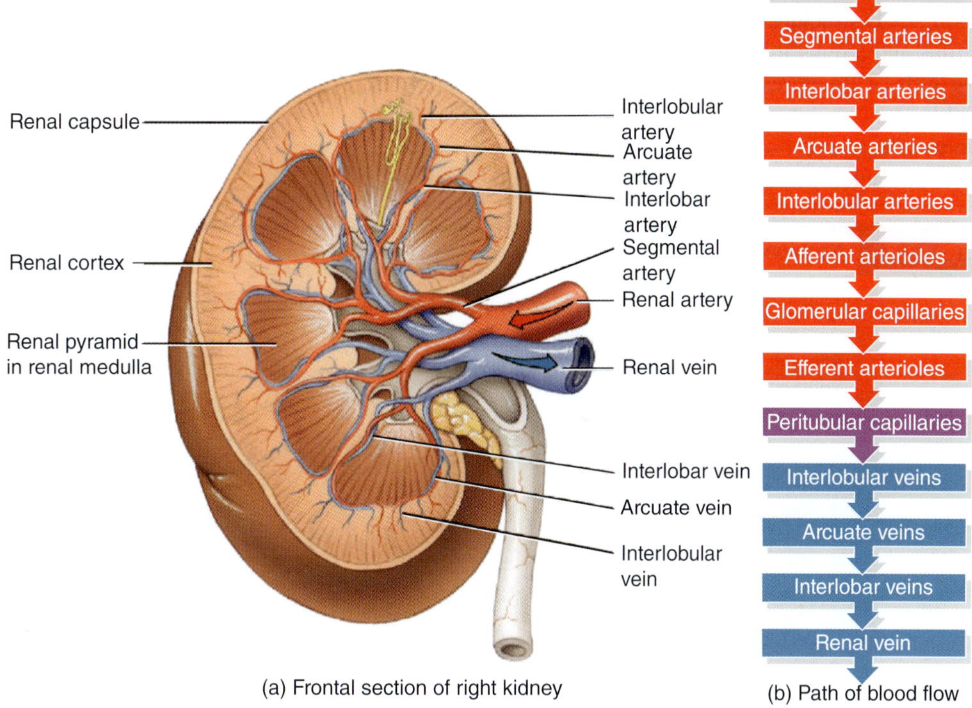

(a) Frontal section of right kidney

(b) Path of blood flow

Source: Tortora and Derrickson (2009). Reproduced with permission of John Wiley & Sons.

FIGURE 11.4 Internal structures

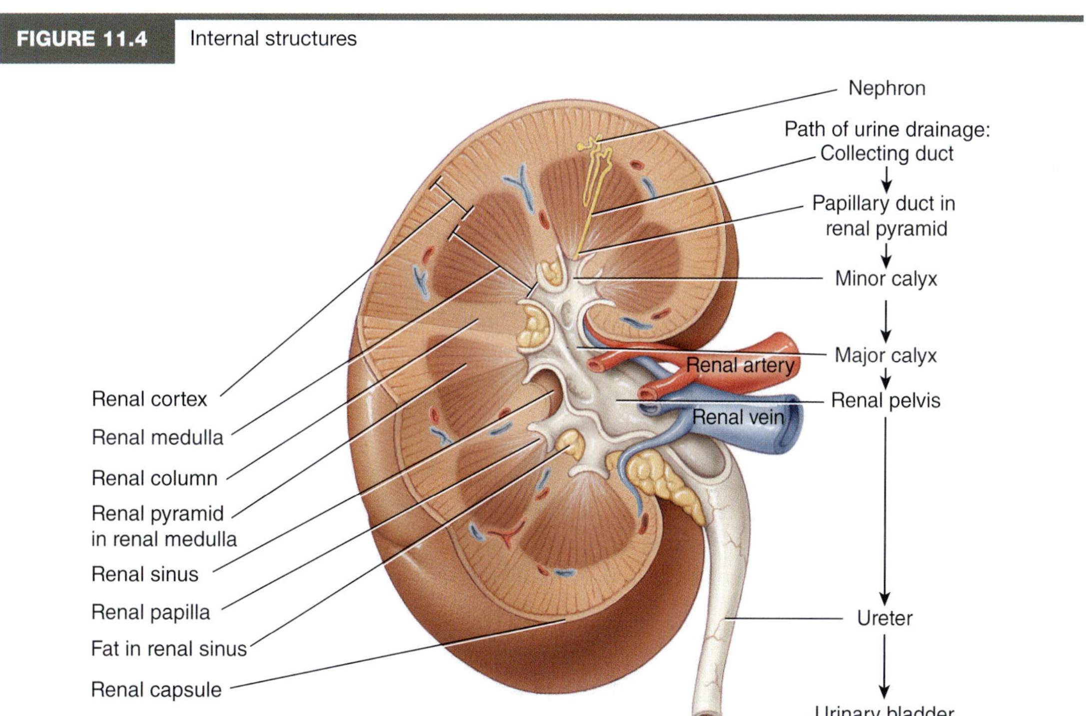

Source: Tortora and Derrickson (2009). Reproduced with permission of John Wiley & Sons.

11.3 Nephrons

LEARNING OBJECTIVE 11.3 Describe the microscopic structures of the kidney.

These are small structures and they form the functional units of the kidney. The nephron consists of a glomerulus and a renal tubule (see figure 11.5). There are approximately 1 million nephrons per kidney, and it is in these structures where urine is formed. The nephrons:

- filter blood
- perform selective reabsorption
- excrete unwanted waste products from the filtered blood.

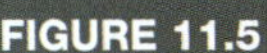

FIGURE 11.5 Nephron

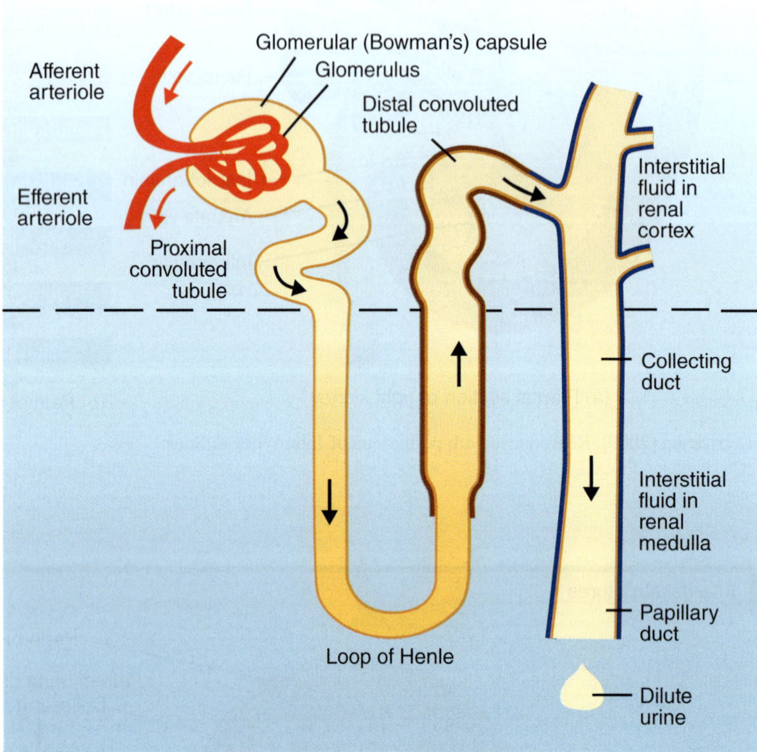

Source: Tortora and Derrickson (2009). Reproduced with permission of John Wiley & Sons.

The nephron is part of the homeostatic mechanism of the body. This system helps regulate the amount of water, salts, glucose, urea and other minerals in the body. The nephron is a filtration system located in the kidney and is responsible for the reabsorption of water and salts. The nephron is divided into several sections:

- Bowman's capsule
- proximal convoluted tubule
- loop of Henle
- distal convoluted tubule (DCT)
- the collecting ducts.

Each section performs a different function; these will be discussed in the following sections.

Bowman's capsule

Also known as the glomerular capsule (see figure 11.6), Bowman's capsule is a cup-like sac and is the first portion of the nephron. Bowman's capsule is part of the filtration system in the kidneys. When blood reaches the kidneys for filtration, it enters Bowman's capsule first, with the capsule separating the blood into two components: a filtrated blood product and a filtrate that is moved through the nephron, another structure in the kidneys. The glomerular capsule consists of visceral and parietal layers (see figure 11.6). The visceral layer is lined with epithelial cells called podocytes, while the parietal layer is lined with simple squamous epithelium and it is in Bowman's capsule that the network of capillaries called the glomerulus (Marieb 2016) is found. Filtration of blood takes place in this portion of the nephron.

FIGURE 11.6 Bowman's capsule

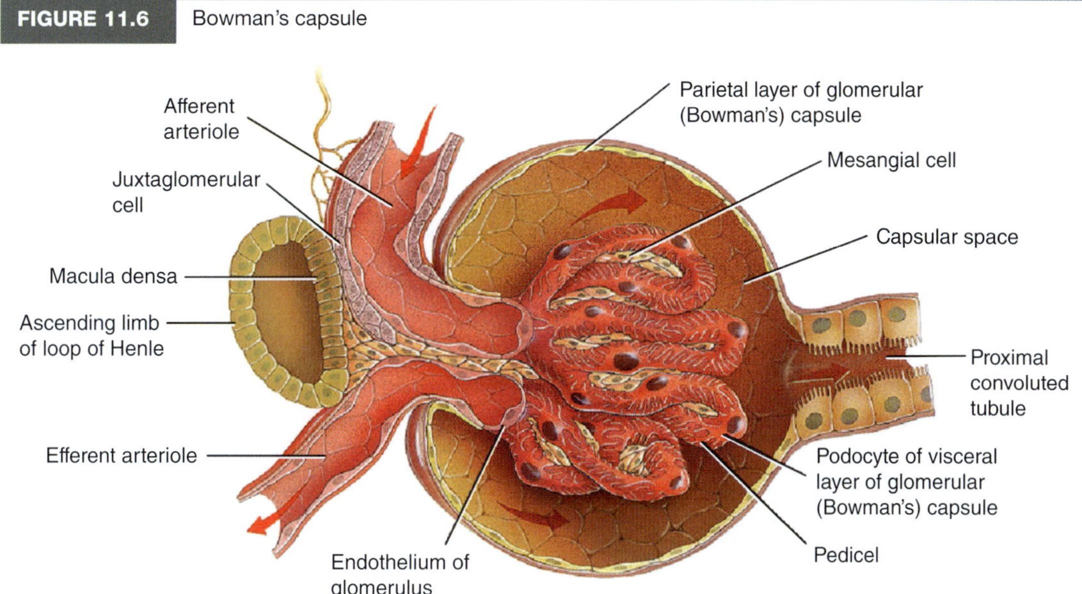

Source: Tortora and Derrickson (2009). Reproduced with permission of John Wiley & Sons.

Proximal convoluted tubule

From Bowman's capsule, the filtrate drains into the proximal convoluted tubule (see figure 11.6). The surface of the epithelial cells of this segment of the nephron is covered with densely packed microvilli. The microvilli increase the surface area of the cells, thus facilitating their resorptive function. The infolded membranes forming the microvilli are the site of numerous sodium pumps. Resorption of salt, water and glucose from the glomerular filtrate occurs in this section of the tubule; at the same time, certain substances, including uric acid and drug metabolites, are actively transferred from the blood capillaries into the tubule for excretion.

Loop of Henle

The proximal convoluted tubule then bends into a loop called the loop of Henle (see figure 11.6). The loop of Henle is the part of the tubule that dips or 'loops' from the cortex into the medulla (descending limb), and then returns to the cortex (ascending limb). The loop of Henle is divided into the descending and ascending loops. The ascending loop of Henle is much thicker than the descending portion. The main function of the loop of Henle is to generate a concentration gradient that creates a region of a high concentration of sodium in the medulla of the kidney. The descending portion of the loop of Henle is highly permeable to water and has low permeability to ions and urea. The ascending loop of Henle is permeable to ions but not to water. When required, urine is concentrated in this portion of the nephron. This is possible because of the high concentration of solute in the substance or interstitium of the medulla. Different parts of the loop of Henle have different actions.

- The descending loop of Henle is relatively impermeable to solute but permeable to water, so that water moves out by osmosis and the fluid in the tubule becomes hypertonic.
- The thin section of the ascending loop of Henle is virtually impermeable to water, but permeable to solute, especially sodium and chloride ions. Thus, sodium and chloride ions move out down the concentration gradient; the fluid within the tubule first becomes isotonic and then hypotonic as more ions leave. Urea, which was absorbed into the medullary interstitium from the collecting duct, diffuses into the ascending limb. This keeps the urea within the interstitium of the medulla, where it also has a role in concentrating urine.
- The thick section of the ascending loop of Henle and early distal tubule are virtually impermeable to water. However, sodium and chloride ions are actively transported out of the tubule, making the tubular fluid very hypotonic.

Distal convoluted tubule

The thick ascending portion of the loop of Henle leads into the distal convoluted tubule (DCT) (see figure 11.6). The DCT is lined with simple cuboidal cells, and the lumen of the DCT is larger than the proximal convoluted tubule lumen because the proximal convoluted tubule has a brush border (microvilli). The DCT is an important site as:

- it actively secretes ions and acids
- it plays a part in the regulation of calcium ions by excreting excess calcium ions in response to calcitonin hormone
- it selectively reabsorbs water
- arginine vasopressin receptor 2 proteins are also located there
- it plays a role in regulating pH by absorbing bicarbonate and secreting protons (H^+) into the filtrate.

The final concentration of urine, in this section, is dependent on a hormone called antidiuretic hormone (ADH). If ADH is present, the distal tubule and the collecting duct become permeable to water. As the collecting duct passes through the medulla with a high solute concentration in the interstitium, the water moves out of the lumen of the duct and concentrated urine is formed. In the absence of ADH the tubule is minimally permeable to water, so a large volume of dilute urine is formed.

Collecting ducts

The DCT then drains into the collecting ducts (see figure 11.6). Several collecting ducts converge and drain into a larger system called the papillary ducts, which in turn empty into the minor calyx (plural: calices). From here the filtrate, now called urine, drains into the renal pelvis. This is the final stage where sodium and water are reabsorbed. When a person is dehydrated, approximately 25 per cent of the water filtered is reabsorbed in the collecting duct. The cells of the collecting ducts are impermeable to water, but with the aid of the ADH and aquaporins water is reabsorbed from the collecting ducts. Aquaporins are proteins embedded in the cell membrane that regulate the flow of water. Aquaporins selectively transport water molecules in and out of the cell while preventing the passage of ions and other solutes. Aquaporin 1 is abundant in the proximal convoluted tubule and the descending thin limb of the loop of Henle, and aquaporins 2, 3 and 4 are present in the collecting ducts; however, aquaporin 4 is predominantly found in the brain.

CLINICAL CONSIDERATIONS

Chronic kidney disease and contrast procedures

Chronic kidney disease is the progressive and irreversible loss of functioning nephrons. This damage to the nephrons in the kidney can be caused by multiple factors including hypertension, diabetes and heart disease. Urea and creatinine in the blood can be used to identify how well the kidneys are working. Glomerular filtration rate is an estimated measurement of how well the kidneys are working, and it represents the amount of blood filtering through the glomeruli each minute.

When a patient requires an MRI, CT scan or angiogram procedure, a contrast dye may be used to help enhance the tests. This dye can cause problems with the kidney and patients with reduced renal function have an increased risk of developing contrast-induced acute kidney injury. Therefore, the patient may require increased monitoring of their renal function, extra fluid and, in some rare cases, haemodialysis or peritoneal dialysis may be instigated straight after the procedure.

MEDICINES MANAGEMENT

Nephrotoxic drugs

Renal impairment may be acute or chronic — both of which can result in problems with medications. Renal impairment may be the result of a variety of renal or systemic diseases, such as diabetic nephropathy or systemic lupus erythematosus. Normal ageing results in a decline in renal function due to loss of nephrons. When prescribing and administering drugs for elderly patients, it should therefore be assumed that some degree of renal impairment exists.

Reasons for problems with medications in renal failure include:

- failure to excrete a drug or its metabolites

- many side effects being poorly tolerated by patients in renal failure
- some drugs ceasing to be effective when renal function is reduced.

Prescribing any drug that increases potassium level is potentially very dangerous — for example, potassium supplements and potassium-sparing diuretics. Other products that contain potassium include ispaghula husk (also known as psyllium husk) laxatives. Non-steroidal anti-inflammatory drugs (NSAIDs), such as ibuprofen and diclofenac, given over a short period of time can cause acute kidney injury as a result of renal under-perfusion. ACE inhibitors can also cause a deterioration in renal function. However, this is a problem only in patients with compromised renal perfusion, particularly those with renal artery stenosis. Care should be taken when an ACE inhibitor and NSAID are prescribed together, as this combination may precipitate an acute deterioration in renal function.

Drugs that may cause interstitial nephritis include penicillins, cephalosporins, sulphonamides, thiazide diuretics, furosemide, NSAIDs and rifampicin.

Therefore, care should be taken when administering medications to patients with renal problems. Always check with the pharmacist or consult the Australian Medicines Handbook for drug interactions before administering medications.

See Azhar et al. (2019).

The branches of the interlobular artery enter the nephrons as afferent arterioles. Each nephron receives one afferent arteriole, which further subdivides into a tuft of capillaries called the glomerulus. The glomerular capillaries reunite and leave Bowman's capsule as efferent arterioles. Efferent arterioles unite to form peritubular capillaries and then interlobular veins that unite to form the arcuate veins and finally interlobar veins. Blood leaves the kidneys through the renal vein, which then flows into the inferior vena cava. The diameter of the afferent arteriole is larger than the diameter of the efferent arteriole.

11.4 Filtration

LEARNING OBJECTIVE 11.4 Explain glomerular filtration.

Three processes are involved in the formation of urine:

- filtration
- selective reabsorption
- secretion.

Urine formation begins with the process of filtration, which goes on continually in the renal corpuscles. Filtration takes place in the glomerulus which lies in Bowman's capsule. The blood for filtration is supplied by the renal artery. In the kidney the renal artery divides into smaller arterioles. The arteriole entering Bowman's capsule is called the afferent arteriole, which further subdivides into a cluster of capillaries called the glomerulus.

As blood passes through the glomeruli, much of its fluid, containing both useful chemicals and dissolved waste materials, soaks out of the blood through the membranes (by osmosis and diffusion) where it is filtered and then flows into Bowman's capsule. This process is called glomerular filtration. The water, waste products, salt, glucose and other chemicals that have been filtered out of the blood are known collectively as glomerular filtrate.

The fluid from the filtered blood is protein free but contains electrolytes such as sodium chloride, potassium and waste products of cellular metabolism; for example, urea, uric acid and creatinine (McCance & Huether 2018). The filtered blood then returns into circulation via the efferent arteriole and finally into the renal vein.

Selective reabsorption

Selective reabsorption processes ensure that any substances in the filtrate that are essential for body function are reabsorbed into the plasma. Substances such as sodium, calcium, potassium and chloride are reabsorbed to maintain fluid and electrolyte balance and the pH of blood. However, if these substances are in excess to body requirements, they are excreted in the urine. Only 1 per cent of the glomerular filtrate actually leaves the body; 99 per cent is reabsorbed into the bloodstream. The reabsorption occurs via three processes:

- osmosis
- diffusion
- active transport.

See table 11.3 for a summary.

TABLE 11.3 Summary of filtration, reabsorption and excretion in the nephron and collecting ducts

Reabsorption	Excretion
Proximal convoluted tubule	
Water, approximately 65% Sodium and potassium, 65% Glucose, 100% Amino acids, 100% Chloride, approximately 50% Bicarbonate, calcium and magnesium Urea	Hydrogen ions Urea Creatinine Ammonium ions
Loop of Henle	
Water Sodium and potassium, approximately 30% Chloride, approximately 35% Bicarbonate, approximately 20% Calcium and magnesium	Urea
Distal convoluted tubule	
Water, approximately 15% Sodium and chloride, approximately 5% Calcium Some urea	Potassium, depending on serum values Hydrogen ions, depending on pH of blood
Collecting duct	
Bicarbonate, depending on serum values Urea Water, approximately 9% Sodium, approximately 4%	Potassium, depending on serum values Hydrogen ions, depending on pH of blood

Source: Adapted from Tortora et al. (2014)

Blood glucose is entirely reabsorbed into the blood from the proximal tubules. In fact, it is actively transported out of the tubules and into the peritubular capillary blood. None of this valuable nutrient is wasted by being lost in the urine. Sodium (Na^+) and other ions are only partially reabsorbed from the renal tubules into the blood. For the most part, however, sodium ions are actively transported back into blood from the tubular fluid. The amount of sodium reabsorbed varies; it depends largely on how much salt we take in from the foods that we eat.

As a person increases the amount of salt intake into the body, kidneys decrease the amount of sodium reabsorption into the blood. That is, more sodium is retained in the tubules. Therefore, the amount of salt excreted in the urine increases. The process works the other way as well. The less the salt intake, the greater the amount of sodium reabsorbed into the blood, and the amount of salt excreted in the urine decreases.

Excretion

Any substances not removed through filtration are secreted into the renal tubules from the peritubular capillaries (see figure 11.7) of the nephron (Martini et al. 2017); these include drugs and hydrogen ions. Tubular secretion mainly takes place by active transport. Active transport is a process by which substances are moved across biological membranes. Tubular secretion occurs from epithelial cells lining the renal tubules and the collecting ducts. Substances secreted into the tubular fluid include:

- potassium ions (K^+)
- hydrogen ions (H^+)
- ammonium ions (NH_4^+)
- creatinine
- urea
- some hormones.

It is the tubular secretion of hydrogen and ammonium ions that helps to maintain the pH of blood. See table 11.3 for a summary.

FIGURE 11.7 Nephron with capillaries

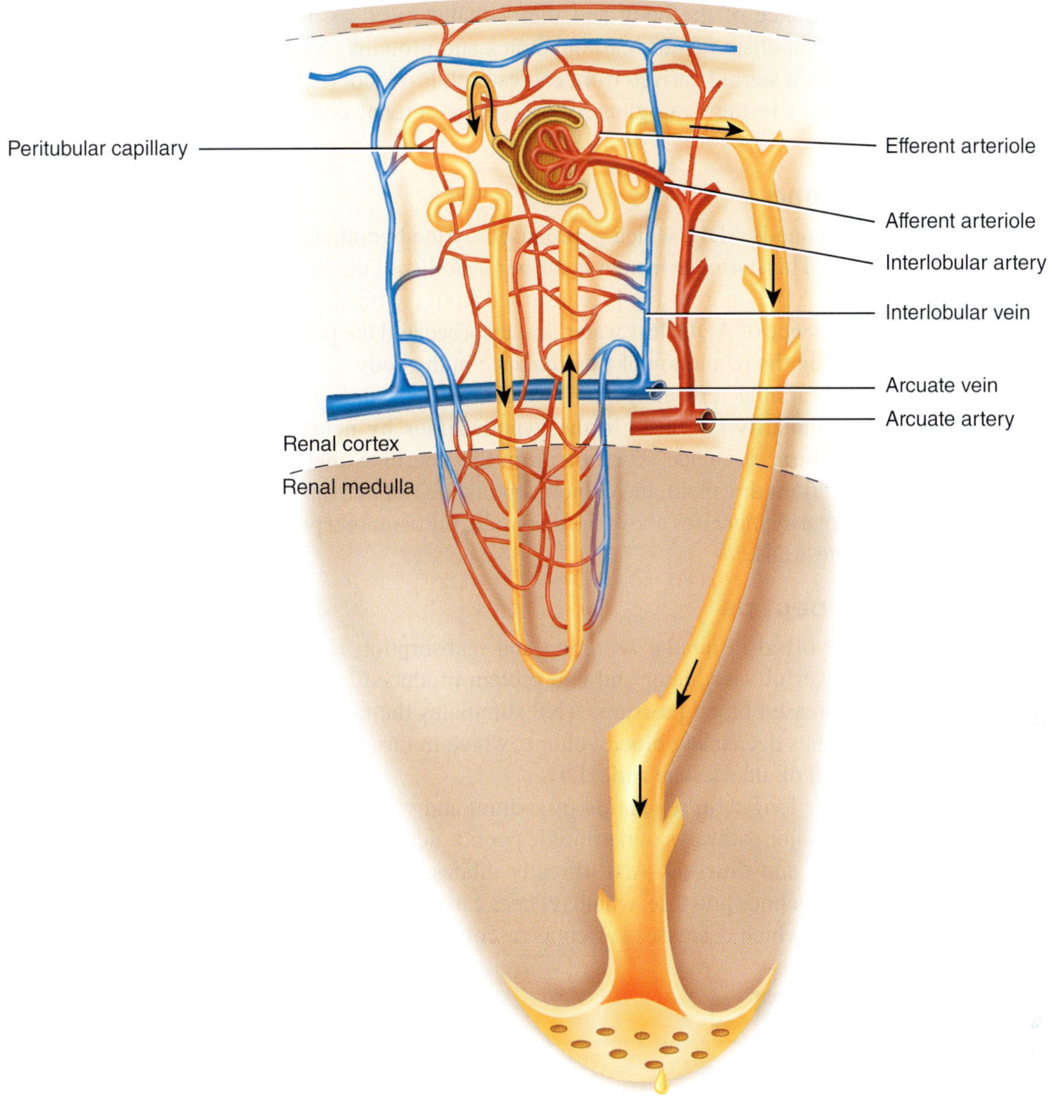

Source: Tortora and Derrickson (2009). Reproduced with permission of John Wiley & Sons.

Hormonal control of tubular reabsorption and secretion

Four hormones play a role in the regulation of fluid and electrolytes:

- angiotensin II
- aldosterone
- antidiuretic hormone (ADH)
- atrial natriuretic peptide (ANP).

Angiotensin and aldosterone

As the blood volume and blood pressure decrease, the juxtaglomerular cells secrete a hormone called renin. Juxtaglomerular cells are found near the glomerulus, and these cells synthesise, store and secrete the hormone renin. Renin acts on a plasma protein called angiotensinogen and converts it into angiotensin I. Angiotensinogen is produced by the hepatocytes of the liver. Angiotensin I is transported by the blood to the lungs. In the lung capillaries there are enzymes called ACE. ACE is predominantly found in the lung capillaries, but this enzyme is also found throughout the body. ACE converts angiotensin I into angiotensin II. Angiotensin II is a short-acting, powerful vasoconstrictor, thus increasing blood pressure.

Angiotensin II promotes the reabsorption of sodium, chloride and water in the proximal convoluted tubule. It also has an effect on the release of aldosterone.

Aldosterone is a steroid hormone secreted by the adrenal glands. It serves as the principal regulator of the salt and water balance of the body and thus is categorised as a mineralocorticoid. It also has a small effect on the metabolism of fats, carbohydrates and proteins. Aldosterone is synthesised in the body from corticosterone, a steroid derived from cholesterol. Production of aldosterone (in adult humans, about 20–200 μg per day) in the zona glomerulosa of the adrenal cortex is regulated by the rennin–angiotensin system.

Antidiuretic hormone

The third principal hormone is ADH, which is produced by the hypothalamus gland and is stored by the posterior pituitary gland. This hormone increases the permeability of the cells in the DCT and the collecting ducts. In the presence of ADH, more water is reabsorbed from the renal tubules; therefore the patient will pass less urine. In the absence of ADH, less water is reabsorbed and the patient will pass more urine. Thus, ADH plays a major role in the regulation of fluid balance in the body.

The most important variable regulating ADH secretion is plasma osmolarity, or the concentration of solutes in blood. Osmolarity is sensed in the hypothalamus by neurones known as osmoreceptors, and those neurones, in turn, stimulate secretion from the neurones that produce ADH. When plasma osmolarity is below a certain threshold, the osmoreceptors are not activated and the secretion of ADH is suppressed. When osmolarity increases above the threshold, the osmoreceptors recognise this and stimulate the neurones that secrete ADH.

Atrial natriuretic peptide

The fourth hormone involved in tubular secretion and reabsorption is atrial natriuretic peptide (ANP) hormone. ANP is a powerful vasodilator and is a protein produced by the myocytes of the atria of the heart in response to increased blood pressure. ANP stimulates the kidneys to excrete sodium and water from the renal tubules, thus decreasing blood volume, which in turn lowers blood pressure. The hormone also inhibits the secretion of aldosterone and ADH.

ANP is involved in the long-term regulation of sodium and water balance, blood volume and arterial pressure. There are two major pathways of natriuretic peptide actions: vasodilator effects and renal effects, which lead to natriuresis and **diuresis**. ANP directly dilates veins (increases venous compliance) and thereby decreases central venous pressure, which reduces cardiac output by decreasing ventricular preload. ANP also dilates arteries, which decreases systemic vascular resistance and systemic arterial pressure.

MEDICINES MANAGEMENT

Polypharmacy

Polypharmacy is the term that is used to describe patients who take several medications concurrently (Page et al. 2019). It is identified that people over the age of 65 are more likely to have multiple medications due to multimorbidity. There are some drugs that can be bought over the counter — including paracetamol, ibuprofen and aspirin — which can interact with some medications such as warfarin and prednisolone. Problems can occur in patients when multiple healthcare professionals are involved, especially if there is no oversight of what is being prescribed.

Common drug interactions in patients with renal disease include cardiovascular agents, antibiotics, anticholinergics and non-steroidal anti-inflammatory drugs.

Chronic conditions and multimorbidity are complex and significantly affect a person's quality of life. They require long-term self-management and health professional support. Thus, for health service providers:

> multimorbidity can make treatment more complex and can require ongoing management and coordination of specialised care across multiple parts of the health system. This places a heavy demand on Australia's healthcare system, and requires substantial economic investment. A key focus of the Australian health system, therefore, is the prevention and better management of chronic conditions to improve health outcomes. (Department of Health 2019)

11.5 Composition of urine

LEARNING OBJECTIVE 11.5 List the chemical compositions of urine.

Urine is a sterile and clear fluid of nitrogenous waste and salts. It is translucent with an amber or light yellow colour. Its colour is due to the pigments from the breakdown of haemoglobin. Concentrated urine tends to be darker in colour than normal urine. However, other factors, such as diet, medications and certain diseases, may affect the colour of the urine. It is slightly acidic, and the pH may range from 4.5 to 8. The pH is affected by an individual's dietary intake and state of health. Diet that is high in animal protein tends to make the urine more acidic, while a vegetarian diet may make the urine more alkaline. The volume of urine produced depends on the circulating volume of blood. ADH regulates the amount of urine passed by the individual. If the person is dehydrated, more ADH is released from the posterior pituitary gland, resulting in water reabsorption and less urine being produced. On the other hand, if the person has consumed a large amount of fluid, which increases the circulating volume, less ADH is released and more water is passed as urine.

Urine is 96 per cent water and approximately 4 per cent solutes derived from cellular metabolism. The solutes include organic and inorganic waste products and unwanted substances such as drugs. Normally there is no protein or blood present in the urine; if these are present, then the person may have a medical condition.

Characteristics of normal urine

The volume produced is one of the physical characteristics of urine. The normal amount of urine produced is 1–2 mL/kg/hour and is influenced by fluid intake and other factors such as blood pressure, medications, body temperature and general health (Health Engine 2021). Other physical characteristics that can apply to urine include colour, turbidity (transparency), smell (odour), pH (acidity/alkalinity) and density.

- *Colour.* Typically yellow–amber, but varies according to recent diet, medication and the concentration of the urine. Drinking more water generally tends to reduce the concentration of urine, and therefore causes it to have a lighter colour. However, if a person does not drink a large amount of fluid, this may increase the concentration and the urine will have a darker colour (see figure 11.8). See table 11.4 for foods, medications and illnesses that may affect the colour of the urine.
- *Smell.* The smell, or odour, of urine may provide health information. For example, the urine of diabetics may have a sweet or fruity odour due to the presence of ketones (organic molecules of a particular structure). Generally, fresh urine has a mild smell, but stale urine or infected urine has a stronger odour, similar to that of ammonia. Cloudy urine can indicate infection in the urine, whereas foamy urine can indicate the presence of protein and glucose.
- *Acidity.* The pH is a measure of the acidity (or alkalinity) of a solution. The pH of a substance (solution) is usually represented as a number in the range 0 (strong acid) to 14 (strong alkali, also known as a 'base'). Pure water is 'neutral', in the sense that it is neither acid nor alkali; it therefore has a pH of 7. The pH of normal urine is generally in the range 4.5–8, a typical average being around 6.0. Much of the variation is due to diet. For example, high protein diets result in more acidic urine, but vegetarian diets generally result in more alkaline urine.
- *Specific gravity.* Specific gravity is also known as 'relative density'. This is the ratio of the weight of a volume of a substance compared with the weight of the same volume of distilled water. Given that urine is mostly water, but also contains some other substances dissolved in the water, its relative density is expected to be close to, but slightly greater than, 1.000.

FIGURE 11.8 Urine colour chart

Urine varies in appearance, depending principally on your level of hydration.
Normal urine is a transparent solution ranging from colourless to amber but is usually a pale yellow.
Strange colours could be harmless or could indicate serious issues.
Seek medical advice for actual diagnosis of unusual colours.

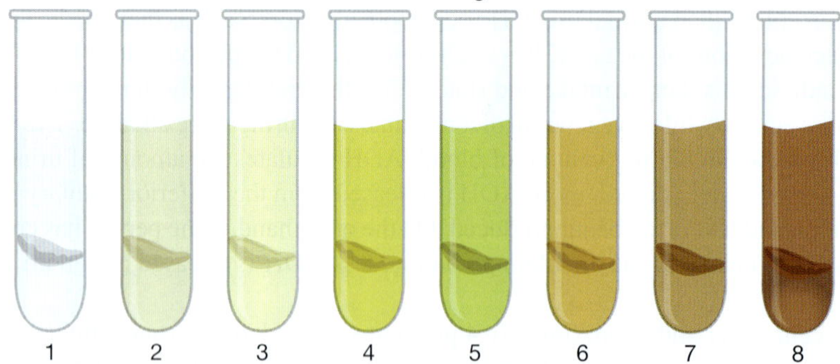

If your urine matches the colours numbered 1 to 3, you are hydrated. If your urine matches the colours numbered 4 up to 8, you are dehydrated and need to drink more fluid.

TABLE 11.4 **Colours of urine**

Food that changes colour of urine	
Dark yellow or orange:	Carrots
Green:	Asparagus
Pink or red:	Beetroot, blackberries, rhubarb
Brown:	Broad beans, rhubarb
Medicines and vitamins that may change the colour of urine	
Yellow or yellow–green:	Cascara, sulfasalazine, the B vitamins (especially B2- riboflavin)
Orange:	Rifampicin, sulfasalazine, vitamin B, vitamin C
Pink or red:	Phenolphthalein, propofol, rifampicin, laxatives containing senna
Green or blue:	Amitriptyline, cimetidine, indomethacin, promethazine, propofol, triamterene, several multivitamins
Brown or brownish-black:	Levodopa, metronidazole, nitrofurantoin, some antimalarial agents, methyldopa, laxatives containing cascara or senna
Medical conditions that may change the colour of urine	
Yellow:	Concentrated urine caused by dehydration
Orange:	A problem with the liver or bile duct
Pink or red:	Blood in the urine, haemoglobinuria (a condition linked to haemolytic anaemia), myoglobinuria (a condition linked to the destruction of muscle cells)
Deep purple:	Porphyria, a rare inherited red blood cell disorder
Green or blue:	Urinary tract infection may cause green urine if caused by *Pseudomonas* bacteria; familial hypercalcaemia, a rare genetic condition, can cause blue urine
Brown or dark brown:	Blood in the urine, a liver or kidney disorder

Source: Mayo Clinic Staff (2019)

SKILLS IN PRACTICE

Taking a urine sample for urinalysis

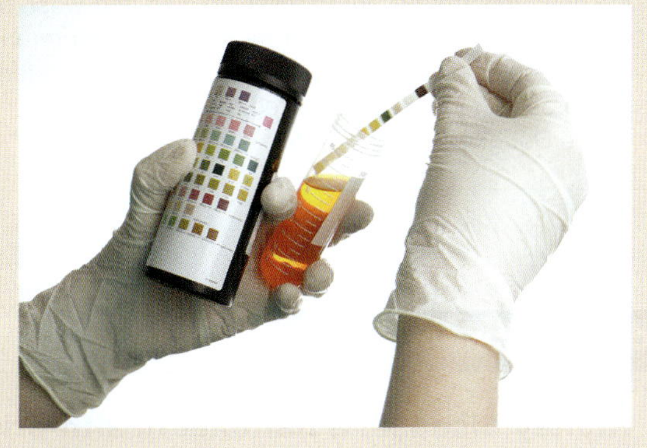

When undertaking a urinalysis, it is important to understand the relevance of certain findings (see figure 11.9). There are many reasons to undertake a urinalysis but importantly it can help aid in diagnosis of certain conditions such as urinary tract infection (under 65 years of age), diabetes and kidney disease.

Urine should be inspected for colour, clarity and odour (Watt 2017). Urine should appear clear and pale straw to amber in colour depending on urine concentration. Frothy or foamy urine could indicate the presence of protein or glucose in the urine. Cloudy urine could indicate the presence of bacteria (Watt 2017). Urinalysis can be undertaken with a reagent strip or an electronic urinalysis device. Standard infection control procedures should be used when collecting urine samples.

FIGURE 11.9 Chart for a urine dipstick analysis test

Test								Units
Leukocytes 120s	Neg.			Trace 15	Small 70	Moderate 125	Large 500	Cacells/µl
Nitrite 60s	Neg.				Positive — Any degree of uniform pink colour			
Urobilinogen 60s	3.2	Normal	16		32 +	64 ++	128 +++	µmol/l
Protein 60s	Neg.		Trace ±	0.3 +	1.0 ++	3.0 +++	>20.0 ++++	g/l
pH 60s	5.0	6.0	6.5	7.0	7.5	8.0	8.5	
Blood 60s	Neg.	Non hemolysed 10Trace		Hemolysed 10Trace	25 Small	80 Moderate	200 Large	Cacells/µl
Specific Gravity 45s	1.000	1.005	1.010	1.015	1.020	1.025	1.030	
Ketone 40s	Neg.		Trace 0.5	Small 1.5	Moderate 4.0	8.0 Large	16	mmol/l
Bilirubin 30s	Neg.				Small 17	Moderate 50	Large 100	µmol/l
Glucose 30s	Neg.		5 Trace	15 +	30 ++	60 +++	110 +++	mmol/l

Source: LaboratoryInfo (2020).

Taking a urine sample for microscopy and culture

When collecting a sample for microscopy, it is advised to take a midstream sample (MSU) to avoid contamination of the sample. A midstream specimen is used to determine the presence of bacteria (microculture) and to determine antibiotic sensitivity (Watt 2017).

To collect an MSU, ask the patient to wash their hands and to clean the urethral meatus (using mild soap and warm water). Use a wipe to clean front to back (to avoid faecal contamination). Ask the patient to begin voiding and use a sterile container to collect the middle stream of urine without interrupting the flow. Ask the patient to finish voiding and wash hands. The urine sample should be sent as soon as possible to the laboratory for microscopy, culture and sensitivity (MC&S). This will aid in identifying the type of bacteria causing an infection and administering appropriate antibiotics. At all times local policy and procedure must be adhered to.

See Dougherty et al. (2015).

CLINICAL CONSIDERATIONS

Kidney disease: a national health crisis

While kidney disease (both acute and chronic) is not currently listed as one of Australia's national health priority areas, Australia is facing a kidney disease crisis (KHA 2019). One in ten adults have early signs of kidney disease, and one in three are at risk of chronic kidney disease (CKD) (ABS 2019, cited in KHA 2019). Around 17 500 deaths per year are caused by CKD. Aboriginal and Torres Strait Islander peoples are disproportionately more vulnerable to CKD than non-Indigenous Australians. There is currently no cure for CKD, a disease that costs the Australian economy more than $5 billion a year (KHA 2019). End-stage kidney disease (ESKD) is crippling and often accompanied by financial hardships; treatment can be debilitating, significantly impacting on the person's quality of life. ESKD's debilitating nature also places significant burden on family and caregivers (KHA 2019).

CLINICALLY REASONED EPISODE OF CARE

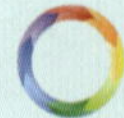

Chronic kidney disease

Consider the patient situation

Mohammed is a 56-year-old man who was diagnosed with chronic kidney disease (CKD) 3 years ago after a routine blood test. Over the last year his blood levels of urea and creatinine have been getting worse and as a result his renal team have advised that he will need to commence dialysis in the next 6 months. He has weekly blood tests to monitor his renal function.

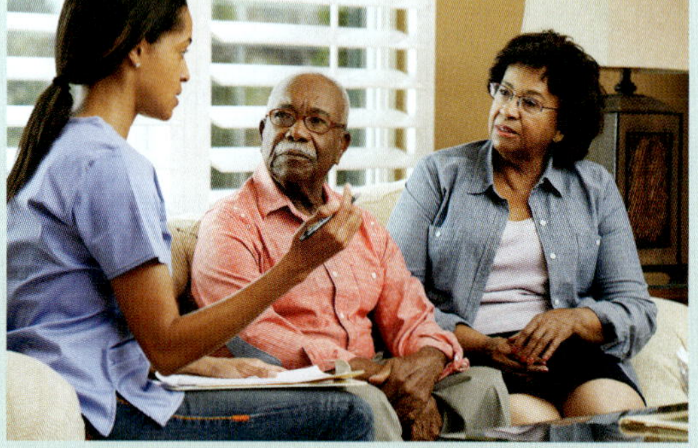

Collect cues and information

- Estimated glomerular filtration rate (eGFR): 18 mL/min/1.73 m^2 ; haemoglobin (Hb): 85 g/L.
- Itchy skin (pruritus), headaches, lethargy and disinterest.

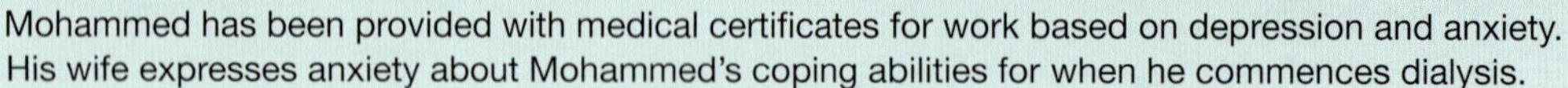

Mohammed has been provided with medical certificates for work based on depression and anxiety. His wife expresses anxiety about Mohammed's coping abilities for when he commences dialysis.

Process information

The most common cause of CKD in Australia is diabetes (36%) (AIHW 2020). Regardless of cause, however, CKD is a result of irreparable damage to the kidneys. It develops slowly and often goes undetected until up to 90 per cent of renal function is lost.

Based on his eGFR, Mohammed is assessed as being in stage 4 CKD (see table 11.5). The eGFR is calculated on the clearance of creatinine by the kidney from the bloodstream and provides an estimate of kidney function.

TABLE 11.5 **Kidney function stage based on eGFR**

Kidney function stage	eGFR (mL/min/1.73 m²)
1	≥ 90
2	60–89
3a	45–59
3b	30–44
4	15–29
5	< 15 or on dialysis

Source: Adapted from Kidney Health Australia (KHA) (n.d.).

The kidney produces a hormone called erythropoietin, which stimulates the bone marrow to produce red blood cells. A decline in this hormone secretion is part of CKD and results in a low haemoglobin level.

When urea is not excreted by the kidneys, it accumulates in the bloodstream. This is called uraemia, and the symptoms can include pruritus, lethargy and apathy.

Nursing action

1. Collaborate with Mohammed and his wife to develop a plan to manage his condition and the therapeutic interventions. The foci of support and education will be the disease, its course, and therapeutic interventions; medications, diet and fluid restrictions, and physical activity; possible complications (e.g. oedema and infections); and community resources and support groups.

   Rationale:
   - Patient education supports the minimisation of impact of ill health in the person's life and also concordance with recommended therapies which will promote good outcomes for the person.

Evaluate outcomes

Mohammed and his wife are able to articulate an appropriate level of understanding of CKD, its likely progression and management plans.

Source: Based on the Clinical Reasoning Cycle, Levett-Jones (2013).

Ureters

The ureters are tubular organs that run from the renal pelvis to the posterolateral base of the urinary bladder. The ureters are approximately 25–30 cm in length and 5 mm in diameter (Martini et al. 2017). The ureters terminate at the bladder and enter obliquely through the muscle wall of the bladder. They pass over the pelvic brim at the **bifurcation** of the common iliac arteries (see figure 11.10).

FIGURE 11.10 Common iliac vessels and ureter

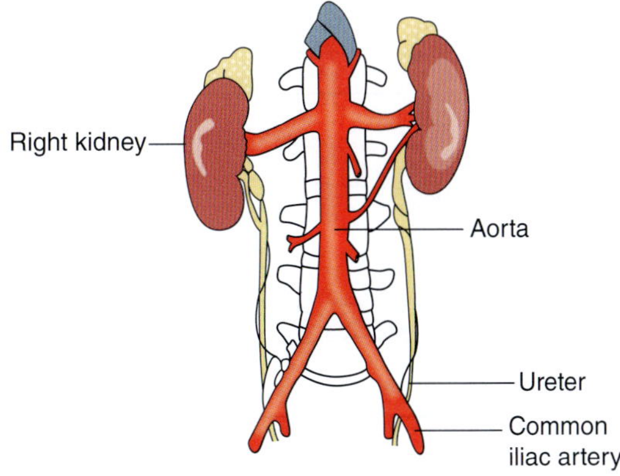

Source: Nair and Peate (2009). Reproduced with permission of John Wiley & Sons.

The ureters have three layers:

- transitional epithelial mucosa (inner layer)
- smooth muscle layer (middle layer)
- fibrous connective tissue (outer layer).

Urine is transported through the ureters via muscular movements of the urinary tract's peristaltic muscular waves. When the renal pelvis becomes laden with urine, the peristaltic wave action encourages urine to leave the body. The amount of urine in the renal pelvis determines the frequency of the peristaltic wave action, which can range from one to every few minutes to one to every few seconds. This action creates a pressure force that moves the urine through the ureters and into the bladder in small spurts.

Urinary bladder

The urinary bladder is a hollow muscular organ and is located in the pelvic cavity posterior to the symphysis pubis. In the male the bladder lies anterior to the rectum, and in the female it lies anterior to the vagina and inferior to the uterus (Martini et al. 2017); it is a smooth muscular sac that stores urine. Although the shape of the bladder is spherical, the shape is altered from pressure of surrounding organs. When the bladder is empty, the inner section of the bladder forms folds, but as the bladder fills with urine the walls of the bladder become smoother. As urine accumulates, the bladder expands without a significant rise in the internal pressure of the bladder. The bladder normally distends and holds approximately 350–750 mL of urine. In females the bladder is slightly smaller because the uterus occupies the space above the bladder.

The inner lining of the urinary bladder is a mucous membrane of transitional epithelium that is continuous with that in the ureters. When the bladder is empty, the mucosa has numerous folds called rugae. The rugae and transitional epithelium allow the bladder to expand as it fills. The second layer in the walls is the submucosa, which supports the mucous membrane. It is composed of connective tissue with elastic fibres.

The inner floor of the bladder includes a triangular section called the trigone. The trigone is formed by three openings in the floor of the urinary bladder. Two of the openings are from the ureters and form the base of the trigone. Small flaps of mucosa cover these openings and act as valves that allow urine to enter the bladder but prevent it from backing up from the bladder into the ureters. The third opening, at the apex of the trigone, is the opening into the urethra (see figure 11.11). A band of the detrusor muscle encircles this opening to form the internal urethral **sphincter**.

FIGURE 11.11 Layers of the urinary bladder

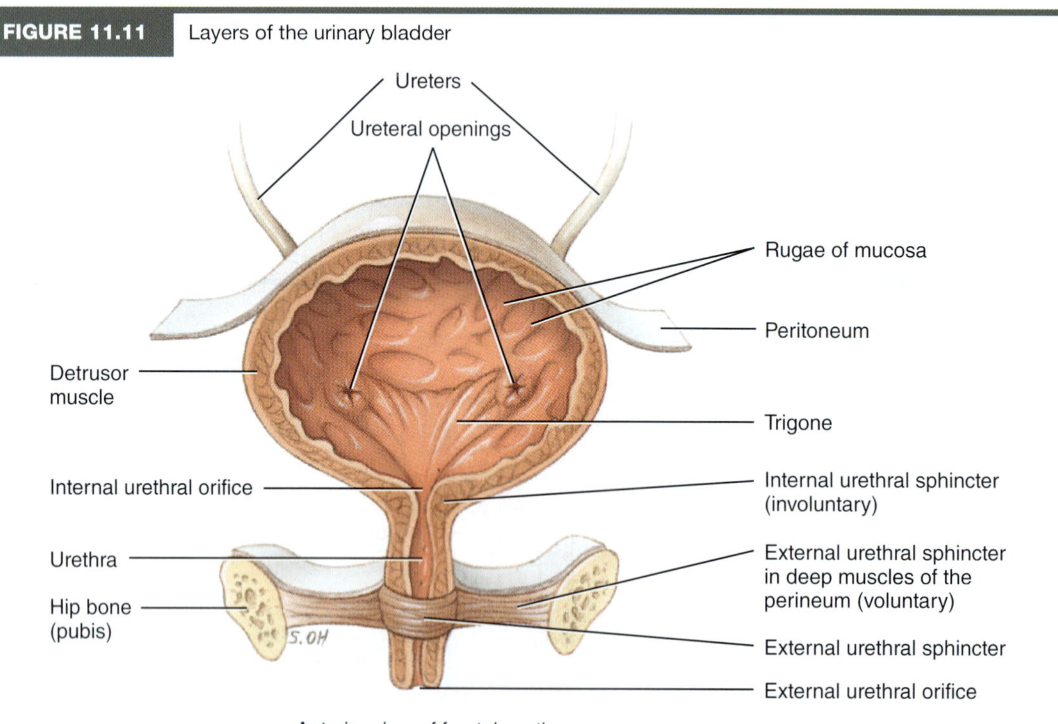

Source: Tortora and Derrickson (2009). Reproduced with permission of John Wiley & Sons.

The walls of the bladder consist of muscle fibres:

- transitional epithelial mucosa
- a thick muscular layer
- a fibrous outer layer.

The urinary tract can become blocked or obstructed (e.g. from a kidney stone, tumour, expanding uterus during pregnancy or enlarged prostate gland). The build-up of urine can lead to infection and injury of the kidney. With a kidney stone, the blockage is often painful. Other obstructions may produce no symptoms and be detected only when a blood or urine test is abnormal or when an imaging procedure, such as an X-ray or ultrasound, detects it.

Urinary tract infections, such as cystitis (an infection of the bladder), can lead to more serious infections further up the urinary tract. Symptoms include pyrexia, frequent urination, sudden and urgent need to urinate, and pain or a burning feeling during urination (dysuria). There is often pressure or pain in the lower abdomen or back. Sometimes the urine has a strong or foul odour or is bloody. Pyelonephritis is an infection of kidney tissue; most often, it is the result of cystitis that has been transmitted to the kidney. An obstruction in the urinary tract can make a kidney infection more likely. Infections elsewhere in the body, including streptococcal infections, the skin infection impetigo or a bacterial infection in the heart, can also be carried through the bloodstream to the kidney and cause a problem there.

CLINICALLY REASONED EPISODE OF CARE

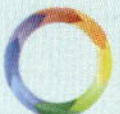

Paediatric urinary tract infection

Consider the patient situation

Beatrice is a 3-year-old female, presenting to the GP with her mother.

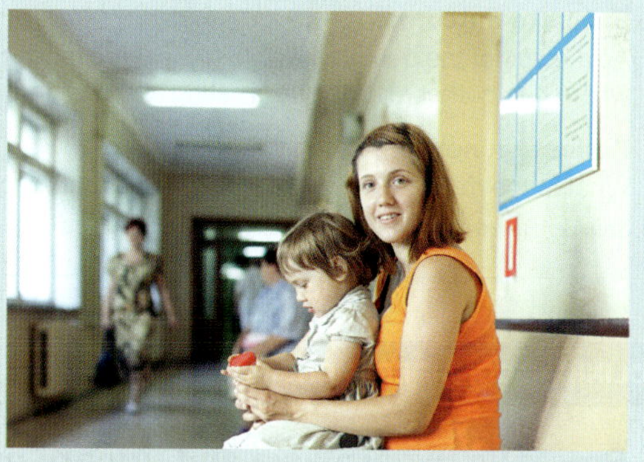

Collect cues and information

Beatrice is observed to be lethargic, febrile and clammy. Beatrice has not had anything to eat or drink in the last 24 hours and becomes distressed and upset upon passing urine.

Beatrice has presented to the GP office, where the practice nurse assists with her care and treatment.

Process information

A urinary tract infection (UTI) is an infection of the urethra, bladder or kidneys. UTIs occur in approximately 1 in 10 girls and 1 in 50 boys aged seven years or younger.

UTIs are caused by bacteria in the urinary tract. Signs and symptoms of a UTI include burning or stinging when passing urine, a pungent urine smell, abdominal or back pain, and feeling the need to pass urine more frequently. Children with a UTI will often have a range of symptoms including fever, lethargy, being unsettled and decreased oral intake.

A UTI is diagnosed via a clean urine sample which is tested for several enzymes. Beatrice's urine analysis is positive for leucocytes and nitrites. Leucocyte esterase is an enzyme present in white blood cells. When a urine analysis is positive for leucocytes it is indicative of inflammation in the urinary tract or kidneys. Nitrite is present in urine when a bacterium converts nitrate — which is normal in urine — to nitrite. A positive result for leucocytes and for nitrite, in conjunction with clinical symptoms, usually indicates a UTI.

Treatment for a UTI will usually involve antibiotic therapy, pain and fever relief, and oral fluids.

Establish goals

1. Manage pain and fever
2. Collect urine sample
3. Commence treatment
4. Educate family

Nursing actions

1. Administer pain and fever medication.
   Rationale:
   - Burning and stinging while urinating is a common symptom of a UTI, therefore the comfort of the individual is an important consideration.
   - Pain relief such as paracetamol can reduce both pain and fever and make the collection of a urine sample more achievable for the patient.
2. Collect urine sample for analysis.
   Rationale:
   - A 'clean catch' is important for an accurate urine analysis, because a foreign body, such as bacteria from surrounding skin, can contaminate the sample and therefore the test results.
   - A urine analysis can detect certain enzymes which will confirm a diagnosis and treatment plan for a UTI.
3. Encourage oral fluid intake.
   Rationale:
   - Children with a UTI are reluctant to urinate due to pain and often reduce their oral intake, placing them at risk of dehydration and further concentrating the urine.
   - Children should take regular small sips of fluids, such as water or diluted apple juice.
   - Parents are encouraged to record their child's oral intake and urine output during treatment.
4. Educate family on treatment, management and future prevention of UTIs.
   Rationale:
   - Nurses are well placed to educate patient and families on treatments such as antibiotics and taking regular sips of fluid. Nurses can educate patient and families on how and when to take antibiotics.
   - Nurses can also assist patients and family in understanding how to prevent UTIs including managing constipation; drinking fluids regularly; and for girls, wiping front to back and wearing breathable underwear fabric.

Evaluate outcomes

As a result of the treatments above, Beatrice recovers after five days of antibiotics. She returns to the GP where her mother reports she is eating and drinking well, going to the toilet with no pain, and without fever.

Reflect on new processes and learning

What is the role of the practice nurse in educating patients and families?

Source: Based on the Clinical Reasoning Cycle, Levett-Jones (2013).

CLINICAL CONSIDERATIONS

Prostatic hyperplasia and urinary problems

Enlargement of the prostate gland is a common condition in older men. The prostate is located beneath the bladder with the urethra passing directly through it. As the prostate enlarges it can partially or fully occlude the urethra leading to urinary symptoms.

These symptoms may include frequency, urgency and difficulty in commencing urination. Occasionally the occlusion can lead to an inability to urinate. This will need to be managed urgently to relieve the pressure and prevent damage to the kidney. A catheter may be inserted into the bladder to allow urine to be excreted. Prolonged retention of urine can lead to the development of AKI.

Urethra

The urethra is a muscular tube that drains urine from the bladder and conveys it out of the body. It contains three coats, and they are muscular, erectile and mucous; the muscular is the continuation of the bladder muscle layer. The urethra is encompassed by two separate urethral sphincter muscles. The internal urethral sphincter muscle is formed by involuntary smooth muscles, while the lower voluntary muscles make up the external sphincter muscles. The internal sphincter is created by the detrusor muscle. The urethra is longer in males than in females. Sphincters keep the urethra closed when urine is not being passed. The internal urethral sphincter is under involuntary control and lies at the bladder–urethra junction. The external urethral sphincter is under voluntary control.

Male urethra

The male urethra passes through four different regions:

- prostatic region — passes through the prostate gland
- membranous portion — passes through the pelvis diaphragm
- bulbar urethra — located inside the perineum and scrotum, extends from the external distal urinary sphincter to the peno-scrotal junction, and is surrounded by the corpus spongiosum; it contains the opening of the ducts of the Cowper glands, and differs in length from person to person
- penile region — extends the length of the penis.

In the male, the urethra not only excretes fluid waste products but is also part of the reproductive system. Rather than the straight tube found in the female body, the male urethra is S-shaped to follow the line of the penis. It is approximately 20 cm long. The male urethra can be segregated into various portions: the spongy portion, the prostatic portion and the membranous portion. The spongy urethra can be subdivided into fossa navicularis, pendulous urethra and bulbous (bulbar) urethra. The proximal portion, which is also the prostatic portion, is only about 2.5 cm long and passes along the neck of the urinary bladder through the prostate gland. This section is designed to accept the drainage from the tiny ducts within the prostate and is equipped with two ejaculatory tubes (see figure 11.12).

FIGURE 11.12 Male urethra

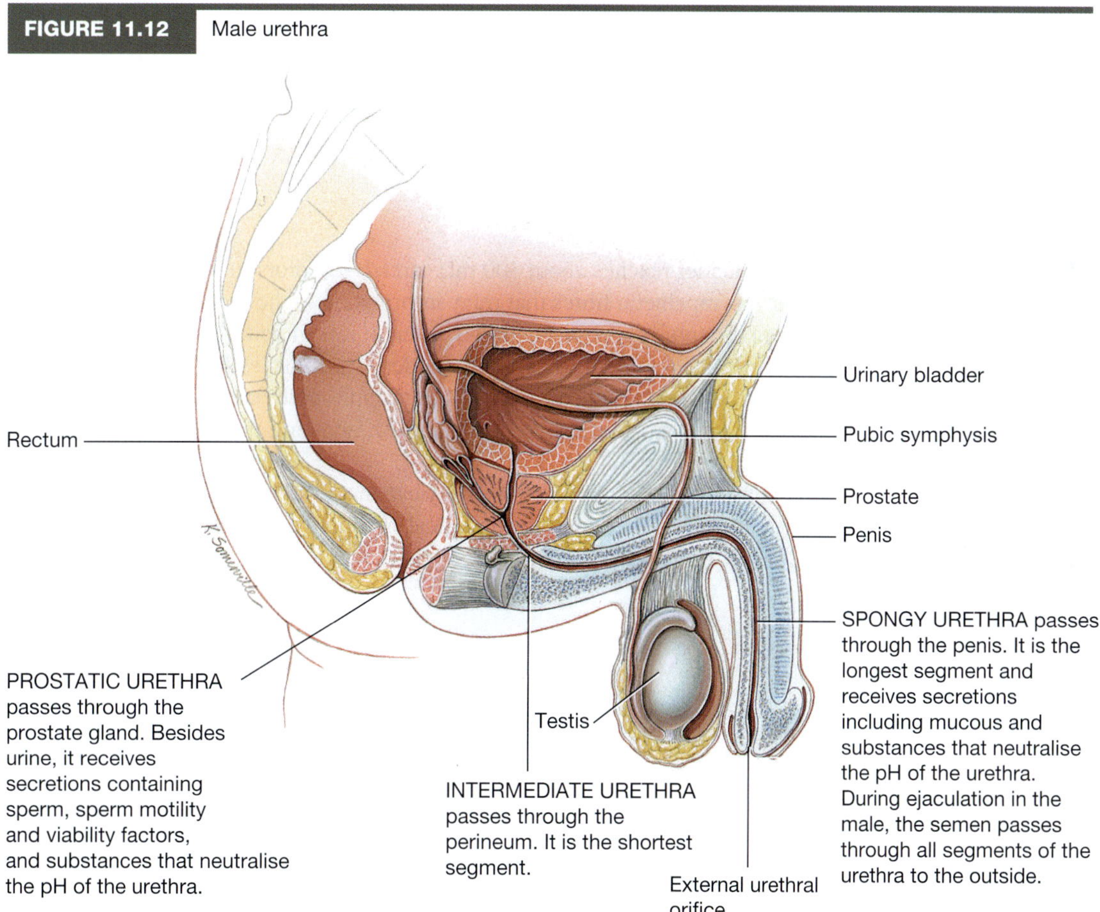

Source: Tortora et al. (2019).

Female urethra

The female urethra is bound to the anterior vaginal wall. The external opening of the urethra is anterior to the vagina and posterior to the clitoris. In the female, the urethra is approximately 4 cm long and leads out of the body via the urethral orifice. In the female, the urethral orifice is located in the vestibule in the labia minora. This can be found located in between the clitoris and the vaginal orifice. In the female body the urethra's only function is to transport urine out of the body (see figure 11.13).

FIGURE 11.13 Location of female urethra

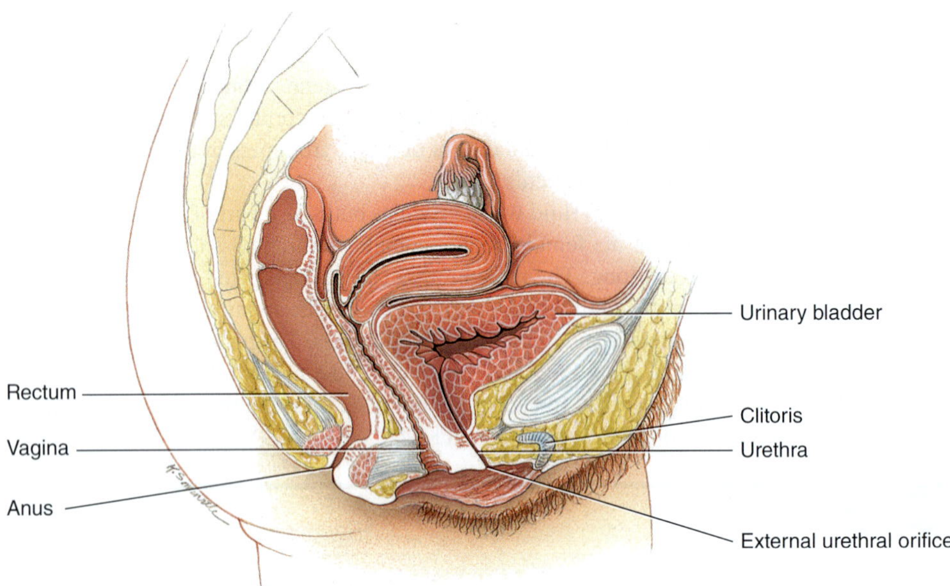

Source: Nair and Peate (2013). Reproduced with permission of John Wiley & Sons.

Micturition

When the volume of urine in the bladder reaches about 300 mL, stretch receptors in the bladder walls are stimulated and excite sensory parasympathetic fibres that relay information to the sacral area of the spine. This information is assimilated in the spine and relayed to two different sets of neurones. Parasympathetic motor neurones (in the pons) are excited and act to contract the detrusor muscles in the bladder so that bladder pressure increases and the internal sphincter opens. At the same time, somatic motor neurones supplying the external sphincter via the pudendal nerve are inhibited, allowing the external sphincter to open and urine to flow out, assisted by gravity.

A person usually has great control over bladder function. They can increase or decrease the rate of flow of urine, and stop and start at will (unless there are physiological problems), thus making micturition a simple reflex action.

SUMMARY

The renal system consists of the kidneys, ureters, urinary bladder and the urethra. These systems collectively play an important role in maintaining homeostasis. They remove the waste products of metabolism, secrete hormones, regulate fluid balance and maintain homeostasis. Some of the functions it carries out include:

- regulating blood volume through urine production and blood pressure by releasing renin
- regulating the electrolyte balance in the body through hormones such as aldosterone
- maintaining the acid–base balance by regulating the secretion of hydrogen and bicarbonate ions
- excreting waste products (e.g. urea and uric acid) and conserving valuable nutrients essential for the body.

Urine is formed by filtration, selective reabsorption and secretion. The selectivity of the glomerular filtrate is determined by the size of the opening of the filter and blood pressure. There are other factors that regulate urine production and electrolyte balance; they include hormone regulation such as ADH, aldosterone and ANP hormones and neuronal regulation through the autonomic nervous system.

The urinary bladder is a storage organ for urine and is located in the pelvic cavity. It contains three layers: the muscular, erectile and mucous layers. Urine is stored in the bladder until the person gets the urge to empty their bladder. The process of micturition is under the control of the sympathetic and parasympathetic system. During micturition, strong muscles in the bladder walls (the detrusor muscles) compress the bladder, pushing its contents into the urethra, thus voiding urine.

KEY TERMS

anterior Front.
bifurcation Dividing into two branches.
calyces Small, funnel-shaped cavities formed from the renal pelvis.
diuresis Excess urine production.
erythropoietin Hormone produced by the kidneys that regulates red blood cell production.
excretion The elimination of waste products of metabolism.
filtration A passive transport system.
glomeruli A network of capillaries found in Bowman's capsule.
hilum (hilus) An indention near to the centre of the concave area of the kidney, where its vessels, nerves and ureter enter/leave.
kidneys Organs situated in the posterior wall of the abdominal cavity.
nephron Functional unit of the kidney.
posterior Behind.
renal arteries Blood vessel that takes blood to the kidney.
renal cortex The outermost part of the kidney.
renal medulla The middle layer of the kidney.
renal pelvis The funnel-shaped section of the kidney.
renal pyramids Cone-shaped structures of the medulla.
renal veins Blood vessel that returns filtered blood into circulation.
renin A renal hormone that alters systemic blood pressure.
sphincter A ring-like muscle fibre that can constrict.
ureters Membranous tube that drains urine from the kidneys to the bladder.
urethra Muscular tube that drains urine from the bladder.

CONDITIONS

The following is a list of conditions that are associated with the renal system. Take some time and write notes about each of the conditions. You may make the notes taken from textbooks or other resources (e.g. people you work with in a clinical area), or you may make the notes as a result of people you have cared for. If you are making notes about people you have cared for, you must ensure that you adhere to the rules of confidentiality.

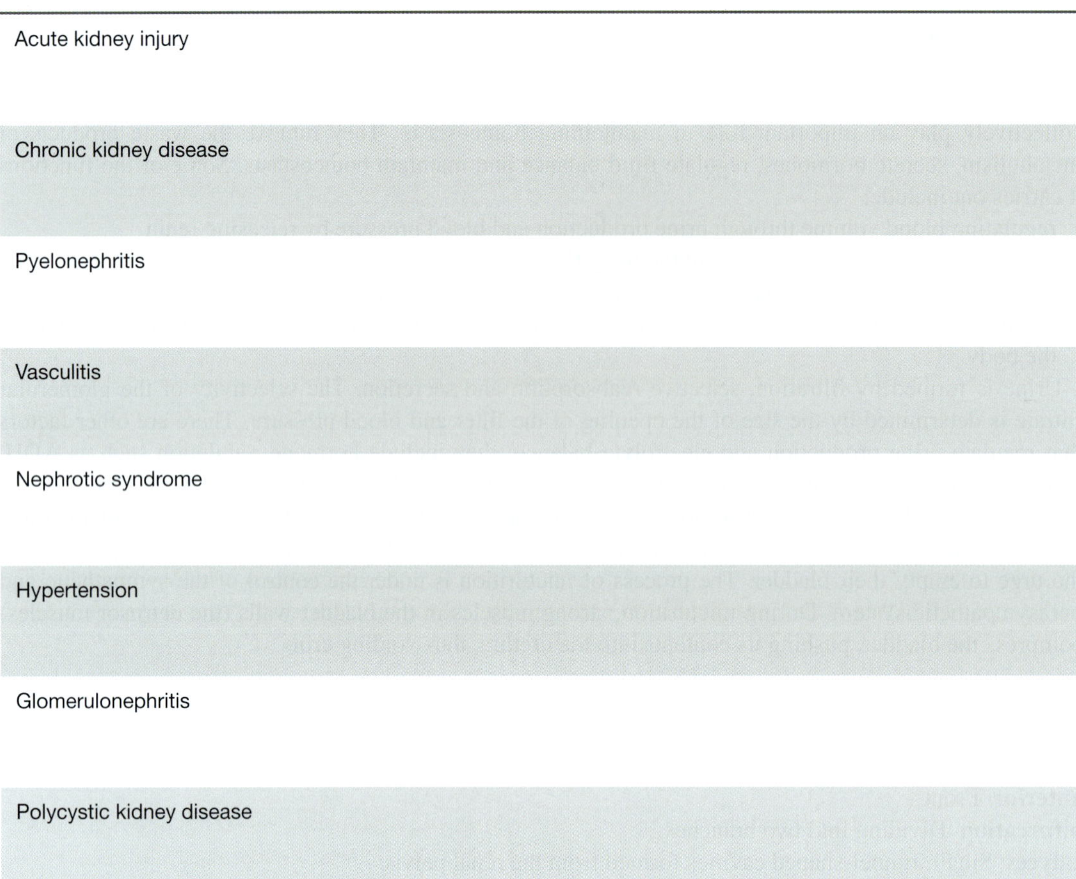

Acute kidney injury
Chronic kidney disease
Pyelonephritis
Vasculitis
Nephrotic syndrome
Hypertension
Glomerulonephritis
Polycystic kidney disease

REFERENCES

Australian Institute of Health and Welfare (2015) Acute kidney injury in Australia: a first national snapshot. www.aihw.gov.au/reports-data/health-conditions-disability-deaths/chronic-kidney-disease/overview (accessed February 2021).

Australian Institute of Health and Welfare (2020) Chronic kidney disease. www.aihw.gov.au/reports-data/health-conditions-disability-deaths/chronic-kidney-disease/overview (accessed February 2021).

Australian Medicines Handbook (2020) Antihypertensives. https://amhonline-amh-net-au.ezp01.library.qut.edu.au/chapters/cardiovascular-drugs/antihypertensives?menu=vertical (accessed 31 December 2020).

Azhar, A., Hussain, K. and Majid, A. (2019) Drug management in patients with reduced kidney function. *Prescriber* (February):18–22.

Department of Health (2019) Chronic conditions and multimorbidity www.aihw.gov.au/reports/australias-health/chronic-conditions-and-multimorbidity (accessed February 2021).

Dougherty, L., Lister, S. and West-Oram, A. (2015) *The Royal Marsden Manual of Clinical Nursing Procedures: Student Edition.* Hoboken, NJ: John Wiley & Sons, Incorporated.

Health Engine (2021) Polyuria (production of large amounts of urine). https://healthengine.com.au/info/polyuria-production-of-large-amounts-of-urine#:~:text=Normal%20urine%20production%20in%20an,mental%20state%20and%20general%20health (accessed February 2021).

Kidney Health Australia (KHA) (2019) National strategic action plan for kidney disease. https://kidney.org.au/get-involved/advocacy/national-strategic-action-plan-for-kidney-disease (accessed February 2021).

Kidney Health Australia (KHA) (n.d.) Stages of kidney disease. https://kidney.org.au/your-kidneys/what-is-kidney-disease/stages-of-kidney-disease (accessed February 2021).

LaboratoryInfo (2020) Urinalysis (urine testing) — types, process, results interpretation, reference charts. https://laboratoryinfo.com/urinalysis-urine-test (accessed March 2021).

Levett-Jones, T. (2013). *Clinical Reasoning: Learning to Think Like a Nurse*. Pearson Australia.

Marieb, E.N.H.K. (2016) *Human Anatomy and Physiology.* Boston: Pearson Education.

Martini, F., Nath, J.L. and Bartholomew, E.F. (2017) *Fundamentals of Anatomy and Physiology, Global Edition.* Boston: Pearson Education.

Mayo Clinic Staff (2019) Urine color. www.mayoclinic.org/diseases-conditions/urine-color/basics/causes/con-20032831 (accessed 26 February 2020).

McCance, K.L. and Huether, S.E. (2018) *Pathophysiology — E-Book: The Biologic Basis for Disease in Adults and Children.* St Louis: Mosby.

Nair, M. and Peate, I. *Fundamentals of Applied Pathophysiology: An Essential Guide for Nursing Students.* Chichester: John Wiley & Sons.

Page, A.T., Falster, M.O., Litchfield, M., Pearson, S-A., and Etherton-Beer, C. (2019) Polypharmacy among older Australians, 2006–2017; a population-based study. *The Medical Journal of Australia*, June 2019. doi:10.5694/mja2.50244

Tortora, G.J. and Derrickson, B.H. (2009) *Principles of Anatomy and Physiology*, 12th edn. Hoboken, NJ: John Wiley & Sons, Inc.

Tortora, G.J., Derrickson, B. and Tortora, G.J. (2014) *Principles of Anatomy and Physiology.* Hoboken, NJ: Wiley.

Tortora, G. J., Derrickson, B., Burkett, B., Peoples, G., Dye, D., Cooke, J., Diversi, T., McKean, M., Samalia, L. and Mellifont, R. (2019) *Principles of Anatomy and Physiology*, 2nd Asia–Pacific edn. Milton: Wiley.

Watt, E. (2017) Maintaining urinary elimination. In Crisp, J. Douglas, C. Rebeiro, G. and Waters, D. (eds) *Potter and Perry's Fundamentals of Nursing (Australia and New Zealand Edition)*, 5th edn, Elsevier: Chatswood.

FURTHER READING

Australia and New Zealand Society of Nephrology (2017) Renal resources. www.nephrology.edu.au/renalresources/index.asp (accessed February 2021).

Cass, A. and Hughes, J.T. (2019) Acute kidney injury in Indigenous Australians: an unrecognised priority for action. *Medical Journal of Australia* 211(1): 14–15.

Johnson, D.W., Atai, E., Chan, M., Phoon, R., Scott, C., Toussaint, N.D., Turner, G.L., Usherwood, T. and Wiggins, K.J. (2013) KHA-CARI guideline: early chronic kidney disease —detection, prevention and management. *Nephrology* 18, 340–350.

Langham, R.G., Bellomo, R., D'Intini, V., Endre, Z., Hickey, B.B., McGuinness, S., Phoon, R.K.S., Salamon, K., Woods, J., Gallagher, M.P., Kidney Health Australia Caring for Australasians with Renal Impairment; Kidney Disease Improving Global Outcomes (2014) KHA-CARI guidelines: KHA-CARI adaptation of the KDIGO Clinical Practice Guideline for Acute Kidney Injury, *Nephrology* (Carlton), 19(5): 261–265.

Levey, A.S. and James, M.T. (2017) Acute kidney injury: screening and prevention, diagnosis and treatment. *Annals of Internal Medicine*, 7 Nov 2017. doi:10.7326/AITC201711070

Makris, K. and Spanou, L. (2016) Acute kidney injury: definition, pathophysiology and clinical phenotypes. *Clinical Biochemist Reviews* 37(2): 85–98.

Nair, M. and Peate, I. (2013) *Fundamentals of Applied Pathophysiology — an Essential Guide for Nursing and Healthcare Students*, 2nd edn. Chichester: John Wiley & Sons, Ltd.

Renal Society of Australasia (2020) *Renal Society of Australasia Journal*. https://journals.cambridgemedia.com.au/rsaj (accessed February 2021).

Royal Australian College of General Practitioners (2020) National guide to a preventive health assessment for Aboriginal and Torres Strait Islander people. www.racgp.org.au/clinical-resources/clinical-guidelines/key-racgp-guidelines/view-all-racgp-guidelines/national-guide/chapter-13-chronic-kidney-disease-prevention-and-m (accessed February 2021).

Think Kidneys (2017) Acute kidney injury best practice guidance for undergraduate nurse educators. www.thinkkidneys.nhs.uk/aki/wp-content/uploads/sites/2/2016/05/Guidance_for_UG-nurse-educators-FINAL.pdf (accessed February 2021).

Thomas, N. (2019) *Renal Nursing: Care and Management of People with Kidney Disease.* London: Wiley.

RegisteredNurseRN (2017) Kidney and nephron anatomy structure — function renal system [YouTube video]. www.youtube.com/watch?v=0qZxw0Nd1lI (accessed February 2021).

ACKNOWLEDGEMENTS

Photo: © sirtravelalot / Shutterstock.com
Photo: © Tetra Images / Alamy Stock Photo
Photo: © EsHanPhot / Shutterstock.com
Photo: © Monkey Business Images / Shutterstock.com
Photo: © Iakov Filimonov / Shutterstock.com
Figure 11.8: © Sergey Shenderovsky / Shutterstock.com
Table 11.2: © Australian Medicines Handbook (2020), Antihypertensives.

CHAPTER 12

The respiratory system

TEST YOUR PRIOR KNOWLEDGE

- List five major structures of the upper and lower respiratory tract.
- What is the main function of the respiratory system?
- Describe the physiological process of breathing — which muscles are utilised?
- How is oxygen transported to body tissue?
- What factors may increase or decrease a person's rate and depth of breathing?

LEARNING OUTCOMES

After reading this chapter you will be able to:

12.1 list the main anatomical structures of both the upper and lower respiratory tract
12.2 describe the events of pulmonary ventilation
12.3 explain how the body is able to control the rate and depth of breathing
12.4 discuss the principles of external respiration
12.5 describe how oxygen and carbon dioxide are transported around the body.

Body map

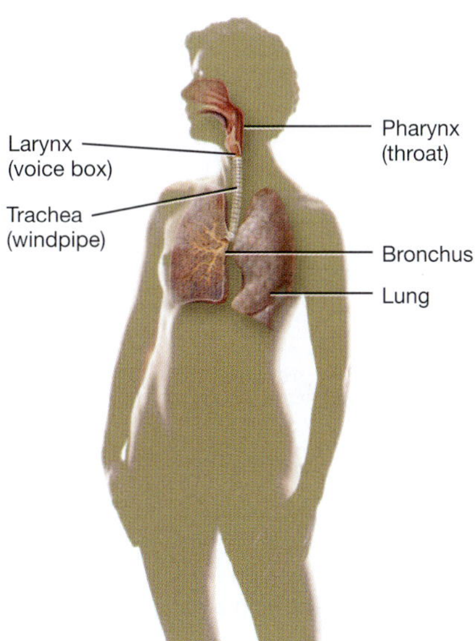

Introduction

Human cells can only survive if they receive a continuous supply of oxygen. As cells use oxygen, carbon dioxide is generated as a waste product. If allowed to build up, carbon dioxide can disrupt cellular activity and disturb homeostasis. The principal function of the respiratory system, therefore, is to ensure that the body extracts enough oxygen from the atmosphere and disposes of the excess carbon dioxide. The collection of oxygen and removal of carbon dioxide is referred to as respiration. Respiration involves the following four distinct processes: **pulmonary ventilation**, **external respiration**, **transport of gases** and **internal respiration**. Although all four are examined in this chapter, only pulmonary ventilation and external respiration are the sole responsibility of the respiratory system. As oxygen and carbon dioxide are transported around the body in blood, effective respiration is also reliant upon a fully functioning cardiovascular system.

12.1 Organisation of the respiratory system

LEARNING OBJECTIVE 12.1 List the main anatomical structures of both the upper and lower respiratory tract.

The respiratory system is divided into the upper and **lower respiratory tract** (see figure 12.1). All structures found below the **larynx** form part of the lower respiratory tract. The respiratory system can also be said to be divided into conduction and **respiratory regions**. The **upper respiratory tract** and the uppermost sections of the lower respiratory tract form the **conduction region**, in which air is conducted through a series of respiratory passages. The respiratory region is the functional part of the lungs, in which oxygen diffuses into blood. The structures within the respiratory region are microscopic, very fragile and easily damaged by infection. For this reason, both the upper and lower respiratory tracts are equipped to fight off any invading airborne bacterial or viral pathogens.

FIGURE 12.1 Major structures of the upper and lower respiratory tract

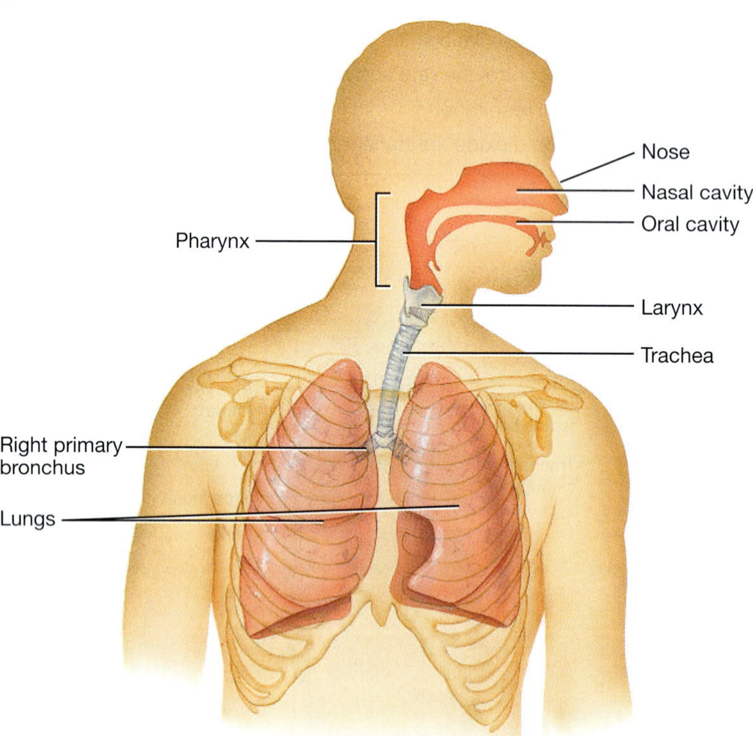

Anterior view showing organs of respiration

***Source*:** Tortora and Derrickson (2017). Reproduced with permission of John Wiley & Sons.

The upper respiratory tract

Air enters the body via the nasal and oral cavities. The **nasal cavity** is divided into two equal sections by the **nasal septum**, a structure formed out of the **ethmoid bones** and the **vomer** of the skull. The space where air enters the nasal cavity just inside the nostrils is referred to as the **vestibule**. Beyond each vestibule the nasal cavities are subdivided into three air passageways, the **meatuses**, which are formed by three shelf-like projections called the superior, middle and inferior **nasal conchae** (see figure 12.2). The region around the superior conchae and upper septum contains **olfactory** receptors, which are responsible for our sense of smell. The **pharynx** connects the nasal and oral cavity with the larynx. The pharynx is divided into three regions called the **nasopharynx**, the **oropharynx** and the **laryngopharynx**. The nasopharynx sits behind the nasal cavity and contains two openings that lead to the auditory (Eustachian) tubes. The oropharynx and laryngopharynx sit underneath the nasopharynx and behind the oral cavity. The oropharynx and oral cavity are divided by the **fauces** (see figure 12.2). Both the oropharynx and the laryngopharynx are passageways for food and drink as well as air. To protect them from abrasion by food particles they are lined with **non-keratinised stratified squamous epithelium** (see the chapter on tissue).

FIGURE 12.2 Structures of the upper respiratory tract

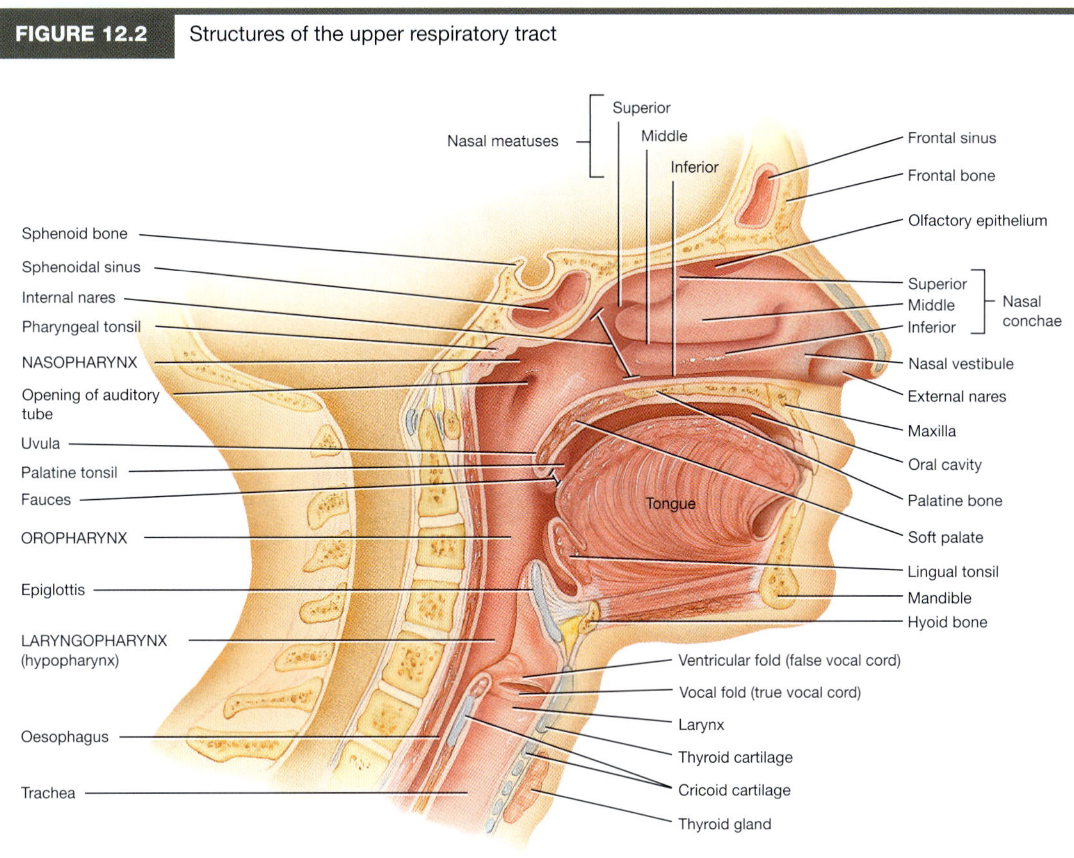

Sagittal section of the left side of the head and neck showing the location of respiratory structures

Source: Tortora and Derrickson (2017). Reproduced with permission of John Wiley & Sons.

As well as providing the sense of smell, the upper respiratory tract also ensures that the air entering the lower respiratory tract is warm, humidified and clean. The vestibule is lined with coarse hairs that filter incoming air, ensuring that large dust particles do not enter the airways. The conchae are lined with a mucous membrane made from **pseudostratified ciliated columnar epithelium**, which contains a network of capillaries and a plentiful supply of mucus-secreting **goblet cells**. The blood flowing through the capillaries warms the passing air, while the mucus moistens it and traps any passing dust particles. The mucus-covered dust particles are then propelled by the **cilia** towards the pharynx, where they can be swallowed or expectorated.

To add further protection, the upper respiratory tract is lined with irritant receptors, which when stimulated by invading particles (e.g. dust or pollen) force a sneeze, ensuring the offending material is ejected through the nose or mouth. The pharynx also contains five **tonsils**. The two tonsils visible when the mouth is open are the **palatine tonsils**; behind the tongue lie the **lingual tonsils**, and the **pharyngeal tonsil** or adenoid sits on the upper back wall of the pharynx. Tonsils are **lymph nodules** and part of the body's defence system. The epithelial lining of their surface has deep folds, called crypts. Inhaled bacteria or particles become entangled within the crypts and are then engulfed and destroyed.

The lower respiratory tract

The lower respiratory tract includes the larynx, the trachea, the right and left primary bronchi and all the constituents of both lungs (see figure 12.3). The lungs are two cone-shaped organs that almost fill the **thorax**. They are protected by a framework of bones, the **thoracic cage**, which consists of the ribs, **sternum** (breastbone) and vertebrae (spine). The tip of each lung, the **apex**, extends just above the **clavicle** (collarbone), and their wider bases sit just above a concave muscle called the **diaphragm**. The larynx (voice box) connects the trachea and the laryngopharynx. The remainder of the lower respiratory tract divides into branches of airways. For this reason, the structure of the lower respiratory tract is often referred to as the **bronchial tree**.

FIGURE 12.3 Gross anatomy of the lower respiratory tract

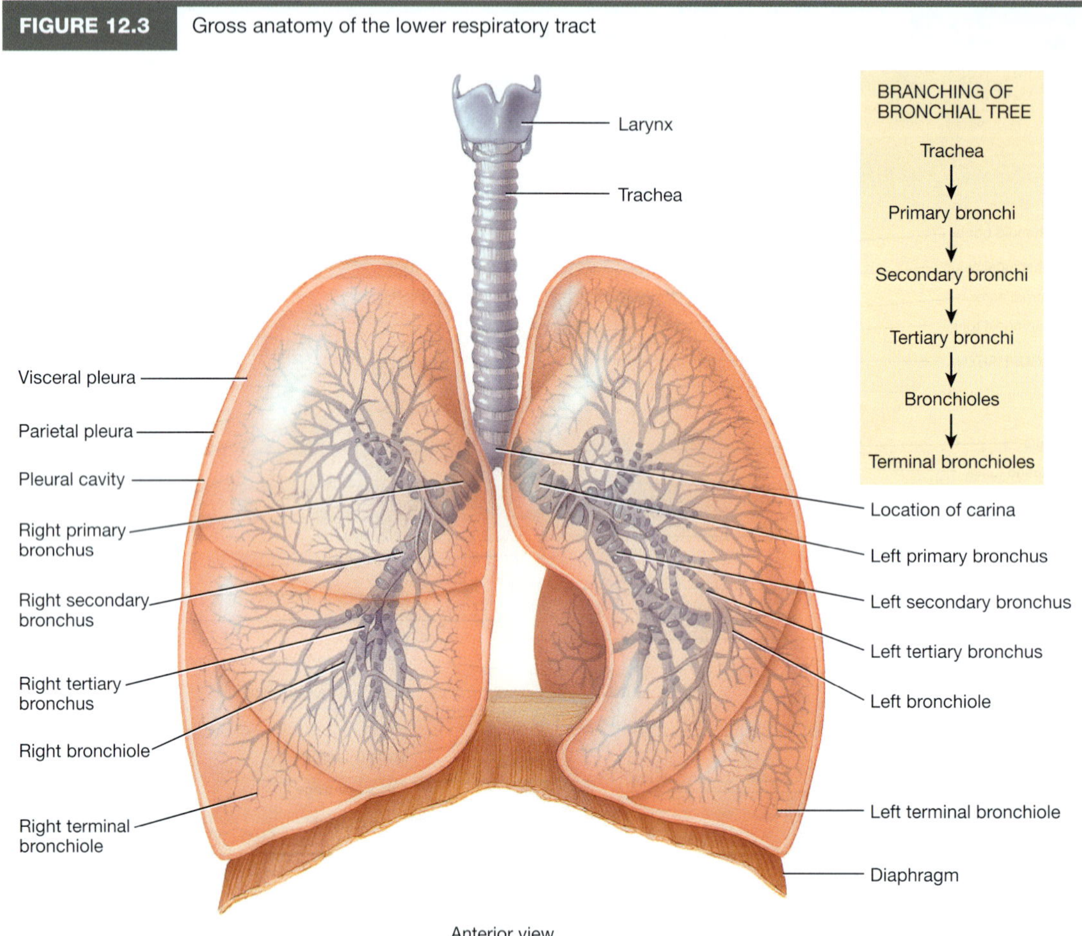

Source: Tortora and Derrickson (2017). Reproduced with permission of John Wiley & Sons.

Larynx

The larynx consists of nine pieces of **cartilage** tissue: three single pieces and three pairs (see figure 12.4). The single pieces of cartilage are the **thyroid cartilage**, the **epiglottis** and the **cricoid cartilage**. The thyroid cartilage is more commonly known as the Adam's apple and, together with the cricoid cartilage, protects the vocal cords. The **cricothyroid ligament**, which connects the thyroid and cricoid cartilage, is the landmark of an emergency airway or **tracheostomy** (McGrath 2014). The epiglottis is a leaf-shaped piece of elastic cartilage attached to the top of the larynx. Its function is to protect the airway from food and water. On swallowing, the epiglottis blocks entry to the larynx and food and liquids are diverted towards the **oesophagus**, which sits nearby. Inhalation of solid or liquid substances can block the lower respiratory tract and cut off the body's supply of oxygen — this medical emergency is referred to as **aspiration** and necessitates the swift removal of the offending substance.

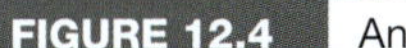

FIGURE 12.4 Anatomy of the larynx

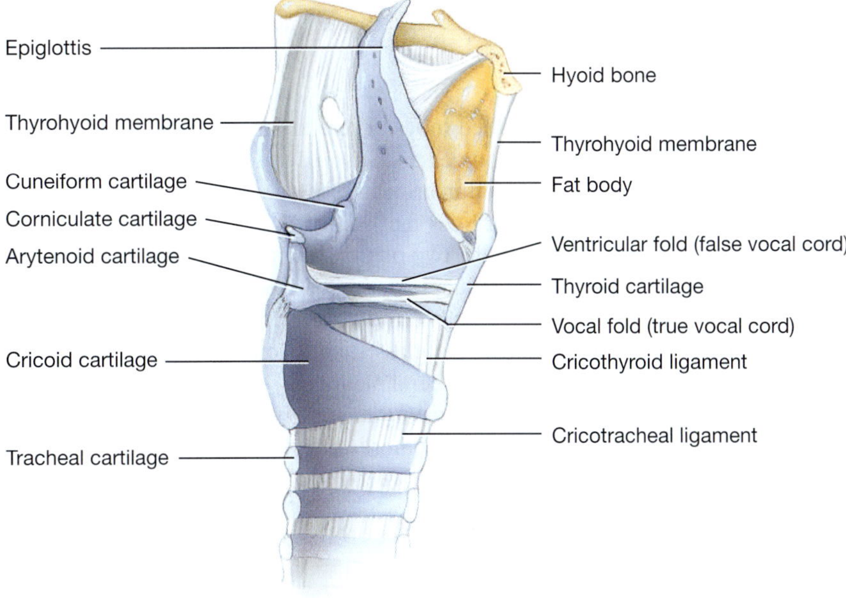

Source: Tortora and Derrickson (2017). Reproduced with permission of John Wiley & Sons.

The three pairs of cartilage are the **arytenoid cartilage**, **cuneiform cartilage** and **corniculate cartilage** (see figure 12.4). The arytenoid cartilages are the most significant as they influence the movement of the mucous membranes (true vocal folds) that generate the voice. Speaking, therefore, is reliant upon a fully functioning respiratory system. Many obstructive lung disorders, such as **asthma**, reduce a person's ability to speak a full sentence without drawing a new breath (Wheatley 2018).

Trachea

The trachea (or windpipe) is a tubular vessel that carries air from the larynx down towards the lungs. The trachea is also lined with pseudostratified ciliated columnar epithelium so that any inhaled debris is trapped and propelled upwards towards the oesophagus and pharynx to be swallowed or expectorated. The trachea and the bronchi also contain irritant receptors, which stimulate a cough, forcing larger invading particles upwards. The outermost layer of the trachea contains connective tissue that is reinforced by a series of 16–20 C-shaped cartilage rings. The rings prevent the trachea from collapsing during an active breathing cycle.

SKILLS IN PRACTICE

Removal of bronchial secretions (suction)

The insertion of a tracheostomy will irritate the airways and stimulate the production of bronchial secretions, which the patient will find difficult to **expectorate**. Suction is a method of removing bronchial secretions and keeping the airways clear.

When clearing bronchial secretions via a tracheostomy, the nurse inserts a sterile catheter, which is attached to suction, into the stoma. The suction then removes the bronchial secretions. It is paramount that the procedure is executed quickly and aseptically and with care to minimise the chances of trauma and **hypoxia**.

Before suctioning can commence the nurse must select an appropriate catheter size and ensure the suction pressure is set at a safe level (ideally 11–16 kPa). Once the procedure has been explained to the patient, the nurse, using aseptic technique, gently inserts the suction catheter into the tracheostomy and pushes it down the airway until the patient coughs or resistance is felt. The nurse should then withdraw the catheter by 1–2 cm before applying the suction. The suction catheter is then withdrawn while continually suctioning until it is removed. While the catheter is in place, the suction pressure will remove excess secretions and dispose of them safely. The process should not take more than 15 seconds and twisting and pushing back and forth should be avoided. Oxygen saturations must be monitored throughout the procedure and if the patient is receiving oxygen it must be replaced immediately afterwards. Local policy and procedures must be adhered to at all time.

Bronchial tree

The lungs are divided into distinct regions called **lobes**. There are three lobes in the right lung and two in the left. The heart, along with its major blood vessels, sits in a space between the two lungs called the **cardiac notch**. Each lung is surrounded by two thin protective membranes called the parietal and **visceral pleura** (see figure 12.3). The **parietal pleura** lines the wall of the thorax, whereas the visceral pleura lines the lungs themselves. The space between the two pleurae, the **pleural space** or cavity, is minute and contains a thin film of lubricating fluid. This reduces friction between the two pleurae, allowing the two layers to slide over one another during breathing. The fluid also helps the visceral and parietal pleura to adhere to each other, in the same way two pieces of glass stick together when wet. However, should any substance enter the pleural space the parietal and visceral pleura may separate, causing the lung to collapse (**atelectasis**). Substances that can enter the pleural cavity include blood or fluid, and in most cases air. A collection of air in the pleural cavity is called a pneumothorax or collapsed lung. Blood in the pleural cavity is referred to as a haemothorax and fluid collecting between the pleura is called a pleural effusion.

SKILLS IN PRACTICE

Nursing care and management of a chest drain

A chest drain is a plastic tube inserted into the pleural cavity to remove air or fluid that may have collected there as a result of disease or trauma. The plastic tube is connected to a container, which collects the air or fluid. When chest drains are used to collect air, the container will contain water, which provides a seal or valve that allows gas to exit the lungs but not to re-enter. When used to extract air, chest drains can be attached to suction pressure to aid lung reinflation.

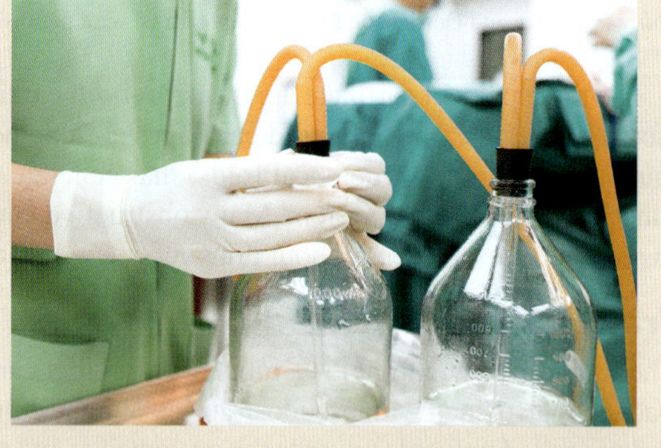

The main care responsibilities when nursing a person with a chest drain are monitoring both the individual and the drain. Attention should be paid to the position of both the patient and the chest drain. The patient should, wherever possible, remain in an upright position to encourage drainage and chest expansion. The position of the drain itself is equally important as it must be kept below the patient's chest level to prevent fluid re-entering the pleural space. The nurse must also check that the drain is not coiled or looped as this will impede drainage.

The nurse must monitor the chest drain closely and observe for signs of 'swinging' and 'bubbling'. The level of the water seal in the container should fluctuate between 5 and 10 cm, in sync with the patient's breathing. This movement is referred to as swinging and absence of swinging could indicate that there is a kink or blockage in the tubing. 'Bubbling' is the presence of bubbles in the water seal. Bubbling normally occurs when the patient coughs or exhales. Continuous bubbling, however, could indicate a problem with the drain or insertion site.

Chest drain insertion can be very painful and nurses must talk with their patients about their pain and administer prescribed analgesics to keep pain levels to a minimum. Furthermore, nurses must regularly assess for signs of infection, such as redness, swelling and heat around the insertion site.

Within the lungs the primary bronchi divide into the secondary bronchi, each serving a lobe (three secondary bronchi on the right and two on the left). The secondary bronchi split into tertiary bronchi (see figures 12.3 and 12.5), of which there are 10 in each lung. Tertiary bronchi continue to divide into a network of **bronchioles**, which eventually lead to a terminal bronchiole. The section of the lung supplied by a terminal bronchiole is referred to as a **lobule**, and each lobule has its own arterial blood supply and **lymph vessels**. The bronchial tree continues to subdivide, with the terminal bronchiole leading to a series of respiratory bronchioles, which in turn generate several alveolar ducts. The airways terminate with numerous sphere-like structures called alveoli, which are clustered together to form alveolar sacs (see figure 12.6). Human lungs contain an average of 480 million alveoli (Ochs et al. 2004). The transfer of oxygen from air to blood only occurs from the respiratory bronchiole onwards. The airways found between the trachea and the respiratory bronchioles form the conduction region of the lungs. The airways found beyond the respiratory bronchioles constitute the functional, respiratory region of the lungs. This region accounts for two-thirds of the lungs' surface area (Tortora & Derrickson 2017).

FIGURE 12.5 The bronchial tree

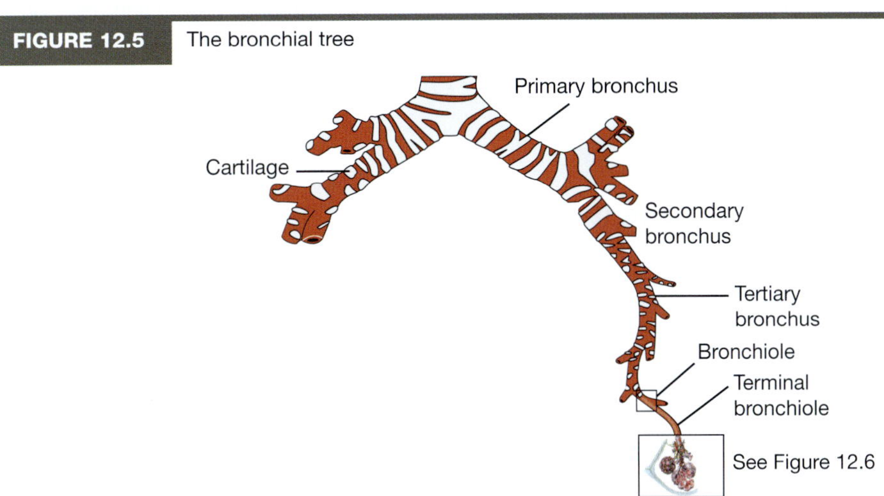

Source: Peate (2017). Reproduced with permission of John Wiley & Sons.

FIGURE 12.6 Microscopic anatomy of a lobule

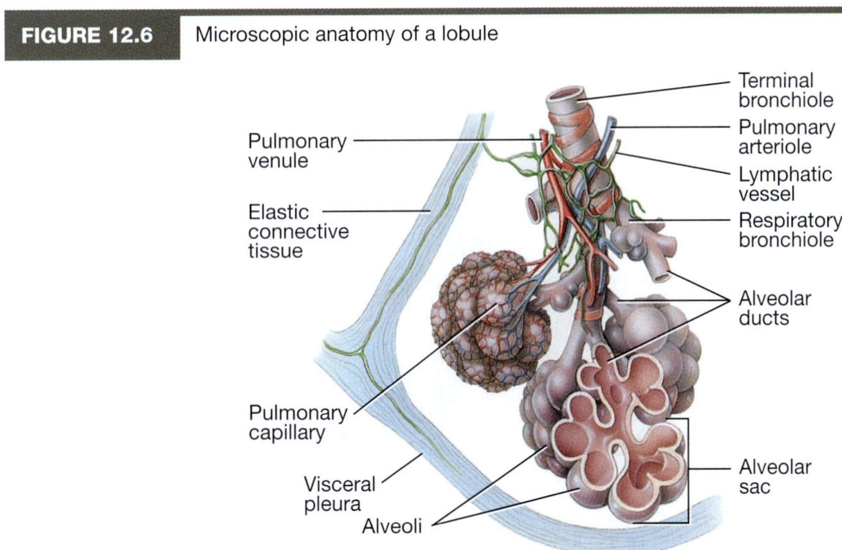

Diagram of a portion of a lobule of the lung

Source: Tortora and Derrickson (2017). Reproduced with permission of John Wiley & Sons.

CLINICAL CONSIDERATIONS

Bronchiectasis: a national health priority

Bronchiectasis is a progressive and permanent dilation and thickening of the airways caused by chronic bacterial and viral infection. This damage and inflammation leads to increased mucous production and decreased mucous clearance from the lungs, causing a persistent and productive cough, shortness of breath and wheezing. Excluding patients with cystic fibrosis, bronchiectasis is relatively rare in the developed world but occurs at disproportionately higher rates within the Aboriginal communities of the Northern Territory (1–2%) (Davey 2021; Chang et al. 2002).

Respiratory disease is the leading cause of preventable death in Indigenous infants and is the second most common cause of death in Indigenous adults (Chang et al. 2002). The burden of respiratory disease is significantly higher in the Aboriginal community with a fortyfold increase in the prevalence of bronchiectasis in children under 15 years when compared with the wider Australian community (Davey 2021). As with many of the health issues facing Indigenous communities, the root cause appears to be linked to high rates of domestic overcrowding in the Northern Territory coupled with reduced access to adequate nutrition, medical care and an increased risk of respiratory infection (Davey 2021; Chang et al. 2002).

CLINICAL CONSIDERATIONS

Asthma: a national health priority

Currently, 11 per cent of Australians suffer from asthma, with 3–10 per cent of those affected suffering from severe asthma. Severe asthma has significant effects on quality of life due to both the persistent nature of the symptoms and the constant threat of life-threatening episodes. Many of these patients are also refractory to standard treatment options and, as a result, have poor management of their symptoms (McDonald et al. 2018).

The severity and frequency of asthmatic episodes has serious social, financial and mental health impacts for sufferers and places a profound financial burden on both healthcare providers and the Australian population in general. For these reasons, asthma has been identified as one of Australia's national health priorities (McDonald et al. 2018).

CLINICALLY REASONED EPISODE OF CARE

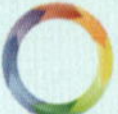

Asthma

Consider the patient situation

Amy is 4 years old and she has had a troublesome cough for 4 weeks. At first her mother and father thought she had a common cold, but the cough remained after the symptoms of the cold abated. Amy's father takes her to the health clinic and explains that the cough is worse at night and it stops Amy from sleeping. He also says that Amy's cough is exacerbated by running and playing with her friends.

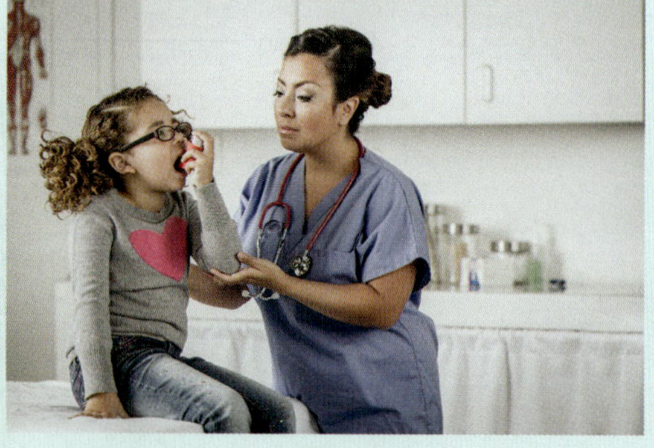

Collect cues and information

The nurse practitioner listens to Amy's chest and asks her to blow into a peak flow meter. The nurse concludes that Amy has asthma-like symptoms.

Process information

Asthma is a chronic inflammatory disorder of the lungs. It causes the bronchi and bronchioles to become inflamed and constricted. As a result, airflow becomes obstructed, often resulting in a characteristic wheeze and a cough.

Asthma is triggered by exposure to substances or situations that wouldn't normally cause airway irritation. Substances such as pollen and dust are common triggers, but asthma can be caused by situations such as inhaling cold air, exercise, stress, and upper airway infections such as the common cold. Asthma can develop at any stage of life but is common in childhood.

An estimated 10 per cent of Australian children aged 0–14 have asthma as a long-term condition (AIHW 2020). However, asthma is very difficult to diagnose in children, especially when they are under 5, as the symptoms may be caused by other common childhood conditions, such as rhinitis, sinusitis or reflux. When caring for a child under the age of 5, GPs and nurse practitioners are advised to use their clinical judgement and treat the child as having asthma if they have asthma-like symptoms.

Children should be closely monitored, and if they still have asthma-like symptoms when they turn 5, GPs should consider diagnostic tests such as spirometry, or peak flow.

Nursing actions

1. Prescribe a short acting beta2 agonist.
   Rationale:
   - This drug will cause the smooth muscle of airways to relax, dilating the respiratory passages and increasing airflow to and from the alveoli.
2. Provide education to Amy and her father on the correct use of the inhaler and spacer.
   Rationale:
   - Correct use of the inhaler and spacer will ensure accurate dose delivery of the drug to Amy's airways.
3. Educate Amy's father about monitoring the effectiveness of the medicine, and how frequently it is required.
   Rationale:
   - This information will be used to determine if Amy requires progression to extra medicines to effectively manage her condition.
4. Schedule a follow-up appointment in 4–6 weeks to review Amy's progress.
   Rationale:
   - If Amy's cough remains, she will require prescription of an inhaled corticosteroid to suppress airway inflammation — refer to AMH (2021a).
5. Provide education on best management of exercise-induced bronchoconstriction in children as advised by the National Asthma Council (2021).
   Rationale:
   - An understanding of the triggers of bronchoconstriction can help minimise the need for medications.

Evaluate outcomes

Amy and her father articulate an appropriate level of understanding of asthma, the triggers and the therapy prescribed to Amy.

Source: Based on the Clinical Reasoning Cycle, Levett-Jones (2013).

MEDICINES MANAGEMENT

Salbutamol

Salbutamol is a beta2 (β_2) agonist bronchodilator therapy used to reverse airway constriction caused by obstructive airways diseases, such as asthma. Asthma is a chronic inflammatory airway disease in which individuals are said to have hypersensitive or hyper-responsive airways. People living with asthma experience periods of reversible inflammation and constriction in the bronchi and bronchioles, which cause breathlessness and a characteristic wheeze. When encountering a trigger (e.g. allergy, infection or stress), mast cells on the walls of the bronchi and bronchioles release several cytokines (chemical messengers) that cause increased mucous production and increased capillary permeability. Very soon the airways become full of mucus and fluid leaking from blood vessels and airflow becomes obstructed. β_2 agonists such as salbutamol stimulate β_2 receptor cells on the walls of the bronchi and bronchioles, causing bronchodilation.

Salbutamol can be inhaled, injected or taken orally. The most common route is via an inhaler, and given its effectiveness in reducing airway constriction it is often referred to by health professionals as a 'reliever'. In emergency situations, salbutamol can be nebulised. A nebuliser forces a jet stream of air or oxygen through a liquid preparation of salbutamol, producing a mist that the patient inhales via a special mask or pipe. While salbutamol is an effective pharmacological treatment, the nurse must be aware of the following side effects, especially when nebulised:

- tachycardia and other arrhythmias
- hand shaking and tremors
- headache
- nervous tension.

Other β_2 agonist therapies include terbutaline, fenoterol and salmeterol.

See Correll et al. (2015).

MEDICINES MANAGEMENT

Corticosteroid therapy

Corticosteroids are potent anti-inflammatory agents that are often used to reduce bronchial hyperactivity in people living with chronic inflammatory airway diseases, such as asthma and **chronic obstructive pulmonary disease**. Corticosteroids reduce airway inflammation and are therefore very effective in the treatment of airway obstruction. Corticosteroids are a first-line treatment for moderate, severe and life-threatening asthma. Common corticosteroids include:

- prednisolone
- hydrocortisone.

Patients taking the above corticosteroids will need careful monitoring as they may cause the following side effects:

- osteoporosis
- diabetes
- mood swings
- weight gain
- increased body hair.

Inhaled corticosteroids are used very effectively for the prophylaxis of asthma and are often referred to as 'preventers' by healthcare professionals. Preparations such as beclamethasone, budesonide and fluticasone are often prescribed for patients living with asthma to be used daily to minimise the potential for exacerbation.

See Correll et al. (2015).

Blood supply

The conduction and respiratory regions of the lungs receive blood from different arteries. Deoxygenated blood is delivered to the lobules via capillaries that originate from the right and left **pulmonary arteries**. Once reoxygenated, blood is sent back to the left-hand side of the heart via one of four **pulmonary veins**, ready to be ejected into **systemic circulation** (see figure 12.7). The conduction region of the lungs receives oxygenated blood from capillaries that stem from the **bronchial arteries**, which originate from the **aorta**. Some of the bronchial arteries are connected to the pulmonary arteries, but most blood returns to the heart via the pulmonary or **bronchial veins**.

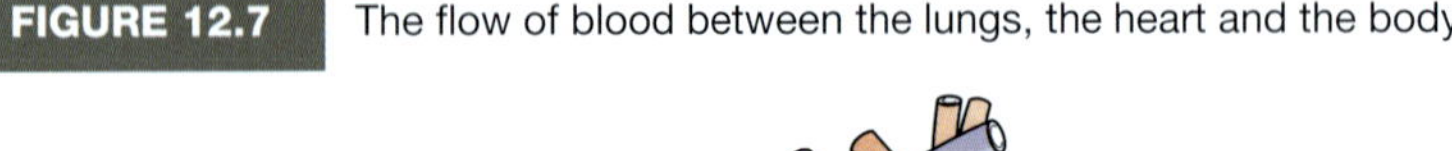

FIGURE 12.7 The flow of blood between the lungs, the heart and the body

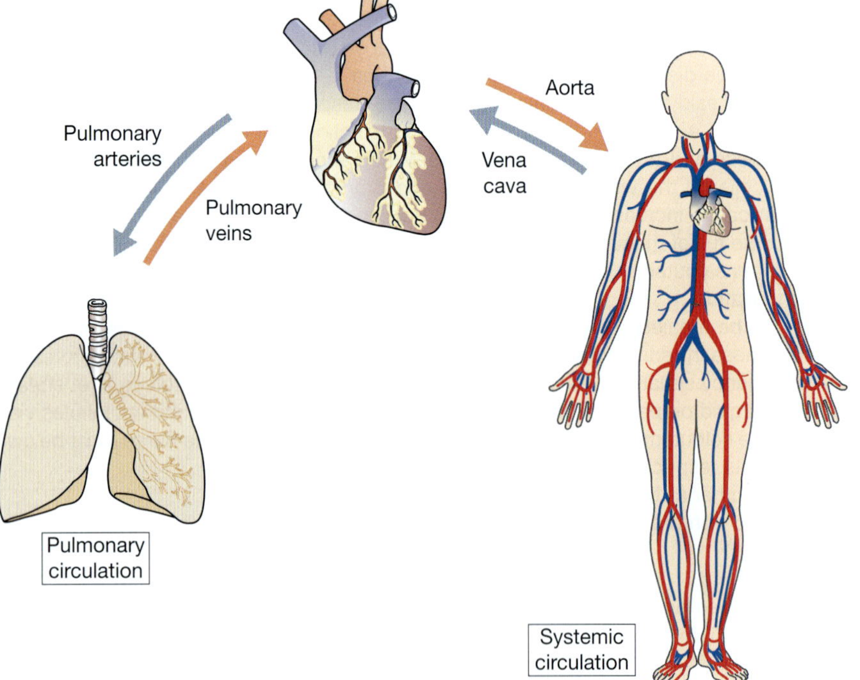

Respiration

The process by which oxygen and carbon dioxide are exchanged between the atmosphere and body cells is called respiration. Respiration follows the following four distinct phases:

- pulmonary ventilation — how air gets in and out of the lungs
- external respiration — how oxygen diffuses from the lungs to the bloodstream and how carbon dioxide diffuses from blood and to the lungs
- transport of gases — how oxygen and carbon dioxide are transported between the lungs and body tissues
- internal respiration — how oxygen is delivered to and carbon dioxide collected from body cells.

The understanding of all four processes is reliant upon the appreciation of a series of gas laws, which are summarised in table 12.1.

TABLE 12.1 Summary of important gas laws

Gas law	Summary	Clinical application
Boyle's law	At a fixed temperature the pressure exerted by gas is inversely proportional to its volume	As the thorax expands, **intrapulmonary pressure** falls below atmospheric pressure
Dalton's law	In a mixture of gases each gas will exert its own individual pressure, as if no other gases are present	Differences in partial pressure govern the movement of oxygen and carbon dioxide between the atmosphere, the lungs and blood
Henry's law	The quantity of gas that will dissolve in a liquid is proportional to its pressure and its solubility	Oxygen and carbon dioxide are soluble in water and are transported in blood. Nitrogen is highly insoluble and, despite accounting for 79% of the atmosphere, very little is dissolved in blood
Fick's law	The rate a gas will diffuse across a permeable membrane will depend upon pressure difference, surface area, **diffusion** distance and molecular weight and solubility	Helps explain how altitude, exercise and respiratory disease can influence the amount of oxygen that is diffused into blood

Source: Adapted from Davies and Moores (2010).

12.2 Pulmonary ventilation

LEARNING OBJECTIVE 12.2 Describe the events of pulmonary ventilation.

The mechanics of breathing

Pulmonary ventilation describes the process more commonly known as breathing. For air to pass in and out of our lungs, a change in pressure needs to occur. Before inspiration the intrapulmonary pressure, the pressure within the lungs, is the same as atmospheric pressure. During inspiration the thorax expands, and the intrapulmonary pressure falls below atmospheric pressure. Because intrapulmonary pressure is now less than atmospheric pressure, the air will naturally enter our lungs until the pressure difference no longer exists. This phenomenon is explained by Boyle's law and Dalton's law. Gases exert pressure, and Boyle's law states that at a fixed temperature the amount of pressure exerted by a given mass of gas is inversely proportional to the size of its container. Larger volumes provide greater space for the circulation of gas molecules, and therefore less pressure is exerted. In smaller volumes the gas molecules are more likely to collide with the walls of the container and exert a greater pressure as a result (see figure 12.8). Dalton's law explains that in a mixture of gases each gas exerts its own individual pressure proportional to its size. For example, atmospheric air contains a mixture of gases. Each individual gas will exert its own pressure dependent upon its quantity. Nitrogen, for example, will exert the greatest pressure as it is the most abundant gas. Collectively, all the gases in the atmosphere exert a pressure, atmospheric pressure, which is 101.3 kPa (kilopascals) at sea level (see table 12.2). On inhalation the thorax expands, intrapulmonary pressure falls below 101.3 kPa and, because air flows from areas of high pressure to low pressure, air enters the lungs (Hickin et al. 2015).

FIGURE 12.8 Boyle's law: the volume of a gas varies inversely with its pressure

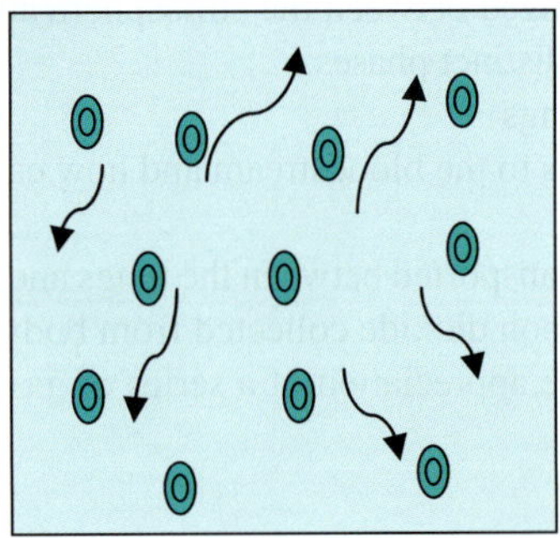

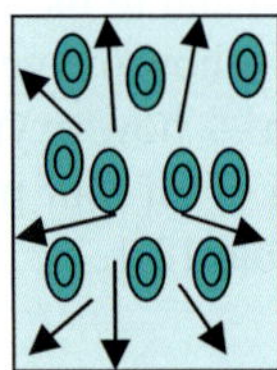

TABLE 12.2 **The proportion of gases that constitute the atmosphere (partial pressures are expressed as P_{gas})**

Gas	Volume (%)	Pressure (KPA)
Nitrogen (P_{N_2})	78.084	79.055
Oxygen (P_{O_2})	20.946	21.218
Carbon dioxide (P_{CO_2})	0.035	0.0355
Argon (PAr)	0.934	0.946
Other gases[a]	0.001	0.001
Total atmospheric pressure (PB)	100	101.3

[a]Neon, helium, methane, krypton, nitrous oxide, hydrogen, ozone, xenon.

Sources: Adapted from Lutgens and Tarbuck (2018); Lumb (2016); and Brimblecombe (1995).

A range of respiratory muscles are used to achieve thoracic expansion during inspiration (see figure 12.9). The major muscles of inspiration are the diaphragm and external intercostal muscles. The diaphragm is a dome-shaped skeletal muscle found beneath the lungs at the base of the thorax. There are 11 external intercostal muscles, which sit in the **intercostal spaces** — the spaces between the ribs. During inspiration the diaphragm contracts downwards, pulling the lungs with it. Simultaneously, the external intercostal muscles pull the rib cage outwards and upwards. The thorax is now bigger than before, and intrapulmonary pressure is reduced below atmospheric pressure as a result. The most important muscle of inspiration is the diaphragm; 75 per cent of the air that enters the lungs is as a result of diaphragmatic contraction. Expiration is a more passive process. The external intercostal muscles and the diaphragm relax, allowing the natural elastic recoil of the lung tissue to spring back into shape, forcing air back into the atmosphere (see figure 12.10).

FIGURE 12.9 The muscles involved in pulmonary ventilation

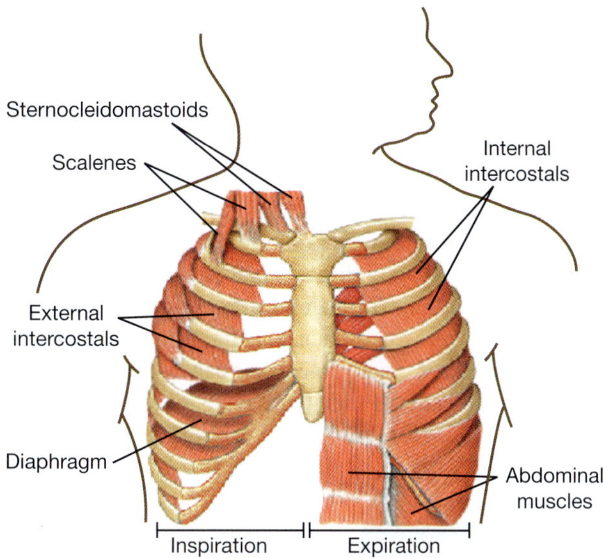

Source: Peate (2017). Reproduced with permission of John Wiley & Sons.

FIGURE 12.10 Movements of inspiration and expiration

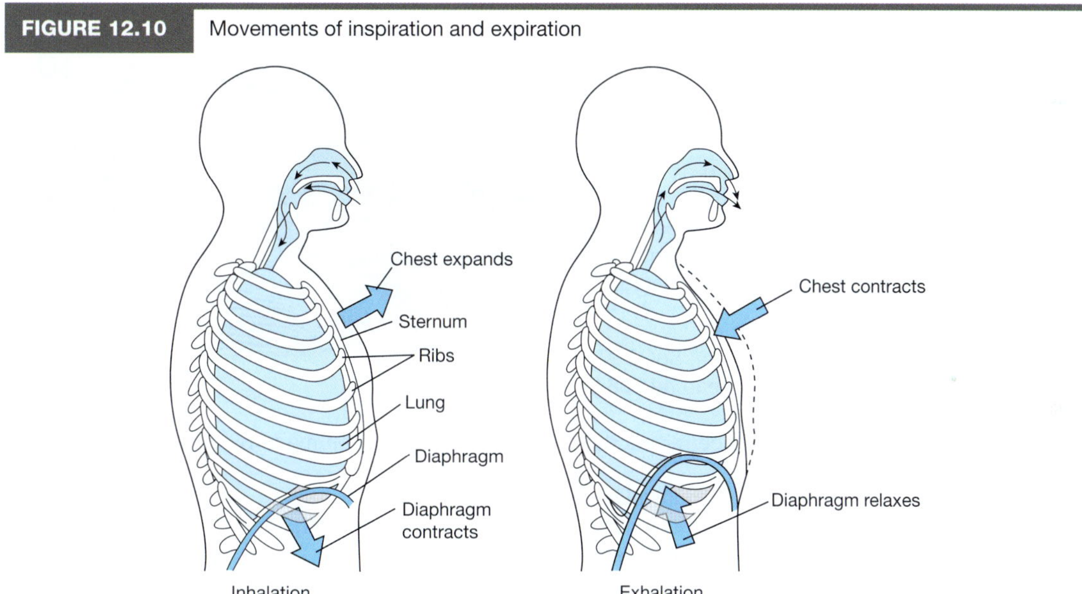

Source: Peate (2017). Reproduced with permission of John Wiley & Sons.

Other respiratory muscles can also be utilised. The abdominal wall muscles and internal intercostal muscles, for instance, are utilised to force air out beyond a normal breath; for example, when playing a musical instrument or blowing out candles on a birthday cake. The sternocleidomastoids, the scalenes and the pectoralis can also be used to produce a deep forceful inspiration. These muscles are referred to as **accessory muscles**, so called because they are rarely used in normal, quiet breathing (Rolfe 2019).

Work of breathing

During inspiration, respiratory muscles must overcome various factors that hinder thoracic expansion. The natural elastic recoil of lung tissue, the resistance to airflow through narrow airways and the surface tension forces at the liquid–air interface in the lobule all oppose thoracic expansion. The energy required by the respiratory muscles to overcome these hindering forces is referred to as work of breathing. The amount of energy expended is kept to a minimum by the ease with which lungs can be stretched. This ease of stretch is called **lung compliance**. Because of lung compliance, an inhalation of around 500 mL of air is achievable without any noticeable effort. Blowing a similar amount of air into a balloon would take a much greater effort. Lung compliance is aided by the production of a detergent-like substance called **surfactant**. Whenever a liquid and gas come into close contact with one another, surface tension is generated. Surfactant reduces the surface tension that occurs where the alveoli meet pulmonary capillary blood flow in the lobule, thereby reducing the amount of energy required to inflate the alveoli. Surfactant is manufactured by type II alveolar cells, found in the alveoli.

Work of breathing is also required to overcome airway resistance. As air flows through the bronchial tree, resistance to airflow occurs as the gas molecules begin to collide with one another in the increasingly narrow airways. Despite these opposing forces, work of breathing accounts for less than 5 per cent of total body energy expenditure. However, many lung diseases can affect lung compliance and airway resistance and, therefore, increase work of breathing. In asthma, for example, airway inflammation reduces the diameter of the airways and increases airway resistance. If the diameter of an airway is halved, resistance increases sixteenfold. Lung diseases that damage lung tissue can also affect lung compliance. Any increase in airway resistance and lung compliance will inevitably increase work of breathing. In acute respiratory disease, work of breathing could account for up to 30 per cent of total body energy expenditure (Levitzky et al. 1990).

CLINICALLY REASONED EPISODE OF CARE

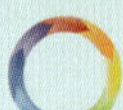

Pneumonia

Consider the patient situation

Howard is a 30-year-old man who has Down syndrome. Howard has been brought into the health clinic by Mike, a care support worker who works at Howard's supported accommodation. He is seen by the nurse practitioner.

Mike is concerned about Howard as his mood has changed significantly over the past week. Instead of being his happy and cheerful self, Howard is much quieter than normal, isn't eating or drinking, and becomes angry and agitated.

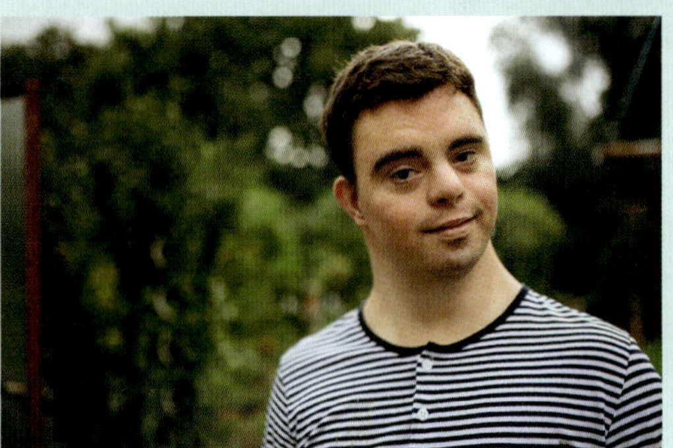

Collect cues and information

- Vital signs: respiratory rate 20 bpm; SpO2 97%; blood pressure 130/80 mmHg; heart rate 88 bpm; temperature 37.9 °C.
- Respiratory assessment:
  - Auscultation — right lower lobe rales (crackling sound thought to be made by air opening closed air spaces)
  - Percussion — dullness over the right lower lobe.
- Pain assessment: Howard reports that it hurts when he takes a deep breath.
- Other information: Howard states that he feels very tired.

Process information

Howard's presentation is indicative of lobar pneumonia.

Pneumonia is an infection of the alveoli and small airways. Inflammation and oedema cause the alveoli to fill with debris and exudate until a solid mass called consolidation is formed. The consolidation can be patchy and spread throughout both lungs or concentrated in one mass, affecting one or more lobes. Symptoms of pneumonia include fever, painful breathing, cough, expectoration of sputum, dehydration and lethargy. Community-acquired pneumonia is most commonly treated in the community, but it can develop into a severe infection, which will require admission to hospital.

Respiratory disease is the most common cause of death in people with a learning disability. This is due to differences in the structure and function of the airways associated with poor muscle tone. Pneumonia is also common in people with Down syndrome, which is thought to be due to their underdeveloped immune system. Pneumonia is treatable with antibiotics, analgesia, bed rest and fluids, but if left untreated, people can develop a severe infection, which could lead to hospital admission. Early detection is key. However, patients with a learning disability often find communicating or understanding their health difficult, which can make accessing health services challenging.

Nursing actions

1. Prescribe a 5-day course of amoxicillin.
   Rationale:
   - This is the first-choice therapy for community-acquired pneumonia — refer to AMH (2021b).
2. Provide education about the safe and effective use of the medicine.
   Rationale:
   - The completion of courses of antibiotics is an important factor in reducing anti-microbial resistance (see NCAS, www.ncas-australia.org).
3. Provide education about general care for the person with pneumonia.
   Rationale:
   - Coughing and deep breathing for ineffective airway clearance is important as the removal of secretions will assist recovery.
   - Rest and appropriate exercise for activity intolerance is important because pneumonia impairs gas exchange and results in reduced carbon dioxide removal and reduced oxygen delivery to tissues. There is an imbalance between oxygen demand and oxygen delivery which reduces energy available to undertake activities of daily living.
   - Adequate fluid intake will assist with liquefying secretions to aid clearance. Fluid intake will assist hydration if the person is experiencing fever.
   - Adequate nutritional intake is important because immunological response increases metabolic (kilojoule) demand.
   - Monitoring for deterioration is required as pneumonia is a common cause of sepsis.

Evaluate outcomes

After 2–3 doses of antibiotic therapy, Howard shows no further deterioration and begins to show an improvement in his health, including increased energy levels and nil pain on inspiration.

On physical examination, Howard has nil adventitious sounds (sounds heard in addition to the expected breath sounds) on auscultation of his lungs and resonance on percussion, as well as a respiratory rate less than 20 bpm and temperature less than 37 °C.

Source: Based on the Clinical Reasoning Cycle, Levett-Jones (2013).

Volumes and capacities

Lung volumes and capacities measure or estimate the amount of air passing in and out of the lungs. Everyone has a **total lung capacity (TLC)**, which is the total amount of air their lungs are capable of housing. Everyone's TLC will be dependent upon their age, sex and height. TLC can be subdivided into a range of potential or actual volumes of air. For example, the amount of air that passes in and out of the lungs during one breath is called the **tidal volume (V_T)**. After a normal, quiet breath the lungs will still have room for a deeper inspiration that could fill the lungs. This potential capacity for inspiration is referred to as **inspiratory reserve volume** (IRV). Likewise, after a normal, quiet breath, there remains the potential for a larger exhalation. This potential capacity of exhalation is referred to as **expiratory reserve volume** (ERV). If tidal volume increases, due to exercise for example, IRV and ERV would be reduced. Tidal volume, IRV and ERV can all be measured. However, because a small volume of air always remains in the lungs — even after maximal exhalation — TLC can only be estimated. This small volume of remaining air is called **residual volume (RV)**. Because RV cannot be exhaled, the total amount of air that could possibly pass in and out of an individual's lungs is a combination of tidal volume, IRV and ERV, which collectively is referred to as **vital capacity** (see figure 12.11).

Other important measures of lung volume include **minute volume (V_E)**, **alveolar minute ventilation** (V_A) and **anatomical dead space** (V_D) (see table 12.3). V_E is the amount of air breathed in each minute and is calculated by multiplying V_T by respiration rate. In health, minute volume is around 6–8 mL per minute. However, only the air that travels beyond the terminal bronchioles will take part in gaseous exchange. For this reason, the air present in the rest of the lungs is referred to as V_D. Therefore, in order to ascertain exactly how much air is available for gaseous exchange, anatomical dead space must be accounted for. V_A is calculated by subtracting anatomical dead space from minute volume, which in health would be approximately 4–6 mL per minute (Hickin et al. 2015).

FIGURE 12.11 Diagrammatic description of the major lung volumes and capacities

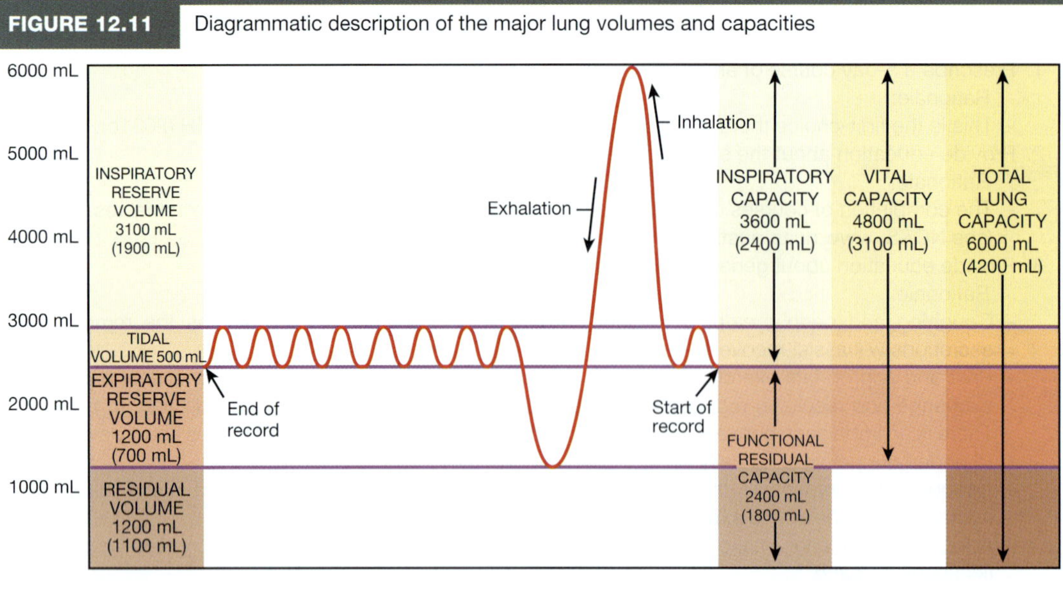

Source: Tortora and Derrickson (2017). Reproduced with permission of John Wiley & Sons.

TABLE 12.3 **Important lung volumes**

Volume	Calculation
Minute volume (V_E)	Tidal volume (V_T) × Respiration rate, e.g. 500 (V_T) × 12 = 6000 mL (V_E)
Alveolar minute ventilation (V_A)	[Tidal volume (V_T) – Anatomical dead space (V_D)] × Respiration rate, e.g. [500 (V_T) – 150 (V_D)] × 12 = 4000 mL (V_A)

Source: Martini and Nath (2018). Reproduced with permission of Pearson Education Limited.

CLINICALLY REASONED EPISODE OF CARE

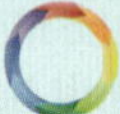

Chronic obstructive pulmonary disease (COPD)

Consider the patient situation

Leonard is a 77-year-old man living with chronic obstructive pulmonary disease (COPD). Recently, Leonard has been experiencing increased levels of breathlessness, fatigue and general feelings of being unwell. Leonard's daughter has made an appointment with the respiratory nurse as she is increasingly concerned about his wellbeing, low mood and general lack of interest in his garden, which is normally his pride and joy.

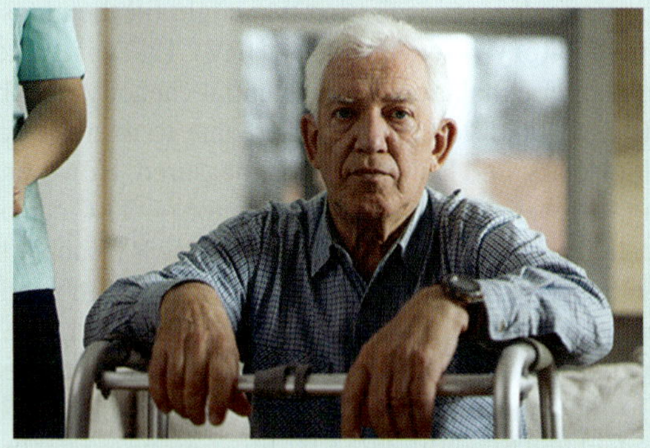

Collect cues and information

- Respiratory assessment: breathlessness (dyspnoea) and reduced exercise tolerance noted, but no signs of infection or exacerbation.
- Mental state assessment: Leonard reports often feeling sad and a loss of interest in 'most things'; he says that he feels as though he has become a burden on his daughter and that he now prefers to stay home more and more.

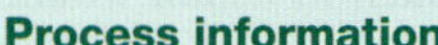

Process information

COPD has been defined as airflow obstruction that is progressive, is not fully reversible and does not change markedly over several months. It has one major cause: smoking. COPD is a term now used to describe the traditional diagnosis of chronic bronchitis or emphysema. People with chronic asthma are also at risk of developing fixed airway obstruction as airways become remodelled over time; these symptoms may be indistinguishable from COPD, and many COPD patients may also have asthma.

Depression is very common in people living with long-term respiratory diseases. However, diagnosing depression in people with COPD can be challenging as many of the symptoms, such as disturbed sleep and lack of appetite, can overlap. One of the main nursing considerations for the management of depression in people living with COPD is the promotion of coping strategies and fostering self-management techniques.

Nursing actions

1. Recommend that Leonard attend pulmonary rehabilitation sessions.
   Rationale:
   - Pulmonary rehabilitation has been positively evaluated and shown to effectively reduce depression and anxiety in patients like Leonard (Lung Foundation Australia 2021b).
   - Pulmonary rehabilitation aims to help people reduce symptoms of breathlessness, manage their condition, increase fitness, reduce frequency of exacerbations and therefore reduce hospital admissions (Lung Foundation Australia 2021b).
2. Recommend peer support programs and groups to connect Leonard with those sharing his lived experience of COPD.
   Rationale:
   - Peer support may 'contribute to giving people hope, which can lead to confidence, self-esteem and ultimately autonomy' and 'help to combat feelings of isolation by connecting people in similar situations and building networks' (Lung Foundation Australia 2021a).

Evaluate outcomes

Leonard reports a reduction in dyspnoea and increased exercise tolerance. He reports feeling less sad and has an increased level of interest in daily life and the activities he used to enjoy.

Source: Based on the Clinical Reasoning Cycle, Levett-Jones (2013).

CLINICAL CONSIDERATIONS

Lung cancer in Indigenous communities: a national health priority

Lung cancer (squamous cell carcinoma and small cell carcinoma) is twice as common in the Aboriginal community than in the non-Indigenous community. This is largely due to the fivefold increase in tobacco exposure in these communities (Davey 2021). Diagnosis and treatment are further complicated due to the remoteness of many Aboriginal communities, entrenched racism, decreased funding and other socioeconomic factors (Davidson et al. 2013). As a national health priority there is a pressing need to reduce the burden of disease in these communities and to address the inequalities that provide barriers to effective management, treatment and prevention of lung cancer.

CLINICAL CONSIDERATIONS

Spirometry and peak flow

Spirometry measures the force and volume of a maximum expiration after a full inspiration. The air the patient forces out is referred to as forced vital capacity (FVC). The volume the patient expires after 1 second is called forced expiratory volume in the first second (FEV_1). By comparing FEV_1 with FVC — the FEV_1 : FVC ratio — the severity of airway obstruction can be ascertained. An FEV_1 : FVC ratio of less than 80 per cent is indicative of obstructive airway disease (Scanlon & Heuer 2017).

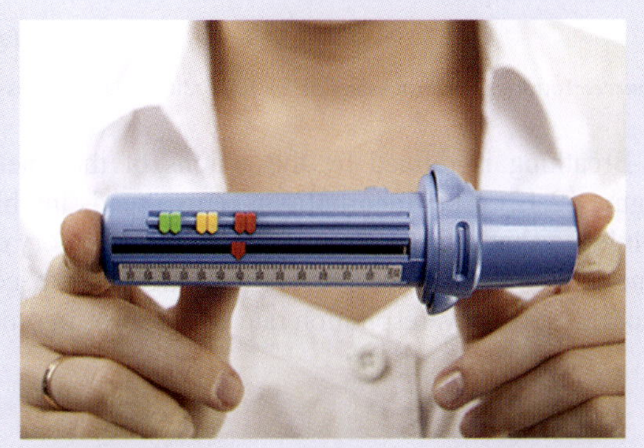

Peak expiratory flow rate (PEFR), or 'peak flow', measures the extent of airway resistance. PEFR is the force of expiration in litres per minute. It measures the patient's maximum expiratory flow rate via their mouth. An inability to meet a predicted value based on age, sex and height could indicate increased airway resistance, as occurs during an asthma attack. PEFR provides a quick and simple assessment of the airways; however, regular peak flow measurements are more revealing than single arbitrary readings, and nurses should be mindful that PEFR is effort dependent (Talley & O'Connor 2017).

12.3 Control of breathing

LEARNING OBJECTIVE 12.3 Explain how the body is able to control the rate and depth of breathing.

The rate and depth of breathing are controlled by the respiratory centres, which are found in the brainstem, within the areas called the **medulla oblongata** and **pons** (see figure 12.12). The rate of breathing is set by the inspiratory centre of the medulla oblongata. The expiratory centre is thought to play a role in forced expiration. Also within the medulla oblongata are specialised **chemoreceptors** that continually analyse carbon dioxide levels within **cerebrospinal fluid**. As levels of carbon dioxide rise, messages are sent via the **phrenic nerve** and **intercostal nerves** to the diaphragm and intercostal muscles instructing them to contract more frequently and harder, increasing respiratory rate and depth. Another set of chemoreceptors found in the aorta and **carotid arteries** analyse levels of oxygen as well as carbon dioxide. If oxygen falls or carbon dioxide rises, messages are sent to the respiratory centres via the **glossopharyngeal nerve** and **vagus nerve**, stimulating further contraction to produce faster, deeper breathing. An increase in CO_2 levels has a more powerful effect on respiratory rate than a reduction in oxygen level.

FIGURE 12.12 The respiratory centres of the brainstem

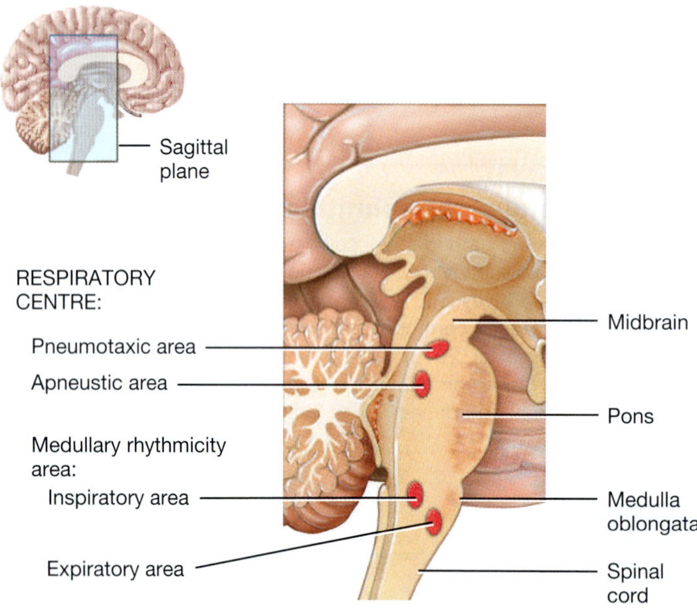

Source: Tortora and Derrickson (2017). Reproduced with permission of John Wiley & Sons.

Breathing is refined by the actions of the pneumotaxic and **apneustic centres** of the pons (see figure 12.12). The **pneumotaxic centre** sends inhibitory signals to the medulla to slow breathing down, while the apneustic centre stimulates the inspiratory centres, lengthening inspiration. Both of these actions fine-tune breathing and prevent the lungs from becoming overinflated. Throughout the day, whether at work, rest or play, respiration rate will change in order to meet the body's oxygen needs.

CLINICAL CONSIDERATIONS

Respiratory rate

In health, an adult's respiratory rate is normally between 12 and 16 respirations per minute. Although breathing is essentially a subconscious activity, the rate and depth of breathing can be controlled voluntarily or even stopped altogether, when swimming underwater for example. However, this voluntary control is limited, as the respiratory centres have a strong urge to keep breathing. Breathing can also be influenced by state of mind. The inspiratory area of the respiratory centres can be stimulated by both the **limbic system** and **hypothalamus**, two areas of the brain responsible for processing emotion. Fear, anxiety or even the anticipation of stressful activities can cause an involuntary increase in the rate and depth of breathing. Other factors that can influence breathing include **pyrexia** and pain. In summary, while the rate and depth of breathing can be consciously altered, subconscious respiratory centre control will override voluntary control in order to maintain homeostasis. Any changes in respiratory rate are, therefore, clinically significant (Hogan 2006).

12.4 External respiration

LEARNING OBJECTIVE 12.4 Discuss the principles of external respiration.

Gaseous exchange

External respiration only occurs beyond the respiratory bronchioles. External respiration is the diffusion of oxygen from the alveoli into pulmonary circulation (blood flow through the lungs) and the diffusion of carbon dioxide in the opposite direction. Diffusion occurs because gas molecules always move from areas of high concentration to low concentration. Each lobule of the lung has its own arterial blood supply; this blood supply originates from the pulmonary artery, which stems from the right ventricle of the heart. The blood present in the pulmonary artery has been collected from systemic circulation and is therefore low in oxygen and relatively high in carbon dioxide. The amount (and therefore pressure) of oxygen in the alveoli is far greater than in the passing arterial blood supply. Oxygen, therefore, moves passively out of the alveoli and into pulmonary circulation and on towards the left-hand side of the heart. Because there is less carbon dioxide in the alveoli than in pulmonary circulation, carbon dioxide transfers into the alveoli ready to be exhaled (see figure 12.13).

FIGURE 12.13 External respiration: exchange of oxygen and carbon dioxide within the lungs

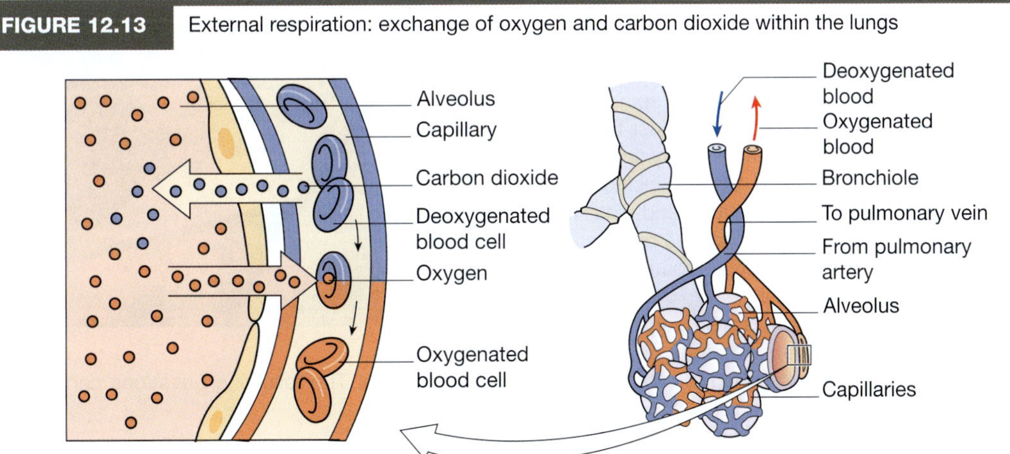

Factors influencing diffusion

It takes approximately 0.25 s for an oxygen molecule to diffuse from the alveoli into pulmonary circulation. However, there are various influencing factors that determine the rate by which oxygen and carbon dioxide diffuse between alveoli and pulmonary circulation. This is best explained using Fick's law of diffusion, which uses an equation to determine the rate of diffusion (see the box on Fick's law of diffusion). According to Fick's law, the rate of diffusion is determined by gas solubility/molecular weight, surface area, concentration difference and membrane thickness. The more soluble a gas is in water, the easier it is for diffusion to occur. Oxygen and carbon dioxide are both soluble in water and therefore easily diffused; indeed, carbon dioxide is 20 times more soluble than oxygen. The most abundant gas in the atmosphere is nitrogen; however, nitrogen is highly insoluble in water and therefore very little diffuses into the bloodstream. The larger the surface area available for diffusion, the greater the rate of diffusion will be. Large inhalations will recruit more alveoli, and a greater rate of diffusion occurs as a result. The greater the gas concentration difference between the alveoli and pulmonary circulation, the faster that gas will diffuse. Because blood travelling towards the alveoli is deoxygenated, there always remains a large difference in concentration of oxygen between the alveoli and pulmonary circulation. However, the rate of diffusion can be enhanced if this concentration difference is increased, by administering prescribed oxygen therapy, for example. The final factor for consideration is membrane thickness. The further the distance gases must travel, the slower the diffusion will be. Conditions such as **pulmonary oedema**, in which fluid collects in the alveoli, result in an increased membrane thickness. The distance between alveoli and pulmonary circulation slows the rate of diffusion.

Fick's law of diffusion

$$J = \frac{S}{\mathrm{wt}_{mol}} \times A \times \frac{\Delta C}{t}$$

where

J is the rate of diffusion

S is the solubility

wt_{mol} is the molecular weight

A is the surface area

ΔC is the concentration difference

t is the membrane thickness.

Source: Hickin et al. (2015).

CLINICAL CONSIDERATIONS

Sputum

Often, the nurse has the responsibility to examine and observe the sputum (sometimes this is called phlegm, secretions or expectorate) that a person may produce. At times the nurse is required to obtain a specimen of the person's sputum for microbiological analysis. The nurse must be able to carry out these important tasks safely and effectively. The skills required to do this include the ability to determine what is sputum and what are oral secretions (saliva), the application of infection control protocols and the ability to document findings and concerns accurately.

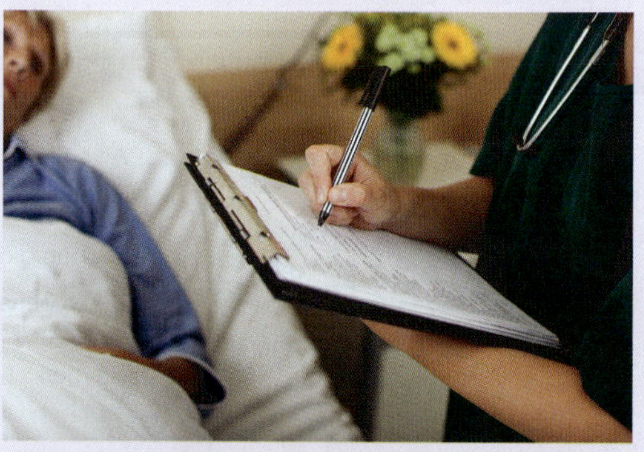

The production of sputum is an important part of a person's immune system. You may be required

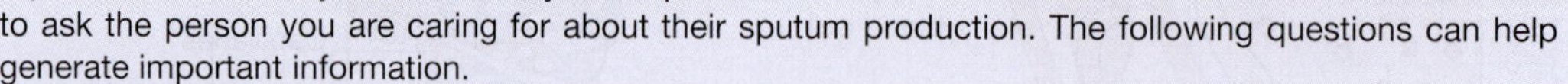

to ask the person you are caring for about their sputum production. The following questions can help generate important information.

- Is there anything that causes (provokes) you to produce sputum?
- When do you produce it?
- How often do you produce it?
- Can you describe it — what does it look like?
- Does your sputum have any smell?
- How much do you produce?
- The sputum you are producing now, has this changed recently? If so, tell me about that.

It can be difficult for the person to provide you with answers concerning their sputum production. You can help them by asking them to measure it in relation to teaspoons, tablespoons or an egg cup. Understanding the sputum produced and describing and reporting its characteristics — for example, the consistency, the amount produced, the odour and its colour — can provide you with much information about the person you are caring for. Also note if the person producing the sputum did this with ease or difficulty, and if, after the specimen was produced, they became breathless or cyanotic.

If the person you are caring for needs to use a sputum pot, you must make sure that it is placed within their reach and that you offer them tissues and a receptacle to dispose of the used tissues. This is particularly important given the potentially infectious nature of sputum, making its safe disposal an important feature of clinical infection control. Care interventions include ensuring that the sputum pot is changed daily and that the lid is firmly closed when it is not in use. Used tissues and sputum pots must be carefully disposed of regardless of the care setting. Disposable, one-use-only sputum pots must be provided. Incineration is needed if sputum is infectious. Local policy and procedures must be adhered to.

MEDICINES MANAGEMENT

Oxygen

Oxygen is a drug, which must be prescribed. Oxygen is used to treat **hypoxaemia**, not breathlessness. There is no evidence that oxygen relieves breathlessness in patients with normal or near normal oxygen saturation readings.

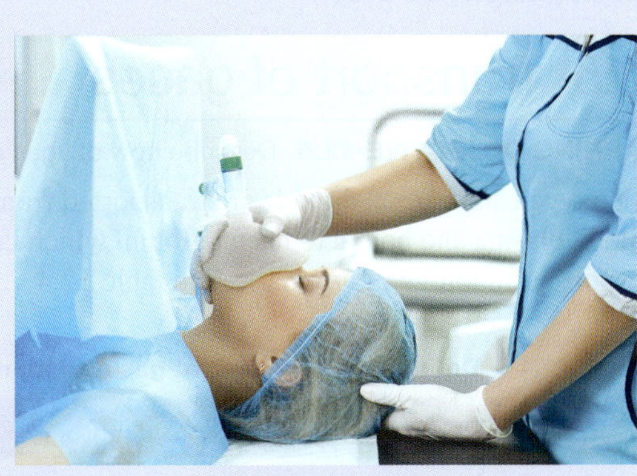

The aim of oxygen therapy is to maintain a normal or near-normal oxygen saturation level and that this should be achieved on the lowest possible concentration of oxygen. The target oxygen saturation levels are 94–98 per cent for acutely ill adults and 88–92 per cent for those at risk of hypercapnic (excess carbon dioxide) failure — that is, patients living with chronic obstructive pulmonary disease.

Oxygen should only be administered by competent clinicians, and each patient receiving oxygen should have their oxygen saturations monitored regularly. For this reason, it is essential that oxygen saturation reading equipment should be within easy reach of patients receiving oxygen therapy.

It is important that nurses use the correct delivery method in order to ensure the patient receives the correct prescription. Many oxygen prescriptions come in the form of a percentage. Venturi masks ensure that the patient receives the correct percentage of oxygen by mixing room air with pure oxygen. Venturi masks are available in the following concentrations — please ensure you include the correct flow rate to ensure the patient receives the correct dose:

24% — 2 L of oxygen per minute
28% — 4 L of oxygen per minute
35% — 8 L of oxygen per minute
40% — 10 L of oxygen per minute
60% — 15 L of oxygen per minute.

Simple oxygen masks do not deliver oxygen with such accuracy. They can deliver between 40 and 60 per cent oxygen with a flow rate of 5–10 L of oxygen per minute. Flow rates of less than 5 L of oxygen per minute may lead to the build-up of carbon dioxide within the mask. Re-breather oxygen masks can deliver up to 90 per cent oxygen and are very effective in emergency situations.

Nasal cannula ensure a steady delivery of oxygen into the nasal cavity. Flow rates between 1 and 4 L of oxygen per minute will provide the patient with 24–40 per cent oxygen. However, the actual volume of oxygen delivered will vary from patient to patient, as mouth breathing may dilute delivery. Flow rates greater than 4 L of oxygen per minute will provide greater concentrations of oxygen, but this may cause nasal dryness and discomfort.

Oxygen in the atmosphere is moist and humidified. Medical oxygen, on the other hand, is dry. Patients on long-term oxygen therapy may encounter nasal or oral dryness, which can cause discomfort. In such situations the team caring for the patient may consider using humidified (passed through water) oxygen.

Documentation and administration must comply with local policy and procedure.

See the Thoracic Society of Australia and New Zealand oxygen guidelines for acute oxygen use in adults (Beasley et al. 2015).

Ventilation and perfusion

External respiration is most effective where there is an adequate supply of both oxygen and blood. In order to ensure a good enough supply of oxygen, the alveoli must be adequately ventilated. In health, a V_A of around 4 L is required. In order to ensure that an adequate supply of blood is reoxygenated, a plentiful supply of blood must be delivered to the lungs from the right ventricle of the heart; in other words, a pulmonary blood flow of around 5 L per minute. This ideal delivery of adequate amounts of both air and blood is referred to as the **ventilation (V_A):perfusion (Q) ratio**. A normal V_A:Q ratio would be 4:5, or 0.8. Any disruption to either ventilation or pulmonary blood flow would lead to a V_A:Q mismatch and less oxygen diffusing into blood. For example, if someone **hypoventilates** and V_A falls below 4 L, then less blood would be reoxygenated. This would be described as a low V_A:Q ratio (i.e. 3:5, or 0.3). Another potential problem would be an inadequate pulmonary blood flow, due to an **embolism**, for example. In such an instance, less blood is available to be reoxygenated and the V_A:Q ratio would become high (i.e. 4:3, or 1.34). However, the V_A:Q ratio differs throughout the lungs and depends upon a person's bodily position (Margereson 2001).

12.5 Transport of gases

LEARNING OBJECTIVE 12.5 Describe how oxygen and carbon dioxide are transported around the body.

Both oxygen and carbon dioxide are transported from the lungs to body tissues in blood. Both gases travel in blood plasma and bound to haemoglobin, which is found within erythrocytes (red blood cells). Key gas transport terminology is summarised in table 12.4.

TABLE 12.4 **Definitions of important gas transport terminology**

Gas transport term	Definition
Oxygen saturation (SaO_2)	The percentage of arterial haemoglobin carrying oxygen molecules SpO_2 = SaO_2 measured by a pulse-oximeter
Partial pressure of arterial oxygen (PaO_2)	The amount of oxygen dissolved in arterial blood plasma measured in kilopascals
Partial pressure of carbon dioxide ($PaCO_2$)	The amount of carbon dioxide dissolved in arterial blood plasma measured in kilopascals
Oxygen capacity	The potential space for oxygen transported by haemoglobin (Hb) per 100 mL of blood Hb × 1.39 = oxygen capacity per 100 mL of blood
Arterial oxygen content (CaO_2)	The actual amount of oxygen in arterial blood carried by haemoglobin per 100 mL of arterial blood Arterial oxygen saturation (SaO_2) × oxygen capacity = oxygen content per 100 mL of arterial blood
Oxygen delivery (DO_2)	The actual amount of oxygen being delivered to body tissues based on cardiac output Arterial oxygen content (CaO_2) × cardiac output = oxygen delivery (DO_2)
Oxygen consumption (VO_2)/ oxygen extraction ratio	The amount of oxygen utilised by body tissues each minute

Transport of oxygen

Most of the oxygen, around 98.5 per cent, is transported attached to haemoglobin in the erythrocyte (red blood cell). Each erythrocyte contains around 280 million haemoglobin molecules and each haemoglobin molecule has the potential to carry four oxygen molecules. The percentage of haemoglobin carrying oxygen is measured as oxygen saturation (SaO_2). The remaining 1.5 per cent of oxygen is dissolved in blood plasma, and is often measured in kilopascals (PaO_2), which in health is around 11–13.5 kPa (82–101 mmHg). The delivery of oxygen, therefore, is also reliant upon the presence of an adequate supply of erythrocytes and haemoglobin. In health, the average male would possess between 15 and 18 g of haemoglobin for every 100 mL of blood. Each gram of haemoglobin can carry approximately 1.3 mL of oxygen. Therefore, a male with a haemoglobin of 16 g per dL would have the capacity to carry 21.44 mL of oxygen for every 100 mL of blood ($16 \times 1.34 = 21.44$). This volume of oxygen is referred to as oxygen capacity. However, it is rare for an individual's haemoglobin to be fully saturated with oxygen. The actual amount of oxygen being transported by haemoglobin is called oxygen content (CaO_2). Oxygen content is determined by oxygen saturation levels. In health, an individual's oxygen saturation level (SaO_2) would normally be between 97 and 99 per cent. Therefore, a male with a haemoglobin of 16 g per dL and an SaO_2 of 98 per cent would have an oxygen content of 21.0 mL (0.98×21.44). CaO_2 only provides the amount of available oxygen per 100 mL of blood. Multiplying CaO_2 by cardiac output will provide the amount of oxygen being delivered to all body tissues each minute. This volume of oxygen is called oxygen delivery (DO_2). In other words, if cardiac output is 5000 mL per minute, the aforementioned individual would have an oxygen delivery (DO_2) of 1050 mL per minute (21.01 mL per 100 mL of blood $\times$ 5000).

The relationship between oxygen attached to arterial haemoglobin (SaO_2) and oxygen dissolved in plasma (PaO_2) is described by the **oxyhaemoglobin dissociation curve** (see figure 12.14). As PaO_2 falls, SaO_2 decreases in an S-shaped curve. If PaO_2 falls as low as 8 kPa (60 mmHg), SaO_2 will remain around 90 per cent. Therefore, natural fluctuations in oxygenation, such as occur when singing, laughing and talking, will not result in dramatic reductions in oxygen saturations. The release of oxygen from haemoglobin can be increased by 2,3-diphosphoglycerate, which is released during hypoxia and high temperatures.

FIGURE 12.14 The oxyhaemoglobin dissociation curve: (a) at normal body temperature, arterial carbon dioxide levels and normal arterial blood pH; (b) with high or low arterial blood pH; (c) with high or low arterial carbon dioxide levels

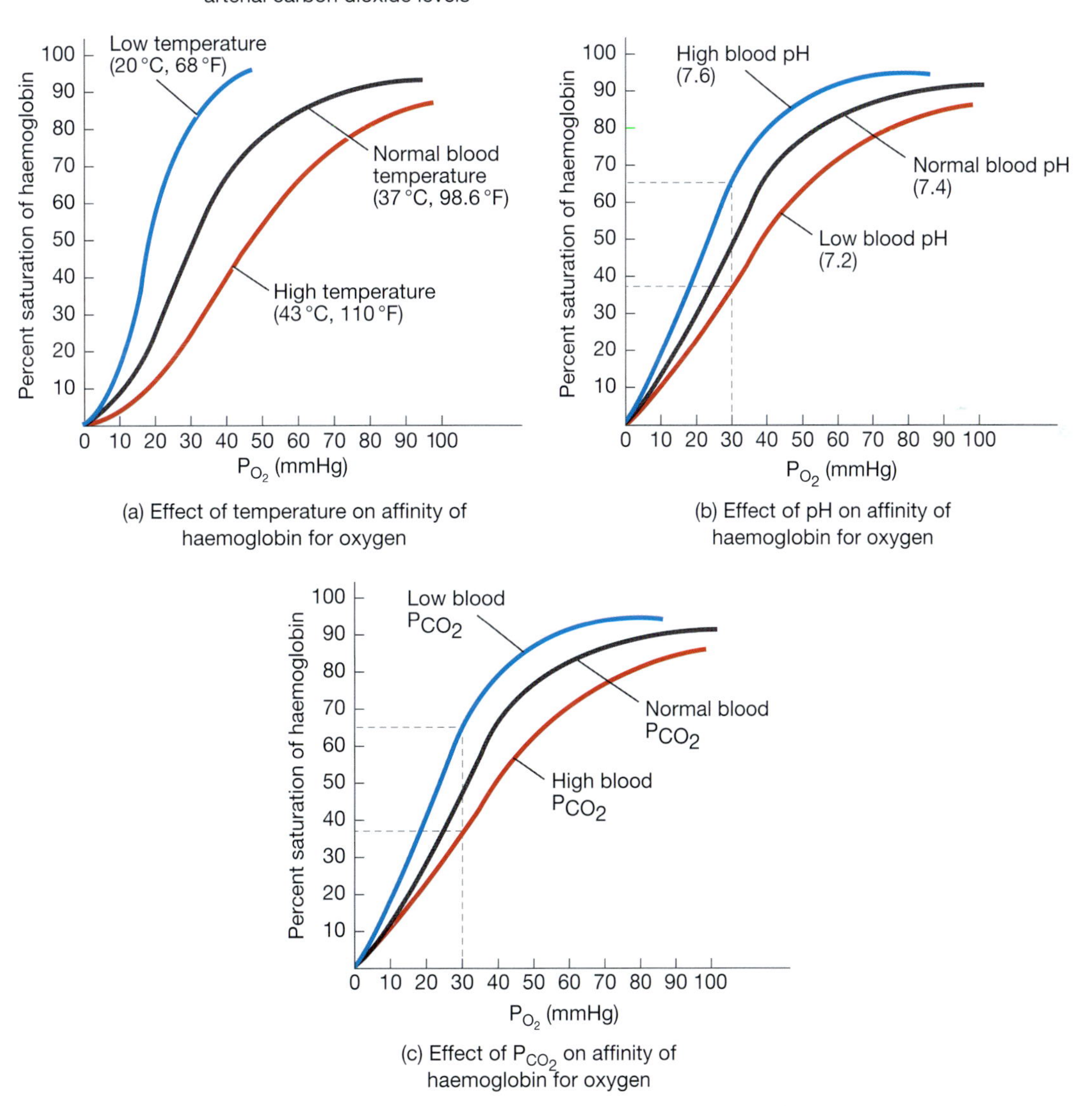

Source: Tortora and Derrickson (2017). Reproduced with permission of John Wiley & Sons.

CLINICAL CONSIDERATIONS

Measuring oxygen levels

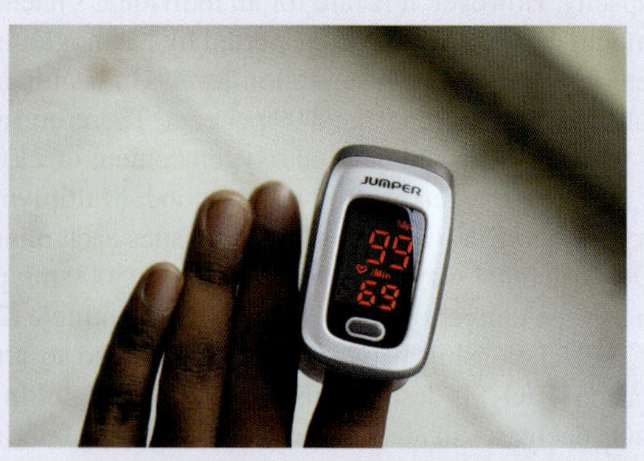

Pulse oximeters measure, via a sensor, the oxygen content of arterial blood flowing through parts of the body that are furthest from your heart (i.e. fingers, feet and earlobes). The oxygen content is expressed as a percentage of haemoglobin carrying oxygen and is called 'oxygen saturation' (SpO_2). In health, SpO_2 should be between 95 and 99 per cent; however, tremors, anaemia, polycythaemia, cold extremities, nail varnish and acrylic nails can all jeopardise an accurate reading. Pulse oximeters also rely on adequate pulsatile blood flow to the area where the sensor is placed. For this reason, SpO_2 should only be used in conjunction with other nursing observations (Clark et al. 2006).

For a more accurate measure, practitioners use an arterial blood gas reading. In such instances a sample of the patient's arterial blood is placed into a blood gas analyser. A printed or visual result is produced within seconds. Arterial blood gas readings provide information on pH, carbon dioxide and bicarbonate as well as oxygen. An oxygen saturation produced via blood gas analysis is referred to as SaO_2. In addition to an oxygen saturation, blood gas analysis measures the pressure exerted by the oxygen dissolved in plasma. In health, arterial oxygen should be around 11–13.5 kPa (82–101 mmHg) and is expressed as PaO_2 (partial pressure of arterial oxygen).

Hypoxia and hypoxaemia

Hypoxia is defined as a lack of oxygen within body tissues. Hypoxaemia is defined as a lack of oxygen within arterial blood. Naturally, hypoxaemia will lead to hypoxia as the tissues are receiving less oxygen. However, as respiration also relies on a fully functioning cardiovascular system, hypoxia can also occur even when arterial blood is fully oxygenated (see table 12.5).

TABLE 12.5 **The major types of hypoxia and their causes**

Type of hypoxia	Cause
Stagnant or circulatory hypoxia	Heart failure, lack of cardiac output, leads to hypoxia
Haemic hypoxia	Lack of blood or haemoglobin (e.g. haemorrhage)
Histotoxic hypoxia	Poisoning (e.g. carbon monoxide inhalation)
Demand hypoxia	May occur when the demand for oxygen is high (e.g. during fever)
Hypoxic hypoxia	Hypoxia as a result of hypoxaemia

Transport of carbon dioxide

Just like oxygen, a small amount of carbon dioxide, around 10 per cent, is transported in plasma. Carbon dioxide is also transported attached to haemoglobin, although only around 30 per cent is transported that way. Nevertheless, haemoglobin has a greater affinity for carbon dioxide than for oxygen. Within the tissues this facilitates the release of oxygen as carbon dioxide is being created. However, as carbon dioxide levels increase (hypercapnia), the amount of oxygen binding to haemoglobin will be reduced. Any build-up of carbon dioxide will affect the oxyhaemoglobin dissociation curve by pulling the natural curve to the right, resulting in a greater risk of hypoxaemia. Conversely, a fall in carbon dioxide (hypocapnia) has the opposite effect (see figure 12.14).

Acid–base balance

The majority of carbon dioxide is transported as bicarbonate ions (HCO_3^-). As carbon dioxide enters the erythrocyte it combines with water to form carbonic acid (H_2CO_3). H_2CO_3 then quickly dissociates into hydrogen ions (H^+) and bicarbonate ions (HCO_3). The formation of H_2CO_3 is very slow in plasma; in the red blood cell this reaction is speeded up by the presence of the enzyme carbonic anhydrase. The newly produced H^+ combines with haemoglobin, whereas HCO_3^- leaves the erythrocyte and enters blood plasma. For this reason, increased and decreased levels of H^+ can also influence the oxyhaemoglobin dissociation curve (see figure 12.14). Within the lungs, as carbon dioxide leaves the pulmonary circulation and enters the alveoli this process is reversed. The transport of carbon dioxide as HCO_3^- is summarised by the following equation:

$$\underset{\text{carbon dioxide}}{CO_2} + \underset{\text{water}}{H_2O} \leftrightarrow \underset{\text{carbonic acid}}{H_2CO_3} \leftrightarrow \underset{\text{hydrogen ions}}{H^+} + \underset{\text{bicarbonate ions}}{HCO_3^-}$$

Note that the arrow symbols indicate that the equation moves both ways. For example, at a tissue level the equation moves from left to right, whereas within the lungs it moves in the opposite direction.

Arterial blood pH is mainly influenced by the levels of H^+. If blood pH falls out of its optimum range of 7.35–7.45, an acid–base imbalance may occur. The respiratory system can help to maintain **acid–base balance** by controlling the expulsion and retention of carbon dioxide. When pH falls (acidosis), respiratory rate increases and more carbon dioxide is expelled. This results in greater amounts of hydrogen ions H^+ and HCO_3^- combining to form carbonic acid (H_2CO_3), which is then broken down to water and CO_2. In other words, the above equation moves from right to left. H^+ levels are reduced, and as a result pH increases. H_2CO_3 is a weak acid and has only a minimal effect on blood pH. If blood pH rises, respiratory rate and depth may fall, resulting in the retention of carbon dioxide. The above equation will now move from left to right and more H^+ will be created.

Internal respiration

Internal respiration describes the exchange of oxygen and carbon dioxide between blood and tissue cells, a phenomenon governed by the same principles as external respiration. Cells utilise oxygen when manufacturing the cells' prime energy source, adenosine triphosphate (ATP). In addition to ATP the cells produce water and carbon dioxide. Because cells are continually using oxygen, its concentration within tissues is always lower than within blood. Likewise, the continual use of oxygen ensures that the level of carbon dioxide within tissue is always higher than within blood. As blood flows through the capillaries, oxygen and carbon dioxide follow their pressure gradients and continually diffuse between blood and tissue (see figure 12.15). The concentration of oxygen in blood flowing away from the tissues back towards the heart is described as deoxygenated. In reality, if measured, the oxygen saturation of venous blood would probably be around 75 per cent. This means that only around 25 per cent of oxygen content (CaO_2) leaves the bloodstream, leaving a plentiful supply. The actual amount of oxygen used by the tissues every minute is referred to as oxygen consumption (VO_2) or oxygen extraction ratio (see table 12.4).

FIGURE 12.15 (a, b) External and internal respiration: oxygen and carbon dioxide follow their pressure gradients (Hb: haemoglobin).

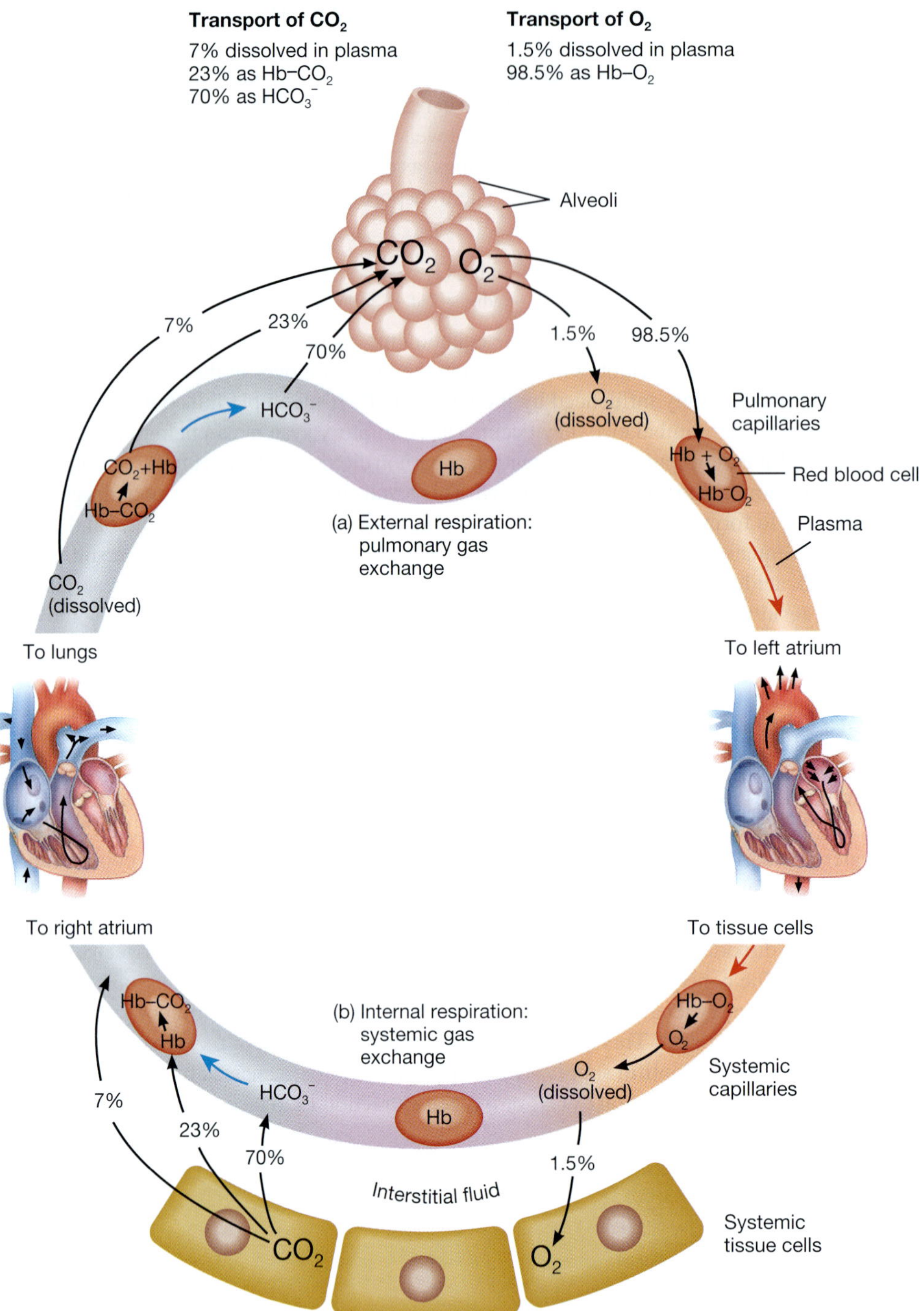

Source: Tortora and Derrickson (2017). Reproduced with permission of John Wiley & Sons.

SUMMARY

This chapter has examined the anatomy and physiology of the respiratory system. The respiratory system is divided into the upper and lower respiratory tracts. The lower respiratory tract consists of lung tissue and major airways. The structures within the lower respiratory tract are fragile and susceptible to infection, the main function of the upper respiratory tract therefore is the protection of the lower respiratory tract. The main function of the lower respiratory tract is the reoxygenation of arterial blood and the expulsion of excess carbon dioxide — a process called respiration. Respiration involves four distinct physiological processes: pulmonary ventilation (breathing), external respiration (gaseous exchange), transport of gases and internal respiration. Only the first two processes are the sole responsibility of the respiratory system, and effective respiration is also reliant upon a fully functioning cardiovascular system.

KEY TERMS

accessory muscles Muscles not normally involved in respiration that can be utilised to increase inspiration.
acid–base balance The mechanisms by which the body maintains arterial blood pH between 7.35 and 7.45.
alveolar minute ventilation The amount of air reaching the respiratory portion of the lungs each minute.
anatomical dead space The portion of the airway not involved in the exchange of oxygen and carbon dioxide (also referred to as the conducting zone).
aorta First major blood vessel of arterial circulation. Emerges from the left ventricle of the heart.
apex The tip or highest point of a structure.
apneustic centres Area of the pons (brainstem), which influences inspiration.
arytenoid cartilage Cartilage tissue involved in the production of the voice.
aspiration The inhalation of solid or liquid substances.
asthma A chronic inflammatory disorder of the lungs. It causes the bronchi and bronchioles to become inflamed and constricted. As a result, airflow becomes obstructed, often resulting in a characteristic wheeze.
atelectasis Complete or partial lung collapse.
bronchial arteries Arteries that deliver oxygenated blood from the aorta to the bronchi and bronchioles.
bronchial tree The lower respiratory tract.
bronchial veins Veins that carry deoxygenated blood from the bronchi and bronchioles to the superior vena cava.
bronchioles Sections of the lower respiratory tract found beyond the tertiary bronchus.
cardiac notch The space between the right and left lung occupied by the heart and its major blood vessels.
carotid arteries Major arteries supplying the brain, stemming from the aorta.
cartilage Type of connective tissue that contains collagen and elastic fibres. Cartilage can stand up to both tension and compression.
cerebrospinal fluid Fluid found within the brain and spinal cord.
chemoreceptors Sensory cells sensitive to specific chemicals.
chronic obstructive pulmonary disease An umbrella term that encompasses chronic bronchitis, emphysema and chronic asthma — respiratory diseases which obstruct airflow.
cilia Hair-like extensions to the plasma membrane.
clavicle Anatomical term for the collarbone.
conduction region Section of the airways which plays no part in the exchange of oxygen and carbon dioxide (also referred to as anatomical dead space).
corniculate cartilage Cartilage tissue involved in the production of the voice.
cricoid cartilage Ring of cartilage that forms the lower part of the larynx (voice box).
cricothyroid ligament Tissue that connects the thyroid cartilage and the cricoid cartilage, the main structures found in the larynx (voice box).
cuneiform cartilage Cartilage tissue involved in the production of the voice.
diaphragm Concave respiratory muscle that separates the lungs and the abdomen.

diffusion The passive movement of molecules or ions from a region of high concentration to low concentration until a state of equilibrium is achieved.
embolism Blockage of a blood vessel by a foreign substance or blood clot.
epiglottis Leaf-shaped piece of cartilage that sits atop the larynx.
ethmoid bones Sponge-like bones found in the skull. Form part of the nasal septum.
expectorate To cough up and spit out mucus or sputum.
expiratory reserve volume The potential capacity for exhalation beyond a normal breath out.
external respiration The process by which oxygen and carbon dioxide are exchanged between the lungs and blood.
fauces The opening into the pharynx from the oral cavity.
glossopharyngeal nerve Cranial nerve IV — nerve that communicates with tongue and pharynx. Also transmits information on oxygen and carbon dioxide levels.
goblet cells Mucus-secreting cells found in epithelial tissue.
hypothalamus Region of the diencephalon area of the brain. Responsible for the maintenance of homeostasis.
hypoventilates Decreased ventilation — lack of air entering the alveoli.
hypoxaemia A reduced amount of oxygen within arterial blood.
hypoxia A reduced amount of oxygen within the tissues.
inspiratory reserve volume (IRV) The potential capacity for inspiration beyond a normal breath in.
intercostal nerves Nerves that link the respiratory centre in the brainstem with the intercostal muscles.
intercostal spaces The anatomical spaces found between the ribs.
internal respiration The process by which oxygen is exchanged for carbon dioxide within the tissues.
intrapulmonary pressure The pressure exerted by all the gases present within the lungs.
laryngopharynx The lower section of the pharynx (throat).
larynx The physiological term for the voice box.
limbic system Part of the functional brain, which processes emotion.
lingual tonsils Tonsils found underneath the tongue.
lobes Distinct regions of the lungs. There are three lobes in the right lung and two in the left lung.
lobule Minute portion of lung tissue served by its own capillary.
lower respiratory tract All respiratory passages found below the larynx.
lung compliance The ease with which the lungs can be inflated.
lymph nodules Egg-shaped masses of lymph tissues that provide an immune response.
lymph vessels Vessels that carry lymphatic fluid. Part of the lymphatic system which forms part of the immune system.
meatuses Three passageways found within the nasal cavity.
medulla oblongata Area of the brainstem.
minute volume (V_E) The amount of air breathed in one minute.
nasal cavity Anatomical space within the nose.
nasal conchae Bones found within the nasal cavity.
nasal septum Structure that divides the nose into two nostrils.
nasopharynx The upper section of the pharynx (throat).
non-keratinised stratified squamous epithelium Cuboid or columnar-shaped cells that line and protect wet surfaces such as the mouth, oesophagus, epiglottis, tongue and vagina.
oesophagus Tubular vessel that carries food and liquid from the pharynx to the stomach.
olfactory Pertaining to the sense of smell.
oropharynx The middle section of the pharynx (throat).
oxyhaemoglobin dissociation curve An S-shaped curve that describes the relationship between the volume of oxygen attached to haemoglobin and the amount of oxygen dissolved in plasma.
palatine tonsils Tonsils found towards the rear of the oral cavity. Usually visible when the mouth is open.
parietal pleura Protective membrane which attaches the walls of the thorax to the lungs.
pharyngeal tonsil Tonsil that sits on the back wall of the pharynx. Also known as the adenoid.
pharynx Passageway for food and air, which links the nasal and oral cavity with the larynx. More commonly called the throat.
phrenic nerve Nerve that links the diaphragm to the respiratory centre in the brainstem.
pleural space The minute space between the visceral and parietal pleura.
pneumotaxic centre Portion of the medulla oblongata (brainstem) that influences inspiration.

pons Area of the brainstem.
pseudostratified ciliated columnar epithelium Covering or lining of internal body surface that contains cilia and mucus-secreting goblet cells.
pulmonary arteries Arteries that carry deoxygenated blood from the right-hand side of the heart towards the lungs.
pulmonary oedema A condition characterised by the leakage of fluid into the alveoli.
pulmonary veins Veins that carry oxygenated blood from the lungs back to the left-hand side of the heart.
pulmonary ventilation The process by which air enters and exits the lungs (breathing).
pyrexia Elevated temperature associated with fever.
residual volume (RV) A small amount of air that permanently remains in the lungs.
respiratory regions The portion of lung tissue involved in the exchange of oxygen and carbon dioxide.
sternum Flat bone which forms part of the thoracic cage. Protects the heart and lungs. Commonly referred to as the breastbone.
surfactant A detergent-like substance manufactured by cells of the alveoli, which reduces surface tension and increases lung compliance.
systemic circulation The flow of blood from the left ventricle and right atrium delivering oxygen to and collecting carbon dioxide from body tissues.
thoracic cage Framework of bones, which consists of the ribs, sternum (breastbone) and vertebrae (spine).
thorax The body trunk above the diaphragm and below the neck.
thyroid cartilage The outer wall of the larynx (voice box).
tidal volume (V_T) The volume of air that passes in and out of the lungs during one breath.
tonsils Lymph nodules found within the upper respiratory tract. They form part of the body's defence.
total lung capacity (TLC) The maximum amount of air that a person's lungs can accommodate.
tracheostomy A procedure in which an incision is made in the trachea to facilitate breathing.
transport of gases The process by which oxygen and carbon dioxide are delivered between the lungs and the tissues.
upper respiratory tract All structures of the respiratory system situated between the oral and nasal passageways and the larynx.
vagus nerve Cranial nerve X — major nerve in parasympathetic function. Also transmits information on oxygen and carbon dioxide levels.
ventilation (V_A): perfusion (Q) ratio The ratio of blood and air delivery to the lungs every minute. Ideally 4 L of air to 5 L of blood.
vestibule The space inside the nasal cavity, just inside the nostrils.
visceral pleura Protective membrane that lines the lungs.
vital capacity The maximum potential for inspiration and expiration, measured in litres.
vomer Triangular-shaped bone that forms the base of the nasal cavity.

CONDITIONS

The following is a list of conditions that are associated with the respiratory system. Take some time and write notes about each of the conditions. You may make the notes taken from textbooks or other resources (e.g. people you work with in a clinical area), or you may make the notes as a result of people you have cared for. If you are making notes about people you have cared for, you must ensure that you adhere to the rules of confidentiality.

Asthma
Chronic obstructive pulmonary disease

(continued)

Pneumoconiosis

Lung cancer

Cystic fibrosis

REFERENCES

Australian Institute of Health and Welfare (2020) Australia's children: asthma prevalence among children. www.aihw.gov.au/reports/children-youth/australias-children (accessed 23 January 2021).

Australian Medicines Handbook (2021a). https://amhonline.amh.net.au/chapters/respiratory-drugs/drugs-asthma-chronic-obstructive-pulmonary-disease/asthma (accessed 23 January 2021).

Australian Medicines Handbook (2021b). https://amhonline.amh.net.au/chapters/anti-infectives/tables/respiratory-infections-table (accessed 23 January 2021).

Beasley, R., Chien, J., Douglas, J., Eastlake, L., Farah, C., King, G., Moore, R., Pilcher, J., Richards, M., Smith, S. and Walters, H. (2015) Thoracic Society of Australia and New Zealand oxygen guidelines for acute oxygen use in adults: 'swimming between the flags'. *Respirology* 20(8): 1182–1191.

Brimblecombe, P. (1995) *Air Composition and Chemistry,* 2nd edn. Cambridge: Cambridge University Press.

Chang, A.B., Grimwood, K., Mulholland, E.K. and Torzillo, P.J. (2002) Bronchiectasis in Indigenous children in remote Australian communities. *Medical Journal of Australia* 177(4): 200–204.

Clark, A.P., Giuliano, K. and Chen, H. (2006) Pulse oximetry revisited: 'but his O_2 sat was normal!' *Clinical Nurse Specialist* 20(6): 268–272.

Correll, P.K., Poulos, L.M., Ampon, R., Reddel, H.K. and Marks, G.B. (2015) *Respiratory medication use in Australia 2003–2013: treatment of asthma and COPD. Cat. no. ACM 31.* Canberra: AIHW.

Davey, R.X. (2021) Health disparities among Australia's remote-dwelling Aboriginal people: a report from 2020. *JALM* 126: 125–141.

Davidson, P.M., Jiwa, M., Digiacomo, M.L., McGrath, S.J., Newton, P.J., Durey, A.J., Bessarab, D.C. and Thompson, S.C. (2013) The experience of lung cancer in Aboriginal and Torres Strait Islander peoples and what it means for policy, service planning and delivery. *Australian Health Review* 37(1): 70–78.

Davies, A. and Moores, C. (2010) *The Respiratory System: Basic Science and Clinical Conditions,* 2nd edn. Edinburgh: Churchill Livingstone.

Hickin, S., Renshaw, J. and Williams, R. (2015) *Crash Course: Respiratory System,* 4th edn. Edinburgh: Mosby.

Hogan, J. (2006) Why don't nurses monitor the respiratory rates of patients? *British Journal of Nursing* 15(9): 489–492.

Levett-Jones, T. (2013). *Clinical Reasoning: Learning to Think Like a Nurse.* Pearson Australia.

Levitzky, M.G., Cairo J.M. and Hall, S.M. (1990) *Introduction to Respiratory Care.* London: W.B. Saunders.

Lumb, A.B. (2016) *Nunn's Applied Respiratory Physiology,* 8th edn. Edinburgh: Elsevier.

Lung Foundation Australia (2021a) Peer support overview. https://lungfoundation.com.au/patients-carers/support-services/peer-support (accessed 23 January 2021).

Lung Foundation Australia (2021b) Pulmonary rehabilitation. https://lungfoundation.com.au/health-professionals/clinical-information/pulmonary-rehabilitation (accessed 23 January 2021).

Lutgens, F.K. and Tarbuck, E.J. (2018) *The Atmosphere: An Introduction to Meteorology,* 14th edn. New York: Pearson.

Margereson, C. (2001) Anatomy and physiology. In Esmond, G. (ed.), *Respiratory Nursing.* Edinburgh: Baillière Tindall.

Martini, F.H. and Nath, J.L. (2018) *Fundamentals of Anatomy and Physiology,* 11th edn. Harlow: Pearson.

McDonald, V.M., Hiles, S.A., Jones, K.A., Clark, V.L. and Yorke, J. (2018) Health-related quality of life burden in severe asthma. *Medical Journal of Australia* 209(S2): S28–S33.

McGrath, B. (2014) *Comprehensive Tracheostomy Care: The National Tracheostomy Safety Project Manual.* Chichester: John Wiley & Sons, Ltd.

National Asthma Council (2021) Managing exercise-induced bronchoconstriction in children www.asthmahandbook.org.au/clinical-issues/exercise/eib/management/children (accessed February 2021).

Ochs, M., Nyengaard, A.J., Knudsen, L. Voigt, M., Wahlers, T., Richter, J. and Gundersen, H.J. (2004) The number of alveoli in the human lung. *American Journal of Respiratory and Critical Care Medicine* 169: 120–124.

Peate, I. (2017) *Fundamentals of Applied Pathophysiology: An Essential Guide for Nursing Students,* 3rd edn. Oxford: John Wiley & Sons, Ltd.

Rolfe, S. (2019) The importance of respiratory rate monitoring. *British Journal of Nursing* 28(8): 504–508.

Scanlon, C.L. and Heuer, A.J. (2017) *Wilkin's Clinical Assessment in Respiratory Care,* 8th edn. St Louis: Elsevier.

Talley, N.J. and O'Connor, S. (2017) *Clinical Examination: A Systematic Guide to Physical Diagnosis,* 8th edn. Chatswood: Elsevier.

Tortora, G.J. and Derrickson, B.H. (2017) *Principles of Anatomy and Physiology,* 15th edn. Hoboken, NJ: John Wiley & Sons, Inc.
Wheatley, I. (2018) Respiratory rate 3: How to take an accurate measurement. *Nursing Times* 114(7): 21–22.

FURTHER READING

AUSTRALIAN LUNG FOUNDATION

https://lungfoundation.com.au

The Australian Lung Foundation website provides a wealth of information for patients withrespiratory disease.

THE THORACIC SOCIETY OF AUSTRALIA AND NEW ZEALAND

www.thoracic.org.au

The Thoracic Society of Australia and New Zealand website provides a range of information and clinical guidance that is based on best available evidence. The guidance is essential for all health professionals who wish to provide gold-standard care for their respiratory patients.

ACKNOWLEDGEMENTS

Photo: © ChaNaWiT / Shutterstock.com
Photo: © Terry Vine / Blend Images LLC
Photo: © Halfpoint / Shutterstock.com
Photo: © Photographee.au / Shutterstock.com
Photo: © Denis Mironov / Shutterstock.com
Photo: © ESB Professional / Shutterstock.com
Photo: © Serhii Bobyk / Shutterstock.com
Photo: © Yasin Hasan / Shutterstock.com

CHAPTER 13

The reproductive systems

TEST YOUR PRIOR KNOWLEDGE

- Where does fertilisation occur?
- What is the inner layer of the uterus called?
- What is the role of the hormone testosterone?
- A woman is most fertile at what stage of the menstrual cycle?
- What is the function of the prostate gland and the testes?

LEARNING OUTCOMES

After reading this chapter you will be able to:

13.1 describe the male reproductive organs and understand the role and functions of the male reproductive system

13.2 provide an overview of the role and functions of the various hormones associated with the male reproductive system

13.3 describe the female reproductive organs and understand the role and functions of the female reproductive system

13.4 provide an overview of the role and functions of the various hormones associated with the female reproductive system

13.5 outline the phases of the uterine cycle.

Body map

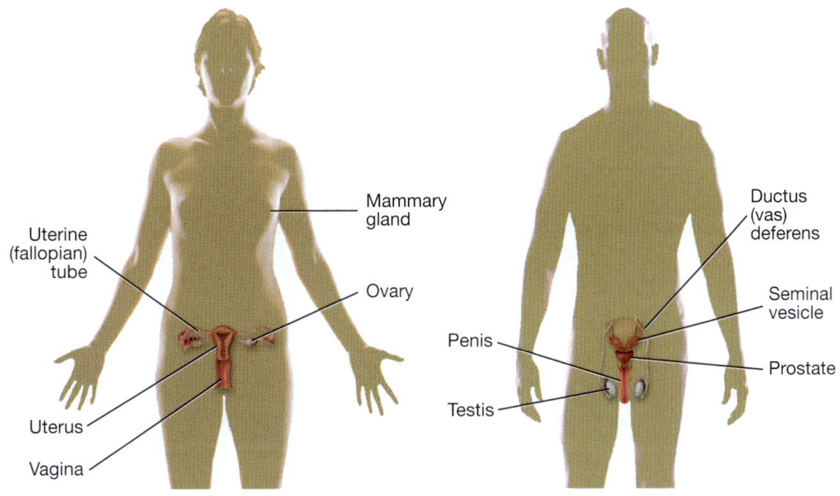

Introduction

Reproduction is one of the most important and essential attributes of living organisms; all living organisms reproduce to create new individuals of their own kind, thereby giving rise to the next generation. Although not necessary for survival of the individual, reproduction is essential for survival of the species. Human reproduction is sexual; the male **gamete** (sperm) and female gamete (**ovum**) combine at fertilisation resulting in a new and unique combination of parental genes. The structure and function of the reproductive systems is a major point of difference between men and women.

The gametes are produced by **gonads**; **testes** produce sperm in the male, and the **ovaries** produce ova in the female. The gonads also produce **hormones** required for the development, upkeep and performance of the reproductive organs and other sexual characteristics. Fertilisation occurs inside the body of the female to form a zygote, which goes on to develop into an embryo and then a **foetus**. The female reproductive organs take on the responsibility for nurturing the developing foetus until birth. After birth, the mother continues to provide nutritional support for the child through lactation and breastfeeding.

This chapter provides an overview of the structure and functions of the male and female reproductive systems, which includes the gonads and a number of accessory organs and structures. The male reproductive system includes the testes, accessory ducts, accessory glands and the **penis**. The female reproductive system includes the **uterus**, Fallopian tubes, ovaries, **vagina**, **vulva** and mammary glands.

13.1 The male reproductive system

LEARNING OBJECTIVE 13.1 Describe the male reproductive organs and understand the role and functions of the male reproductive system.

The male reproductive system, being located partially outside of the body cavity, is more visually obvious than the female reproductive system; there are, however, internal and external structures. Testes are the male gonads that, working in unison with other body systems (e.g. the neuroendocrine system), produce the hormones that are essential for development of the male reproductive tract, sexual behaviour, performance and actions. The male reproductive tract shares some structures with the urinary system including the **urethra** and penis. The male reproductive system is shown in figure 13.1.

FIGURE 13.1 The male reproductive system

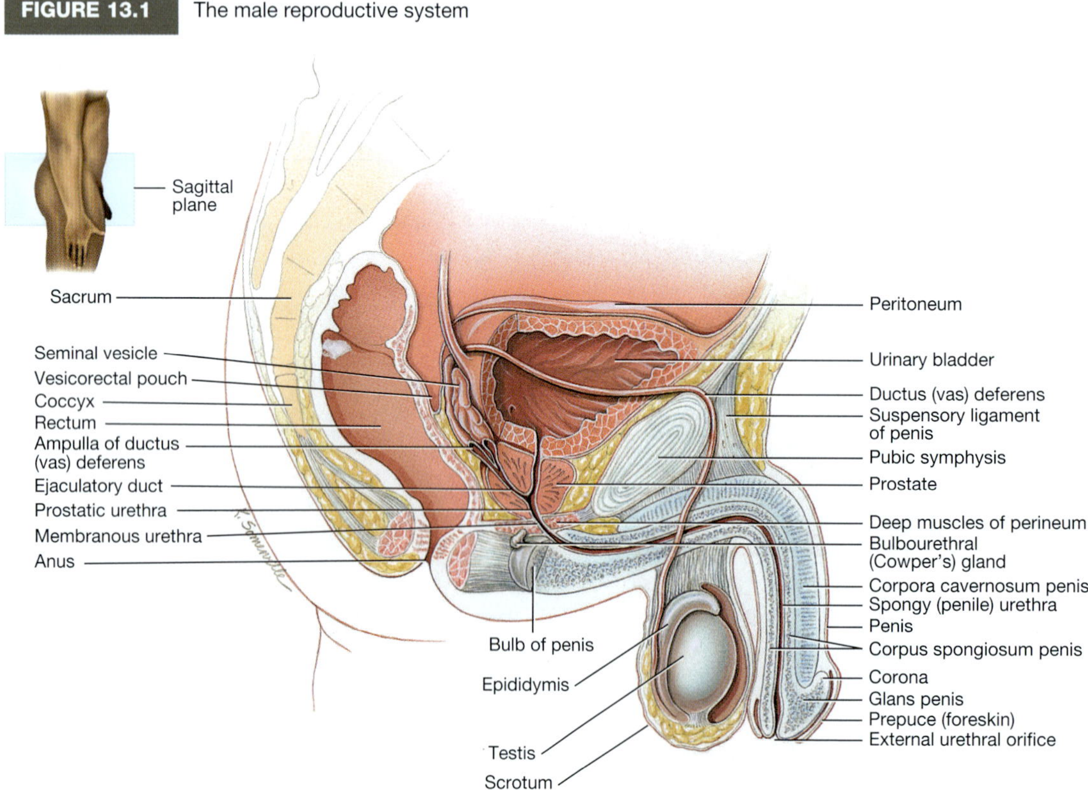

Source: Tortora and Derrickson (2009). Reproduced with permission of John Wiley & Sons.

The functions associated with the male reproductive system include:

- production, maintenance and transport of sperm (the male reproductive cells)
- production of the fluid components of **semen**
- ejection of sperm from the penis
- production and secretion of the male sex hormones.

The major structures of the male reproductive system include the testes and other external genitalia (penis and **scrotum**); a number of ducts responsible for the transportation of the sperm from the testes to the penis (epididymis and **vas deferens**) and outside the body (ejaculatory duct and urethra); and two seminal vesicles, bulbourethral glands and the prostate gland.

The scrotum

The scrotal sac can be likened to a loose bag of skin suspended from the root of the penis. From the outside, the scrotum usually appears as a single sac of skin that is separated into two portions by a ridge in the middle known as the raphe. From the inside, the scrotum is divided into two sacs separated by a scrotal septum with a testicle in each (see figure 13.2).

FIGURE 13.2 The scrotum and testes

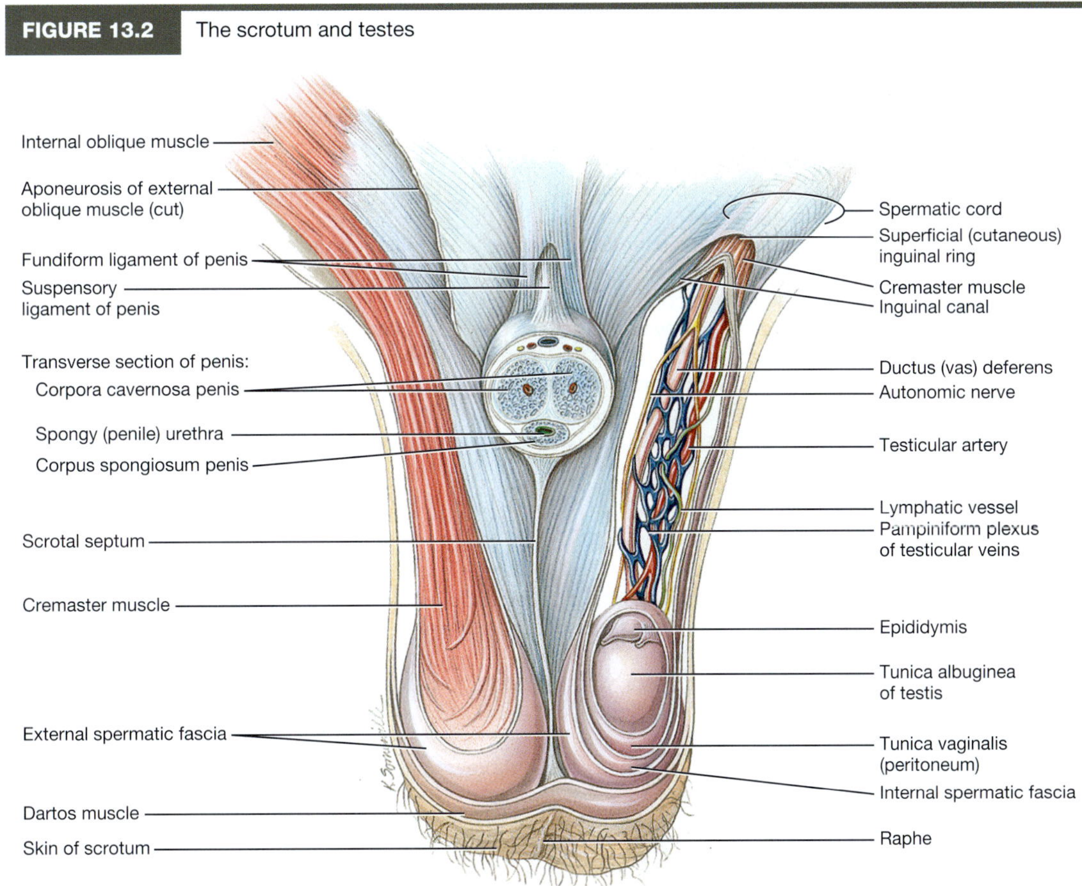

Anterior view of scrotum and testes and transverse section of penis

Source: Tortora and Derrickson (2009). Reproduced with permission of John Wiley & Sons.

The location of the scrotum outside of the pelvic cavity, and its association with muscle fibres, assists with maintaining the temperature of the testes at approximately 2–3 °C below core body temperature, which is the most favourable temperature for sperm production. The cremaster and dartos muscles respond to changes in temperature to regulate the temperature of the testes. In response to cold temperatures, the cremaster muscle contracts, moving the testes upwards towards the body where more body heat can be absorbed. Contraction of the dartos muscle tightens the scrotum around the testes to reduce heat loss. Conversely, when cooling is required, the cremaster muscle loosens and the testes are subsequently moved away from the heat of the body and cool down. The dartos muscle also loosens allowing for increased heat exchange and cooling.

CLINICALLY REASONED EPISODE OF CARE

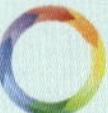

Testicular torsion

Consider the patient situation

Anil, a 17-year-old, is playing squash. During the game, his opponent's racquet hits him in the groin with some force, which winds Anil. He falls to the ground but recovers in order to continue playing the game.

After the game, Anil goes to have a shower. The pain in his scrotal region is excruciating. He then notices his left testicle is swollen and very tender to touch. He starts vomiting and his lower abdomen 'feels like it is going to burst'. He is taken to the accident and emergency department.

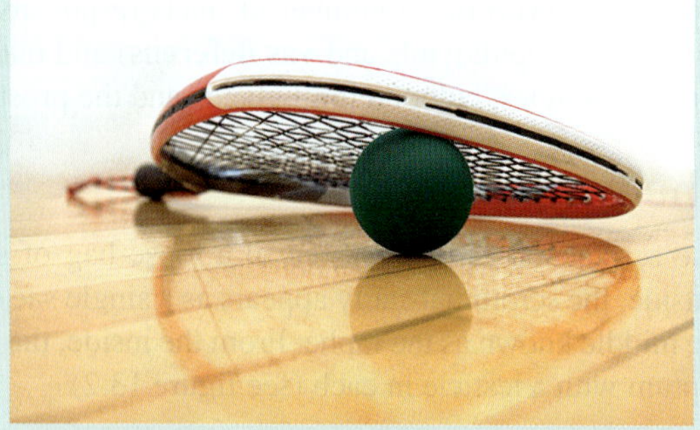

Collect cues and information

Anil is examined by a nurse practitioner who tries to manually rotate what he thinks is torsion of the left testicle.

However, the pain is so intense that a colour Doppler examination is performed to observe blood flow in the scrotum. The findings confirm the nurse's diagnosis of left testicular torsion.

Process information

Testicular torsion is twisting of the spermatic cord. Review figure 13.2 to see how this will result in compression of the arteries that supply the testicle.

This can happen spontaneously but most often occurs when trauma ruptures the gubernaculum, which is the tissue anchoring the testis to the scrotum. The testis then becomes mobile and is able to rotate, simultaneously twisting the spermatic cord.

Loss of blood supply (ischaemia) to any tissue causes pain and inflammation. Prolonged ischaemia will result in necrosis (death of tissue), which means that testicular torsion is a medical emergency if function and fertility are to be preserved. Complications of an untreated or delayed torsion include infarction of the testicle along with subsequent atrophy, infection and cosmetic deformity. There is evidence that the contralateral testis (the testis on the opposite side) can also be negatively affected after unilateral testicular torsion and detorsion (Shimizu et al. 2016).

Nursing actions

1. Administer prescribed pain relief and an antiemetic.
   Rationale:
   - There is a physiological and moral imperative to treat acute pain (Schug et al. 2020, p. iii).
   - Intense pain can result in severe nausea as chemicals released by the pain pathways can trigger emetic (vomiting) centres in the brain.
2. Provide perioperative nursing care for Anil who will undergo detorsion and **orchidopexy** (securement of the testicle to the scrotal wall).
   Rationale:
   - Detorsion will restore blood supply to the testis and prevent necrosis and infarction. Securement of the testis will reduce the risk of reoccurrence.

Evaluate outcomes

Anil reports reduction of pain level and nausea. He recovers from the surgical procedure with no complications.

Source: Based on the Clinical Reasoning Cycle, Levett-Jones (2013).

The testes

During the development of male foetuses **in utero**, the testes first appear in the abdominal cavity, then before birth they traverse the **inguinal canal** and enter the scrotal sac. The testes are suspended in the scrotal sac, hanging one on either side of the penis, usually with one hanging lower than the other. Production of viable sperm requires a temperature approximately 2 °C lower than the normal body temperature, and for this reason the testes in the scrotal sac are external to the body.

The key functions of the testes are to:

- produce sperm (spermatozoa)
- produce the male sex hormones (e.g. **testosterone**).

The testes are small oval-shaped organs measuring approximately 5 cm long and 2.5 cm wide with a layer of serous fibrous **connective tissue** surrounding them. The three layers that cover the testes are the:

1. tunica vaginalis
2. tunica albuginea
3. tunica vasculosa.

The testes are divided into approximately 250–300 compartments or lobules. Inside each compartment is a collection of tightly coiled hollow tubes known as the seminiferous tubules, which are the site of sperm production (see figure 13.3). There are spaces located between the tubules, and in these spaces is a cluster of cells called the interstitial or **Leydig cells** that synthesise and secrete the hormone testosterone, as well as other **androgens**.

FIGURE 13.3 A testicle demonstrating seminiferous tubules

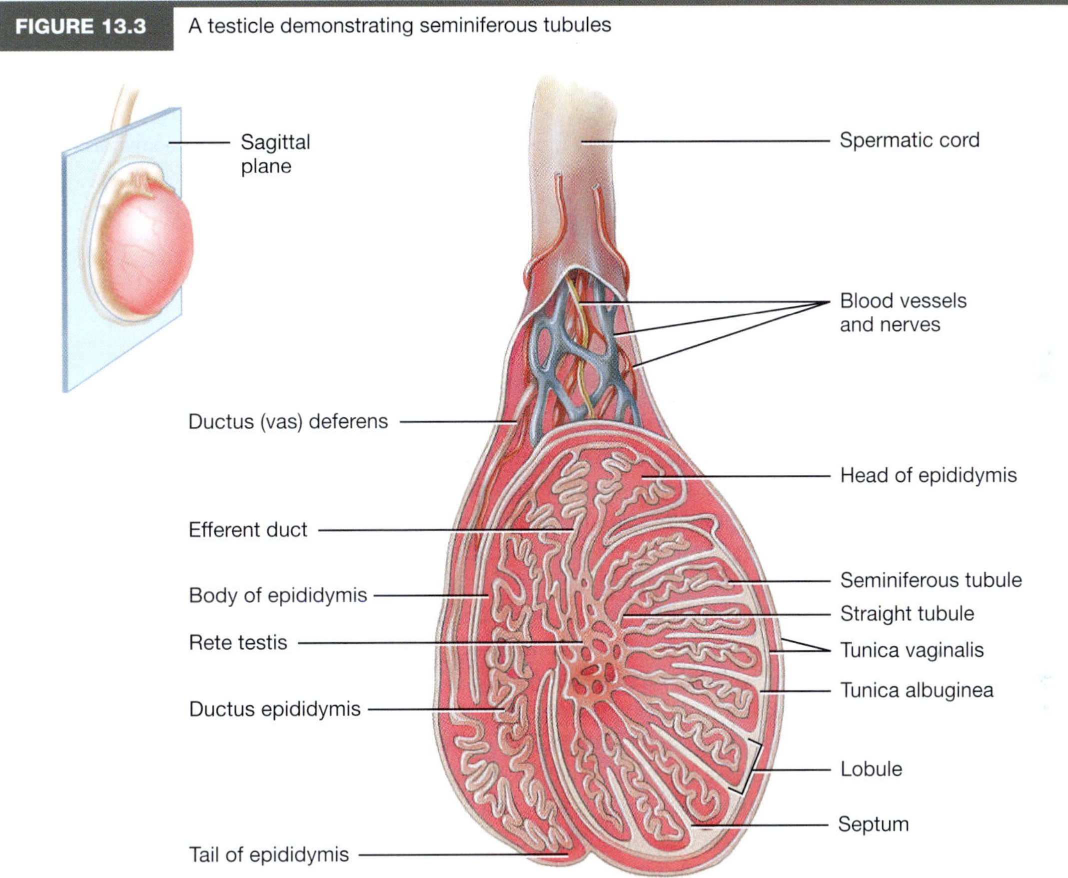

Source: Tortora and Derrickson (2009). Reproduced with permission of John Wiley & Sons.

The seminiferous tubules have an outer layer of smooth muscle and an inner layer composed of Sertoli cells and developing sperm cells. Sperm cells, in their various stages of development, slowly make their way through the spaces between adjacent Sertoli cells until they are released into the lumen of the seminiferous tubule. Sertoli cells nurture and control the developing sperm, and are therefore sometimes referred to as the nurse cells or mother cells. Some of the key functions of Sertoli cells include stimulation of sperm proliferation and differentiation, provision of nutrients for developing sperm, **phagocytosis** of defective sperm, and secretion of fluid and proteins into the lumen of the seminiferous tubule.

Spermatogenesis

Sperm production occurs in the seminiferous tubules of the testes and is called **spermatogenesis** (see figure 13.4). Spermatogenesis usually commences around puberty and continues for the rest of a man's life, with most men producing 50–200 million sperm every day.

FIGURE 13.4 Stages of spermatogenesis

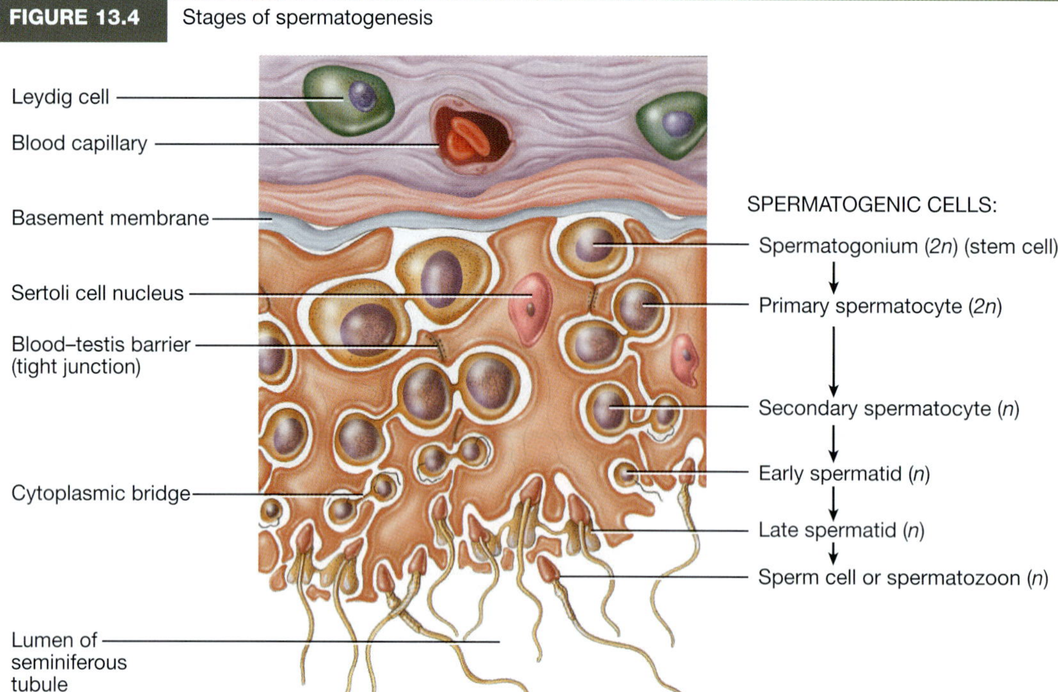

Source: Tortora and Derrickson (2009). Reproduced with permission of John Wiley & Sons.

Spermatogenesis is a complex activity that takes approximately 74 days in humans. Spermatogenesis begins with the mitotic division of spermatogonia, undifferentiated stem cells that are located close to the basement membrane. Spermatogonia contain the diploid ($2n = 46$) number of chromosomes and divide continually by mitosis to produce primary spermatocytes that are also diploid ($2n = 46$). Some spermatogonia remain close to the basement membrane of the seminiferous tubule, acting as a pool of undifferentiated stem cells for future sperm production.

Primary spermatocytes (with 46 chromosomes) then undergo the first division of **meiosis** to form **haploid** secondary spermatocytes with 23 chromosomes each. Each secondary spermatocyte then undergoes a second meiotic division to form spermatids. As a result of these meiotic divisions, each primary spermatocyte (containing 46 chromosomes) has gone on to produce four spermatids, each containing 23 chromosomes. The final stage of spermatogenesis is the differentiation of round spermatids into elongated sperm cells that are released into the lumen of the seminiferous tubule.

The sperm cells have 23 chromosomes each, which is half the number of a normal human cell. When the sperm unites with an ovum (also containing 23 chromosomes) at fertilisation, the result of conception (conceptus) will have the required 46 chromosomes.

CLINICAL CONSIDERATIONS

Cryptorchidism

Undescended testes (cryptorchidism) is a common childhood condition where the child is born without both testes in the scrotal sac. In the majority of cases no action will be required, as the testes will migrate down into the scrotum during the first 3–6 months. There are, however, a small number of cases where the testes remain undescended unless treated. Current recommendations are that a diagnosis of congenital cryptorchidism should be confirmed at 3–6 months of age and orchidopexy done at 6–12 months of age (Holland et al. 2016).

In utero the testes develop inside the child's abdomen prior to slowly moving down into the scrotal sac from about 2 months before birth. The exact reason why some boys are born with undescended testes is not fully understood, but risk factors that have been identified include a relationship with low birth weight, being born prematurely (before the 37th week of pregnancy) and having a family history of undescended testicles.

Boys with undescended testicles may have problems associated with fertility, and there is also an increased risk of developing testicular cancer.

Sperm

There are approximately 200 million sperm produced every day (Tortora & Derrickson 2012). Each sperm cell is equipped with structural specialisations that allow it to reach the site of fertilisation and penetrate the ovum; the elongated tail assists with movement, the midpiece contains the mitochondria necessary to provide energy, and the head contains the genetic material and is covered by an acrosomal cap that contains enzymes to assist the sperm with penetration of the egg cellular and non-cellular coverings that surround the ovum (see figure 13.5).

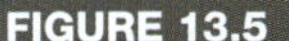
FIGURE 13.5 Components of a sperm

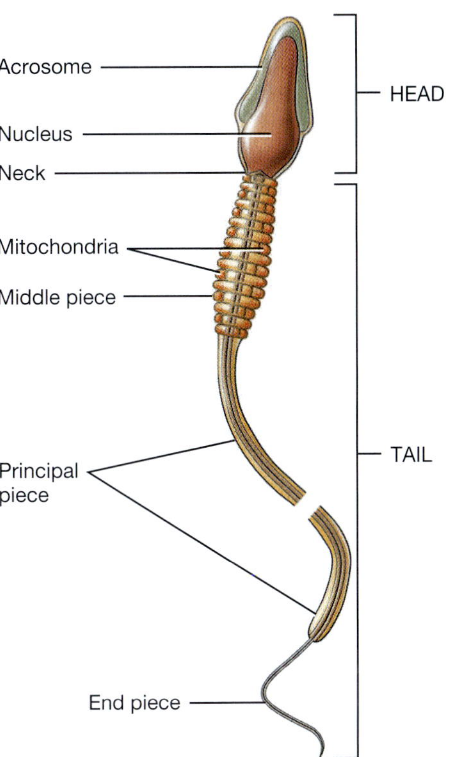

Source: Tortora and Derrickson (2009). Reproduced with permission of John Wiley & Sons.

After sperm are released into the lumen of the seminiferous tubules, they move towards the **rete** testes, a network of interconnected tubes that empty into a single tube called the epididymis.

Epididymis

The epididymis is a long and highly coiled duct that is loosely attached to the testis; it is lined with pseudostratified columnar epithelium and surrounded by a layer of smooth muscle. If it were fully uncoiled, each human epididymis would stretch to approximately 5 metres in length. As sperm travel, they travel through highly coiled duct that constitutes the epididymis and they develop the ability to move spontaneously and actively (motility).

Transport of sperm through the epididymis usually takes 1–2 weeks in humans and is required in order for sperm to develop motility and the ability to fertilise an ovum. Sperm can also be stored in the epididymis and then released via peristaltic activity as the smooth muscle contracts during sexual arousal, moving the sperm along the epididymis into the vas deferens. Sperm stored in the epididymis can remain there for several weeks; those sperm that are not ejaculated are eventually reabsorbed.

The epididymis leads to the larger and more muscular duct called the vas deferens.

The vas deferens, spermatic cord and ejaculatory duct

The vas deferens (plural vasa deferentia), also referred to as the ductus deferens, is less convoluted than the epididymis and has a larger diameter, and the length of the vas deferens is approximately 45 cm (Tortora & Derrickson 2012). This tube contains ciliated epithelium and is surrounded by a thick muscle layer. The vas deferens carries sperm from the scrotum, through a slit-like passage in the abdominal wall called the inguinal canal, to the abdominal cavity. Between the scrotal sac and the inguinal canal is the spermatic cord, a supporting structure consisting of the vas deferens as it ascends through the scrotum, blood vessels and nerves (Colbert et al. 2012).

There are two vasa deferentia, one arising from each testicle, that join at the base of the urinary bladder. Each vas deferens merges with one seminal vesicle to form the ejaculatory ducts. The ejaculatory ducts connect to the urethra, where the sperm will be ejaculated during orgasm as a result of sexual intercourse or masturbation. After the sperm are ejaculated it is unusual for it to survive longer than 48 hours within the female reproductive tract.

The seminal vesicles and prostate gland

The seminal vesicles and prostate gland also secrete most of the fluids that are found in the ejaculate. The fluid secreted is a milky alkaline fluid providing a friendly environment for sperm to survive, preparing them for survival in the acidity of the vagina.

There are a pair of seminal vesicles, each about 5 cm in length, that lie at the base of the urinary bladder. Secretions from the seminal vesicles are released into the ejaculatory duct and account for approximately two-thirds of the volume of semen. The secretions include fructose (a sugar) as an energy source for sperm and a clotting protein that helps semen to coagulate after ejaculation.

The prostate is a single doughnut-shaped gland approximately the size of a walnut, measuring about 4 cm. It goes around the urethra under the urinary bladder and is made of 20–30 glands enclosed in smooth muscle (Marieb 2018).

The prostate consists of three distinct zones:

- the central zone
- the peripheral zone
- the transition zone.

Secretions of the prostate gland comprise approximately one-third of the volume of the semen; the fluid helps sperm motility and to maintain viability. Prostatic fluid is slightly acidic (**pH** 6.5). Prostatic secretions enter the urethra via a number of ducts during ejaculation.

The penis

The penis is the male copulatory organ. The penis encloses the urethra and is a highly vascular organ. This organ is the passageway for excretion of urine as well as the ejaculation of semen. The penis has a shaft and a tip known as the glans, and in the uncircumcised male this is covered by the prepuce (also called the foreskin). The attached portion of the penis is known as the root, and the freer moving part is called the shaft or the body.

The penis is cylindrical in shape, composed of three cylindrical masses of tissues surrounded by fibrous tissue called the tunica albuginea. There are two masses of corpora cavernosa, and the corpus spongiosum which contains the spongy urethra (see figure 13.6).

The penis is usually flaccid and hangs down, but during sexual excitation it becomes erect (an erection), swollen, engorged with blood, firmer and straighter. The erection reflex depends upon stimulation of the parasympathetic nervous system and can be incited by sight, touch, pressure, sounds, smells or visions of a sexual encounter. Following parasympathetic stimulation, the penis becomes erect as a result of blood filling erectile tissue in the corpora cavernosa and corpus spongiosum, permitting the penis to penetrate the vagina and deposit sperm (ejaculation) as close to the site of fertilisation as possible.

When ejaculation has occurred, the arterioles vasoconstrict and the penis becomes flaccid.

FIGURE 13.6 The anatomy of the penis

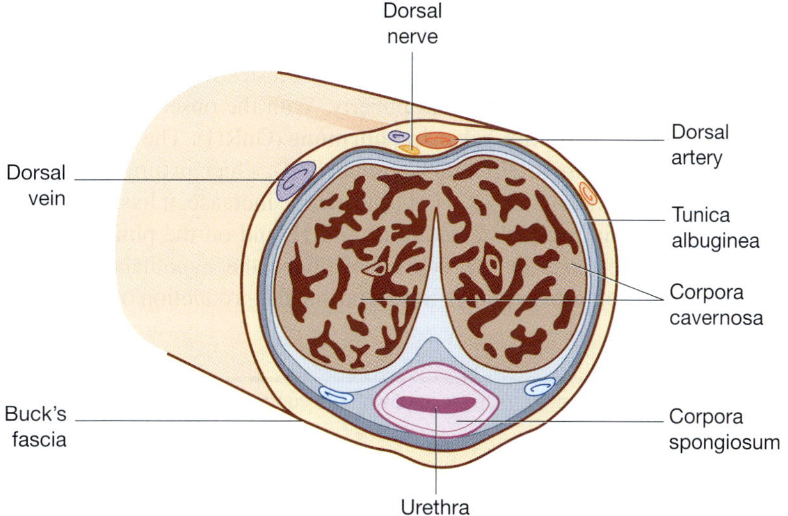

Source: Peate (2009). Reproduced with permission of John Wiley & Sons.

MEDICINES MANAGEMENT

Erectile dysfunction

Erectile dysfunction occurs when a man cannot get or maintain an erection that allows sexual activity with penetration. There are a number of treatments for this condition. One works by preventing the action of a chemical in the body called phosphodiesterase type 5. Viagra (sildenafil) is one example; it improves the blood flow to the penis following sexual stimulation. Before taking sildenafil, the prescriber needs to know if the person has:

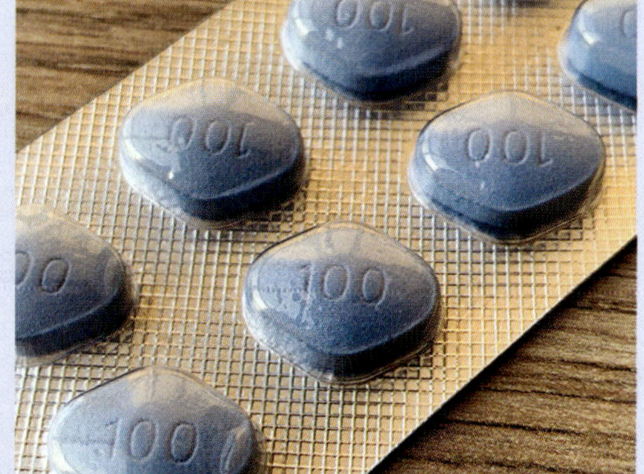

- any disease, injury or deformity of the penis
- any heart or blood vessel disease
- a gastric condition that causes bleeding
- an eye condition causing loss of vision
- hypotension or angina
- liver or kidney problems
- had a stroke or a heart attack
- sickle-cell disease
- ever had an allergic reaction to sildenafil or to any other medicine.

Sildenafil should be taken as prescribed: one (25–100 mg) tablet should be taken 1 h before the man plans to have sex. The medication can be taken before or after food, but may take longer to work if taken with food. Sildenafil should not be taken more frequently than once a day.

See McMahon (2019); and Australian Medicines Handbook (2019).

13.2 Hormonal control of male reproduction

LEARNING OBJECTIVE 13.2 Provide an overview of the role and functions of the various hormones associated with the male reproductive system.

Testicular functions, including sperm production, are under hormonal control.

The male sex hormones are known as androgens. The majority of androgens are produced in the testes, although the cortical region of the adrenal gland is also responsible for producing a small amount.

Testosterone is the main androgen produced by the testes. This hormone is essential for the growth and maintenance of the male sexual organs as well as the secondary sex characteristics (e.g. pitch of voice, musculature and body hair) and for effective spermatogenesis. It also encourages metabolism, growth of muscles and bone, as well as libido (sexual desire).

Apart from a small amount of testosterone secreted by the testes in utero, testosterone levels remain low throughout childhood, until the male reaches puberty. With the onset of puberty the hypothalamus intensifies its secretion of **gonadotrophin-releasing hormone** (GnRH). The release of GnRH stimulates the **anterior** pituitary gland to release **luteinising hormone** (LH), which in turn stimulates the Leydig cells in the testis to produce testosterone. As the levels of testosterone increase, it has a negative feedback effect on the hypothalamus resulting in reduced secretion of GnRH, and on the pituitary resulting in reduced secretion of LH. This negative feedback mechanism involving the hypothalamus, pituitary and testes controls the levels of secretion of testosterone in the blood and the production of sperm (spermatogenesis) (see figure 13.7).

FIGURE 13.7 Negative feedback system associated with the control of testosterone in the blood

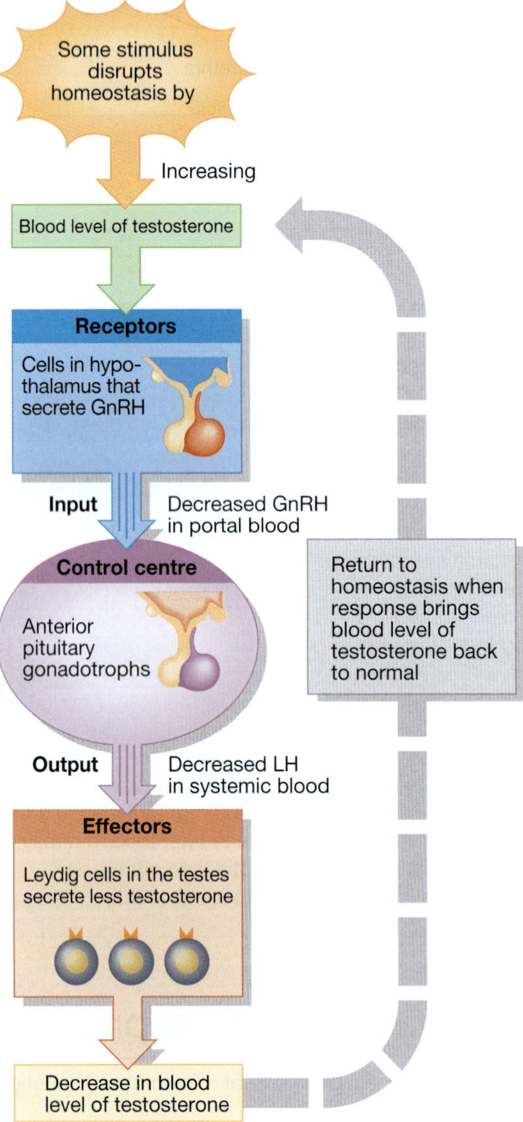

Source: Tortora and Derrickson (2009). Reproduced with permission of John Wiley & Sons.

13.3 The female reproductive system

LEARNING OBJECTIVE 13.3 Describe the female reproductive organs and understand the role and functions of the female reproductive system.

The female reproductive system is designed to produce ova, receive the penis during intercourse and the sperm that has been ejaculated, store, contain and nourish a foetus, and feed the newborn after birth with breastmilk. Usually, each month, a woman's body (during puberty to **menopause**) prepares itself to become pregnant. If pregnancy does not happen then a menstrual period occurs and the cycle recommences.

The organs of the female reproductive system include the ovaries, Fallopian tubes (oviducts), uterus, vagina, and the external genitalia known collectively as the vulva.

The breasts are also a part of the female reproductive organs. Unlike in men, the urethra and urinary **meatus** are not part of the reproductive organs in women; nevertheless, they are very close in proximity and, as such, health problems that may affect one can often affect the other. Figure 13.8 demonstrates the location of the female reproductive organs.

FIGURE 13.8 The female reproductive system

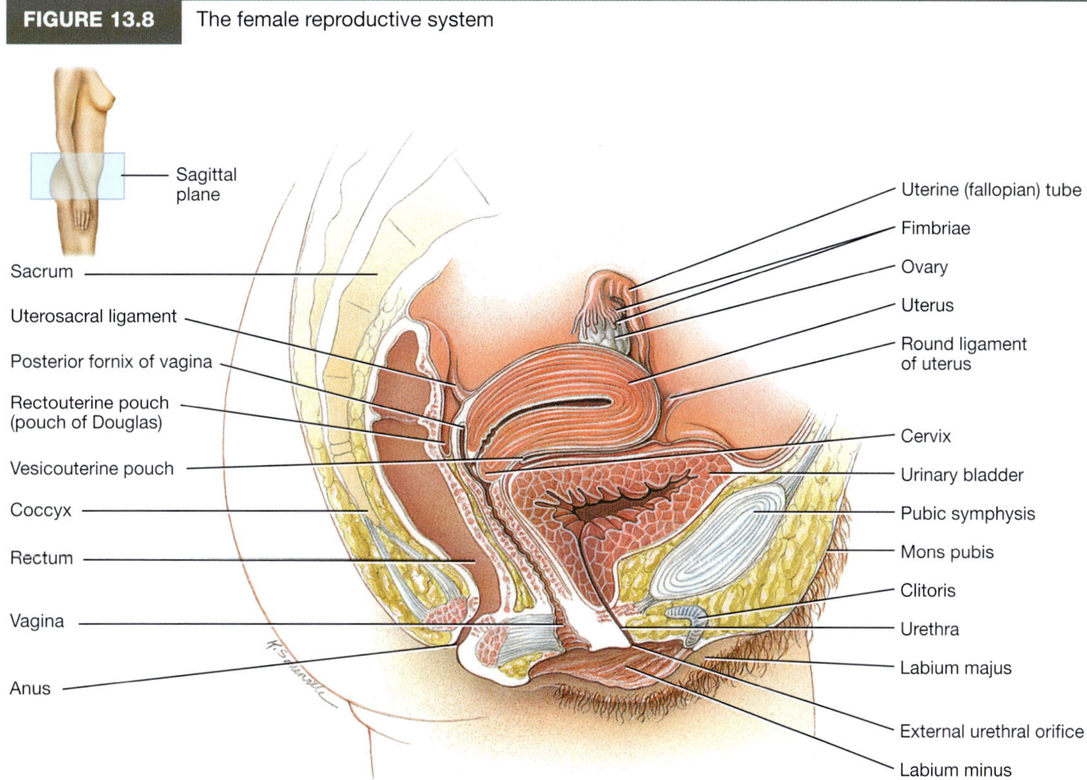

Source: Tortora and Derrickson (2009). Reproduced with permission of John Wiley & Sons.

The ovaries

The ovaries are the female gonads; they are paired almond-shaped glands located on either side of the uterus. A collection of **ligaments** holds them in position; the ovarian ligament attaches the ovaries to the uterus, and the suspensory ligament attaches them to the pelvic wall. The ovaries provide a space of storage for the female germ cells; they also produce the female hormones **oestrogen** and **progesterone**. A woman's total number of ova is present at her birth; when a girl reaches puberty she usually ovulates each month.

The ovary contains a number of small structures called **ovarian follicles**. Each **follicle** contains an immature ovum, called an **oocyte**. Monthly, follicles are stimulated by two hormones, **follicle-stimulating hormone** (FSH) and luteinising hormone (LH), which stimulate the follicles to mature, leading to the release of a mature ovum at **ovulation**.

Follicles are not evenly distributed throughout the ovary; they are restricted to the ovarian cortex or outer region of the ovary, surrounded by dense irregular connective tissue. The ovarian medulla, or inner portion of the ovary, contains blood vessels, nerves and lymphatic tissues surrounded by loose connective tissue. There is an unclear border between the ovarian cortex and medulla.

Oogenesis and follicular development

The term **oogenesis** refers to the formation of the female gametes in the ovary. Oogonia are diploid ($2n$) stem cells (Stanfield 2017) that form during foetal development; they go on to increase in size to form primary oocytes that begin the first stage of meiosis before birth (figure 13.9). Females are therefore born with their entire lifetime supply of gametes, unlike males that continue to produce spermatozoa throughout their adult life. Primary oocytes remain arrested in the first stage of meiosis until puberty, when the correct hormonal conditions are established for further development of the follicle and the ovum that it contains. At this stage the primary oocyte is surrounded by a single layer of follicle cells, and the structure is known as a primordial follicle (see figure 13.10).

FIGURE 13.9 Oogenesis

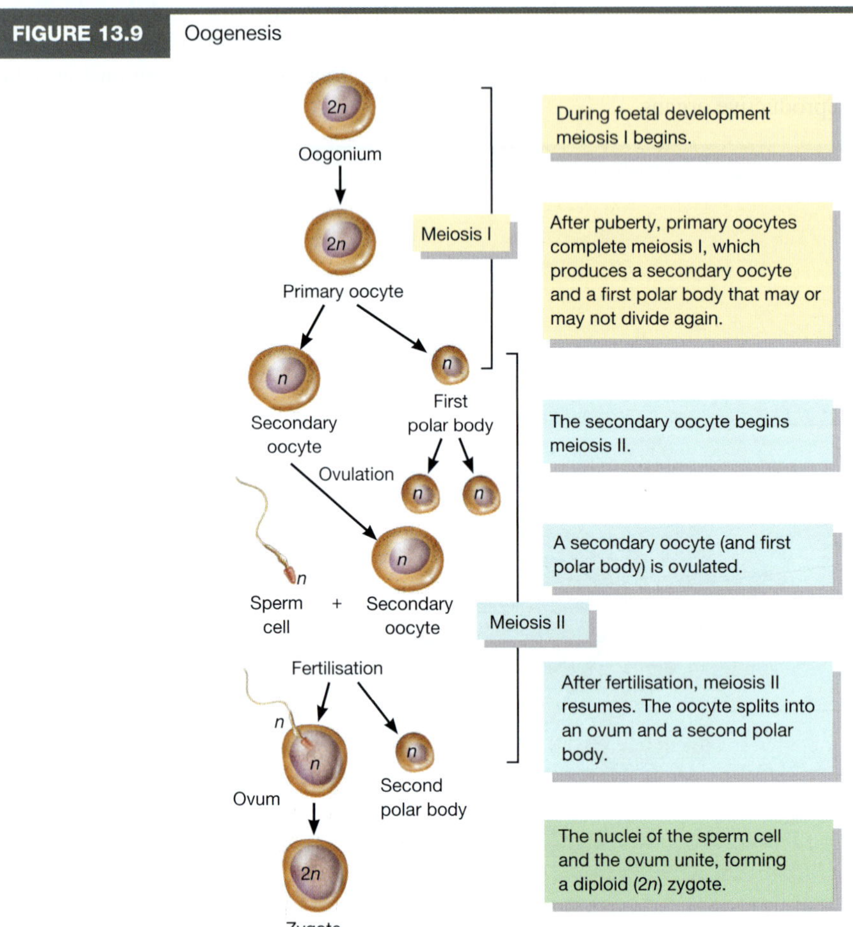

Source: Tortora and Derrickson (2009). Reproduced with permission of John Wiley & Sons.

Every month, from puberty until menopause, FSH and LH are released by the anterior pituitary gland and stimulate follicle growth and maturation. A few primordial follicles start growing each month in response to FSH and LH, developing into a secondary follicle with increased numbers of follicle cells that secrete fluid that builds up in a cavity within the follicle (figure 13.10). The fluid-filled cavity within the developing follicle is called an antrum. Follicles at this stage of development are called Graafian follicles. It is at this stage, just before ovulation, that the diploid primary oocyte completes the first meiotic division to produce a haploid secondary oocyte and a polar body. The polar body contains very little cytoplasm, and essentially acts as a dumping site for the nuclear material not required by the developing ovum. The secondary oocyte becomes arrested during the second meiotic division, which is only completed if the ovum becomes fertilised.

The Graafian follicle also manufactures oestrogen; this stimulates the growth of **endometrium**. Usually only one Graafian follicle will reach the maturity required to release an oocyte each month. This is called ovulation.

FIGURE 13.10 (a–f) The developmental sequences associated with maturation of an ovum

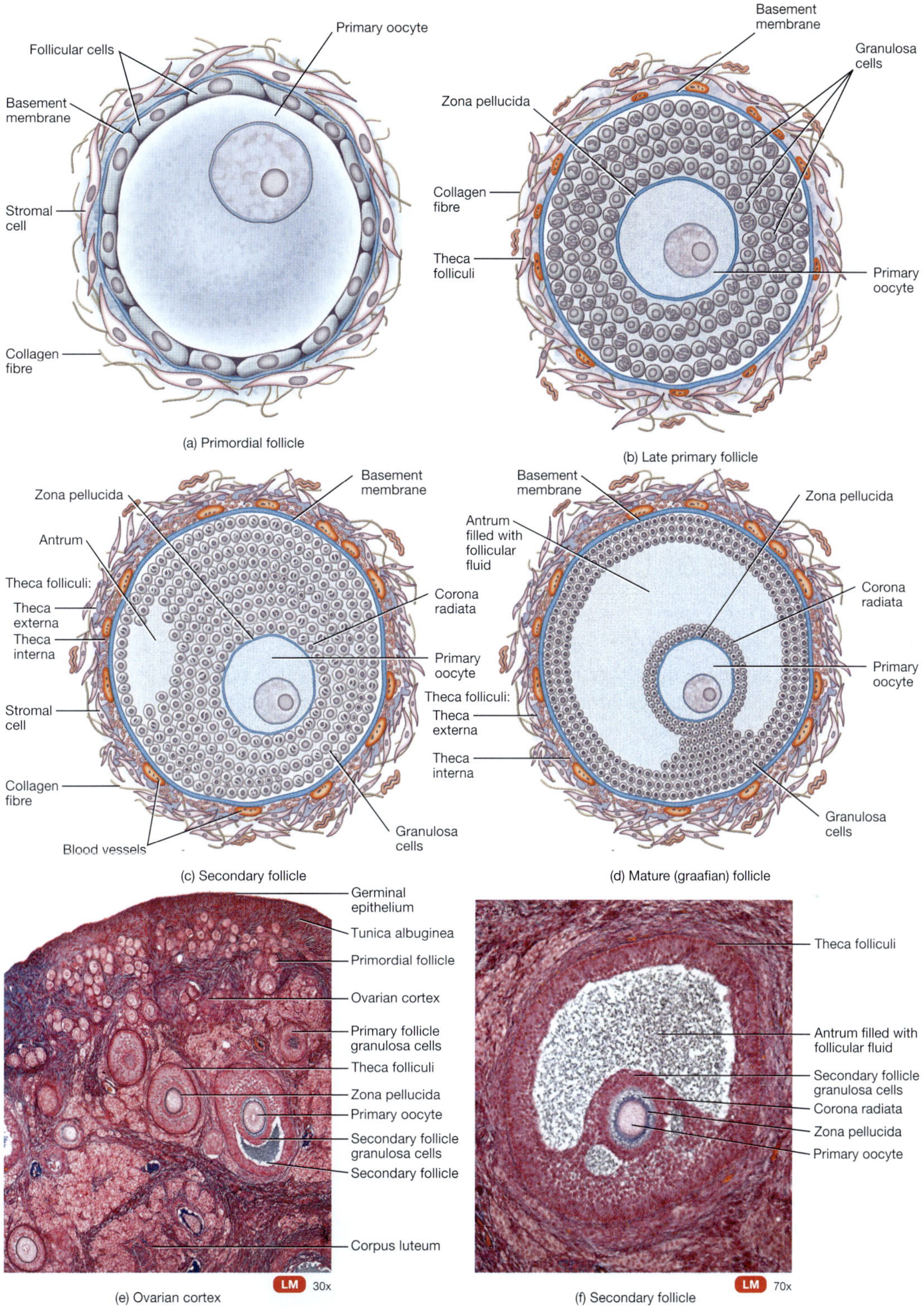

Follicular cells
Basement membrane
Stromal cell
Collagen fibre
Primary oocyte

(a) Primordial follicle

Basement membrane
Granulosa cells
Zona pellucida
Collagen fibre
Theca folliculi
Primary oocyte

(b) Late primary follicle

Zona pellucida
Antrum
Theca folliculi:
Theca externa
Theca interna
Stromal cell
Collagen fibre
Blood vessels
Basement membrane
Corona radiata
Primary oocyte
Granulosa cells

(c) Secondary follicle

Basement membrane
Antrum filled with follicular fluid
Theca folliculi:
Theca externa
Theca interna
Zona pellucida
Corona radiata
Primary oocyte
Granulosa cells

(d) Mature (graafian) follicle

Germinal epithelium
Tunica albuginea
Primordial follicle
Ovarian cortex
Primary follicle granulosa cells
Theca folliculi
Zona pellucida
Primary oocyte
Secondary follicle granulosa cells
Secondary follicle
Corpus luteum
LM 30x

(e) Ovarian cortex

Theca folliculi
Antrum filled with follicular fluid
Secondary follicle granulosa cells
Corona radiata
Zona pellucida
Primary oocyte
LM 70x

(f) Secondary follicle

Source: Tortora and Derrickson (2009). Reproduced with permission of John Wiley & Sons.

Corpus luteum

The remnants of a large ruptured follicle become a new structure called the **corpus luteum**.

The corpus luteum produces two hormones, oestrogen and progesterone, with the aim of supporting the endometrium until conception takes place or the cycle starts again. The corpus luteum gradually disintegrates and a scar is left on the outside of the ovary that is called the **corpus albicans**.

CLINICAL CONSIDERATIONS

Cancer: a national health priority

Cancer control remains a top national health priority in Australia (AIHW 2018). In Australia, one in two men and one in three women can expect to be diagnosed with cancer in their lifetime (Australian Government Cancer Australia 2014). Aboriginal and Torres Strait Islander peoples are 6 per cent more likely to be diagnosed with cancer than non-Indigenous people, and are 50 per cent more likely to die from cancer than non-Indigenous Australians (Australian Government Cancer Australia 2014).

Breast cancer was estimated to be the most commonly diagnosed cancer in 2020 (Australian Government Cancer Australia 2021b). Gynaecological cancers, as a group, represent 9.5 per cent of all cancers in Australian women, with uterine cancer being the most common (Australian Government Cancer Australia 2021c). Prostate cancer is the most commonly diagnosed cancer in males in Australia, and was the second most commonly diagnosed cancer in Australia in 2020 (Australian Government Cancer Australia 2021d).

13.4 The role of the female sex hormones

LEARNING OBJECTIVE 13.4 Provide an overview of the role and functions of the various hormones associated with the female reproductive system.

Oestrogens, progesterone and androgens are produced by the ovaries in a repetitive pattern. Although oestrogens are secreted all the way through the menstrual cycle, they are at their highest level just prior to the ovulation stage of the cycle.

Oestrogens are essential for the development and maintenance of secondary sex characteristics; and, working in combination with a number of other hormones, they stimulate the female reproductive system to prepare for growth of a foetus (LeMone & Burke 2011). Oestrogens have a key role to play in the usual structure of the skin and blood vessels. They also help to reduce the rate of bone resorption (bone breakdown), enhance increased high-density lipoproteins, decrease cholesterol levels and increase blood clotting.

MEDICINES MANAGEMENT

Contraception

The combined oral contraceptive pill (the pill) contains two hormones: an oestrogen and a progestogen. If taken correctly, it is a very effective form of contraception.

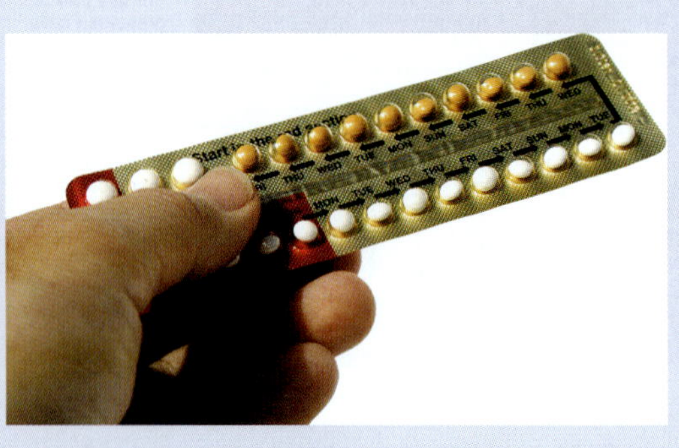

The pill alters the body's hormone balance so that ovulation does not occur. It causes the mucus made by the cervix to thicken and form a mucous plug. This makes it difficult for sperm to get through to the uterus to fertilise an egg. The pill also makes the lining of the uterus thinner. This makes it less likely that a fertilised egg will be able to attach to the uterus. Before taking the combined oral contraceptive pill the prescriber needs to know if the person:

- has unexplained vaginal bleeding
- has current or recent breast cancer
- has migraines, with or without aura
- has diabetes mellitus
- is smoking
- has a BMI > 30

- has systemic lupus erythematosus
- has antiphospholipid syndrome
- has hereditary angiodema
- has recently given birth.

The pill should be taken at the same time every day.
See Australian Medicines Handbook (2019).

The internal organs

The internal organs of the female reproductive system are the vagina and cervix, uterus, Fallopian tubes (also known as oviducts or uterine tubes) and ovaries. The ovaries (discussed earlier) are the primary reproductive organs in women and produce female sex hormones. The vagina, uterus and Fallopian tubes act as an accessory channel for the ovaries and the growing foetus.

The uterus

This hollow organ is also known as the womb. It is a very muscular organ lying in the pelvic cavity posterior and superior to the urinary bladder; it lies anterior to the rectum (figure 13.11).

FIGURE 13.11 The uterus and associated structures

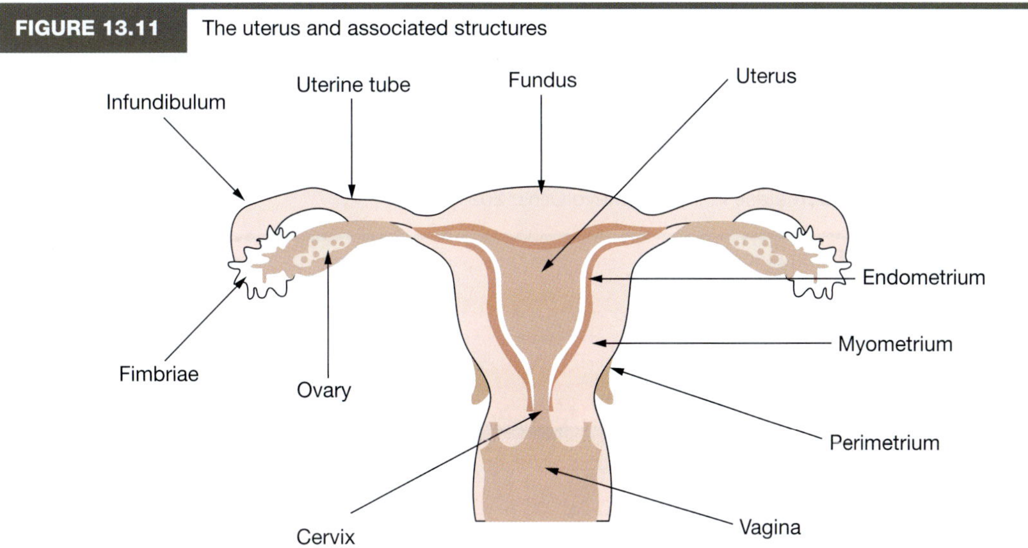

Source: Nair and Peate (2009). Reproduced with permission of John Wiley & Sons.

The uterus is approximately 7.5 cm long. There are three principal parts associated with the uterus:

- fundus — a thick muscular region situated above the Fallopian tubes
- body — the main portion of the uterus, joined to the cervix by an **isthmus**
- cervix — the narrowest part of the uterus opening out into the vagina.

As well as having three aspects or parts, the uterus also has three layers. The perimetrium is the outer serous layer, merging with the peritoneum. The middle layer is the **myometrium** and comprises most of the uterine wall. There are a number of muscle fibres in this layer running in a number of various directions; this arrangement allows contractions to occur during menstruation or childbirth and an increase in size as the foetus grows. The endometrium, the innermost layer, lines the uterus, and this layer is shed during menstruation. The three layers are summarised in table 13.1.

TABLE 13.1 **The layers of the uterus**

Layer	Comments
Perimetrium	A serous membrane enveloping the uterus; this is the outer layer. It provides support to the uterus located within the pelvis. This may also be known as the parietal peritoneum.

(continued)

TABLE 13.1 *(continued)*

Layer	Comments
Myometrium	This layer is the middle layer and is composed of smooth muscle. During pregnancy and childbirth, the uterus is required to stretch and the muscular layer allows this to happen. The muscle will contract during labour, and postnatally this muscular layer contracts forcefully to force out the **placenta**. The contractions also help to control potential blood loss after birth.
Endometrium	The endometrium is the mucous membrane lining the inside of the uterus. The endometrium changes throughout the menstrual cycle. It becomes thick and rich with blood vessels to prepare for pregnancy. If the woman does not become pregnant then, part of the endometrium is shed, resulting in menstrual bleeding.

Source: Adapted from McGuinness (2010); and Waugh and Grant (2018).

HOMEOSTATIC IMBALANCE

Endometriosis

Endometriosis is characterised by the growth of endometrial-like tissue outside the uterine cavity and can be found in the ovaries, Fallopian tubes and the intestines (see figure 13.12). This condition affects approximately 1 in 10 women of reproductive age (Marquardt et al. 2019). Symptoms include pain, heavy bleeding, and bladder and bowel problems (e.g. constipation, diarrhoea and urine urgency), bloating and infertility (Jean Hailes for Women's Health 2021). Pain is a significant issue with this condition and includes dysmenorrhoea (painful periods), dyspareunia (pain experienced during sexual intercourse) and pain with bowel movements or urination (Mayo Clinic 2021). Treatment for endometriosis focuses on pain management, hormonal contraceptives, gonadotropin-releasing hormone agonists and antagonists, progestin therapy or araomatase inhibitors (Mayo Clinic 2021).

FIGURE 13.12 Endometriosis

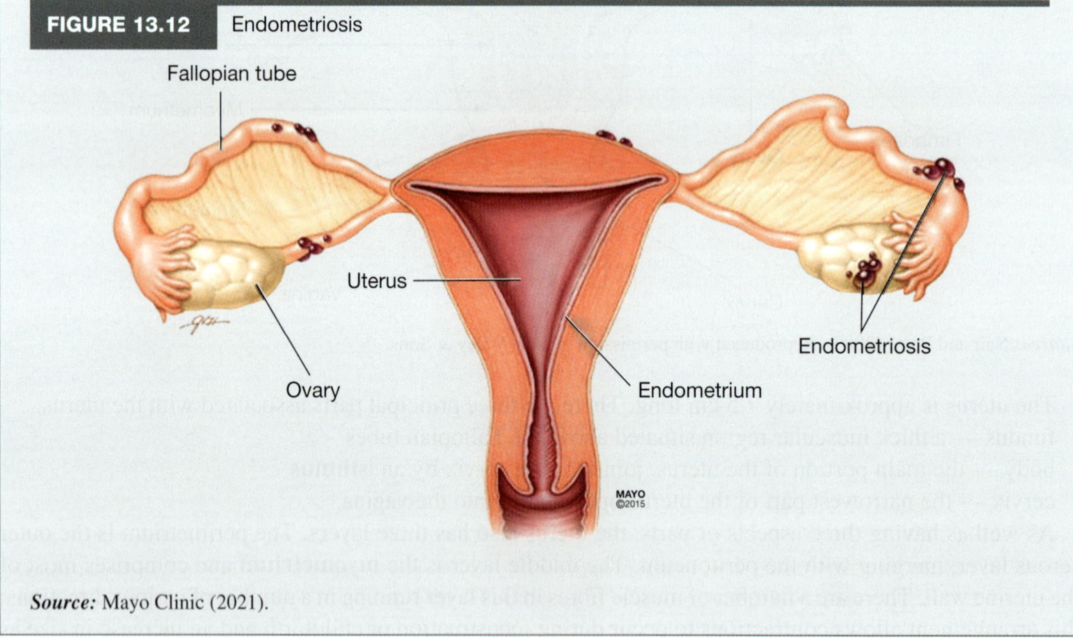

Source: Mayo Clinic (2021).

The Fallopian tubes

The paired Fallopian tubes (also known as oviducts, salpinges or uterine tubes) are delicate, thin cylindrical structures approximately 8–14 cm long (Marieb 2018). They are affixed to the uterus at one end and are supported by the **broad ligaments**. The **lateral** ends of the Fallopian tubes are open and made of projections called **fimbriae** that drape over the ovary. The fimbriae pick up the ovum after it is discharged from the ovary.

The Fallopian tubes have a layer of smooth muscle and are lined with ciliated, mucus-producing epithelial cells. The actions of the cilia and contractions of the smooth muscle transport the ovum along the tubes onwards to the uterus. It is in the end of the Fallopian tube closest to the ovary where the fertilisation of the ovum by the sperm usually occurs.

The term adnexa is used collectively when discussing the Fallopian tubes, ovaries and supporting tissues.

CLINICAL CONSIDERATIONS

Insertion of intrauterine contraceptive device

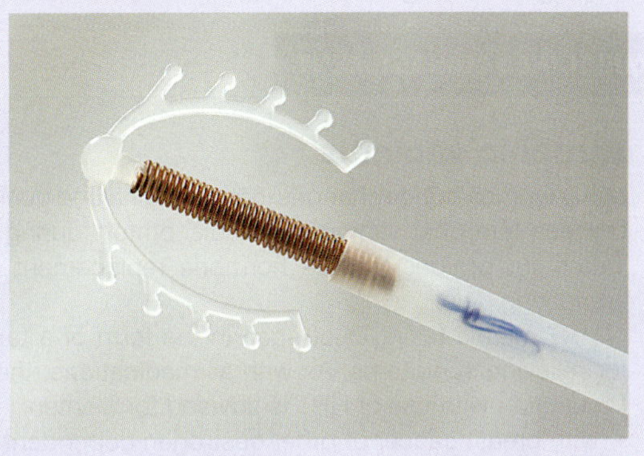

An intrauterine device (IUD) is a small T-shaped plastic and copper device that is inserted into the uterus by a specially trained nurse or a doctor. The IUD works by preventing the sperm and egg from surviving in the uterus or Fallopian tubes; it can also prevent a fertilised egg from implanting in the uterus.

There are different types of IUD; some contain more copper than others. Those IUDs with more copper are more than 99 per cent effective. Copper changes the make-up of the fluids in the uterus and Fallopian tubes. IUDs with less copper will be less effective. There are types and sizes of IUD to suit different women; they can be inserted at the GP surgery, local contraception clinic or sexual health clinic. An IUD can be inserted at any time, though it may be easier when the woman is menstruating, as the cervix is slightly open at that time.

A metal or plastic speculum is gently inserted into the vagina in order to see the cervix. The cervix is wiped with a special cleanser. Next, a small 'sound' (probe-like instrument) is inserted to measure the length of the uterus. The IUD is then inserted using a very small straw. The IUD has a string attached to one end. The nurse or doctor will trim the IUD string that is coming through the cervix into the vagina. The string allows the woman to check that the IUD is in place (see figure 13.13).

FIGURE 13.13 An IUD device in situ

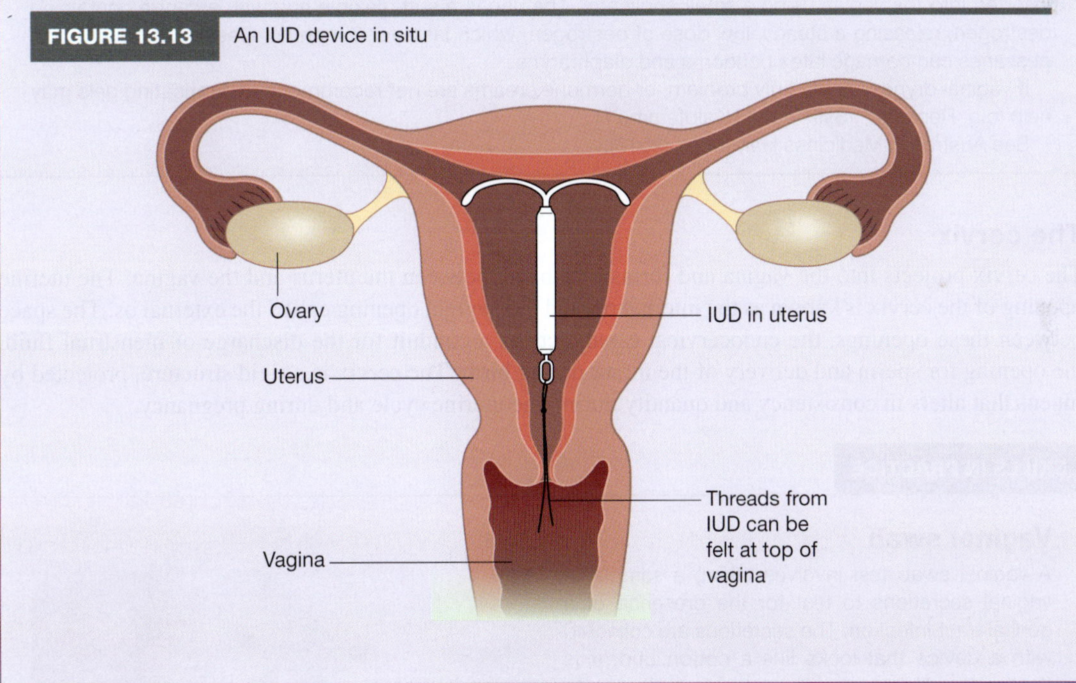

The vagina

The vagina is a tubular, fibromuscular structure approximately 8–10 cm in length (Jenkins & Tortora 2012) with several functions; it is the receptacle for the penis during sexual intercourse, an organ of sexual response, the **canal** that allows the menstrual flow to leave the body, and the passage for the birth of the child. The vagina is situated posterior to the urinary bladder and urethra; it is anterior to the rectum. The upper element contains the uterine cervix in an area that is known as the fornix. The vaginal walls are made of membranous folds of tissue called the rugae. These membranes are made up of mucus-secreting stratified squamous epithelial cells.

Usually, the walls of the vagina are moist and have a pH ranging from 3.8 to 4.2. This pH inhibits the growth of bacteria (it is bacteriostatic) and is maintained by the action of the hormone oestrogen and healthy vaginal microorganisms (the normal vaginal flora). Oestrogen stimulates the growth of vaginal mucosal cells, making them thicken and develop and increase glycogen content. The glycogen is fermented to lactic acid by lactobacilli (organisms that produce lactic acid) that usually live in the vagina, causing slight acidifying of the vaginal fluid (LeMone & Burke 2011).

MEDICINES MANAGEMENT

Atrophic vaginitis

Many women notice changes in their vagina and genital area after menopause. These changes may include dryness (atrophic vaginitis) and discomfort during sex. These can often be improved with treatment. Treatment options include hormone replacement therapy (HRT), oestrogen cream, or pessaries and lubricating gels.

HRT means taking oestrogen in the form of a tablet, gel or patches. This is often the best treatment for relieving symptoms. As with all medications, there are advantages and disadvantages of using HRT. Precaution with use of HRT is advised for women:

- with breast cancer or other oestrogen dependent tumour
- with unexplained vaginal bleeding
- with a history of endometriosis or uterine fibroids
- with migraines
- with diabetes mellitus
- with epilepsy
- who are smokers
- with systemic lupus erythematosus
- with hereditary angioedema.

Sometimes a cream, pessary or vaginal tablet or ring containing oestrogen is prescribed. A pessary is inserted into the vagina using a small applicator. The ring is a soft, flexible ring with a centre containing oestrogen, releasing a steady, low dose of oestrogen, which lasts for 3 months. Oestrogen creams and pessaries can damage latex condoms and diaphragms.

If vaginal dryness is the only problem, or hormone creams are not recommended, lubricating gels may help (e.g. Replens®, Sylk® and Hyalofemme®).

See Australian Medicines Handbook (2019).

The cervix

The cervix projects into the vagina and forms a pathway between the uterus and the vagina. The uterine opening of the cervix is known as the internal os, and the vaginal opening called the external os. The space between these openings, the endocervical canal, acts as a conduit for the discharge of menstrual fluid, the opening for sperm and delivery of the infant during birth. The cervix is a rigid structure, protected by mucus that alters in consistency and quantity during the uterine cycle and during pregnancy.

SKILLS IN PRACTICE

Vaginal swab

A vaginal swab test involves taking a sample of vaginal secretions to test for the presence of a genital tract infection. The secretions are collected with a device that looks like a cotton bud; it is then placed in a special container and sent to the microbiology laboratory for further analysis. This procedure can be used to test for chlamydia and gonorrhea, as well as fungal and bacterial infections such as candida albicans and bacterial vaginosis.

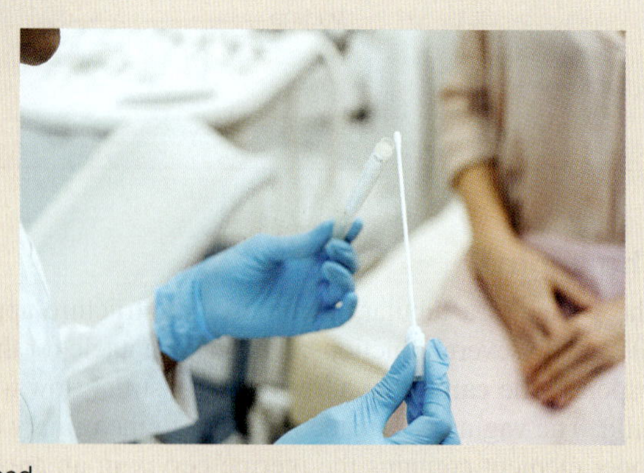

A full medical and sexual history should be obtained, and the procedure must be explained. Offer a chaperone to all women and obtain informed consent before the procedure is commenced.

Ensure that the patient's bladder is empty and position her in a dorsal position with knees flexed and hips abducted. Depending upon local protocols, a speculum may be used. The sterile swab is carefully inserted into the inside opening of the vagina, and gently rotated against the sides of the vagina for 10–30 seconds. The sterile swab is inserted approximately 5 cm into the vagina for a high vaginal swab, and approximately 1–2 cm for a low vaginal swab. The patient may prefer to collect her own low vaginal swab, with instructions from the medical or nursing staff. The swab is then withdrawn without touching the skin and placed into a collection tube containing transport medium. The samples should reach the pathology lab within 24 hours for optimal culture results.

The external genitalia

Collectively, the external genitalia are known as the vulva. They include the mons pubis, the labia, the clitoris, the vaginal and urethral openings, and glands (LeMone & Burke 2011).

The mons pubis is a pad of elevated adipose tissue covered with skin that lies anteriorly to the symphysis pubis to provide cushioning. After puberty, the mons is covered with coarse pubic hair.

The labia are divided into two structures. The labia majora are the outermost folds of skin that begin at the base of the mons pubis and terminate at the anus. They are covered with pubic hair and contain an abundance of adipose tissue. The labia minora, situated between the clitoris and the base of the vagina, are enclosed by the labia majora. They are made of skin, adipose tissue and some erectile tissues with a number of sebaceous glands. They are usually light pink and are devoid of pubic hair.

The clitoris is composed of two small erectile bodies, the corposa cavernosa and several nerves and blood vessels. The glans clitoris is covered by a layer of skin called the clitorial prepuce (or clitoral hood) that is formed where the labia minora unite. The glans clitoris is the exposed portion of the clitoris and is likened to the **glans penis** in the male. This aspect of the external genitalia is capable of enlargement and has a role to play in sexual excitement in the woman.

CLINICALLY REASONED EPISODE OF CARE

Sexual health

Consider the patient situation

Xanthe is a 22-year-old woman who has recently obtained a clitoral hood piercing and attends the sexual health clinic with discharge, pain and swelling. She sees the sexual health nurse.

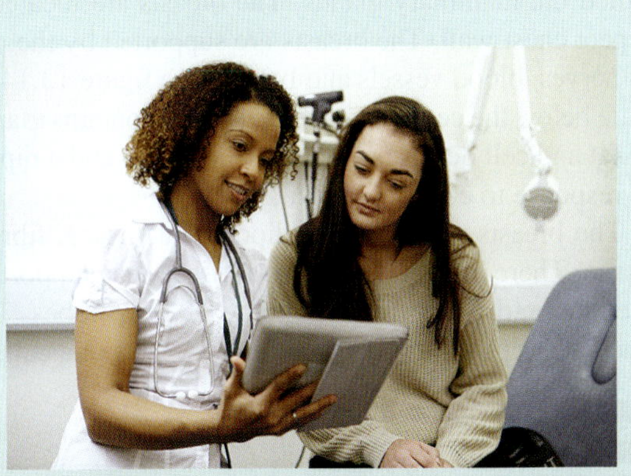

Collect cues and information

Xanthe had her clitoral hood pierced five days ago and is now experiencing discharge, redness at the piercing site, pain, fever, nausea, and generally feeling unwell. On examination, the area is swollen, red and exuding yellow discharge.

Process information

Clitoral piercings are similar to other piercings and are performed by passing a needle through the skin, leaving jewellery in the place of the piercing. Due to the needle passing through the skin, the most common complications are bacterial infection, bleeding, nerve damage, allergic reaction to jewellery and scarring. If a clean needle is not used, there is a risk of contracting diseases such as HIV, and hepatitis B and C.

People with genital piercings should also be educated on the potential risk of damage to condoms.

Establish goals

1. Assessment for infection and other concerns
2. Treatment of infection
3. Education on maintaining piercing and appropriate use of condoms

Nursing actions

1. Conduct assessment.
   Rationale:
   - Sexual health nurses can assess and evaluate the needs of the individual and conduct a thorough sexual health history.
   - Assessment allows for the appropriate management and treatment plan to be implemented.
2. Treat infection.
   Rationale:
   - In conjunction with an appropriate prescriber, such as a medical officer or nurse practitioner, sexual health nurses can recommend treatments such as the removal of the piercing and antibiotics.
   - If not treated, the infection can cause tissue damage and ongoing issues to the area.
3. Educate on piercing healing and sexual health.
   Rationale:
   - Clear education and information on maintaining the piercing includes avoiding sexual intercourse and touching of the area, swimming pools and hot tubs until the piercing heals (usually 6–8 weeks). The area should be cleaned regularly with a diluted saline solution, especially after sexual intercourse.
   - Genital piercings may pose an increased risk to condom tear; therefore the individual should be educated to take care when engaging in sexual intercourse.
   - Respectful and appropriate education and advice is essential to sexual health. Sexual health nurses are well placed to provide information and education on sexual health measures.

Evaluate outcomes

As a result of the assessment and treatment plan implemented by the sexual health team, Xanthe's infection clears. She is able to care for her piercing to avoid further complications.

Reflect on new processes and learning

Reflect on the role of the sexual health nurse. How do nurses in specialist areas work with the multidisciplinary team to achieve positive outcomes for patients?

Source: Based on the Clinical Reasoning Cycle, Levett-Jones (2013).

The breasts

The breasts are dome-shaped protrusions that differ in size between individuals; they are also sometimes called the mammary glands. The breasts are located between the third and seventh ribs on the anterior aspect chest wall. The breasts are supported by the pectoral muscles and are provided with a rich supply of nerves, blood vessels and lymph (see figure 13.14). A pigmented area known as the areola is situated a little below the centre of each breast and contains glands that secrete sebum — a thick substance composed of fat and cell debris (sebaceous glands) — and a nipple. The nipple is usually protruding, becoming erect in response to cold and stimulation.

The breasts are made of adipose (fat) tissue, fibrous connective tissue and milk-producing glandular tissue. There are bands of fibrous tissue that support the breast and extend from the outer breast tissue to the nipple, dividing the breast into 15 to 25 lobes. The lobes are composed of alveolar glands joined by ducts that open out on to the nipple. A hormone called **prolactin** controls the production of milk.

SKILLS IN PRACTICE

Breast examination

A clinical breast examination is an essential step to evaluate any woman with a breast symptom or lump and is therefore an important skill for medical and nursing practitioners. Women who present with breast pain, skin changes, nipple discharge, lumps or changes in size, shape or texture should undergo a thorough breast examination.

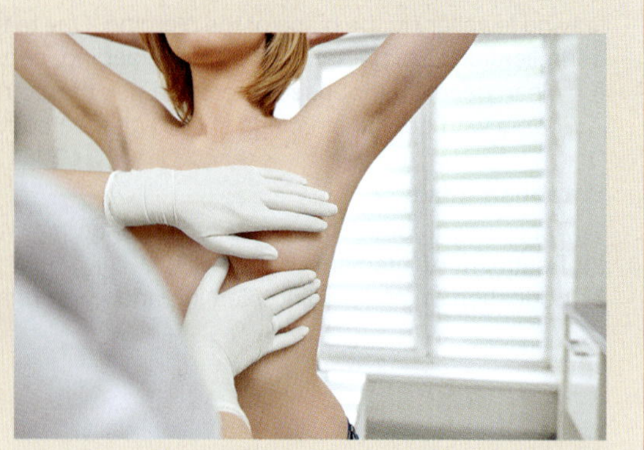

A thorough breast examination requires the woman to be undressed down to the waist, firstly in a seated position for visual inspection followed by laying in a supine position for palpation. The visual inspection is conducted with the woman in several positions (e.g. hands on hips and raised overhead) so that the size, shape, symmetry, texture and colour of the whole breast and nipple can be assessed. The palpation phase requires a meticulous and systematic approach to cover the entire extent of breast tissue, which usually covers most of the anterior chest wall. A variety of techniques exist to ensure complete palpation of the breast tissue including the 'spoke' or 'wagon wheel' method and the concentric circles method. The nipple areolar area should also be palpated for abnormalities, and for expressible nipple discharge.

After examination of the breast, the axilla and supraclavicular area should be palpated for lymph node enlargement.

See Henderson and Ferguson (2019); and Australian Government Cancer Australia (2021a).

FIGURE 13.14 The breast

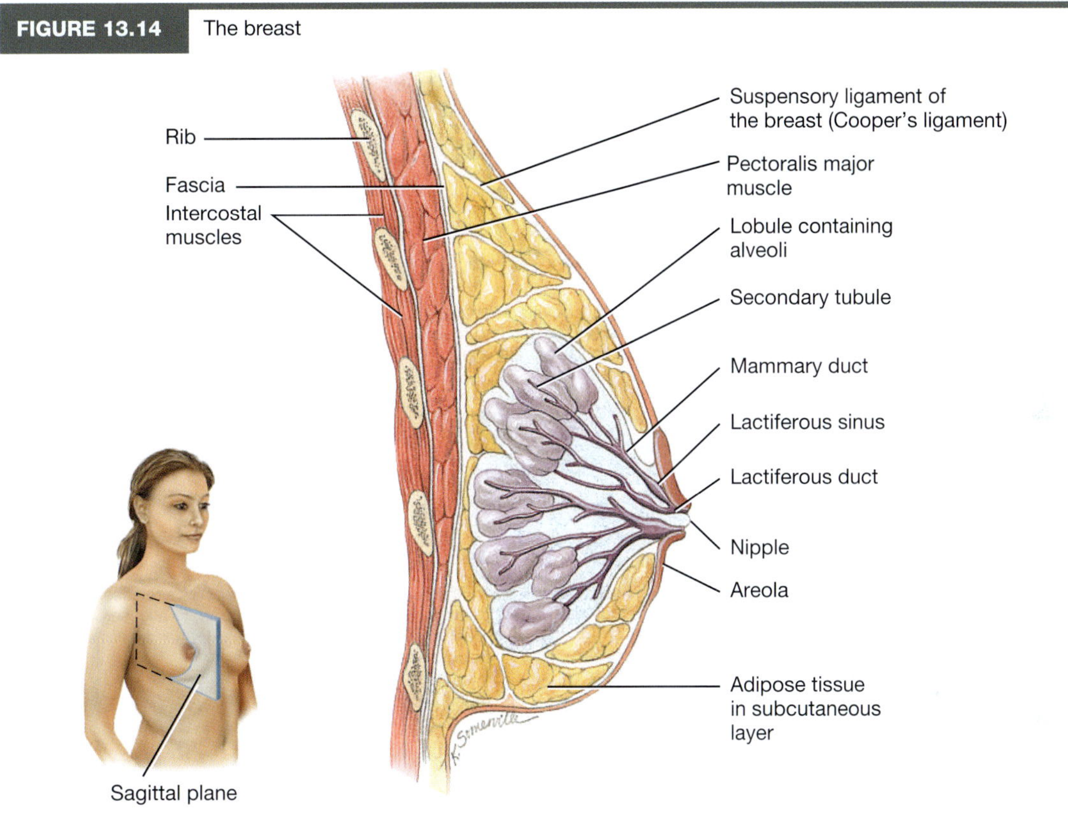

Source: Tortora and Derrickson (2009). Reproduced with permission of John Wiley & Sons.

13.5 The uterine cycle

LEARNING OBJECTIVE 13.5 Outline the phases of the uterine cycle.

The endometrium of the uterus responds to changes in oestrogen and progesterone during the **ovarian cycle** as it prepares for the implantation of a fertilised embryo. The endometrium is receptive to implantation of the embryo for only a brief period every month, coinciding with the time when the embryo would normally reach the uterus from the Fallopian tube (usually 7 days after ovulation).

The menstrual cycle begins with the menstrual phase which lasts from days 1 to 5. During this time the inner functionalis layer of the uterine endometrium is released as menstrual fluid. As the growing follicle in the ovary begins to produce the hormone oestrogen (days 6 to 14), the proliferative phase of the uterine endometrium commences. During this time the functionalis layer thickens while at the same time spiral arteries multiply and tubular glands form (LeMone & Burke 2011). Cervical mucus is produced in increasing amounts and becomes thin and stretchy, enabling sperm to penetrate it easily and travel up into the uterus.

The final phase of the uterine cycle, lasting from days 14 to 28, is the secretory phase. As the corpus luteum produces progesterone, the rising levels act on the endometrium, resulting in an increased vascularity, changing the inner layer to secretory mucosa, stimulating the secretion of glycogen into the uterine cavity. It also causes the cervical mucus to become thick again, blocking the passage of sperm. If an embryo has not implanted into the uterus by this stage, hormone levels will fall. Spasm of the spiral arteries causes hypoxia (lack of oxygen) of the endometrial cells, which begin to degenerate and then slough off. As with the ovarian cycle, the process begins again with the sloughing of the functionalis layer. Figure 13.15 demonstrates the ovarian and uterine cycles.

FIGURE 13.15 The ovarian and uterine cycles

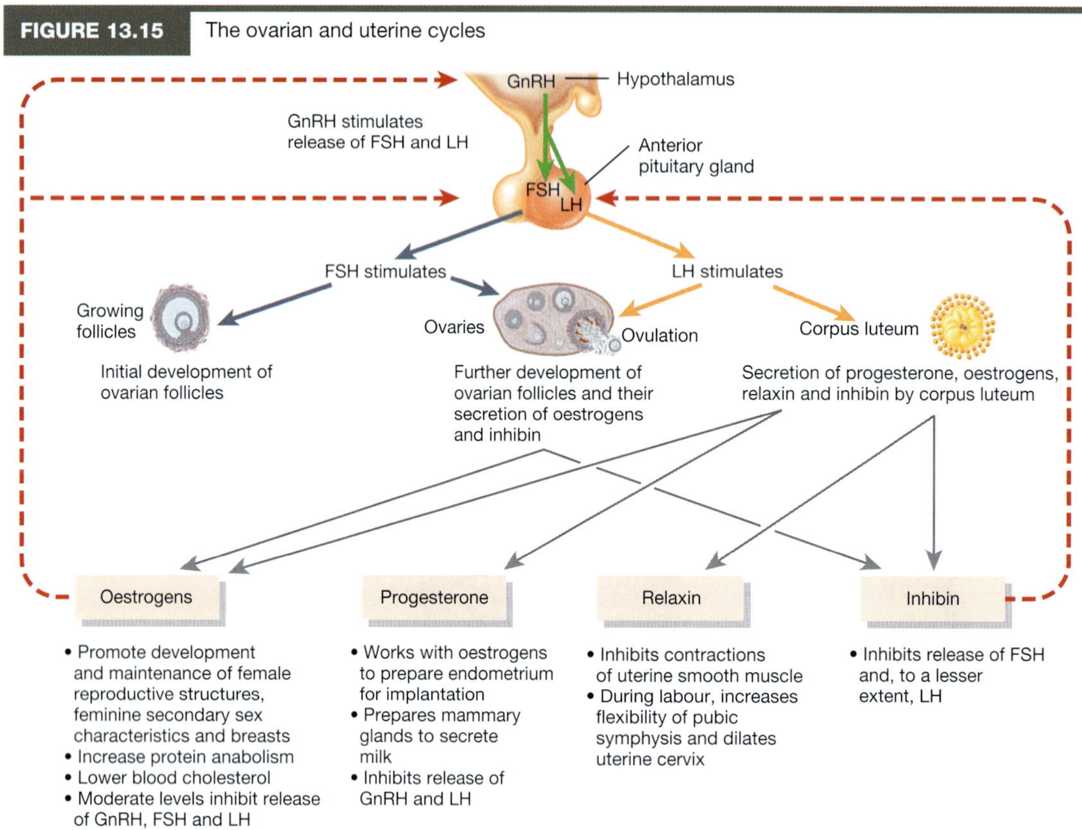

Source: Tortora and Derrickson (2009). Reproduced with permission of John Wiley & Sons.

CLINICALLY REASONED EPISODE OF CARE

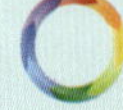

Ectopic pregnancy

Consider the patient situation

Alice is a 27-year-old woman who has recently undergone a salpingectomy. She presents to the GP with abdominal pain.

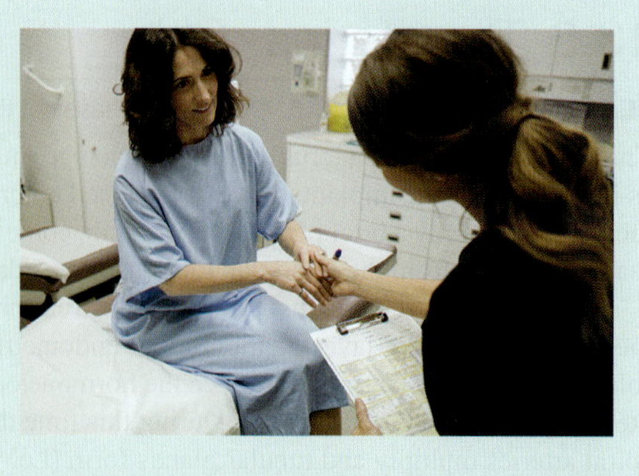

Collect cues and information

Alice was diagnosed with an ectopic pregnancy and underwent a right salpingectomy two days ago. She is currently experiencing right-sided abdominal pain, and neck and shoulder pain.

Process information

An ectopic pregnancy occurs when an embryo implants outside of the uterus, usually in the Fallopian tube. The Fallopian tube is not able to expand to accommodate the pregnancy. As the embryo develops, the Fallopian tube can rupture, causing bleeding and pain. An ectopic pregnancy can be an emergency; therefore the removal of the Fallopian tube (salpingectomy) can be necessary.

A salpingectomy is achieved via laparoscopic surgery under anaesthetic. The abdomen is inflated with carbon dioxide gas to allow space to complete the procedure. The gas used to inflate the abdomen can cause irritation of the diaphragm and phrenic nerve, causing referred pain to the shoulder and neck. Additionally, bleeding can also cause irritation of the phrenic nerve and referred pain.

Unfortunately, ectopic pregnancies are not viable. It can be an emotional and distressing time for patients. Fertility rates for women who have had a salpingectomy will remain good; however, having a previous ectopic pregnancy does pose a risk for future ectopic pregnancies.

Establish goals

1. Clinical assessment
2. Pain management
3. Education and support

Nursing actions

1. Conduct a thorough clinical assessment.
   Rationale:
   - While it is likely that the symptoms Alice is experiencing are due to the laparoscopic procedure, it is important to conduct an assessment to ensure the pain is not secondary to bleeding.
   - The assessment should include vital signs, in particular temperature for infection, hypotension and tachycardia, which may indicate hypovolaemia secondary to bleeding. It should also include the nature of the pain and amount of vaginal blood loss. Any concerns arising from the assessment should be immediately discussed with the general practitioner.
2. Manage pain.
   Rationale:
   - Any surgical intervention can cause pain and discomfort which should be managed.
   - The nature of laparoscopic surgery can cause additional pain such as neck and shoulder pain.
   - Pharmacological and other pain management techniques such as lying down to reduce phrenic nerve irritation should be encouraged.
3. Provide education and support to Alice.
   Rationale:
   - Nurses are well placed to provide education and information on pain management and when to seek help for pain management.
   - Given the nature of the procedure, Alice may require emotional support, education and reassurance about her future fertility.

Evaluate outcomes

As a result of the interventions, Alice is reassured. At her follow-up appointment one week later, Alice reports that her symptoms have resolved.

Reflect on new processes and learning

Reflect on the scenario. What is the benefit of conducting a thorough assessment and examination for Alice? While it is likely that the referred pain is secondary to the procedure, what else could the pain indicate?

Source: Based on the Clinical Reasoning Cycle, Levett-Jones (2013).

SUMMARY

The male and female reproductive systems are complex. All living things reproduce; fundamentally, organisms make more organisms akin to themselves. Without these reproductive systems human life would end; these systems are essential for life. In the human reproductive process, two types of sex cells, or gametes, are required. The male gamete, or sperm, and the female gamete, the egg or ovum, meet in the female's reproductive system to begin the creation of a new individual. Anatomical and physiological processes are required to ensure this marvel works effectively.

Sexual reproduction, the process of producing offspring for the survival of the species and passing on hereditary traits from one generation to the next, is the key function of the male and female reproductive systems. The male and female reproductive systems contribute to the events leading to fertilisation. The female organs take on responsibility for the developing human, birth and nourishment. The systems also provide pleasure, sexual pleasure and sexual excitement; for a number of people this is an important aspect of their being.

KEY TERMS

androgens Masculinising male sex hormones produced by the testes in the male and the adrenal cortex in both sexes.

anterior Near to the front.

broad ligaments A double fold of parietal peritoneum attaching the uterus to the side of the pelvic cavity.

canal A channel or passageway, a narrow tube.

connective tissue The most prominent type of tissue in the body; this tissue provides support.

corpus albicans A whitish fibrous patch in the ovary formed after the corpus luteum regresses.

corpus luteum A yellowish body found in the ovary when a follicle has discharged its secondary oocyte.

endometrium The mucous membrane lining the uterus.

fimbriae Finger-like structures found at the end of the Fallopian tubes.

foetus The developing organism in utero.

follicle A secretory sac or cavity containing a group of cells that contains a developing oocyte in the ovary.

follicle-stimulating hormone Secreted by the anterior pituitary gland; initiates the development of an ovum.

gamete A male or female sex cell.

glans penis The enlarged region at the end of the penis.

gonads A gland that produces hormones and gametes — in men the testes, in females the ovaries.

gonadotrophin-releasing hormone Anterior pituitary hormone affecting the gonads.

haploid Having half the number of chromosomes.

hormones A secretion of endocrine cells that alters the physiological activity of target cells.

inguinal canal Passage in the lower abdominal wall in the male.

in utero Within the uterus.

isthmus A narrow strip of tissue or a narrow passage connecting to bigger parts.

lateral Farthest from the midline of the body.

Leydig cells A type of cell that secretes testosterone.

ligaments Dense regular connective tissue.

luteinising hormone A hormone secreted by the anterior pituitary stimulates ovulation and prepares glands in the breast to produce milk. Stimulates testosterone secretion in the testes.

meatus A passage or opening.

meiosis A kind of cell division occurring during the production of gametes.

menopause The termination of the menstrual cycles.

myometrium The smooth muscle layer of the uterus.

oestrogen A feminising sex hormone produced by the ovaries.

orchidopexy Surgery to move an undescended testicle into the scrotum and permanently fix it there.

oocyte An immature egg cell.

oogenesis Formation and development of the female gametes.

ovarian cycle The ovarian cycle is a series of events in the ovaries that occur during and after the maturation of the oocyte.
ovarian follicles A general name for immature oocytes.
ovaries Female gonads.
ovulation The rupture of a mature Graafian follicle with discharge of a secondary oocyte after penetration by sperm.
ovum The female egg cell.
penis The organ of urination and copulation.
pH A measure of acidity and alkalinity.
phagocytosis The process by which phagocytes ingest and destroy microbes, cell debris and other foreign matter.
placenta An organ attached to the lining of the uterus during pregnancy.
progesterone A female sex hormone produced by the ovaries.
prolactin A hormone secreted by the anterior pituitary that initiates and maintains milk production.
rete The network of ducts in the testes.
scrotum The skin-covered pouch containing the testes.
semen Fluid discharged by ejaculation.
spermatogenesis The maturation of spermatids into sperm.
testes The male gonads.
testosterone Male sex hormone.
urethra The tube from the urinary bladder to the exterior of the body that conveys urine in females and urine and semen in males.
uterus Hollow muscular organ in the female, also called the womb.
vagina A muscular tubular organ in the female leading from the uterus to the vestibule.
vas deferens The main secretory duct of the testicle, through which semen is carried from the epididymis to the prostatic urethra, where it ends as the ejaculatory duct.
vulva The female external genitalia.

FIND OUT MORE

1. What does the surgical procedure circumcision entail?
2. Discuss the various methods of contraception.
3. What advice should be given to a man who is considering using Viagra for the first time?
4. What is the role and function of the nurse in respect to protecting vulnerable people?
5. How can the nurse ensure that the information provided to various communities is appropriate and informative?
6. Outline the barriers that may be encountered when conducting an assessment of a person's sexual health.
7. How may the nurse reduce the impact of the barriers identified above?
8. Describe the changes that can occur in the normal ageing process in relation to the female reproductive system.
9. List the issues a man may have to face post-prostatectomy.
10. Discuss the services and support systems available to young mums in the area where you live.

CONDITIONS

The following is a list of conditions that are associated with the reproductive systems. Take some time and write notes about each of the conditions. You may make the notes taken from textbooks or other resources (e.g. people you work with in a clinical area), or you may make the notes as a result of people you have cared for. If you are making notes about people you have cared for, you must ensure that you adhere to the rules of confidentiality.

Prostatitis	
Cervicitis	
Uterine cancer	
Cervical cancer	
Endometriosis	
Polycystic ovarian syndrome	
Premature ejaculation	
Benign prostate hyperplasia	

REFERENCES

Australian Government Cancer Australia (2014) Cancer Australia Strategic Plan 2014–2019. www.canceraustralia.gov.au/publications-and-resources/cancer-australia-publications/cancer-australia-strategic-plan-2014-2019 (accessed February 2021).

Australian Government Cancer Australia (2021a) Early detection of breast cancer. www.canceraustralia.gov.au/publications-and-resources/position-statements/early-detection-breast-cancer (accessed February 2021).

Australian Government Cancer Australia (2021b) Breast cancer in Australia statistics. www.canceraustralia.gov.au/affected-cancer/cancer-types/breast-cancer/breast-cancer-australia-statistics#:~:text=In%202018%2C%20there%20were%203%2C034,33%20males%20and%202%2C997%20females).&text=In%202018%2C%20the%20age%2Dstandardised,males%20and%2019%20for%20females(accessedFebruary2021).

Australian Government Cancer Australia (2021c) Gynaecological cancers. www.canceraustralia.gov.au/affected-cancer/cancer-types/gynaecological-cancer/gynaecological-cancer-australia-statistics (accessed February 2021).

Australian Government Cancer Australia (2021d) Prostate cancer. www.canceraustralia.gov.au/affected-cancer/cancer-types/prostate-cancer/prostate-cancer-australia-statistics (accessed February 2021).

Australian Institute of Health and Welfare (2018) Improving Australia's burden of disease. www.aihw.gov.au/getmedia/28c917f3-cb00-44dd-ba86-c13e764dea6b/Improving-Australia-s-burden-of-disease-9-01-2019.pdf.aspx (accessed February 2021).

Australian Medicines Handbook (2019) *Australian Medicines Handbook*. Adelaide: Australian Medicines Handbook Pty Ltd.

Colbert, B.J., Ankney, J. and Lee, K.T. (2012) *Anatomy and Physiology for Health Professionals: An Interactive Journey*, 2nd edn. Upper Saddle River, NJ: Pearson.

Henderson, J.A. and Ferguson, T. (2019) *Breast Examination Technique*. Treasure Island FL: StatPeals Publishing.

Holland, A.J., Nassar, N. and Schneuer, F.J. (2016) Undescended testes: an update. *Current Opinion in Pediatrics* 28(3): 388–394.

Jean Hailes for Women's Health (2021) Endometriosis — fact sheet. www.jeanhailes.org.au/resources/endometriosis-fact-sheet?gclid=Cj0KCQiA0fr_BRDaARIsAABw4EvkuWCXRJYpj6xiX4Qq7RZ6KXNrBKr99PaJnviTF7ayXXA2nq_v3rYaAm8BEALw_wcB (accessed February 2021).

Jenkins, G.W. and Tortora, G.J. (2012) *Anatomy and Physiology: From Science to Life*, 3rd edn. Hoboken, NJ: John Wiley & Sons, Inc.

LeMone, P. and Burke, K. (2011) *Medical-Surgical Nursing: Critical Thinking in Client Care*, 5th edn. Upper Saddle River, NJ: Pearson.

Levett-Jones, T. (2013). *Clinical Reasoning: Learning to Think Like a Nurse*. Pearson Australia.

Marieb, E.N. (2018) *Human Anatomy and Physiology*, 11th edn. San Francisco, CA: Pearson.

Marquardt, R.M., Kim, T.H., Shin, J-H. and Jeong, J-W. (2019) Progesterone and estrogen signaling in the endometrium: what goes wrong in endometriosis? *International Journal of Molecular Sciences* 20(15): 3822.

Mayo Clinic (2021) Endometriosis. www.mayoclinic.org/diseases-conditions/endometriosis/diagnosis-treatment/drc-20354661 (accessed February 2021).

McMahon, C. (2019) Current diagnosis and management of erectile dysfunction. *Medical Journal of Australia* 210(10): 469–476.

McGuinness, H. (2018) *Anatomy and Physiology*, 5th ed. London: Hodder.

Nair, M. and Peate, I. (2009) *Fundamentals of Applied Pathophysiology: An Essential Guide for Nursing Students*. Oxford: John Wiley & Sons, Ltd.

Peate, I. (2009) *Men's Health*. Oxford: John Wiley & Sons, Ltd.

Schug, S.A., Scott, D.A., Mott, J.F., Halliwell, R., Palmer, G.M., Alcock, M. and APM:SE Working Group of the Australian and New Zealand College of Anaesthetists and Faculty of Pain Medicine (2020) *Acute Pain Management: Scientific Evidence*, 5th edn, Melbourne: ANZCA & FPM.

Shimizu, S., Tsounapi, P., Dimitriadis, F., Higashi, Y., Shimizu, T. and Saito, M. (2016) Testicular torsion-detorsion and potential therapeutic treatments: a possible role for ischemic postconditioning. *International Journal Urology* 23: 454–463.

Stanfield, C.L. (2017) *Principles of Human Physiology*, 6th edn. Boston, MA: Pearson.

Tortora, G.J. and Derrickson, B.H. (2009) *Principles of Anatomy and Physiology*, 12th edn. Hoboken, NJ: John Wiley & Sons, Inc.

Tortora, G.J. and Derrickson, B.H. (2012) *Essentials of Anatomy and Physiology*, 9th edn (international student version). New York: John Wiley & Sons, Inc.

Waugh, A. and Grant, A. (2018) *Ross and Wilson Anatomy and Physiology in Health and Illness*, 13th edn. Edinburgh: Churchill Livingstone.

FURTHER READING

ENDOMETRIOSIS

www.endometriosisaustralia.org

Endometriosis Australia provides information on and support for those affected by endometriosis.

FAMILY PLANNING

www.fpnsw.org.au

Family Planning NSW provide straightforward information, advice and support on sexual health, sex and relationships.

PROSTATE CANCER

www.ausprostatecancer.com.au

Australian Prostate Cancer (APC) aims to help men survive prostate cancer and enjoy a better quality of life. It offers support to men and provides information, funds research, raises awareness and improves care.

WOMEN'S HEALTH

https://jeanhailes.org.au

Jean Hailes for Women's Health is an Australian not-for-profit organisation dedicated to improving women's knowledge of women's health throughout the various stages of their lives.

MENOPAUSE

www.menopause.org.au

The Australasian Menopause Society seeks to provide accurate and evidenced-based information to the wider community and to healthcare workers who work with women experiencing menopause.

SEXUAL HEALTH

http://ashhna.org.au

The Australian Sexual Health and HIV Nurses Association is the peak Australasian sexual health, reproductive health and HIV nurses professional association.

AUSTRALASIAN SEXUAL HEALTH ALLIANCE

www.sti.guidelines.org.au

ASHA is a group of organisations aiming to improve local and national responses to sexual health issues. This link shows Australian STI management guidelines for use in primary care.

ACKNOWLEDGEMENTS

Photo: © Olga Green / Shutterstock.com
Photo: © Yuriy Maksymiv / Shutterstock.com
Photo: © Getty Images / iStockphoto
Photo: © JPC-PROD / Shutterstock.com

Photo: © Kzenon / Shutterstock.com
Photo: © Monkey Business Images / Shutterstock.com
Photo: © Serhii Bobyk / Shutterstock.com
Photo: © Getty Images / Hero Images
Figure 13.12: © Mayo Foundation for Medical Education and Research. All Rights Reserved.

CHAPTER 14

The nervous system

TEST YOUR PRIOR KNOWLEDGE

- Which other system does the nervous system work closely with?
- List the structures of the central nervous system.
- How many pairs of cranial nerves are there?
- Name the two divisions of the autonomic nervous system.
- Differentiate between sensory information and motor information.

LEARNING OUTCOMES

After reading this chapter you will be able to:

14.1 describe the structures of the nervous system and the functions of each of these structures
14.2 describe the conduction of nerve impulses
14.3 identify the function of different areas of the brain
14.4 understand the structure and function of the spinal cord
14.5 differentiate between the sympathetic and parasympathetic nervous systems.

Body map

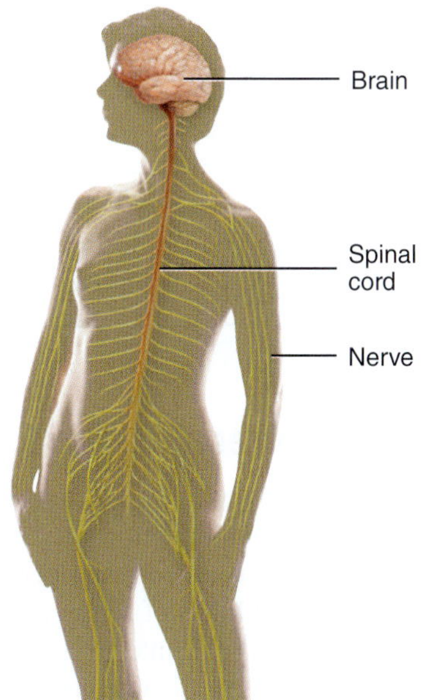

Introduction

The nervous system is a major communicating and control system within the body. It works with the endocrine system to control many body functions. The nervous system provides a rapid and short-acting response, and the endocrine system provides a slower but often more sustained response. The two systems work together to maintain homeostasis.

The nervous system interacts with all of the systems of the body. This system is large and complex. In order to facilitate understanding of the nervous system it has to be divided into smaller functional and anatomical parts. This chapter outlines the divisions of the nervous system; it discusses the structure and function of the nervous system and how it influences other structures of the body. Having such an important role in maintaining homeostasis, the nervous system possesses additional protection, and that too will be investigated.

14.1 Organisation of the nervous system

LEARNING OBJECTIVE 14.1 Describe the structures of the nervous system and the functions of each of these structures.

The nervous system can be divided into two parts: the **central nervous system** and the **peripheral nervous system**. The central nervous system consists of the brain and spinal cord and is the control and integration centre for many body functions.

The peripheral nervous system carries sensory information to the central nervous system and motor information out of the central nervous system. The direction of information flow to and from the nervous system is important and is shown in figure 14.1.

FIGURE 14.1 Organisation of the nervous system

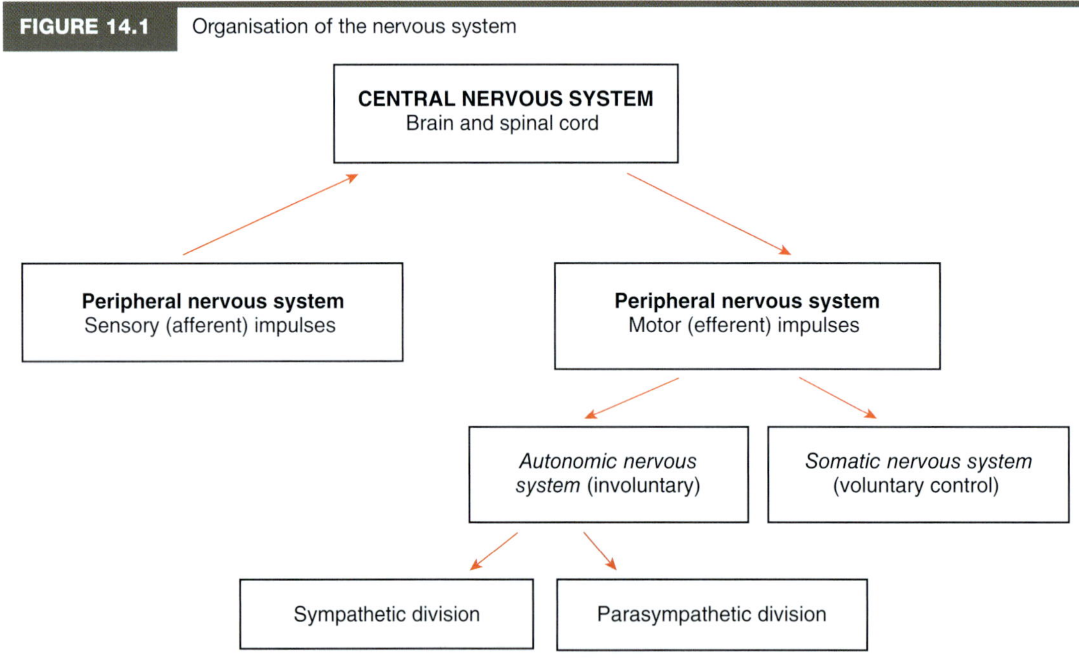

Sensory division of the peripheral nervous system

Sensory information (stimuli) is gathered from both inside and outside of the body. This sensory input is delivered to the central nervous system via the peripheral nerves. **Sensory nerve** fibres are also called **afferent fibres**. Sensory information always travels from the peripheral nervous system towards the central nervous system. There are many different kinds of sensory information, including pain, pressure, temperature, chemical levels and more. Consider the maintenance of body temperature. As warm-blooded animals, it is important that body temperature is maintained between 36.5 and 37.5 °C. Temperature **receptors** in the skin called thermoreceptors detect changes in temperature, and as temperature changes have the potential to cause damage to cells and tissues, this information must be relayed to the central nervous system and, if required, acted upon.

Central nervous system

The central nervous system consists of the brain and spinal cord. The central nervous system processes and integrates sensory information. The received information has to be interpreted, it can be stored to be dealt with later or it can be acted upon immediately with one or more motor responses. For example, the sensation of temperature change would be received and interpreted by the **hypothalamus** (a structure of the central nervous system) and an appropriate action would be initiated.

Motor division of the peripheral nervous system

The motor division of the peripheral nervous system always carries impulses away from the central nervous system, usually to **effector** organs. **Motor nerve** fibres are also called **efferent fibres**. There are two types of motor information: motor information to the **somatic nervous system** or to the **autonomic nervous system**.

Somatic nervous system

The somatic nervous system is under voluntary control, and the effector (tissue or organ responding to instruction from the central nervous system) is skeletal (voluntary) muscle.

The central nervous system's response to sensory information may be to activate the somatic nervous system, eliciting a voluntary response involving skeletal muscle movement. So, from the example of temperature, if an increase in temperature is detected, then it might require the removal of a coat or the opening of a window — this is the motor response that involves the somatic nervous system. It is a voluntary activity that the person chooses to do.

Autonomic nervous system

The central nervous system's response to sensory information may be to activate the autonomic nervous system. This would lead to an involuntary action. The autonomic nervous system is responsible for involuntary motor responses. The effector may be smooth or cardiac muscle (both involuntary muscles) or a gland.

In the example of increased temperature, the involuntary response is to lose heat through the skin — so warm blood is directed to the skin when peripheral blood vessels vasodilate. Vasodilatation is an example of an involuntary autonomic nervous system response. The individual cannot control this response.

The autonomic nervous system is further divided into the sympathetic (fight or flight) and the parasympathetic (rest and digest) divisions. The autonomic nervous system will be discussed later in the chapter. A fine balance between both of these divisions is required for the maintenance of homeostasis.

Neurones

The functional unit of the nervous system is the **neurone** or nerve cell. It has many features in common with other cells, including a nucleus and mitochondria, but because of its vital role it is well protected and has some specialist modifications. Two specialist characteristics of neurones are:

- irritability, in response to a stimulus — the ability to initiate a nerve impulse
- conductivity — the ability to conduct an impulse.

Neurones consist of an **axon**, **dendrites** and a cell body. Their function is to transmit nerve impulses. Nerve impulses only travel in one direction: from the receptive area — the dendrites — to the cell body, and down the length of the axon (see figure 14.2).

Axons bundled together are called nerves. Neurones rely on a constant supply of oxygen and glucose. Once the neurones of the brain and spinal cord have matured after birth they will not be replaced or regenerated if they become damaged. Peripheral neurones can regenerate if the cell body is not damaged and the alignment of the neurone is not disrupted.

Dendrites

Dendrites are short branching processes that receive information and conduct it towards the cell body. Their branching processes provide a large surface area for this function. In sensory neurones the dendrites may form the part of the sensory receptors, and in motor neurones they can form part of the **synapse** between one neurone and the next.

FIGURE 14.2 Motor neurone

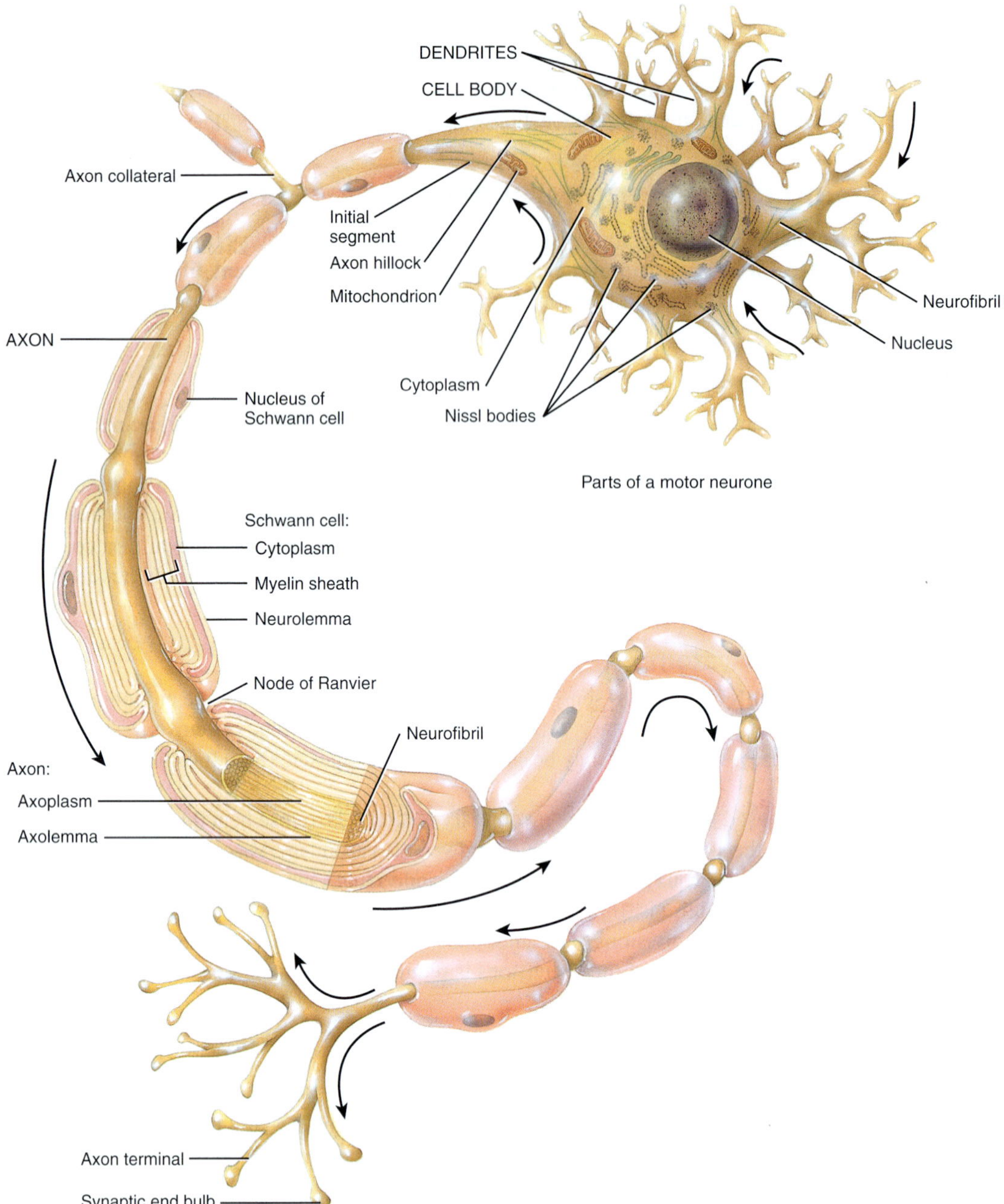

Source: Tortora and Derrickson (2009). Reproduced with permission of John Wiley & Sons.

Cell body

Most of the neurone cell bodies are located inside the central nervous system and form the grey matter. When clusters of cell bodies are grouped together in the central nervous system they are called **nuclei**. Cell bodies located in the peripheral nervous system are called **ganglia**.

Axons

Each neurone has only one axon that conducts information away from the cell body. The axon can branch to form an axon collateral (see figure 14.2). The axon will also branch at its terminal into many axon terminals. The axon delivers the impulse to another neurone or a gland or a muscle.

The axon length can vary quite significantly from very short to 100 cm long (Marieb & Hoehn 2019).

Myelin sheath

Peripheral nerve axons and long or large axons are covered in a **myelin sheath**. Myelin is a fatty material whose purpose is to protect the neurone and to electrically insulate it, speeding up impulse transmission. Within the peripheral nervous system Schwann cells wrapped in layers around the neurone form the myelin sheath. The outermost part of the Schwann cell is its plasma membrane, and this is called the neurilemma. There is a regular gap (about 1 mm) between adjacent Schwann cells. The gaps are called the nodes of Ranvier. Collateral axons can occur at the node (see figure 14.2). Some nerve fibres are unmyelinated, and this makes nerve impulse transmission significantly slower.

CLINICAL CONSIDERATIONS

Multiple sclerosis (MS)

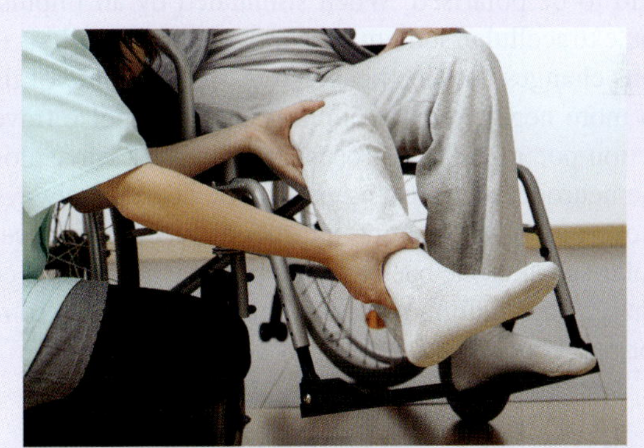

Multiple sclerosis is a condition where areas of demyelination of the **white matter** (myelinated fibres form white matter) can occur. Areas of demyelination are called plaques. Multiple sclerosis affects the 20–40 years age range and is most frequently seen in temperate climates. The cause is unknown but it is suspected that there may be a genetic link; viral infection has also been implicated. Neuronal damage caused by the demyelination leads to:

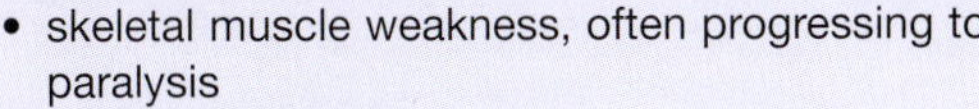

- skeletal muscle weakness, often progressing to paralysis
- visual disturbances
- uncoordinated movements
- burning or tingling sensations.

Multiple sclerosis can be a chronic disease characterised by periods of remission, or the disease can progress rapidly, leading to death.

Sensory (afferent) nerves

The dendrites of sensory neurones are often sensory receptors, and when they are stimulated the impulse generated travels towards the spinal cord and brain. There are different types of sensory receptors:

- special senses (as discussed in the chapter on the senses)
- somatic sensory receptors, located in the skin, such as touch, temperature and pain
- autonomic nervous system receptors, located throughout the body, such as baroreceptors monitoring blood pressure, chemoreceptors monitoring blood pH and visceral pain receptors
- proprioceptors, monitoring muscle movement, stretch and pain.

Motor (efferent) nerves

Information from the central nervous system is delivered to the peripheral nervous system via the motor nerves. Information transmitted through a voluntary somatic nerve may result in skeletal muscle contraction or the information may be autonomic in nature, not under voluntary control, and may lead to smooth muscle contraction or the release of the products of a gland.

14.2 The action potential

LEARNING OBJECTIVE 14.2 Describe the conduction of nerve impulses.

The nervous system is a vast communicating network sending information from the internal and external environment to the central nervous system and from the central nervous system to the muscles and glands. The way that the functional unit, the neurone, achieves this is by the generation and conduction of impulses or **action potentials**.

Generation of the action potential occurs due to the movement of ions into and out of the neurone and the electrical charge associated with this movement.

Two principal ions are involved:

- sodium — normally found outside of the cell (principal extracellular **cation**)
- potassium — normally found inside the cell (principal intracellular cation).

Simple propagation of nerve impulses

When there is no impulse being transmitted the cell is in its resting state — the nerve cell membrane is said to be polarised. When stimulated by an impulse, the cell membrane changes its permeability and the extracellular sodium ions move into the cell — this is called depolarisation. The movement of these ions changes the electrical charge on either side of the cell membrane from more positive extracellularly to more negative extracellularly as the impulse travels the length of the axon. This activity creates the action potential. This process happens in a wave along the length of the neurone from the active part of the neurone to the resting part of the neurone, always in one direction. At the same time, potassium ions move out of the neurone into the extracellular space, returning the electrical charge associated with the polarised neurone back to more positive outside the cell and more negative inside. This is the repolarising phase. The sodium–potassium pump is activated to return sodium to the extracellular space in exchange for potassium (see figure 14.3).

Saltatory conduction

Saltatory conduction occurs in myelinated neurones as the electrical charge associated with the nerve impulse jumps between one node of Ranvier and the next. This occurs much faster than simple propagation. Conduction is also faster when the neurone has a larger diameter.

The refractory period

When the action potential is stimulated, the neurone cannot accept another impulse or generate another action potential no matter how strong the impulse is. This is known as the **refractory period**.

FIGURE 14.3 Action potential

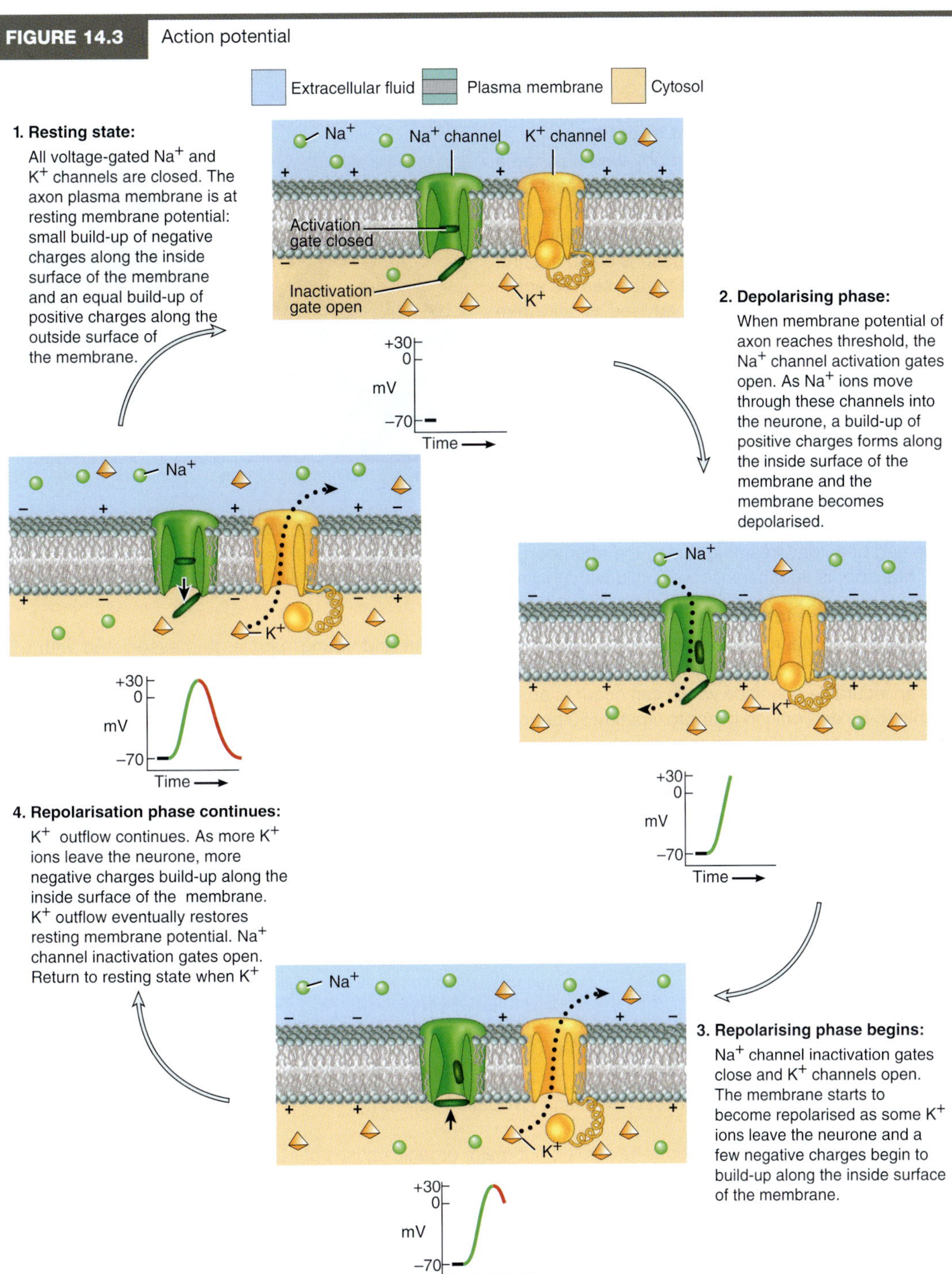

Source: Tortora and Derrickson (2009). Reproduced with permission of John Wiley & Sons.

CLINICALLY REASONED EPISODE OF CARE

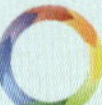

Epilepsy

Consider the patient situation

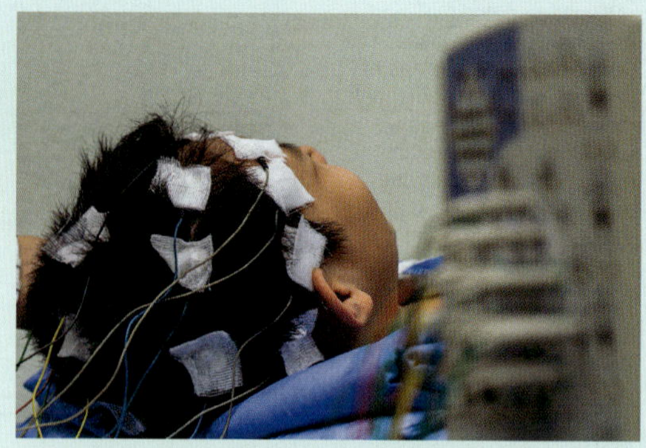

Mansoor Khan is a 6-year-old boy who has had a suspected epileptic seizure. His parents called an ambulance, but the seizure was over by the time the ambulance arrived. Mansoor was admitted to hospital; however, the investigations could not find any abnormalities to account for the seizure activity. Mansoor's parents were advised to take him home and to return to the hospital if there was any further seizure activity.

Mansoor's parents have now noticed periods when he appears vague, so they have returned to the GP for further investigation. Mansoor is seen by the practice nurse as part of the care team.

Collect cues and information

Mansoor had been observed by his parents as having seizure-like activity. Mansoor's teachers noted that he had been daydreaming during the afternoon of the day that he had the seizure.

Mansoor is an otherwise well child with no illnesses and there is no family history of epilepsy.

Process information

Epilepsy is a neurological condition that can affect children and young people. It is associated with a disruption of the electrical activity within the neurones in the brain and affects 1 in 200 children. Epilepsy is an incurable condition which can occur at any stage in a person's life. The cause of epilepsy will not be able to be determined in approximately 50 per cent of cases. More obvious causes include brain tumour, stroke or encephalitis, among others.

Symptoms of epilepsy include staring, loss of consciousness, difficulty breathing, jerky movements of the limbs, and loss of bladder and/or bowel control. Tests to diagnose epilepsy include electroencephalogram (EEG). Some tests (e.g. CT or MRI) are important to carry out as they rule out other conditions such as brain tumour.

Treatments include a modified diet, antiepileptic medication or surgery, depending on the cause of the epilepsy.

A diagnosis of epilepsy can be a frightening time for families, and emotional and educational support is an important part of the care provided.

Establish goals

1. Referral to neurologist
2. Education and support

Nursing actions

1. Refer to a neurologist for investigation and navigation support.
   Rationale:
   - While hospital investigations have ruled out major organic causes of Mansoor's epilepsy, a specialist neurologist is able to conduct an EEG.
   - While the GP will conduct the initial referral, practice nurses are well placed to liaise with the multidisciplinary team and the family to ensure that referrals and appointments are communicated, helping families to navigate the system.
2. Provide education and ongoing support.
   Rationale:
   - Investigation and diagnosis of epilepsy can be a challenging time for patients and families. Practice nurses are well placed to provide support and information to families, in addition to specialist nurse educators.
   - Education about epilepsy, treatment options and when to seek help will help inform Mansoor's parents and family.

Evaluate outcomes

As a result of the actions above, Mansoor is formally diagnosed with epilepsy; however, the cause remains unknown. Mansoor and his family are seen regularly by the general practice and neurologist team. The treatment plan ensures that Mansoor's epilepsy is well managed.

Reflect on new processes and learning

Consider the family situation. What information and advice can Mansoor's family obtain from the practice nurse?

Source: Based on the Clinical Reasoning Cycle, Levett-Jones (2013).

Neurotransmitters

Neurones do not come into contact with one another. Where one neurone ends and another begins, there is a space called the synapse. In order for communication to occur between neurones or between the neurone and a muscle or gland, a chemical messenger called a neurotransmitter is secreted by the neurone into the extracellular space at the synapse. Those effector cells or neurones in close proximity to the neurotransmitter will either be stimulated or inhibited by the neurotransmitter, depending upon which neurotransmitter is secreted. The action of the neurotransmitter is short-lived, and any neurotransmitter not used is absorbed by the neurone to be recycled and used again or deactivated by enzymes.

Some examples of neurotransmitters are:

- acetylcholine, released within the central nervous system and also at the **neuromuscular junction**
- norepinephrine, released within the central nervous system and also at autonomic nervous system synapses
- dopamine, released within the central nervous system and also at autonomic nervous system synapses.

CLINICAL CONSIDERATIONS

Electroencephalogram (EEG)

An electroencephalogram (EEG) records brain activity. It is particularly useful for diagnosing conditions such as epilepsy, dementia and encephalopathy.

Electrodes are placed on the head and attached to an EEG machine. The electrical activity generated by nerve impulses is then measured. During the EEG, the patient may be asked to breathe deeply or blink several times. There are different types of EEG used to ascertain triggers that may lead to seizure activity, and these include sleep EEG, sleep-deprived EEG, ambulatory EEG and strobe lighting EEG.

The test can usually be carried out in an out-patient department (apart from sleep EEG), and the outcome could lead to a treatment plan being implemented or altered.

CLINICALLY REASONED EPISODE OF CARE

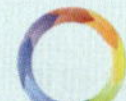

Alzheimer's disease

Consider the patient situation

Grace is a 75-year-old woman. She is experiencing some symptoms of forgetfulness that are concerning her. Her family have brought her to see her GP. Grace and her family liaise with the practice nurse as part of the general practice team.

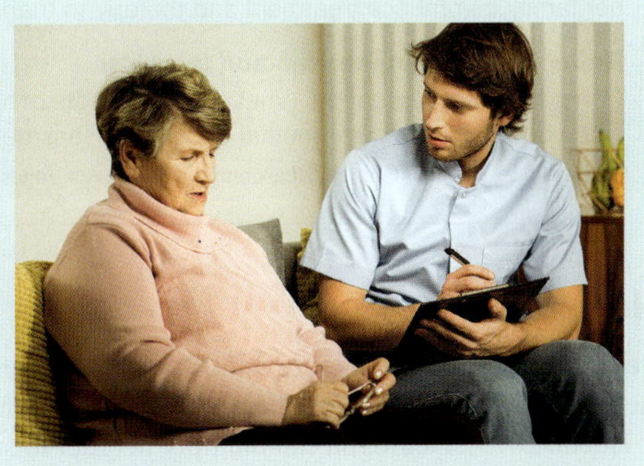

Collect cues and information

Both Grace and her family have noticed a decrease in Grace's memory, with Grace reporting that she frequently forgets family anniversaries and where she has put things. Grace is concerned as her mother developed dementia at a young age and she recognises some of the symptoms she has developed.

Grace sought treatment for depression after her husband died 10 years ago; however, she did not take the prescribed antidepressants and her family suspects that her alcohol consumption increased at this time.

Given Grace's age and symptoms, she is concerned about the potential for Alzheimer's disease.

Process information

Alzheimer's disease is a form of dementia. It is a progressive neurodegenerative disease which affects the brain cells. Neurofibrillary tangles are formed within the neurones and amyloid plaques are formed around the neurones. There is also a reduction in the neurotransmitter acetylcholine. Contributing factors to the condition include being over 65 years of age, having a family history, and having untreated depression or cardiovascular disease. There may also be some association between alcohol consumption and Alzheimer's.

Approximately 459 000 Australians live with dementia and almost 1.6 million Australians are involved in their care. Initial symptoms of Alzheimer's include memory loss, forgetting recent conversations, getting lost in familiar places, losing items, repeating the same conversations, poor spatial awareness, difficulty concentrating and disorientation. These symptoms progress as the disease progresses.

Treatment for Alzheimer's includes the use of acetylcholinesterase inhibitors, which help increase acetylcholine and therefore can help to manage symptoms. Other treatments include antidepressants, cognitive behavioural therapy and cognitive rehabilitation.

Establish goals

1. Conduct assessments and test
2. Liaise with multidisciplinary team, Grace and her family
3. Provide support and education to Grace and her family

Nursing actions

1. Conduct assessment and tests.
   Rationale:
   - It is important to conduct a thorough assessment to rule out organic or other causes of symptoms. Assessment should include a urine analysis, vital signs, blood tests and mental assessments such as the Mini Mental Assessment and the General Practitioner Assessment of Cognition test.
   - Nurses are an essential part of the practice team and are well placed to collect and assess information.
2. Liaise with multidisciplinary team, Grace and her family.
   Rationale:
   - Grace has been referred to a psychiatrist and will have others involved in care. Practice nurses can act as a point of liaison for the practice, with the GP acting as the care coordinator.
   - As Alzheimer's is a progressive disease, the practice nurse can conduct ongoing assessments and tests to track progress and liaise with the team.
3. Provide support and education to Grace and her family.
   Rationale:
   - Nurses are well placed to provide information and education to Grace and her family, including information about the diagnosis, treatment and what to expect long term.
   - A diagnosis of Alzheimer's can be a lifelong challenge for Grace and her family. Having a point of liaison can assist with making and managing appointments and medications, and it can provide ongoing support to the family unit.

Evaluate outcomes

As a result of her examination and assessments, Grace is diagnosed with Alzheimer's disease. Grace and her family commence treatment and therapy to manage the progression of the disease.

Reflect on new processes and learning

Consider Grace's situation. What are the benefits of having a practice nurse as part of the team, particularly when conducting regular mental capacity assessments?

Source: Based on the Clinical Reasoning Cycle, Levett-Jones (2013).

Neuroglia

Neuroglia (see figure 14.4) are cells that support neurones. They are more numerous than neurones. Within the central nervous system the neuroglial cells account for more than half of the weight of the brain (Marieb & Hoehn 2019). Neuroglia can multiply in order to support the neurones. Because of this, nervous system tumours often originate from neuroglia.

FIGURE 14.4 Neuroglia

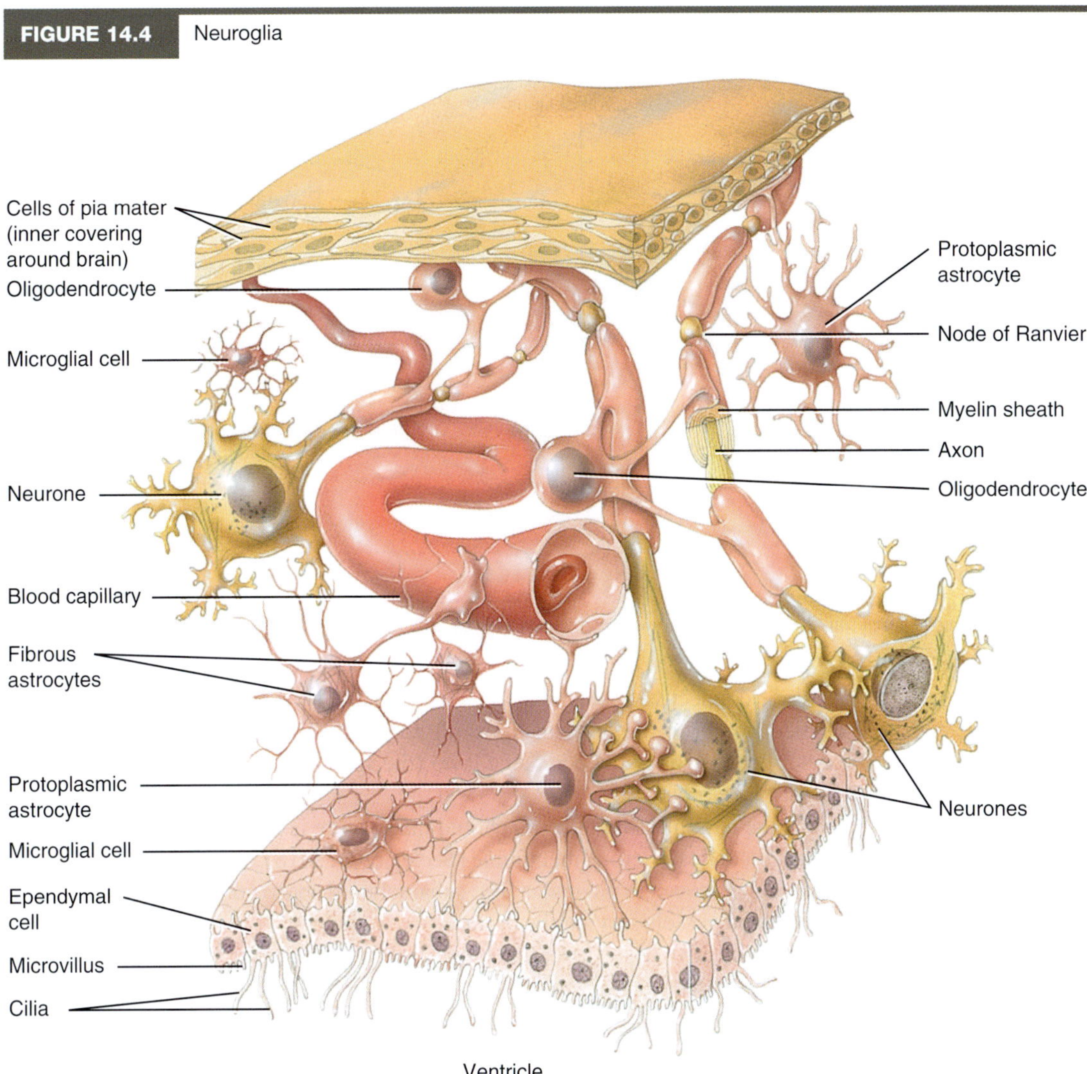

Source: Tortora and Derrickson (2009). Reproduced with permission of John Wiley & Sons.

Within the peripheral nervous system, two types of neuroglia have been identified.

1. *Schwann cells*. These cells are responsible for forming the myelin sheath.
2. *Satellite cells*. The function of satellite cells is not known.

Within the central nervous system; four type of neuroglial cell have been identified.

1. **Astrocytes** are star-shaped cells which occur in large quantities between neurones and blood vessels, supporting and anchoring them to each other. They help form the blood–brain barrier, which gives the neurones an extra layer of protection from any toxic substances within the blood.
2. **Microglia** lie close to neurones and can move closer if they need to fulfil their function as nervous system macrophages. They phagocytose pathogens or cell debris.
3. **Oligodendrocytes** are found close to myelinated neurones. They help to form and maintain the myelin sheath.
4. **Ependymal cells** are often ciliated and are found lining cavities, such as the spinal cord or the **ventricles** of the brain. Their role is to circulate **cerebrospinal fluid** (CSF) (Waugh & Grant 2018).

The meninges

Nervous tissue is easily damaged by pressure and therefore needs to be protected. The hair, skin and bone offer an outer layer of protection. Adjacent to the nervous tissue are the **meninges** (see figure 14.5). The meninges cover the delicate nervous tissue, providing further protection. They also protect the blood vessels that serve nervous tissue and they contain CSF.

FIGURE 14.5 The meninges

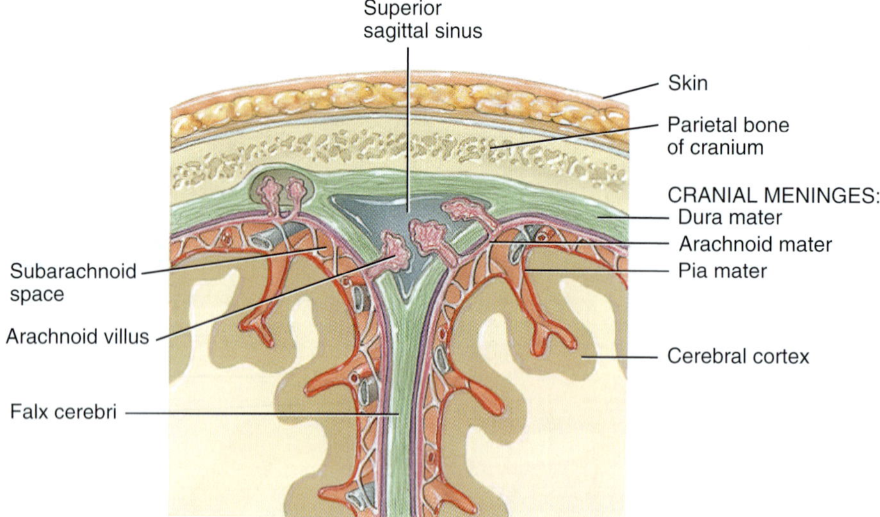

Source: Tortora and Derrickson (2009). Reproduced with permission of John Wiley & Sons.

The meninges consist of three connective tissue layers.

- ***Dura mater***. This layer lies closest to the bone of the skull and is a double layer of tough, fibrous, connective tissue. The outer layer is called the periosteal layer (the spinal cord lacks this layer), and the meningeal layer lies closest to the brain.
- ***Arachnoid mater***. Between the dura mater and the arachnoid mater there is a space called the subdural space. The arachnoid mater is a delicate serous membrane (Seeley et al. 2016). The subarachnoid space is below the arachnoid mater and above the pia mater. The subarachnoid space contains CSF and is also home to some of the larger blood vessels serving the brain.
- ***Pia mater***. This is a delicate connective tissue layer that clings tightly to the brain. It contains many tiny blood vessels that serve the brain.

CLINICAL CONSIDERATIONS

Meningitis

Meningitis is inflammation of the meninges caused by either bacteria or viruses. It can be diagnosed through symptoms that include photophobia, headache, nausea and vomiting and also by a procedure called a lumbar puncture. In lumbar puncture a small amount of CSF is removed and examined in the laboratory for the presence of microbes. A lack of prompt treatment can have fatal consequences.

Cerebrospinal fluid

CSF is produced by the choroid plexus in the ventricles of the brain (see figure 14.6). There is approximately 150 mL of CSF circulating around the brain, in the ventricles and around the spinal cord. The CSF is replaced every 8 h (Marieb & Hoehn 2019). It is a thin fluid similar to plasma and has several important functions.

- It acts as a cushion, supporting the weight of the brain and protecting it from damage.
- It helps to maintain a uniform pressure around the brain and spinal cord.
- There is a limited exchange of nutrients and waste products between neurones and CSF.

There are four ventricles in the brain: the paired lateral ventricles, one in each **cerebral hemisphere**; the third ventricle, situated below this; and the fourth ventricle, located inferior to the third. The third and fourth ventricles communicate via the central canal and CSF circulates through the central canal and into the spinal cord.

Any additional pressure applied to the brain caused by swelling (cerebral oedema), tumour or haemorrhage (through trauma) can lead to a reduced volume of CSF being produced.

FIGURE 14.6 The ventricles (right lateral view of the brain)

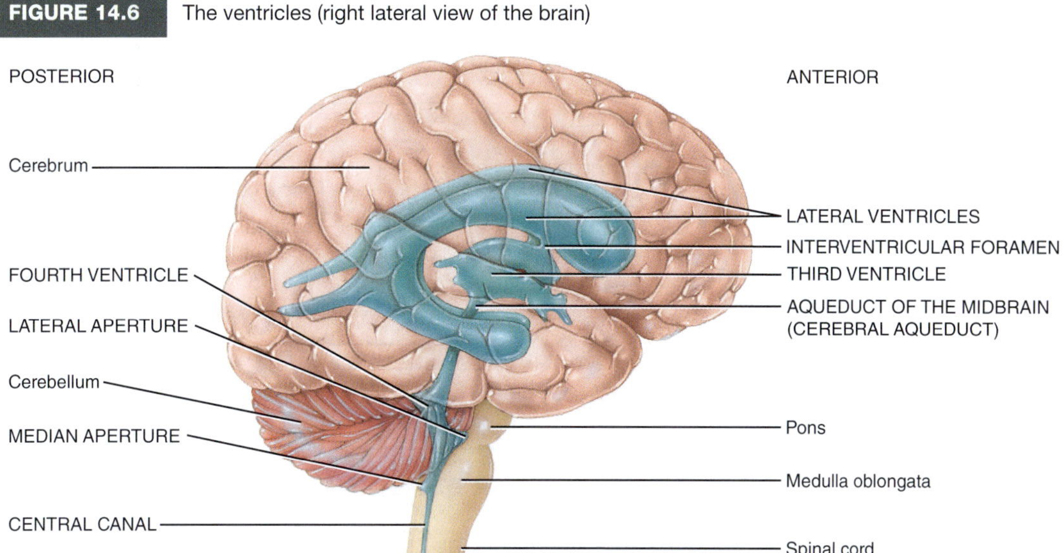

Source: Tortora and Derrickson (2009). Reproduced with permission of John Wiley & Sons.

CLINICAL CONSIDERATIONS

Lumbar puncture

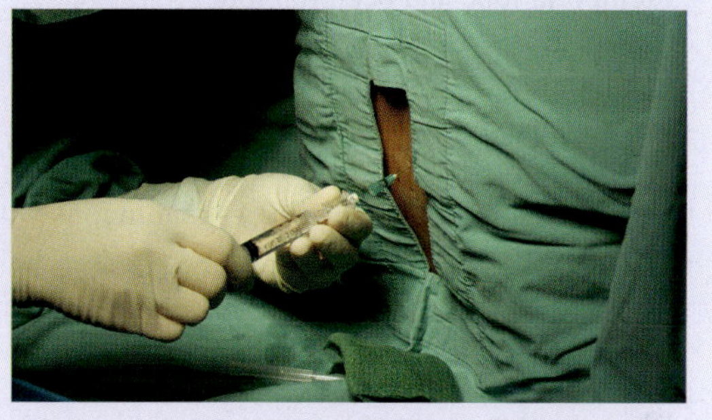

Lumbar puncture is often used to diagnose conditions such as meningitis and multiple sclerosis.

A sample of CSF is removed and sent for laboratory analysis. The sample is taken by inserting a needle between the third and fourth lumbar vertebrae and the CSF is removed from the subarachnoid space. This procedure is usually carried out under local anaesthetic.

The CSF circulates around the brain and spinal cord. The pressure exerted by the CSF is known as intracranial pressure (ICP). Normal ICP is 8–20 cm H_2O. If the ICP is raised this could be for a variety of reasons, including cerebral oedema in the brain as might be seen in head injury, head trauma or meningitis. It could also be raised because of the additional white cells, protein or myelin within the CSF, as in multiple sclerosis.

The CSF should be colourless. Cloudy CSF may indicate the presence of infection. CSF is usually watery in viscosity. If it is more viscous then this could indicate the presence of infection or tumour. Laboratory analysis will give a more accurate interpretation than a visual inspection.

Laboratory analysis will show the amount of glucose protein and immunoglobulins, for example, present in CSF. The white cells can be analysed, and the presence of bacteria and viruses is also investigated.

There are side effects associated with lumbar puncture, and these include back pain from the site of the puncture and headache. The headache is relieved by lying down.

14.3 The brain

LEARNING OBJECTIVE 14.3 Identify the function of different areas of the brain.

The brain lies in the cranial cavity and weighs between 1450 and 1600 g (Marieb & Hoehn 2019). It receives 15 per cent of the cardiac output and has a system of autoregulation ensuring the blood supply is constant despite positional changes. The arrangement of the arteries serving the brain is unique, and they are connected to each other by a structure called the **circle of Willis** (see figure 14.7). This arrangement ensures that blood pressure remains equal in both halves of the brain. Should one of the arteries serving the brain become narrowed by arterial disease or thrombus then there will be an alternative route available, maintaining the essential supply of oxygen and glucose required by the brain.

FIGURE 14.7 Circle of Willis

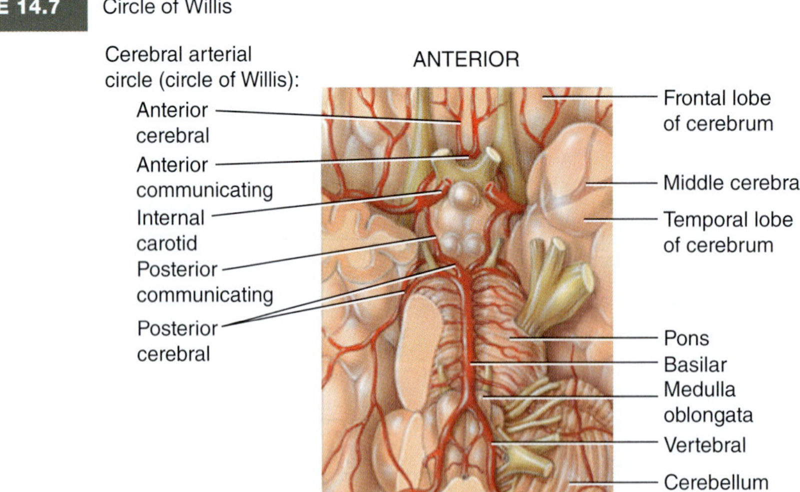

Source: Tortora and Derrickson (2009). Reproduced with permission of John Wiley & Sons.

The brain can be divided into four anatomical regions: **cerebrum**, **diencephalon**, **cerebellum** and **brainstem**. Each region contains one or more structures (see figure 14.8):

- cerebrum (front of the brain)
  - right and left cerebral hemispheres — each hemisphere has four **lobes**: frontal lobe, parietal lobe, temporal lobe and occipital lobe
- diencephalon
  - **thalamus**
  - hypothalamus
  - **epithalamus**
- brainstem (middle of the brain) — continuous with the **spinal cord**
  - **midbrain**
  - pons
  - **medulla oblongata**
- cerebellum (back of brain)
  - vermis; right and left cerebellar hemispheres — each hemisphere consists of anterior, posterior and flocculonodular lobes.

Cerebrum

This is the largest brain structure. It is divided into the left and right hemispheres by the longitudinal cerebral fissure. Each hemisphere can be divided into lobes — occipital, frontal, parietal and temporal. The outer layer of the cerebrum is called the cerebral cortex and is made of grey matter (nerve cell bodies). The layers below this are white matter (nerve fibres). The cerebral cortex is responsible for our conscious mind and consists of interneurones (the neurones that lie between sensory and motor neurones). The cerebral cortex can be divided into functional areas, which were mapped by Brodmann in 1906 (see figure 14.9). The circled numbers on the diagram represent important areas on Brodmann's map. While functional and structural areas of the brain have been identified, it is important to remember that the areas do not function independently from one another, and damage to one structure may have consequences for another.

The first of the functional areas is the **motor area** and it is subdivided as follows:

- the primary motor area — responsible for contraction of skeletal muscles
- the premotor area — involved in fine skeletal muscle movement creating the manual dexterity associated with repetitive or learned motor movement (e.g. tying a shoelace, learning to paint, giving an injection)
- Broca's area — responsible for the motor movement required to produce speech
- the frontal eye field area — controls voluntary movement of the eyes.

FIGURE 14.8 The structures of the brain

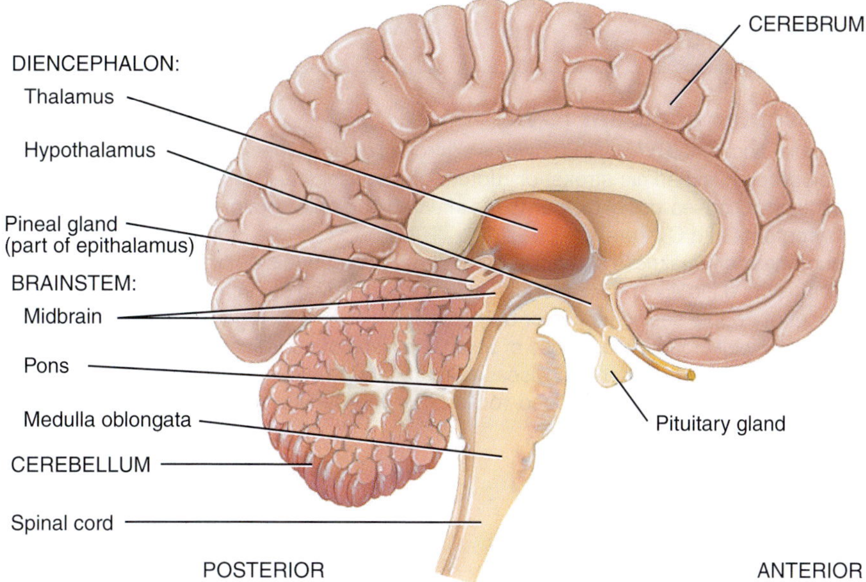

Source: Tortora and Derrickson (2009). Reproduced with permission of John Wiley & Sons.

FIGURE 14.9 Right cerebral hemisphere

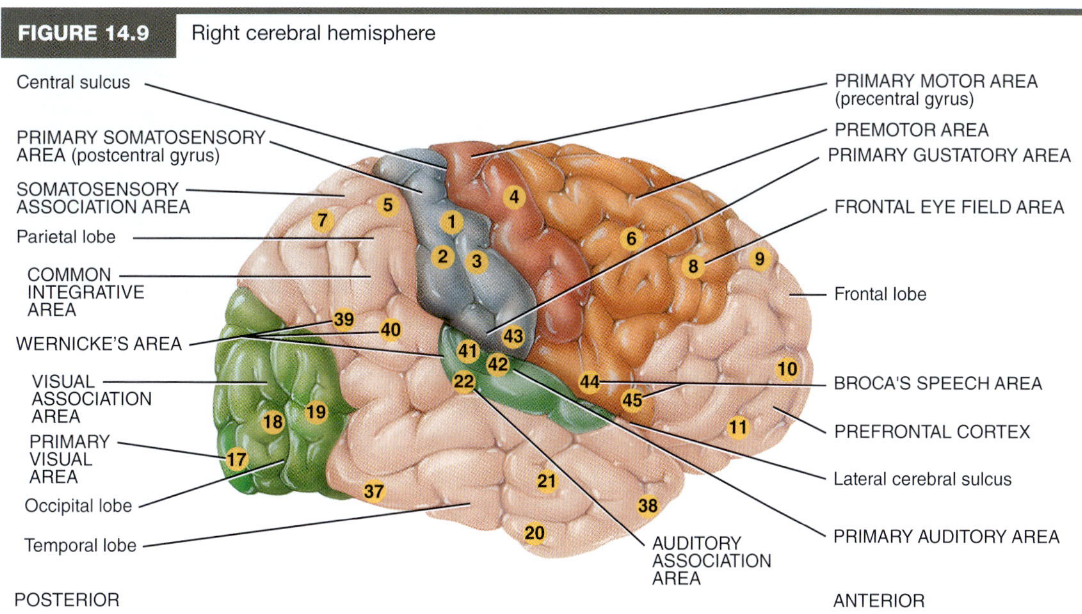

Source: Tortora and Derrickson (2009). Reproduced with permission of John Wiley & Sons.

The second functional area is the **sensory area**, responsible for awareness of sensation. It can be divided as follows:

- the primary somatosensory area — receives sensory information from the skin and also from proprioceptors in skeletal muscles
- the somatosensory association area — integrates the sensory information being relayed to the primary somatosensory area and provides information about size, texture, previous experience
- the visual areas — the primary visual area receives information from the eye and the visual association area helps to connect this information with past visual experiences
- the auditory areas — associated with the interpretation of sounds
- the olfactory area — interprets smell information received from the nose via the olfactory nerves
- the gustatory area — interprets taste information.

There are many other association areas within the cerebrum that act as communication areas between different functional regions in the cerebrum, such as Wernicke's area, which is responsible for understanding written and spoken language and is closely associated with Broca's speech area.

HOMEOSTATIC IMBALANCE

Cerebrovascular accident (CVA)

A cerebrovascular accident (CVA), also known as a 'stroke', occurs when blood flow to the brain is stopped by either a blood clot (ischaemic stroke) or rupture of a vessel (haemorrhagic stroke) (AIHW 2020b). A blockage to the brain causes loss of oxygen to the affected part of the brain, resulting in death of brain cells.

Five key symptoms of a CVA are:

- sudden numbness or weakness in the face, arm or leg (along one side of the body)
- sudden confusion, difficulty speaking or difficulty understanding speech
- sudden onset of trouble seeing (in one or both eyes)
- sudden difficulty walking, dizziness, loss of balance or lack of coordination
- sudden severe headache (Centers for Disease Control and Prevention 2021).

The acronym FAST has been developed to assist in the early diagnosis of stroke (Stroke Foundation 2021).

- **F**ace
- **A**rms
- **S**peech
- **T**ime

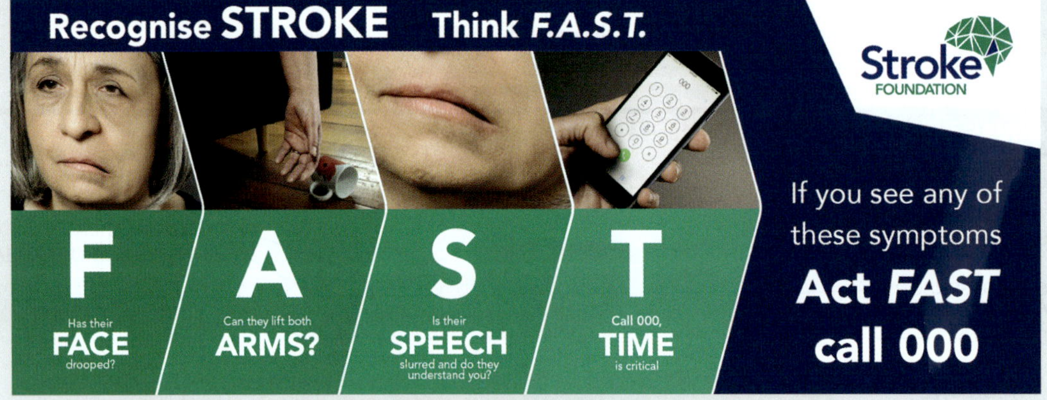

In 2018, approximately 387 000 people in Australia have had a stroke at some time in their lives; and approximately 38 000 stroke events occurred in 2017, which is over 100 per day (AIHW 2020b). Stroke accounted for 8400 deaths in 2018, accounting for 5.3 per cent of all deaths in Australia (AIHW 2020b).

Diencephalon

This part of the brain is surrounded by the cerebrum and contains three paired structures.

- *Thalamus*. The thalamus acts as a relay station for sensory impulses going to the cerebral cortex for integration and motor impulses entering and leaving the cerebral hemispheres. It also has a role in memory.
- *Hypothalamus*. The hypothalamus is closely associated with the **pituitary gland** and produces two hormones: **antidiuretic hormone (ADH)** and oxytocin. The hypothalamus has many functions and these include:
  - control of body temperature
  - control of the autonomic nervous system
  - control of fluid balance and thirst
  - control of appetite
  - those associated with the limbic system dealing with emotional reactions
  - control of sexual behaviours.
- *Epithalamus*. This structure is linked to the **pineal gland**, which secretes the hormone melatonin responsible for sleep–wake cycles.

Brainstem

The structures that form the brainstem are involved in many activities that are essential for life. The brainstem is associated with the **cranial nerves**.

- *Midbrain*. The midbrain is the conduction pathway that connects the cerebrum with the lower brain structures and spinal cord.
- *Pons*. The pons is also a conduction pathway communicating with the cerebellum. The pons works with the medulla oblongata to control depth and rate of respiration.
- *Medulla oblongata*. This is the relay station for sensory nerves going to the cerebrum. The medulla contains autonomic centres such as the cardiac centre, the respiratory centre, the vasomotor centre and the coughing, sneezing and vomiting centre. The medulla is also the site of decussation of the pyramidal tracts — this means that the right side of the body is controlled by the left cerebral hemisphere and vice versa.

CLINICAL CONSIDERATIONS

Concussion

Concussion is a minor head injury and is defined as a brief period of unconsciousness. It is also termed mild traumatic brain injury (VanMeter & Hubert 2014). Signs and symptoms include nausea, headaches, dizziness, impaired concentration, amnesia (memory loss), extreme tiredness, and intolerance to light and noise. The symptoms usually only last for 24 h.

Cerebellum

The cerebellum coordinates voluntary muscle movement, balance and posture. It ensures that muscle movements are smooth, coordinated and precise.

The limbic system and the reticular formation

The limbic system and reticular formation are functional systems as they consist of networks of neurones that can be located close to many anatomical structures.

The limbic system is located close to the cerebrum and the diencephalon. It is known as the emotional brain and is responsible for the interpretation of facial expression, helping identify fear and danger.

The reticular formation is a functional system located in the core of the brainstem and consists of a collection of neurones that have several functions.

- It contains the reticular activating system that is responsible for alertness.
- It filters or blocks repetitive stimuli, such as background noise.
- It regulates skeletal muscle activity.
- It coordinates visceral activity controlled by the autonomic nervous system.

The brain is a well-protected control and integration centre that receives information from the peripheral sensory nervous system and sends motor information to the peripheral nervous system through a comprehensive network of pathways via the spinal cord.

MEDICINES MANAGEMENT

Midazolam

Midazolam is a medication classified as a benzodiazepine. Benzodiazepines act on central nervous system receptors and produce a sedative effect. Midazolam is thought to produce amnesia (Ambulance Australia 2020) and is therefore useful in procedures that require the patient to be awake and cooperative despite the unpleasant nature of the procedure, such as endoscopy (Therapeutic Goods Administration 2018). The intention is that the patient will not remember the procedure.

Midazolam is a short-acting benzodiazepine and has a half-life of 2.5 hours (Ambulance Australia 2020). It is available for administration via a variety of routes, including intravenous and intramuscular. Midazolam has a number of side effects and these include:

- respiratory failure
- respiratory depression

- hypotension
- anaphylaxis
- convulsions
- dry mouth
- constipation
- nausea
- euphoria
- hiccups
- headache.

As benzodiazepines can be addictive, in some instances their use has been abused. An antagonist called flumazenil is available to reverse the effects of the medication. Benzodiazepines should be prescribed with caution.

See Bullock and Manias (2016).

MEDICINES MANAGEMENT

Phenytoin

John is 34 years old and experiences seizures following his recovery from a head injury. He is prescribed phenytoin sodium 100 mg orally three times a day. This medicine works during the action potential. It promotes the removal of sodium during the refractory period, thus reducing the hyperexcitability of neurones that can lead to seizure (McFadden 2019). John is advised to avoid alcohol and to maintain good oral hygiene practices as this medicine has a known side effect of gingival hyperplasia (gum overgrowth).

SKILLS IN PRACTICE

Neurological assessment

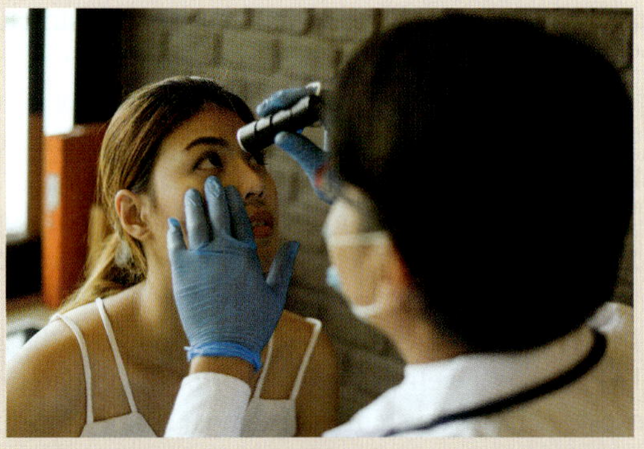

Neurological assessment is an important role for both nurses and paramedics in the assessment of a person's neurological status following a head injury or for patients who have the potential for rapid deterioration in level of consciousness (Calleja et al. 2020). The Glasgow coma scale (GCS) (table 14.1) is an internationally recognised assessment tool for grading neurological responses of the injured or severely ill patient (Calleja et al. 2020). Three parameters of consciousness are assessed using the GCS: 1) eye opening; 2) verbal response; and 3) motor response. Using these parameters the patient is graded a score out of 15, with the higher scores indicating the most positive response of a fully alert and orientated individual. The lower the score, the greater the neurological deficit.

A neurological assessment also includes assessment of pupil size and reaction to light. Pupil size and symmetry are firstly assessed, with normal size pupils ranging from 2 to 6 mm in diameter. Patients with normal neurological status should demonstrate a brisk and consensual pupillary response to light. Pupil response is assessed by briefly shining a penlight from the side of the face into each eye. The procedure is repeated in the other eye and results recorded. The pupils of both eyes should constrict briskly (Douglas 2021).

Assessment of motor function and muscle strength in each limb is also an important part of a neurological assessment. Diminished motor function or strength may indicate a lesion in either the central or peripheral nervous system. During assessment, each limb is assessed for bilateral equality of muscle strength (Douglas 2021).

TABLE 14.1 **The Glasgow coma scale (GCS)**

Behaviour	Response	Score
Eye opening response	Spontaneously To speech To pain No response	4 3 2 1
Best verbal response	Oriented to time, place and person Confused Inappropriate words Incomprehensible sounds No response	5 4 3 2 1
Best motor response	Obeys commands Moves to localised pain Flexion withdrawal from pain Abnormal flexion (decorticate) Abnormal extension (decerebrate) No response	6 5 4 3 2 1
Total score:	*Best response* *Comatose client* *Totally unresponsive*	15 8 or less 3

Source: Teasdale and Jennett (1974).

14.4 The peripheral nervous system

LEARNING OBJECTIVE 14.4 Understand the structure and function of the spinal cord.

The peripheral nervous system includes all the tissues that lie outside of the central nervous system:

- cranial nerves
- **spinal nerves**
- spinal cord
- autonomic nervous system.

The peripheral nervous system is subdivided into the efferent or motor system and the afferent or sensory system. The somatic sensory system serves the skeletal muscles, joints, tendons and the skin and includes the senses of vision, hearing, smell and taste (Logenbaker 2016). The internal organs of the body are supplied by the visceral sensory system. Both the somatic and visceral sensory systems take information from peripheral sensory receptors towards the central nervous system.

Commands from the central nervous system to the skeletal muscles are carried by the somatic motor system. The autonomic motor system predominantly regulates the activity of smooth and cardiac muscles and glands (Logenbaker 2016).

Cranial nerves

There are 12 pairs of cranial nerves that emerge from the brain and supply various structures, most of which are associated with the head and neck. Figure 14.10 provides an overview of the location and function of the cranial nerves.

The 12 pairs of cranial nerves differ in their functions: some are sensory nerves (i.e. contain sensory fibres), some are motor nerves (i.e. contain only motor fibres) and some are mixed nerves (i.e. contain both sensory and motor nerves).

Table 14.2 provides a summary of the cranial nerves, their different components and function.

FIGURE 14.10 Functions of cranial nerves

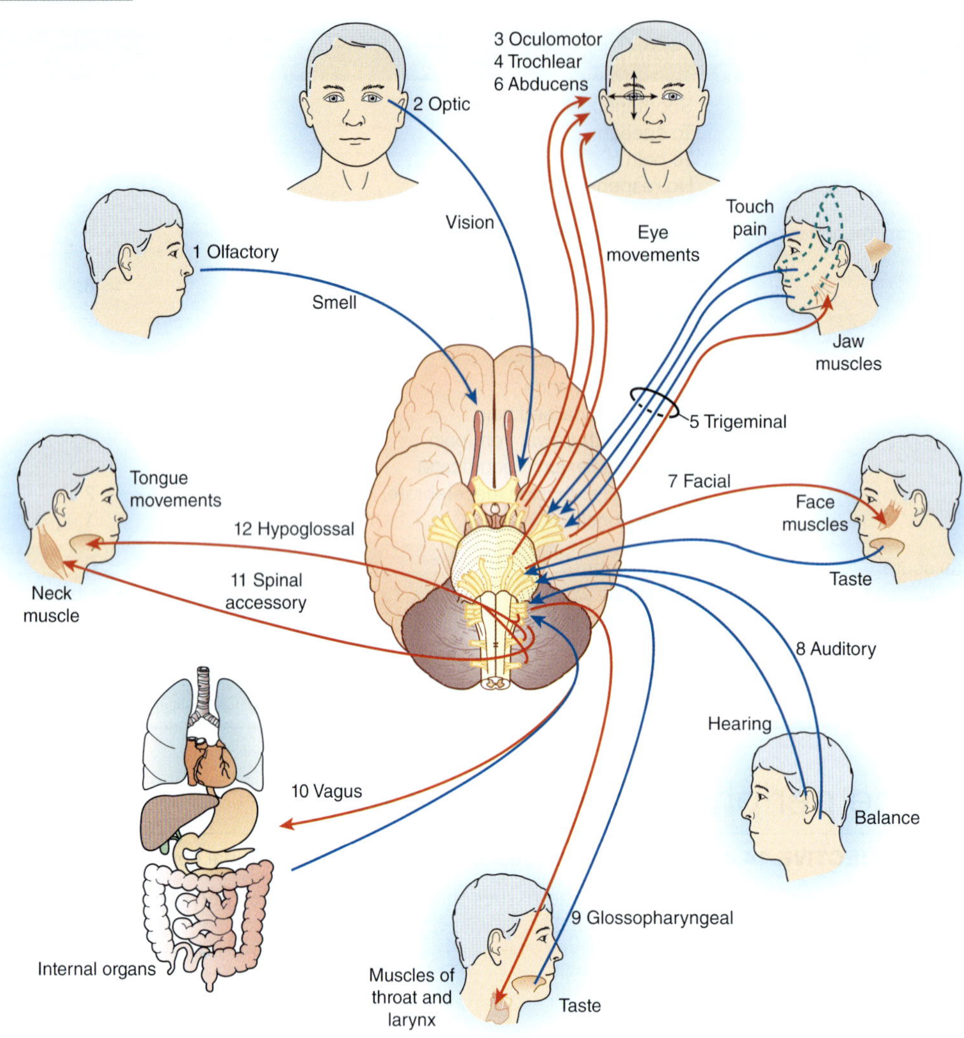

TABLE 14.2 **The cranial nerves**

Number	Name	Components	Location/function
I	Olfactory	Sensory	Olfactory receptors for sense of smell
II	Optic	Sensory	Retina (sight)
III	Oculomotor	Motor	Eye muscles (including eyelids and lens, pupil)
IV	Trochlear	Motor	Eye muscles
V	Trigeminal	Sensory and motor	Teeth, eyes, skin, tongue for sensation of touch, pain and temperature
VI	Abducens	Motor	Jaw muscles (chewing)
			Eye muscles
VII	Facial	Sensory and motor	Taste buds
			Facial muscles, tear and salivary glands

VIII	Vestibulocochlear	Sensory	Inner ear (hearing and balance)
IX	Glossopharyngeal	Sensory and motor	Pharyngeal muscles (swallowing)
X	Vagus	Sensory and motor	Internal organs
XI	Spinal accessory	Motor	Neck and back muscles
XII	Hypoglossal	Motor	Tongue muscles

The spinal cord

The average adult spinal cord (see figure 14.11) is between 42 and 45 cm long and extends from the medulla oblongata (lower part of the brain) to the upper part of the second lumbar vertebra. The spinal cord is enclosed within the vertebral canal, which forms a protective ring of bone around the cord. Other protective coverings include the spinal meninges, which are three layers of connective tissue coverings that extend around the spinal cord. The spinal meninges consist of:

- the pia mater — the innermost layer
- the arachnoid mater — the middle layer
- the dura mater — the outermost layer, which consists of a dense, irregular connective tissue.

FIGURE 14.11 The spinal cord

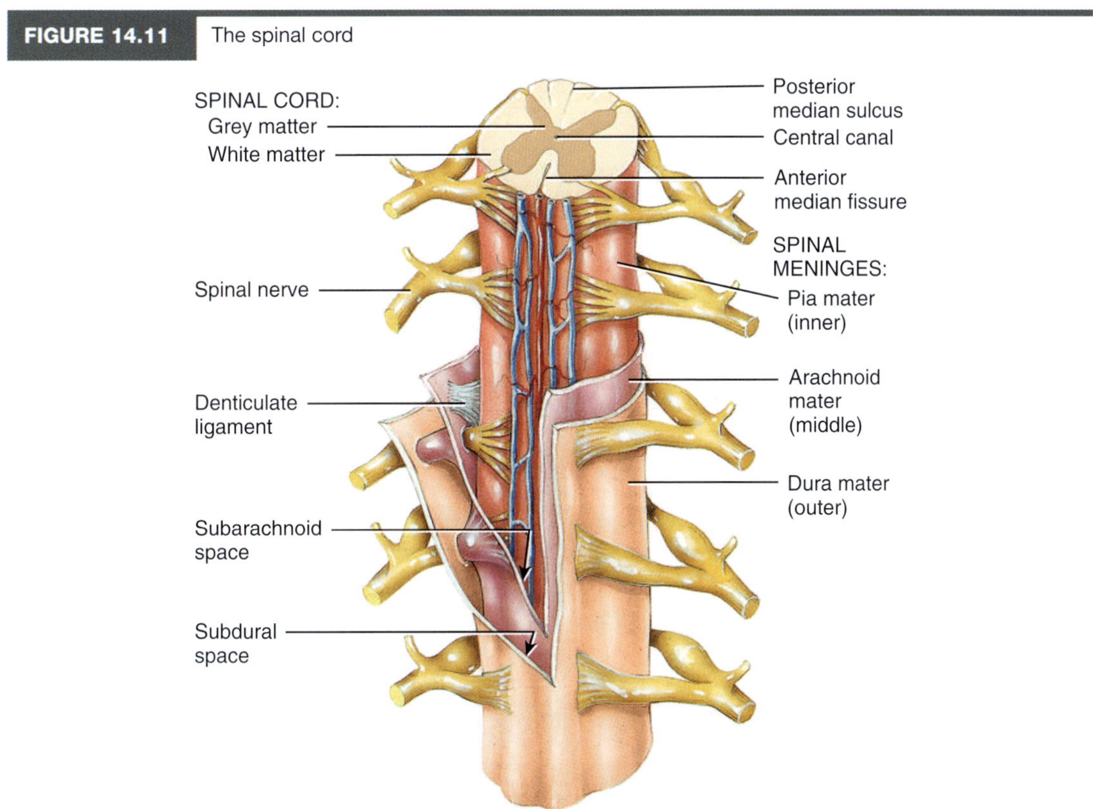

Source: Tortora and Derrickson (2009). Reproduced with permission of John Wiley & Sons.

The spinal cord consists of a central canal and grey and white matter. The central canal and the spinal meninges contain CSF. The grey matter consists mostly of cell bodies and their dendrites, and the whiter areas consist of the axons of neurones, which carry signals up and down the cord via ascending and descending tracts. These tracts cross as they enter and exit the brain, and this explains why the right side of the brain controls the left side of the body and the left side of the brain controls the right side of the body.

The spinal cord is divided into the right and left halves by the deep anterior median fissure and the shallow posterior median sulcus (Tortora & Derrickson 2014).

Functions of the spinal cord

The spinal cord provides a means of communication between the brain and the peripheral nerves that leave the spinal cord (Logenbaker 2016) and has two major functions in maintaining homeostasis (Tortora & Derrickson 2014).

- The tracts of the white matter of the spinal cord carry sensory impulses to the brain and motor impulses from the brain to the skeletal muscles and other effector muscles.
- The grey matter of the spinal cord is a site for integration of reflexes, which is a rapid, involuntary action in relation to a particular stimulus.

Spinal nerves

There are 31 pairs of spinal nerves attached to the spinal cord within the human body, which are named and numbered according to the region and level of the vertebral column from which they emerge (figure 14.12).

FIGURE 14.12 The spinal cord and spinal nerves

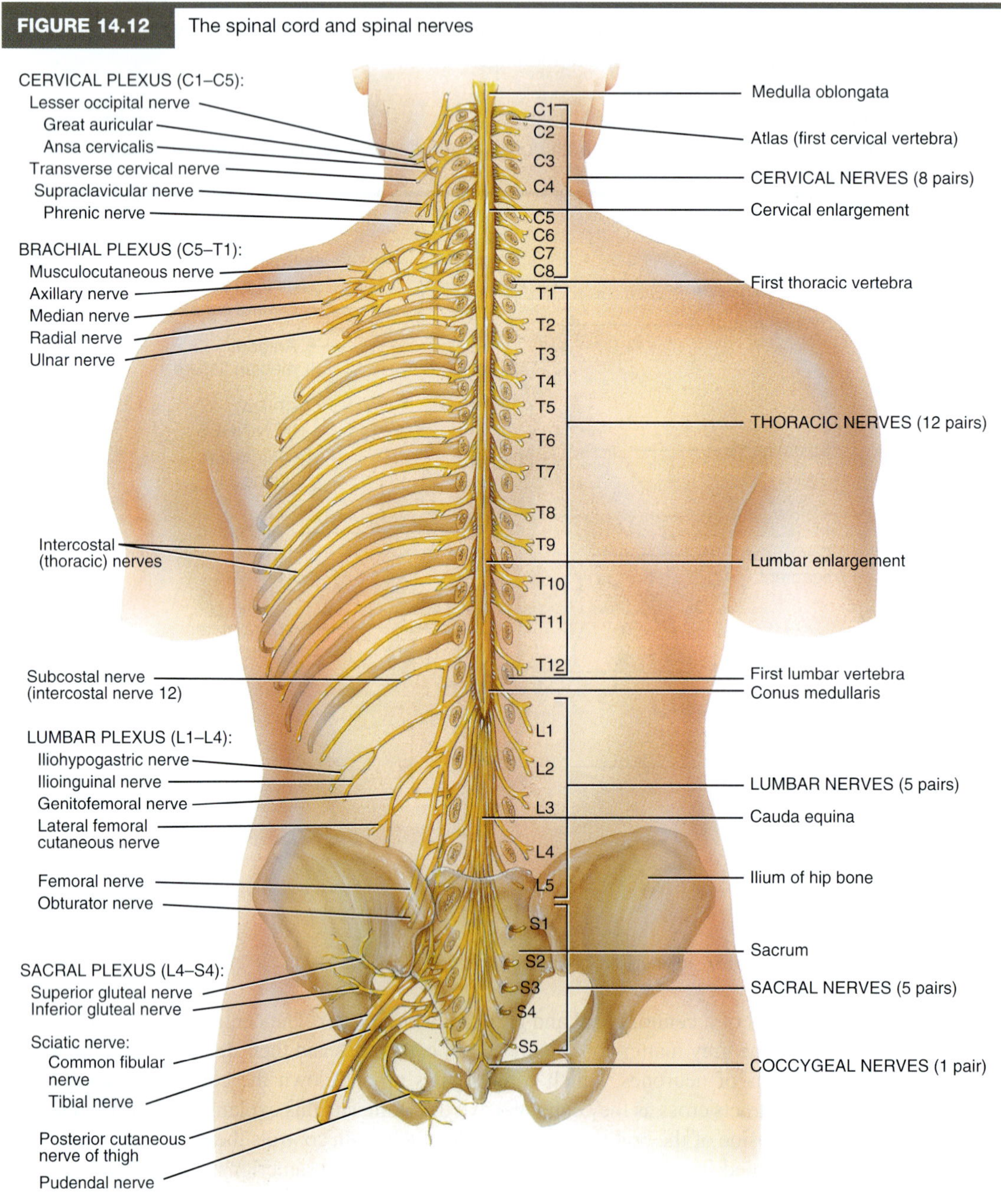

Posterior view of entire spinal cord and portions of spinal nerves

Source: Tortora and Derrickson (2009). Reproduced with permission of John Wiley & Sons.

Each nerve innervates a group of muscles (myotome) and an area of skin (dermatome), and most also innervate some of the thoracic and abdominal organs (figure 14.13).

FIGURE 14.13 The spinal nerves and their areas of innervations

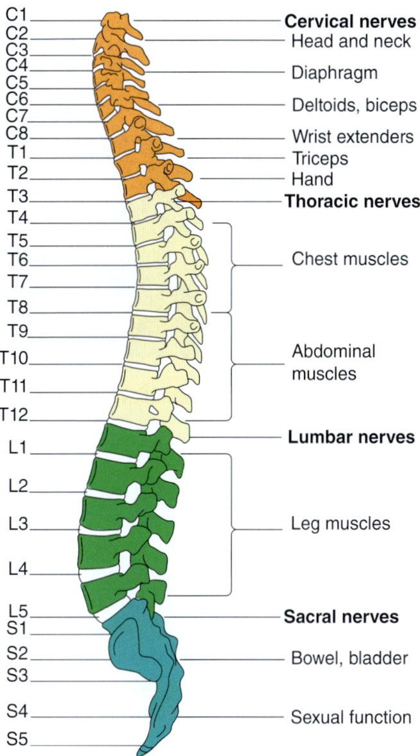

The spinal nerves provide the paths of communication between the spinal cord and specific regions of the body as they connect the central nervous system to sensory receptors, muscles and glands in all the parts of the body. A typical spinal nerve (figure 14.14) has two connections to the spinal cord — a posterior root and an anterior root, which unite to form a spinal nerve at the intervertebral foramen. A spinal nerve is an example of a mixed nerve as it contains both sensory (posterior root) and motor (anterior root) nerves.

FIGURE 14.14 A typical spinal nerve (CNS: central nervous system)

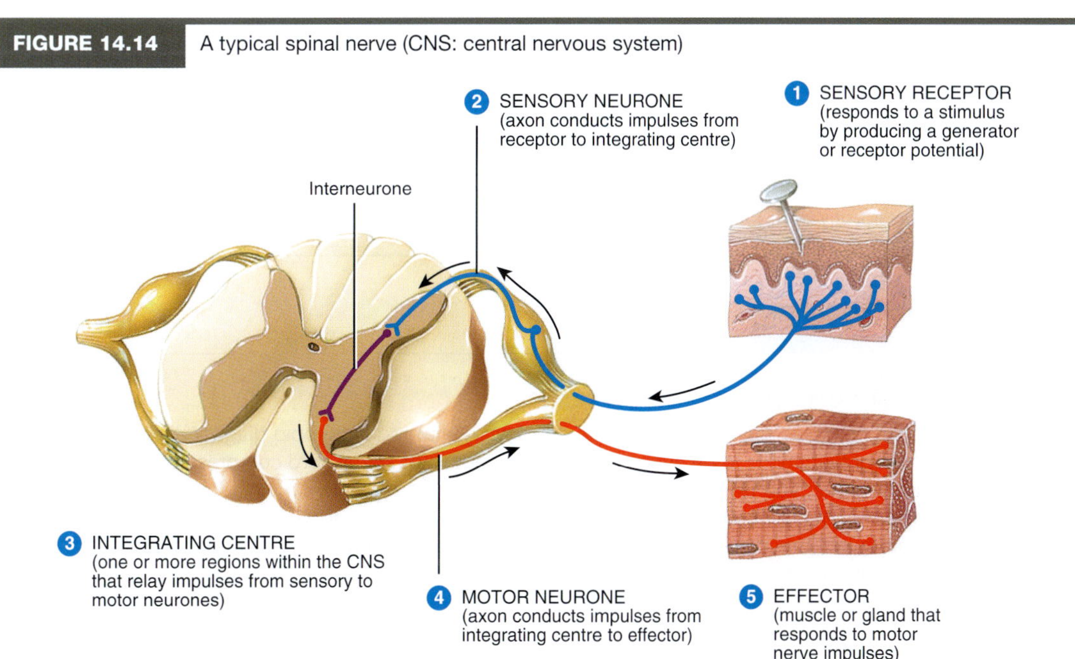

Source: Tortora and Derrickson (2009). Reproduced with permission of John Wiley & Sons.

CLINICALLY REASONED EPISODE OF CARE

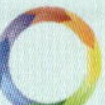

Depression

Consider the patient situation

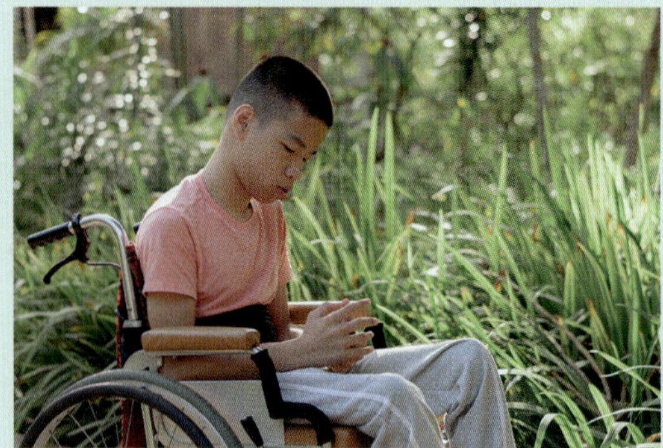

Josh is a 15-year-old with a learning disability who enjoys horseriding and playing horseball for his local club. During a recent match, Josh was thrown from his horse and he landed awkwardly, sustaining a spinal cord injury (SCI) to his thoracic region, which has resulted in paralysis from the waist down. Josh has experienced intense grief because of his condition and has become very depressed. Due to his learning disability, at times Josh cannot communicate clearly and becomes very anxious, frustrated and agitated, often refusing to participate in his usual daily life.

Collect cues and information

Josh is seen and assessed by a psychiatrist and specialist learning disabilities nurse. A diagnosis of exogenous depression is made.

Process information

An SCI is a devastating and life-altering injury that affects nearly all body systems due to them being innervated by the spinal cord.

In Australia, 4 per cent of SCI injuries are horse related. In 2016–17 there were 227 new SCI cases as a result of traumatic injury for those aged 15 years and over, and 80 per cent of cases were male (AIHW 2020a). Approximately more than 15 000 Australians live with an SCI.

The psychosocial needs of the patient with an SCI should never be overlooked and requires skilled interventions by health professionals to improve health and wellbeing. In the case of an individual with a learning disability, the assessment of mental health is fraught with difficulties, and without accurate assessment and diagnosis the selection of appropriate treatment can be very difficult (Gates et al. 2014).

Nursing actions

1. Organise for medication (selective serotonin reuptake inhibitor).
   Rationale:
   - All medications have risks for the person who takes them. Josh and his carers need to be counselled and told that this group of drugs can cause increased suicidal thought, particularly in young people, and to not stop the medication suddenly. People who use these medications need to be monitored frequently and carefully early in treatment (AMH 2021).
2. Support Josh and his family with psychological interventions such as appropriate cognitive behaviour therapy.
   Rationale:
   - There is strong evidence that cognitive behaviour therapy is an effective intervention for persons experiencing depression (Orygen 2017).

Evaluate outcomes

Josh and his family report a positive response to the medication and psychological interventions. Josh feels less frustrated and agitated, and he is more willing to engage with daily life.

Source: Based on the Clinical Reasoning Cycle, Levett-Jones (2013).

CLINICAL CONSIDERATIONS

Acute apinal cord compression

Acute spinal cord compression is a neurological emergency that requires rapid diagnosis and treatment if permanent loss of function is to be avoided. Common causes of spinal cord compression include:

- trauma (car accidents, sports injury and falls)
- tumours, both benign and malignant
- a prolapsed intervertebral disc (L4–L5 and L5–S1 are the most common levels of disc prolapse)
- an epidural or subdural haemorrhage
- inflammatory disease (e.g. rheumatoid arthritis)
- infection.

Signs and symptoms include sensory loss, paraesthesia, disturbance of gait, loss of power or paralysis.

MEDICINES MANAGEMENT

Paracetamol

Paracetamol (acetaminophen) is a common over-the-counter medication used to treat mild to moderate pain and is also effective as a fever reducer. The exact mechanism of action is not known; however, it is thought that the analgesic mechanism of paracetamol involves the metabolites of paracetamol, which act on receptors in the spinal cord and are thought to suppress the signal transduction from the superficial layers of the dorsal horn to alleviate pain (Farquhar-Smith et al. 2018).

In relation to its fever-reducing properties, it has been proposed that the main mechanism of action is the inhibition of the enzyme cyclooxygenase (COX), and recent findings suggest that it is highly selective for COX-2. The COX family of enzymes is responsible for the metabolism of compounds that encourage inflammatory responses. Paracetamol is thought to reduce the oxidised form of the COX enzyme, preventing it from forming pro-inflammatory chemicals. This leads to a reduced amount of prostaglandins S, thus lowering the hypothalamic set-point in the thermoregulatory centre.

Paracetamol is used to treat many conditions, such as headache, muscle aches, arthritis, backache, toothache, colds and fevers.

Overdosage of paracetamol is particularly dangerous as it may cause liver damage, which may not be apparent for 4–6 days after ingestion. Treatment includes infusing acetylcysteine, which protects the liver. However, it is most effective if given within 8 h of ingestion, after which effectiveness declines.

CLINICAL CONSIDERATIONS

Panic attack

A panic attack is a rush of intense psychological and physical symptoms. These symptoms of panic can be frightening and happen suddenly, often for no clear reason. Up to 40 per cent of Australians will experience a panic attack at some time in their life (ReachOut.com 2021).

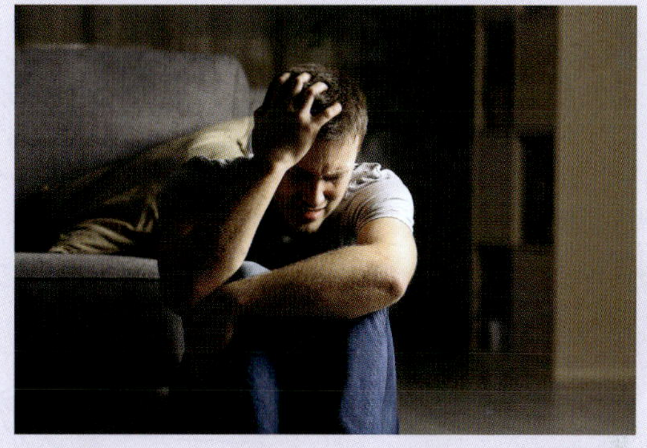

Panic attacks usually last between 5 and 20 minutes, and the individual may experience unpleasant psychological and physical symptoms; however, these are usually short-lived and will not cause harm (NHS Choices 2019). Psychological symptoms can include an overwhelming sense of fear and a sense of unreality, as if the individual is detached from the world around them. Physical symptoms of panic can include sweating, trembling, shortness of breath, a choking sensation, chest pain, a feeling of nausea and palpitations.

The physical symptoms of a panic attack are caused by the body's sympathetic response to something that the individual perceives as a threat and causes the release of hormones, such as adrenaline, resulting in an increased heart rate and muscle tension.

Sufferers of panic attacks can be helped to manage their condition through learning breathing and relaxation techniques and avoiding substances such as caffeine, nicotine and alcohol (NHS Choices 2019). In some cases medication may be recommended (Beyond Blue 2020).

14.5 The autonomic nervous system

LEARNING OBJECTIVE 14.5 Differentiate between the sympathetic and parasympathetic nervous systems.

The autonomic nervous system plays a major role in the maintenance of homeostasis by regulating the body's automatic, involuntary functions. In common with the rest of the nervous system, it consists of neurones, neuroglia and other connective tissue. However, its structure is unique, in that it is divided into two: namely, the sympathetic division and the parasympathetic division. These two divisions have several common features (Logenbaker 2016).

- They innervate all internal organs.
- They utilise two motor neurones and one ganglion to transmit an action potential.
- They function automatically and usually in an involuntary manner.

Sympathetic division (fight or flight)

The sympathetic division (see figure 14.15) includes nerve fibres that arise from the 12 thoracic and first two lumbar segments of the spine; hence, it is also referred to as the thoracicolumbar division. The sympathetic division takes control of many internal organs when a stressful situation occurs. This can take the form of physical stress if undertaking strenuous exercise or emotional stress at times of anger or anxiety. In emergency situations, the sympathetic nervous system releases norepinephrine, which assists in the 'fight or flight' response (Migliozzi 2017).

FIGURE 14.15 Sympathetic nervous system

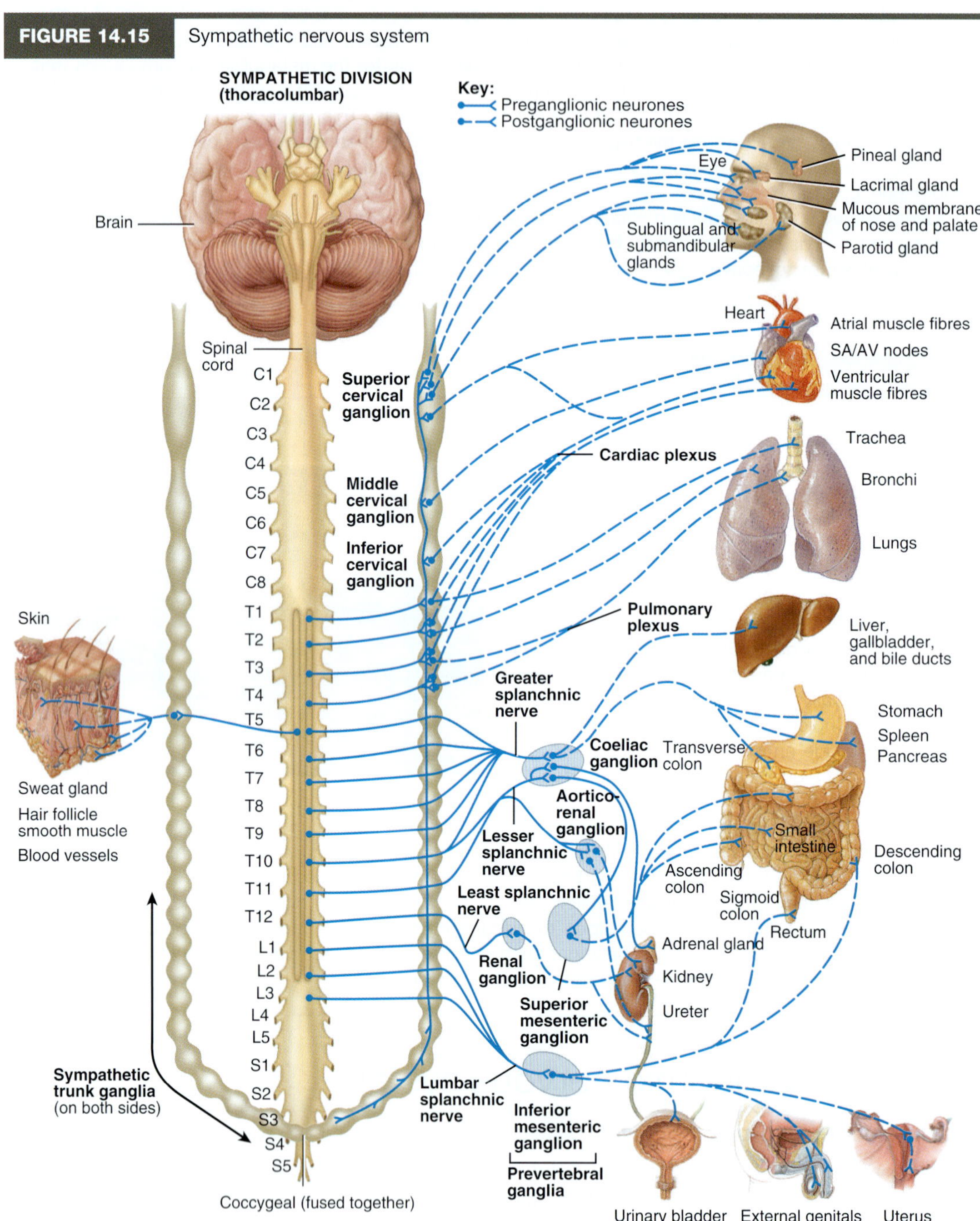

Source: Tortora and Derrickson (2009). Reproduced with permission of John Wiley & Sons.

Parasympathetic division (rest and digest)

The parasympathetic division includes fibres that arise from the lower end of the spinal cord and several cranial nerves; hence, it is often referred to as the craniosacral division. The parasympathetic division is most active when the body is at rest; it utilises acetylcholine to control all the internal responses associated with a state of relaxation (figure 14.16) and, therefore, has many opposite effects on the body to the sympathetic nervous system (Migliozzi 2017).

FIGURE 14.16 Parasympathetic nervous system

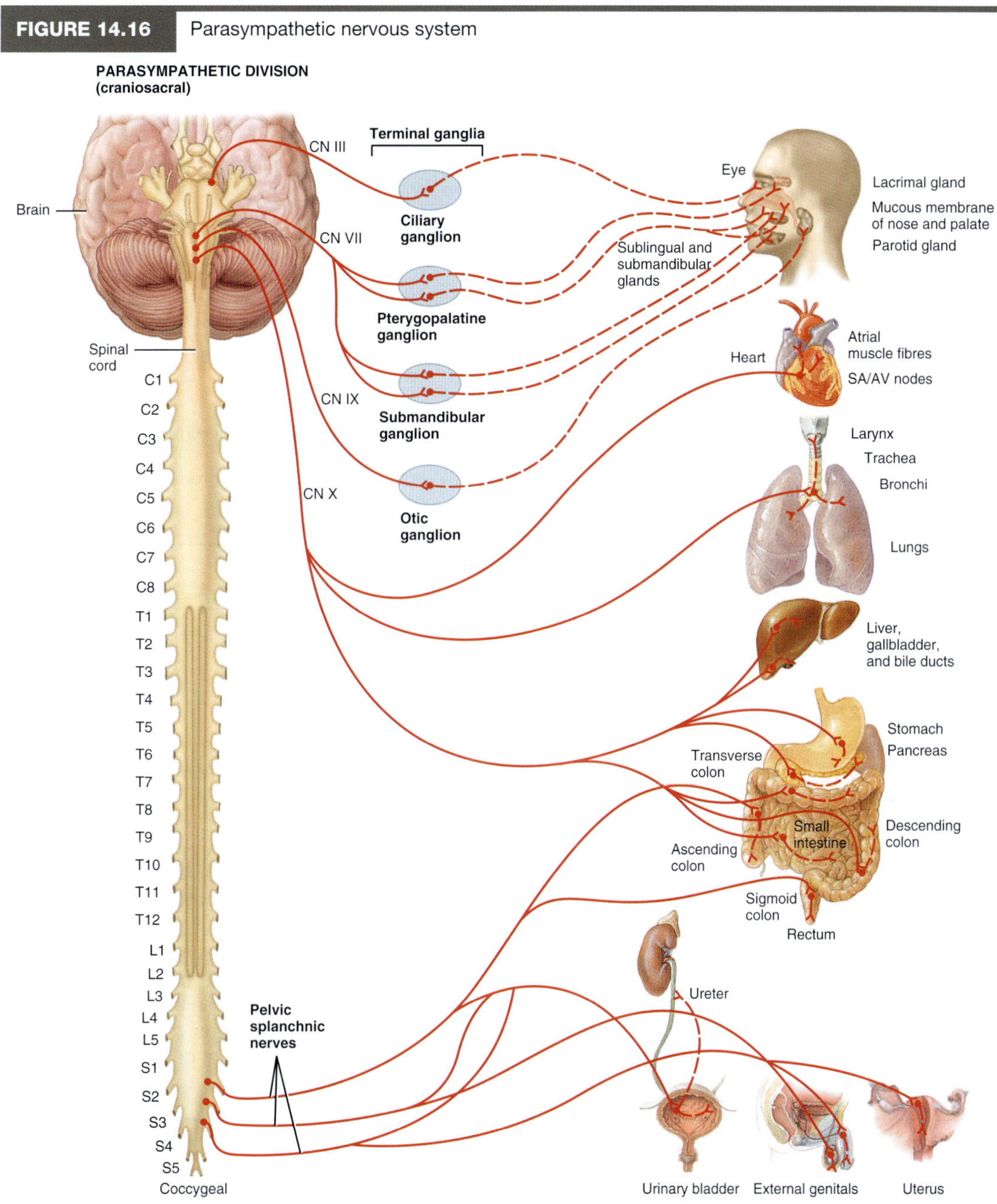

Source: Tortora and Derrickson (2009). Reproduced with permission of John Wiley & Sons.

Table 14.3 provides a summary of the physiological effects of the sympathetic and parasympathetic divisions of the nervous system.

TABLE 14.3 **Effects of the parasympathetic and sympathetic divisions of the autonomic nervous system**

Organ/system	Sympathetic effects	Parasympathetic effects
Cell metabolism	Increases metabolic rate, stimulates fat breakdown and increases blood sugar levels	No effect
Blood vessels	Constricts blood vessels in viscera and skin	
	Dilates blood vessels in the heart and skeletal muscle	No effect
Eye	Dilates pupils	Constricts pupils
Heart	Increases rate and force of contraction	Decreases rate
Lungs	Dilates bronchioles	Constricts bronchioles
Kidneys	Decreases urine output	No effect
Liver	Causes the release of glucose	No effect
Digestive system	Decreases peristalsis and constricts digestive system sphincters	Increases peristalsis and dilates digestive system sphincters
Adrenal medulla	Stimulates cells to secrete **epinephrine** and norepinephrine	No effect
Lacrimal glands	Inhibits the production of tears	Increases the production of tears
Salivary glands	Inhibits the production of saliva	Increases the production of saliva
Sweat glands	Stimulates to produce perspiration	No effect

MEDICINES MANAGEMENT

Carbamazepine

Carbamazepine is an anticonvulsant primarily used in the treatment of epileptic seizures. Carbamazepine works by blocking the sodium channels of nerve cells in the brain and so reduces the increased excitability and firing activity of neurones that occur during an epileptic seizure.

Antiepileptic hypersensitivity syndrome has been associated with some antiepileptic drugs and usually starts between 1 and 6 weeks after commencing treatment, and signs and symptoms include fever, rash, lymphadenopathy liver and haematological dysfunction (Australian Medicines Handbook 2021). If signs of hypersensitivity syndrome occur, the drug should be withdrawn immediately (Joint Formulary Committee 2018) and not restarted (Australian Medicines Handbook 2021).

Patients with epilepsy may drive a car, but commercial vehicle drivers (drivers of heavy vehicles, public passenger vehicles or those with a dangerous goods licence) are not able to drive for a minimum of 10 years since the last seizure (Austroads and National Transport Commission 2017). Patients, however, are advised not to drive during medication changes or withdrawal of antiepileptic drugs, and for 6 months afterwards. Similarly, patients who have had a first or single epileptic seizure must not drive for 6 months after the last seizure (Austroads and National Transport Commission 2017).

SUMMARY

In conclusion, the nervous system is a highly organised network of cells and structures that include the brain and cranial nerves and the spinal cord and spinal nerves, which play a major role in maintaining homeostasis. The nervous system responds to external and internal stimuli through three basic functions: the sensory, integrative and motor functions, which generate responses and create changes in bodily functions as required. Conditions affecting the nervous system can have a devastating effect on the quality of life and the functions essential for survival.

KEY TERMS

action potentials Conductions along a nerve or muscle cell membrane caused by a large, transient depolarisation.
afferent fibres Carry nerve impulses towards the central nervous system.
antidiuretic hormone (ADH) Hormone that acts on the kidneys to reabsorb more water, thus reducing urine output.
arachnoid mater Middle layer of the meninges.
astrocytes Neuroglial cells that help the blood–brain barrier.
autonomic nervous system Involuntary motor division of the motor nervous system.
axon Process of a neurone that carries impulses away from the cell body.
brainstem Collective name given to the pons, medulla and midbrain.
cation An ion with a positive charge.
central nervous system Brain and spinal cord.
cerebellum Anatomical region of the brain responsible for coordinated and smooth skeletal muscle movements.
cerebral hemisphere Division of the cerebrum.
cerebrospinal fluid Fluid that surrounds the central nervous system.
cerebrum Large anatomical region of the brain which is divided into the cerebral hemispheres.
circle of Willis Part of arterial blood supply to the brain.
cranial nerves Twelve pairs of nerves that leave the brain and supply sensory and motor neurones to the head, neck, part of the trunk and the viscera of the thorax and abdomen.
dendrites Parts of a neurone that transmit impulses towards the cell body.
diencephalon Anatomical region of the brain consisting of the thalamus, hypothalamus and epithalamus.
dura mater Tough outer layer of the meninges.
effector Muscle, gland or organ stimulated by the nervous system.
efferent fibres Carry nerve impulses away from the central nervous system.
ependymal cells Neuroglial cells that line the cavities of the central nervous system.
epinephrine Hormone produced by the adrenal medulla that is also a neurotransmitter.
epithalamus Part of the brain that forms the diencephalon.
ganglia A group of neuronal cell bodies lying outside the central nervous system.
hypothalamus Part of the diencephalon with many functions.
lobes A clear anatomical division or boundary within a structure.
medulla oblongata Part of the brainstem.
meninges Three layers of tissue that cover and protect the central nervous system (dura, arachnoid and pia maters).
microglia Neuroglia that has the ability to phagocytose material.
midbrain Part of the brainstem that links the brainstem to the diencephalon.
motor area The area located in the cerebral cortex that controls voluntary motor function.
motor nerve A neurone that conducts impulses to effectors which may be either muscle or glands.
myelin sheath Fatty insulating layer that surrounds nerve fibres responsible for speeding up impulse conduction.
neuroglia Cells of the nervous system that protect and support the functional unit — the neurone.
neuromuscular junction Region where skeletal muscle comes into contact with a neurone.
neurone Functional unit of the nervous system responsible for generating and conducting nerve impulses.

nuclei Cluster of cell bodies within the central nervous system.
oligodendrocytes Glial cell that helps produce the myelin sheath.
peripheral nervous system All nerves located outside of the brain and spinal cord (the central nervous system).
pia mater Innermost layer of the meninges.
pineal gland Part of the diencephalon that has an endocrine function.
pituitary gland An endocrine gland located next to the hypothalamus that produces many hormones.
receptors Sensory nerve endings or cells that respond to stimuli.
refractory period The period immediately after a neurone has fired when it cannot receive another impulse.
reticular formation Area located throughout the brainstem that is responsible for arousal, regulation of sensory input to the cerebrum and control of motor output.
saltatory conduction Transmission of an impulse down a myelinated nerve fibre where the impulse moves from node of Ranvier to node.
sensory area An area of the cerebrum responsible for sensation.
sensory nerve A neurone that carries sensory information from cranial and spinal nerves into the brain and spinal cord.
somatic nervous system Voluntary motor division of the peripheral nervous system.
spinal nerves Thirty-one pairs of nerves that originate on the spinal cord.
synapse Junction between two neurones or neurones and effector site.
thalamus Part of the diencephalon.
ventricles Cavities in the brain.
white matter Myelinated nerve fibres.

FIND OUT MORE

1. Name the two major divisions of the nervous system.
2. Differentiate between the parasympathetic nervous system and the sympathetic nervous system.
3. Identify the functions of the neuroglia.
4. Describe the action potential.
5. Identify the functions of the different regions of the brain.
6. Describe to a patient's relative what the acronym FAST in relation to stoke means.
7. Explain the difference between stroke and transient attacks.
8. Define the term saltatory conduction.
9. What is the difference between the terms afferent and efferent?
10. What is the function of the brainstem?

CONDITIONS

The following is a list of conditions that are associated with the nervous system. Take some time and write notes about each of the conditions. You may make the notes taken from textbooks or other resources (e.g. people you work with in a clinical area), or you may make the notes as a result of people you have cared for. If you are making notes about people you have cared for, you must ensure that you adhere to the rules of confidentiality.

Multiple sclerosis
Botulism
Fibromyalgia

Parkinson's disease

Epilepsy

Raised intracranial pressure

Alzheimer's disease

Glioblastoma

Cerebrovascular accident (CVA)

Dementia

REFERENCES

Ambulance Australia (2020) Drug therapy protocols: midazolam. www.ambulance.qld.gov.au/docs/clinical/dtprotocols/DTP_Midazolam.pdf (accessed February 2021).

Australian Government Department of Health (2005) What is panic disorder and agoraphobia? www1.health.gov.au/internet/publications/publishing.nsf/Content/mental-pubs-p-panic-toc~mental-pubs-p-panic-wha (accessed February 2021).

Australian Institute of Health and Welfare (2020a) Spinal cord injury, Australia 2016–17, Injury research and statistics series, no. 129, Cat. No. INJCAT 209. https://scia.org.au/sci-statistics/ (accessed 6 February 2021).

Australian Institute of Health and Welfare (2020b) Stroke. www.aihw.gov.au/reports/australias-health/stroke (accessed February 2021).

Australian Medicines Handbook (2021) Carbamazepine. https://amhonline-amh-net-au (accessed February 2021).

Austroads and National Transport Commission (2017) Assessing fitness to drive for commercial and private vehicle drivers: 2016 Medical standards for licensing and clinical management guidelines, as amended up to August 2017. https://austroads.com.au/__data/assets/pdf_file/0022/104197/AP-G56-17_Assessing_fitness_to_drive_2016_amended_Aug2017.pdf (accessed February 2021).

Beyond Blue (2020) Panic disorder. https://au.reachout.com/articles/what-are-panic-attacks (accessed February 2021).

Bullock, S. and Manias, E. (2016) *Fundamentals of Pharmacology*, 8th edn. Melbourne: Pearson Education Australia.

Calleja, P., Harvey, T. and Theobald, K. (2020) *Estes Health Assessment and Physical Examination, Australia and New Zealand*, 3rd edn. Sydney: Cengage Learning.

Centers for Disease Control and Prevention (2021) Stroke signs and symptoms. www.cdc.gov/stroke/signs_symptoms.htm (accessed February 2021).

Douglas, C. (2021) Undertaking a focussed assessment: physical assessment of body systems. In Crisp, J., Douglas, C., Rebeiro, G. and Waters, D. (eds), *Potter & Perry's Fundamentals of Nursing, Australia and New Zealand*, 6th edn. Chatswood: Elsevier.

Farquhar-Smith, P., Beaulieu, P. and Jaggar, S. (2018) *Landmark Papers in Pain: Seminal Papers in Pain with Expert Commentaries*. Oxford: Open University Press.

Gates, B., Fearns, D. and Welch, J. (2014) *Learning Disability Nursing at a Glance*. Oxford: Wiley-Blackwell.

Joint Formulary Committee (2018) *BNF 75*. London: Pharmaceutical Press.

Levett-Jones, T. (2013). *Clinical Reasoning: Learning to Think Like a Nurse*. Pearson Australia.

Logenbaker, S.N. (2016) *Mader's Understanding Human Anatomy and Physiology*, 9th edn. London: McGraw-Hill.

Marieb, E.N. and Hoehn, K. (2019) *Human Anatomy and Physiology*, 11th edn. Hoboken NJ: Pearson Education Ltd.

McFadden, R., (2019) *Introducing Pharmacology: For Nursing and Healthcare*, 3rd edn. England: Routledge.

Migliozzi, J.G. (2017) The nervous system and associated disorders. In Nair, M. and Peate, I. (eds) *Fundamentals of Applied Pathophysiology: An Essential Guide For Nursing And Healthcare Students*, 3rd edn. Oxford: John Wiley & Sons, Ltd.

NHS Choices (2019) Panic disorder. www.nhs.uk/conditions/panic-disorder/ (accessed February 2019).

Orygen (2017) Treating depression in young people. www.orygen.org.au/Training/Resources/Depression/Clinical-practice-points/Treating-depression-in-yp (accessed 6 February 2021).
ReachOut.com (2021) What are panic attacks? https://au.reachout.com/articles/what-are-panic-attacks (accessed February 2021).
Seeley, R.R., Stephens, T.D. and Vanputte, C. (2016) *Anatomy and Physiology*, 11th edn. New York: McGraw-Hill.
Teasdale, G. and Jennett, B. (1974) Assessment of coma and impaired consciousness. A practical scale. *Lancet* 2: 81–84. https://doi.org/10.1016/S0140-6736(74)91639-0.
Tortora, G.J. and Derrickson, B.H. (2009) *Principles of Anatomy and Physiology*, 12th edn. Hoboken, NJ: John Wiley & Sons, Inc.
Tortora, G.J. and Derrickson, B.H. (2014) *Principles of Anatomy and Physiology*, 15th edn. Hoboken, NJ: John Wiley & Sons, Inc.
Stroke Foundation (2021) Signs of stroke. https://strokefoundation.org.au/About-Stroke/Learn/signs-of-stroke (accessed February 2021).
Therapeutic Goods Administration (2018) Australian product information — midazolam injection (midazolam). www.ebs.tga.gov.au/ebs/picmi/picmirepository.nsf/pdf?OpenAgent&id=CP-2010-PI-07035-3 (accessed February 2021).
VanMeter, K.C. and Hubert, R.J. (2014). *Gould's Pathophysiology for Health Professions*, 5th edn. St Louis: Elsevier Saunders.
Waugh, A. and Grant, A. (2018) *Ross and Wilson Anatomy and Physiology in Health and Illness*, 13th edn. Edinburgh: Elsevier Churchill Livingstone.

FURTHER READING

DEMENTIA

www.racgp.org.au/download/Daocuments/AFP/2016/December/AFP-Dec-Clinical-Laver-V2.pdf

Clinical practice guidelines and principles of care for people with dementia in Australia.

EPILEPSIES: DIAGNOSIS AND MANAGEMENT

Epilepsy Australia

www.epilepsyaustralia.net

Epilepsy Australia is the national coalition of Australian epilepsy organisations working together to keep our communities informed on the latest medical breakthroughs, social research, publications, news and policy about epilepsy.

Epilepsy Foundation

https://epilepsyfoundation.org.au/understanding-epilepsy/epilepsy-and-seizure-management-tools/epilepsy-plans

The Epilepsy Foundation recommends the use of epilepsy management plans (EMPs).

Epilepsy Society of Australia

www.epileps-society.org.au

The Epilepsy Society of Australia is a professional organisation for clinicians, technologists and scientists involved in the diagnosis, treatment and research of epilepsy in Australia.

HEAD INJURY: ASSESSMENT AND EARLY MANAGEMENT

Clinical guidance on head injury: triage, assessment, investigation and early management of head injury in children, young people and adults.

Adult trauma clinical practice guidelines: initial management of closed head injury in adults

https://aci.health.nsw.gov.au/__data/assets/pdf_file/0003/195150/Closed_Head_Injury_CPG_2nd_Ed_Full_document.pdf

Concussive head injury in children and adolescents

www.racgp.org.au/afp/2016/july/concussive-head-injury-in-children-and-adolescents

Head injury: emergency management in children

www.childrens.health.qld.gov.au/wp-content/uploads/PDF/guidelines/CHQ-GDL-60023-head-injury.pdf

PARKINSON'S DISEASE

Information and advice on Parkinson's disease.

Brain Foundation

https://brainfoundation.org.au/disorders/parkinsons-disease

National Prescriber Service (NPS) Medicinewise: management of Parkinson's disease

www.nps.org.au/australian-prescriber/articles/management-of-parkinsons-disease

Parkinson's Western Australia

www.parkinsonswa.org.au/what-is-parkinsons/information-sheets

STROKE

https://strokefoundation.org.au

The Stroke Foundation is a national Australian charity that partners with the community to prevent, treat and beat stroke.

ACKNOWLEDGEMENTS

Photo: © ESB Professional / Shutterstock.com
Photo: © Chaikom / Shutterstock.com
Photo: © Photographee.eu / Shutterstock.com
Photo: © Casa nayafana / Shutterstock.com
Photo: © Stroke Foundation
Photo: © Peerayut Chan / Shutterstock.com
Table 14.1: © Teasdale, G. and Jennett, B. (1974) Assessment of coma and impaired consciousness. A practical scale. *Lancet* 2: 81–84. https://doi.org/10.1016/S0140-6736(74)91639-0.

CHAPTER 15

The senses

TEST YOUR PRIOR KNOWLEDGE

- Which cranial nerve is responsible for conveying information about perceived smells to the brain?
- Name the main components of the ear involved in the sense of balance.
- What part of the tongue is involved in the sense of taste?
- Name the two substances that fill the eye chambers and help to maintain the shape of the eye.
- What is the name for short-sightedness?

LEARNING OUTCOMES

After reading this chapter you will be able to:

15.1 describe the process by which we perceive smell

15.2 explain the mechanisms responsible for the perception of different tastes

15.3 describe the structural parts of the ear that are necessary for hearing and a sense of balance

15.4 explain the way in which human beings maintain a sense of balance

15.5 explore the mechanisms that lead to sound information being converted into action potentials to be relayed to the brain

15.6 describe the basic anatomical structures of the eye

15.7 describe the retina, and differences between rods and cones in the eye

15.8 explain how a visual image is focused on the retina.

Introduction

The senses are usually thought of as the five senses of smell, taste, hearing, vision and touch. However, in physiology the sense of touch is excluded from the senses as it is considered a somatic sense involved in touch, temperature, pain and proprioception. Thus the 'senses' is a term used to refer to the senses of:

- smell
- taste
- hearing
- sight.

Also included in this list of senses is the sense of:

- **equilibrium**.

This chapter will explore these five senses in three sections:

- the 'chemical' senses of smell and taste
- the senses associated with the ear: those of equilibrium and hearing
- the sense of sight.

Sensory systems in the human body differ vastly in complexity. The chapter on the nervous system described how a sensory input (stimulus) is gathered and delivered to the central nervous system via a sensory receptor. The receptor is a transducer that converts the stimulus into an intracellular signal by evoking a change in membrane potential. If the stimulus is above the threshold value, action potentials are generated and pass along the afferent **neurone** to the central nervous system. In the special senses, the sensory receptors detecting the stimuli are highly sophisticated in multicellular sense organs like the ear and the eye, which are made up of non-neural receptor cells (i.e. ear hair cells, eye **photoreceptors** and tastebuds). These cells **synapse** and release neurotransmitters directly on to sensory neurons initiating action potentials. In all these sections there will be a review of the anatomy of the particular organs involved in these senses, followed by a discussion of the physiology of how these senses are monitored and create action potentials to be transmitted to the brain. Finally, the pathways these action potentials take to the brain will be reviewed, along with a brief discussion of the processing of this information in the brain itself.

15.1 The chemical senses

LEARNING OBJECTIVE 15.1 Describe the process by which we perceive smell.

With regard to the senses, the chemical senses are the senses of smell and taste, which rely on chemoreceptors. There are two main types of chemoreceptor:

- distance chemoreceptors — for instance, the **olfactory** (smell) receptors
- direct chemoreceptors — for instance, the sense of taste, which relies on the tastebuds.

The sense of smell (olfaction)

In evolutionary terms, the sense of smell is one of the oldest senses, and the most primitive vertebrate brains have well-developed regions for processing olfactory information. It is a form of chemoreception. The sense of smell is useful to us for the identification of food that is safe to eat and that which has gone rotten; it helps us to identify dangers such as hazardous chemicals and gives us pleasure through the smell of flowers and perfume. Chemoreceptor inputs travel directly from the nose to the cerebral cortex instead of the **thalamus** like other sensory inputs. **Olfaction** (the sense of smell) is dependent on receptors that respond to airborne particles. In the nasal cavity either side of the nasal septum there are paired olfactory organs made up of two layers (figure 15.1).

- *Olfactory epithelium*. This layer contains the olfactory receptor cells, supporting cells and regenerative basal cells (stem cells) that mature into receptor cells to replace those that die.
- *Lamina propria*. A layer of areolar tissue containing numerous blood vessels and nerves. This layer also contains the olfactory glands, which secrete a **lipid**-rich substance that absorbs water to form a thick mucus that covers the olfactory epithelium.

The olfactory region of each of the two nasal passages is about 2.5 cm^2 (Jenkins & Tortora 2003) and between them they contain approximately 50 million receptor cells high in the nasal cavity. Olfactory cells in the epithelium are short-lived. They remain in the epithelium for 2 months and are then replaced by new cells whose **axons** make their way into the **olfactory bulb**.

FIGURE 15.1 (a, b) Gross and microscopic anatomy of olfaction

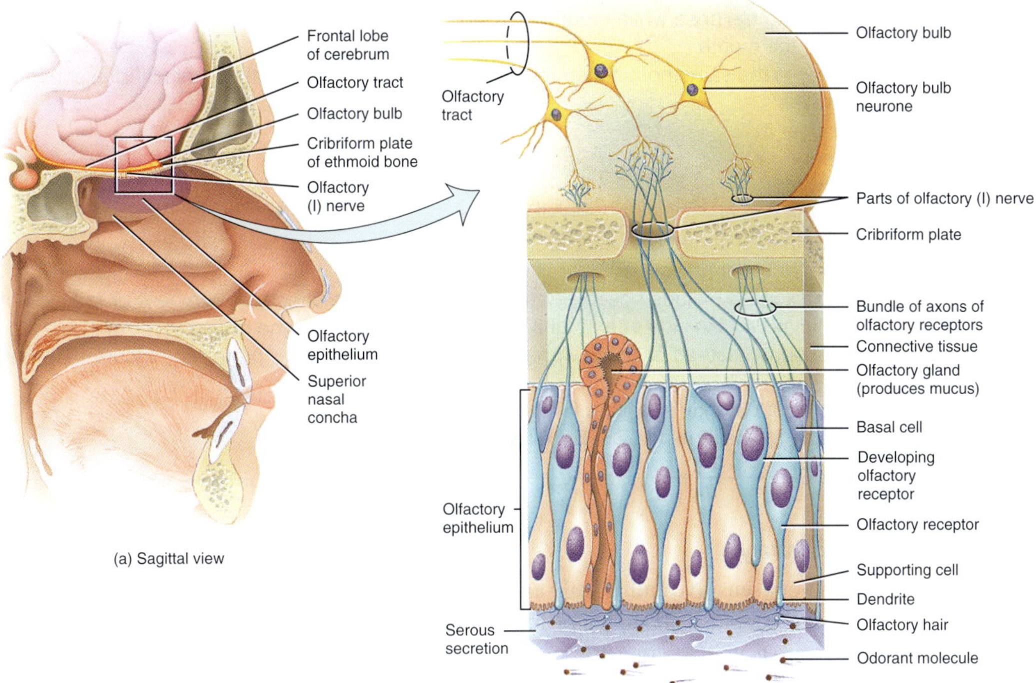

Source: Tortora and Derrickson (2009). Reproduced with permission of John Wiley & Sons.

When air is inhaled through the nose, the air in the nasal cavity is subject to turbulent flow and this ensures that airborne smell particles (odorant molecules) are brought to the olfactory organs. Approximately 2 per cent of the inhaled air in an average inspiration passes the olfactory organs; the act of sniffing increases this percentage by a large amount. The olfactory receptors can only be stimulated by compounds that are soluble in water or lipid and can therefore diffuse through the mucus that overlies the olfactory epithelium.

Olfactory receptors

The olfactory receptors are highly modified neurones contained within the olfactory epithelium. The tip of each receptor projects beyond the surface of the epithelium (figure 15.1). This projection forms the base for up to 20 **cilia** (hair-like structures) that extend into the surrounding mucus. These cilia lie laterally in the mucus (they lie relatively flat rather than upright), thus exposing a larger surface area to any odorant compound that must initially get dissolved into the mucus.

Dissolved chemicals interact with odorant-binding proteins on the surface of the cilia; a local depolarisation occurs by the opening of sodium channels in the cell membrane. If enough local depolarisations occur, then an action potential is generated within the receptor cell, which then travels along the olfactory pathway to the brain.

MEDICINES MANAGEMENT

Flixonase

Flixonase (fluticasone propionate) is a topical glucocorticoid medicine that is commonly used for the treatment of allergic rhinitis (inflammation of the inside of the nose) and nasal polyps.

Flixonase is available as a nasal spray or nasal drops. The methods for instilling nasal drops and nasal sprays vary slightly and are detailed below. The nurse should adhere to local policy and procedure at all times.

Nasal spray technique:

- Blow the nose to clear it.
- Shake the bottle.

- Close off one nostril and put the nozzle in the open nostril.
- Tilt the head forward slightly and keep the bottle upright.
- Squeeze a fine mist into the nose while breathing in slowly. The person should not sniff hard.
- Breathe out through the mouth.
- Take a second spray in the same nostril then repeat this procedure for the other nostril if prescribed.

Nasal drops technique:

- Blow the nose to clear it.
- Shake the container.
- Tilt the head backwards.
- Place the drops in the nostril.
- Keep the head tilted and sniff gently to let the drops penetrate.
- Repeat for the other nostril if prescribed.

The side effects of flixonase include nosebleed (a very common side effect) and dryness or irritation of the nose or throat. Minimising the side effects of flixonase medications can be done by:

- prescribing a nasal spray instead of drops; if nasal drops are indicated or preferred, ensure that they are used correctly
- prescribing the weakest potency possible, for the shortest period of time.

See National Institute for Health and Care Excellence (2015).

The olfactory pathway

The olfactory system is very sensitive and as little as four molecules can lead to the activation of a receptor. However, activation of a receptor cell does not mean there will be awareness of the smell. There is a significant amount of **convergence** along the olfactory nervous pathway and inhibition at intervening synapses can prevent the signal from reaching the olfactory cortex in the brain. However, the olfactory threshold remains very low; for instance, humans can detect very low concentrations of the chemicals added to the odourless natural gas used in the home, making it 'smell' and thus ensuring leaks are detected by the homeowner.

On each side of the nose, axons leaving the olfactory epithelium receptor cells collect into 20 or more bundles that penetrate the cribriform plate of the **ethmoid bone** (figure 15.2); these bundles comprise the right and left olfactory nerves until they reach the olfactory bulbs in the brain. At the olfactory bulbs the axons converge to connect with postsynaptic (mitral) cells in large synaptic structures called **glomeruli**. **Efferent** fibres of cells elsewhere in the brain also innervate the olfactory bulb, thus allowing for the potential inhibition of the signalling pathways — for instance, in central adaptation (see the box on central adaptation).

Central adaptation

Have you ever noticed that when meeting someone during the day you will smell their perfume or aftershave, but having spent some time with them you will no longer be aware of that smell? Humans tend to 'habituate' to persistent smells to the point that they are no longer perceived. This is not due to the local receptors adapting to the persistent stimuli; it is a function of central adaptation. That is, higher centres in the brain are responsible for our reduced perception of a persistent smell. The transmission of the sensory information for that particular smell is inhibited at the level of the olfactory bulb by nerve impulses from the centres in the brain.

Axons exiting from the olfactory bulbs travel along the olfactory nerves (cranial nerve I, which is a paired nerve) to reach the olfactory cortex, the hypothalamus and portions of the **limbic system** via the olfactory tracts. Olfactory stimulation is the only sensory information that reaches the cerebral cortex directly; all other senses are processed by the thalamus first. The fact that the limbic system and hypothalamus receive olfactory input helps to explain the profound emotional response that can be triggered by certain smells.

Olfactory discrimination

The olfactory system can make distinctions among some 2000–4000 chemical stimuli; however, there are no reasons that can be found to explain this in the structure of the receptor cells themselves. Though the epithelium is divided into areas of receptors with particular sensitivity for certain smells, it appears that the central nervous system interprets each smell by analysing the overall pattern of receptor activity (Tortora &

Derrickson 2012). The brain uses inputs from hundreds of different olfactory cells in various combinations to generate perceptions of different smells. It has been proposed that smell is perceived in primary odours (Haehner et al. 2013); the exact number remains a source of contention and estimates vary from 7 to 30. Some of the smells that we perceive are not detected by the olfactory receptors at all; some of what we sense is actually pain. The nasal cavity contains pain receptors that respond to certain irritants such as ammonia, chillies and menthol. As we get older, smell discrimination and sensitivity reduce as we lose receptors compared with the total number we had when younger and the receptors that remain become less sensitive.

FIGURE 15.2 Olfactory pathway

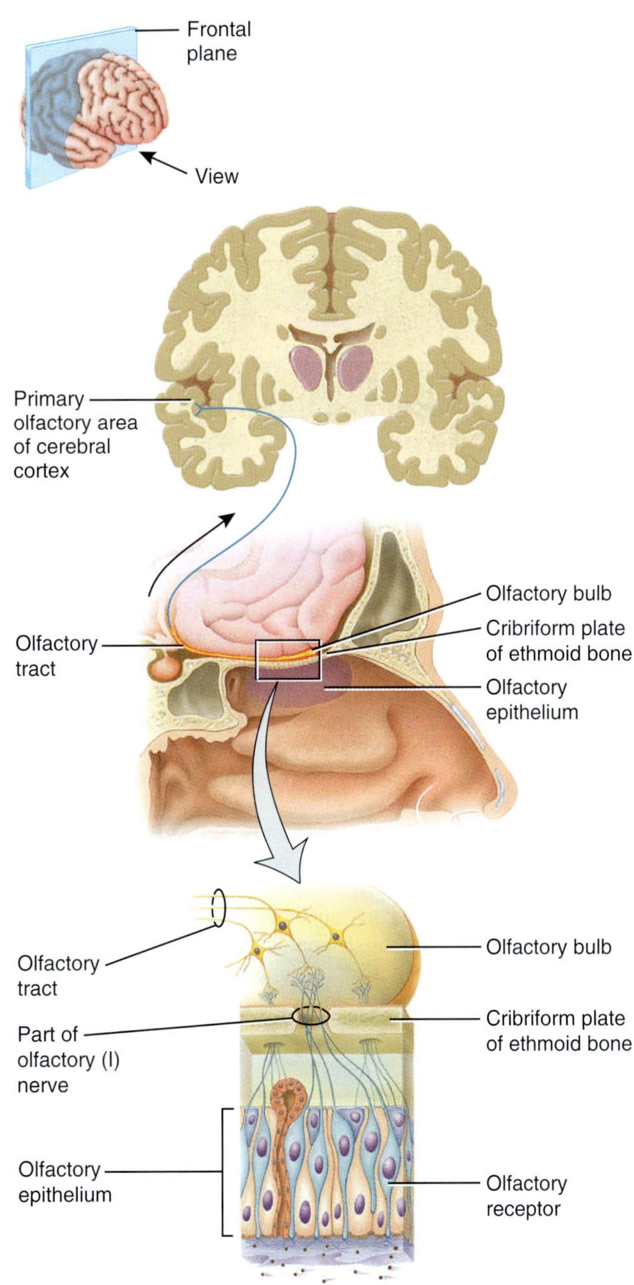

Source: Tortora and Derrickson (2009). Reproduced with permission of John Wiley & Sons.

CLINICAL CONSIDERATIONS

Loss of the sense of smell (anosmia)

The loss of the sense of smell (known as anosmia) is normally an acquired disorder due to either trauma to the nose or brain injury, but some people are born without a sense of smell (congenital anosmia).

While appearing to be a minor problem, the loss of the sense of smell is often associated with feelings of depression and a reduced quality of life (Neuland et al. 2011).

While temporary anosmia is common with conditions such as rhinitis, the common cold and hayfever, permanent anosmia is often related to trauma, surgery and degenerative conditions such as Alzheimer's and Parkinson's disease and dementia with Lewy bodies.

Anosmia is noted to be an early indicator of Parkinson's disease with 95 per cent of patients presenting with anosmia years before motor-related symptoms appear (Haehner et al. 2013). Unfortunately, the available Parkinsonian treatments have not been effective towards anosmia (Haehner et al. 2013).

Patients with anosmia are advised to take certain safety measures such as:

- installing smoke alarms
- clearly marking expiry dates on food and leftovers
- reading the warning labels on chemical agents and cleaners to avoid potentially harmful gases
- switching from gas to electric.

See NHS (2015).

HOMEOSTATIC IMBALANCE

Olfactory dysfunction or anosmia in SARS-CoV-2 (COVID-19) patients

Peer-reviewed studies have reported that loss of smell and taste is a stronger predictor for severe acute respiratory syndrome coronavirus 2 (SARS-CoV-2) infection than fever. Meng and colleagues (2020) stated that patients with SARS-CoV-2 could acquire a sudden onset of anosmia and distorted sense of taste (dysgeusia) approximately 4 days after SARS-CoV-2 infection without presenting other clear symptoms, and this is consistent with data released from several countries. To support this, a large multicentre study reported that 82 per cent of patients with mild forms of SARS-CoV-2 subjectively reported experiencing anosmia; this number increases to 90 per cent when moderate SARS-CoV-2 cases are included. However, the olfactory problems completely resolved in about 80 per cent of patients within the first two months after being diagnosed (Lechien et al. 2021). Strikingly, 20 per cent of SARS-CoV-2 patients remain asymptomatic throughout the infection period, although the viral load has been found to be similar between asymptomatic and symptomatic individuals (Buitrago-Garcia et al. 2020). Recovery time from anosmia suggests that the older dysfunctional olfactory cells are slowly replaced by new cells during the 2-month period. Dysgeusia, impaired taste, was also reported in 56 per cent of SARS-CoV-2 patients (Lechien et al. 2021).

A possible explanation for this high rate of anosmia in mild SARS-CoV-2 cases are high levels of angiotensin-converting enzyme 2 and transmembrane protease serine 2 expression in human olfactory epithelium, which are also the receptors for SARS-CoV-2, thereby raising local olfactory inflammatory reaction only in this area (Lechien et al. 2021). In conjunction, the shorter route supplied to the airway by the olfactory epithelium allows this area to be the diagnostic epicentre of airborne infections (Li et al. 2020). Given the mounting recent evidence for olfactory dysfunction being a stronger predictor for detecting asymptomatic or milder forms of SARS-CoV-2, standardised objective olfactory assessments should be considered as a diagnostic aid (Lechien et al. 2021; Li et al. 2020).

See Melbourne ENT group (n.d.).

15.2 The sense of taste

LEARNING OBJECTIVE 15.2 Explain the mechanisms responsible for the perception of different tastes.

Like the sense of smell, the sense of taste helps to protect us from poisons but also drives our appetite. There are five basic tastes:

- sweet
- sour
- bitter
- salt
- **umami**.

The first four tastes are already common knowledge, but the fifth was relatively unknown in the Western Hemisphere until recently. Umami is the taste associated with the proteins found in meat and fish (Osawa 2012) and has been known as a concept of taste to the Japanese for many years. Umami helps to enhance the flavour in foods by a type of amino acid, glutamate, which is rich in the food additive monosodium glutamate.

The sense of taste is associated with the tastebuds, which are the sensory receptor for taste and found primarily in the oral cavity. There are about 10 000 tastebuds in the adult oral cavity (numbers vary for each individual), which are found mostly on the tongue. However, there are fewer tastebuds on the soft palate, the inner surface of the cheeks, the larynx, the pharynx and epiglottis. Each tastebud consists of a collection of about 100 taste cells, support cells and regenerative basal cells. Due to the damaging effects of temperature, textures and food, the cells have an average lifespan of about 10 days, getting replaced from the basal cell layer. The number of tastebuds starts to decline gradually from 45 years of age, at a rate of about 1 per cent per year, resulting in a progressive reduction in taste sensation. An older adult may only have approximately 5000 or less working tastebuds as they do not get replaced as frequently as before, or even replaced at all.

Most of the tastebuds are found in peg-like projections of the tongue's mucosa. These projections are known as **papillae** (singular is papilla) and give the tongue its slightly rough feel. The papillae are found in four major forms (figure 15.3).

- *Fungiform*. The mushroom-shaped papillae are found scattered over the tongue surface but are most abundant at the tip and sides. They usually contain 1–18 tastebuds, which are located on the top of these papillae.
- *Circumvallate (otherwise known as vallate)*. These are the largest of the papillae and found in the least number. Seven to 12 of them are found in an inverted 'V' shape at the back of the tongue. They contain approximately 250 tastebuds, which are located in the side walls of these papillae.
- *Foliate*. These 'leaf-like' papillae are found on the sides of the rear of the tongue, which contain around 100 tastebuds.
- *Filiform*. These thread-like structures contain no tastebuds. They provide friction to aid the movement of food by the tongue.

FIGURE 15.3 Tongue and the location of the papillae

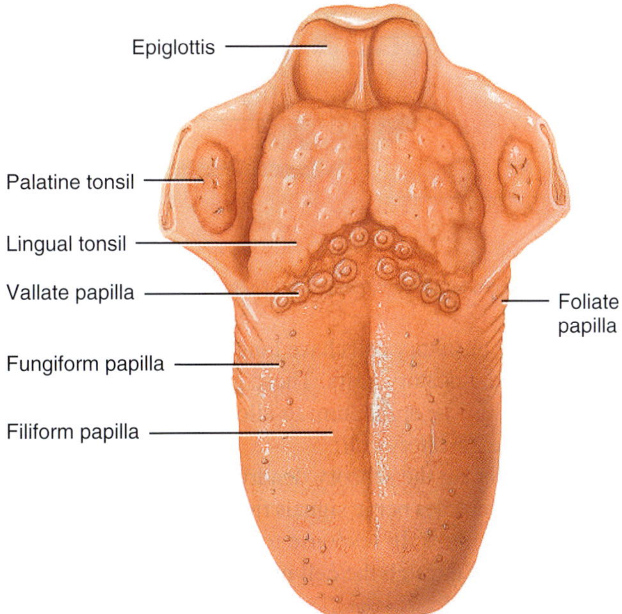

Source: Tortora and Derrickson (2009). Reproduced with permission of John Wiley & Sons.

Tastebuds

Tastebuds are bunches of polarised sensory cells embedded in the stratified oral epithelium. Each tastebud is an onion-shaped end organ that measures 0.03 x 0.06 mm, and consists of roughly 100 cells of three major types (figure 15.4).

- Supporting cells form the greatest part of the tastebud. They help to insulate the receptor cells from each other and the epithelium of the tongue.
- **Gustatory** (or taste) cells are the chemoreceptor responsible for sensing taste.
- Basal cells are stem cells that mature into new cells to replace those that die.

FIGURE 15.4 Cross-section of part of the tongue and microscopic view of a tastebud

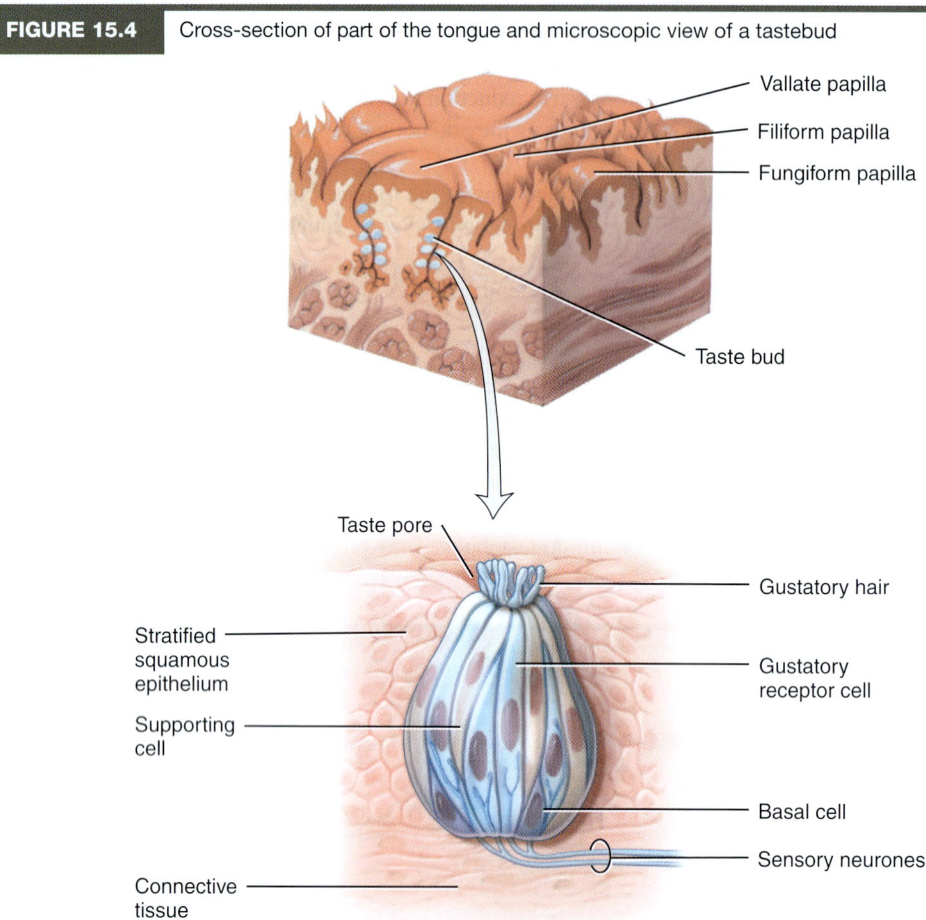

Source: Tortora and Derrickson (2009). Reproduced with permission of John Wiley & Sons.

Both the supporting cells and the gustatory cells have long **microvilli** (protrusions of the cell membrane that increase its surface area) called gustatory hairs. These gustatory hairs project from the tip of the cell and protrude through a 'taste pore' in the epithelium to allow them to be bathed in saliva. The gustatory hairs are the sensitive portion of the gustatory cell.

Coiling around the gustatory cells are the sensory dendrites, which are the initial part of the gustatory pathway. Each **afferent** nerve fibre receives nerve signals from several receptor cells. Several vesicles form beneath the cell membrane near the fibres. In response to taste, stimulation neurotransmitters, which are contained in the vesicles, are released through the cell membrane to excite the nerve fibre endings.

The taste receptor

The activation of the taste receptor requires the chemical compound (known as a tastant; Jenkins & Tortora 2013) that is to be tasted to dissolve in the saliva, then diffuse into the taste pore and come into contact with the gustatory hairs. Depending on the type of taste, this has one of four potential effects (the exact mechanism that is involved in the sensing of umami is unknown):

- salt — salty taste initiates an influx of sodium into the cell
- sour — sour taste leads to a hydrogen ion blockade of sodium and potassium channels in the cell membrane
- bitter — bitter taste leads to an influx of calcium ions into the cell
- sweet — sweet taste leads to an inactivation of potassium channels.

All these effects lead to the depolarisation of the cell and the release of neurotransmitters. Salt taste and sour taste have direct effects on the cell membrane. Bitter taste, sweet taste and umami exert their action on the cell by the use of messenger systems activated by G-protein-coupled receptors.

It appears that we have various sensitivities to different tastes. We are most sensitive to bitter tastes, then sour and then sweet and salty. To an extent this makes evolutionary sense as poisons tend to taste bitter, whereas acids and food that have 'gone off' often taste sour. Thus, we are most sensitive to those tastes that may indicate something that could harm us.

It should be noted that the tastebuds are not the only methods by which we experience the taste of a food. It is clear that the sense of smell is also of vital importance to how we experience taste — just think of how food tastes when your nose is blocked due to a cold; 80 per cent of the sense of taste is actually smell. As with the sense of smell, there are also pain receptors involved with the sense of taste and certain tastes will elicit a pain stimulus as opposed to a gustatory one.

The gustatory pathway

The release of neurotransmitters by the gustatory cells creates an action potential in related afferent nerve fibres. The sensory information from the tongue is transmitted along two cranial nerve pairs:

- chorda tympani — a branch of the facial nerve (cranial nerve VII) relays impulses from the **anterior** two-thirds of the tongue
- lingual branch of the glossopharyngeal nerve (cranial nerve IX) — carries the sensory information of the **posterior** third of the tongue.

Sensory information from the tastebuds in the epiglottis and pharynx is transmitted by the vagus nerve (cranial nerve X). All the afferent fibres terminate in the solitary nucleus of the medulla. The sensory messages are then transmitted, ultimately, to the thalamus and the gustatory cortex in the parietal lobes. Afferent fibres also project into the hypothalamus and limbic system. Ultimately, many of the branches of afferent nerves that divert to various parts of the brain, apart from the cortex, are involved in the triggering of **reflexes** involved with digestion (e.g. salivation).

The gustatory pathway is unique among the senses because if the tastebuds lose their afferent nerve fibres (e.g. they are cut) the tastebud then degenerates. As we get older, we lose the sense of taste as there is a reduction in the number of tastebuds; gustatory cells die and are not replaced at the same rate as they die and those cells that remain become less sensitive.

CLINICALLY REASONED EPISODE OF CARE

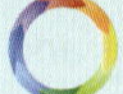

Antidepressants

Consider the patient situation

Jennifer is a 36-year-old woman who is being treated for severe depression. She attends the outpatient department and sees the outpatient nurse as part of the care team.

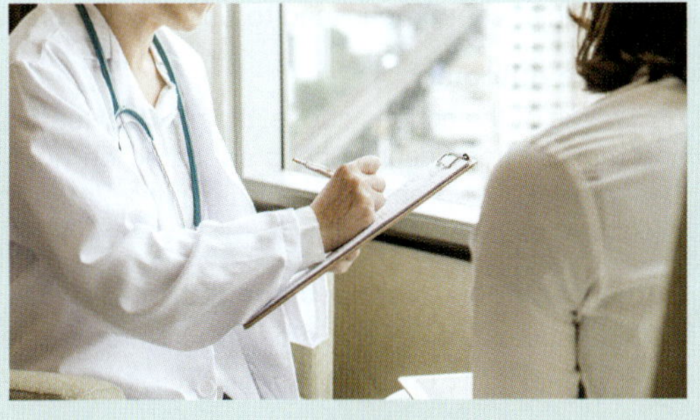

Collect cues and information

Jennifer is being treated for severe depression and is currently taking fluoxetine. She complains about having a constantly dry mouth which is affecting her sense of taste and appetite, and has led to severe halitosis (bad breath) and recurrent gum infections.

Jennifer understands that her dry mouth is a known side effect of fluoxetine. She is unhappy with the side effects of the medication and has reduced how frequently she is taking the medication. She suggests to the nurse that she may stop taking the medication completely.

Process information

Saliva is an essential body fluid that contains substances that lubricate and cleanse the oral mucosa, aid chewing and digestion, and protect the teeth from decay and the mouth and throat from infection. Saliva is also essential for a person's sense of taste.

Dry mouth (xerostomia) is a known side effect of many medications used in the treatment of depression and psychosis including selective serotonin reuptake inhibitors, tricyclic antidepressants, and many antipsychotic medications. The effects of dry mouth are challenging and can exacerbate feelings of depression. The effects include an altered taste sensation, difficulty eating, gum and tooth disease, halitosis, and sores in the mouth. These symptoms can become so distressing that patients may elect to stop taking the medication.

However, ceasing antidepressant medication abruptly can cause additional challenges and risks if it is not adjusted appropriately, causing withdrawal symptoms and relapse of depression symptoms. The reduction or cessation of antidepressants should occur under the supervision of a general practitioner over several weeks and an alternative treatment should be implemented.

Due to the risks associated with ceasing antidepressant medication, the risks and benefits of medication will need to be carefully negotiated between the patient and the medical officer.

If a decision is made to stay on the antidepressants, there are several things patients can do to help symptoms of dry mouth, including drinking water regularly and avoiding acidic drinks and caffeine, chewing sugar-free gum, avoiding alcohol and cigarettes, cleaning teeth regularly and using lip balm, as well as using a humidifier in the bedroom at night.

Establish goals

1. Review of medication and side effects
2. Education and information for medication side effect management
3. Follow-up

Nursing actions

1. Review medications and side effects with the multidisciplinary team and the patient.
   Rationale:
   - Side effects can be challenging and debilitating, impacting on an individual's quality of life.
   - Side effects and medication management discussions must include the patient as a central point in the treatment plan.
   - The challenge for healthcare practitioners is weighing the risks and benefits of treatment and side effects and the potential to decrease the dose.
   - Nurses are well placed to advocate on behalf of and alongside the patient.
2. Provide education on how to manage symptoms of dry mouth.
   Rationale:
   - Should medication continue, education on how to manage the symptoms of dry mouth may help Jennifer. This would include how to manage the symptoms on a daily basis and the importance of continuing medication adherence.
   - Nurses are well placed to provide education and resources to the patient in a way that meets their needs.
3. Follow up with Jennifer.
   Rationale:
   - Nurses must offer ongoing support and education to patients.
   - Nurses can organise for medical review should an individual's circumstances, wants and needs change.
   - Regular support can lead to positive outcomes for patients.

Evaluate outcomes

As a result of the actions above, the medical team and Jennifer decide to decrease her dose of fluoxetine and monitor her closely. She is educated on how to decrease the symptoms of her dry mouth. At her 2-month follow-up appointment, Jennifer states that the symptoms have improved and she has been taking her medications regularly.

Reflect on new processes and learning

How do nurses work within a person-centred framework to provide care to individuals and families?

Source: Based on the Clinical Reasoning Cycle, Levett-Jones (2013).

CLINICAL CONSIDERATIONS

Taste disorders

Taste disorders are relatively common in the general population. Taste abnormalities can contribute to health issues such as anorexia, weight loss and malnutrition. Disorders in taste can be split into three types:

- ageusia — the complete loss of taste; ageusia is rare
- hypogeusia — this is much more common and is the reduced ability to taste the five main tastes of salt, sweet, bitter, sour and umami
- dysgeusia — this is usually characterised as a foul, salty, rancid or metallic taste that persists in the mouth.

The causes of altered taste sensations are varied and include:

- upper respiratory and middle ear infections
- acquired immunodeficiency syndrome caused by HIV infection
- autoimmune and/or inflammatory diseases such as Sjögren's syndrome, systemic lupus erythematosus, bowel diseases, rheumatic arthritis and diabetes
- chemotherapy and radiation therapy for cancers — taste dysfunction is reported in up to two-thirds of cancer patients receiving chemotherapy, and also in head and neck cancer patients receiving radiation therapy
- exposure to certain chemicals, such as insecticides and some medications, including some common antibiotics and antihistamines
- trauma to the peripheral or central nervous system (i.e. head injury)
- some types of surgery to the ear, nose and throat (such as middle ear surgery) or extraction of the wisdom teeth
- poor oral hygiene and dental problems (Feng et al. 2014).

Alteration in taste can affect the appetite and can lead to a reduced food intake, especially in the elderly. The advice for improving appetite for patients with a taste disorder includes:

- preparing foods with a variety of colours and textures
- using aromatic herbs and hot spices to add more flavour; however, avoid adding more sugar or salt to foods
- adding small amounts of cheese, bacon bits, butter, olive oil or toasted nuts on vegetables if the diet permits
- avoiding combination dishes, such as casseroles, that can hide individual flavours and dilute taste.

15.3 The sense of hearing and sense of balance

LEARNING OBJECTIVE 15.3 Describe the structural parts of the ear that are necessary for hearing and a sense of balance.

The ear is the sensory organ necessary for hearing and balance regulation. The sense of hearing is a sophisticated mechanism that conveys the raw incoming sound energy (intensity and frequency) through the air or other mediums towards the brain via the highly adapted ear structures. The brain is able to translate and perceive them as meaningful sounds (e.g. loudness and pitch) after higher-order processing. This then enables us to experience the sound that we hear. The ear structures are also responsible for perception of balance and spatial orientation, also known as the sense of balance.

The structure of the ear

The ear is divided into three sections: external, middle and inner (see figure 15.5).

Each of these three sections is integral in the process of hearing and the inner ear is also essential in the maintenance of the sense of **balance**.

The external ear

The external ear consists of the:

- auricle or pinna
- external auditory canal
- tympanic membrane.

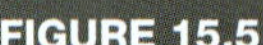

FIGURE 15.5 Structure of the ear

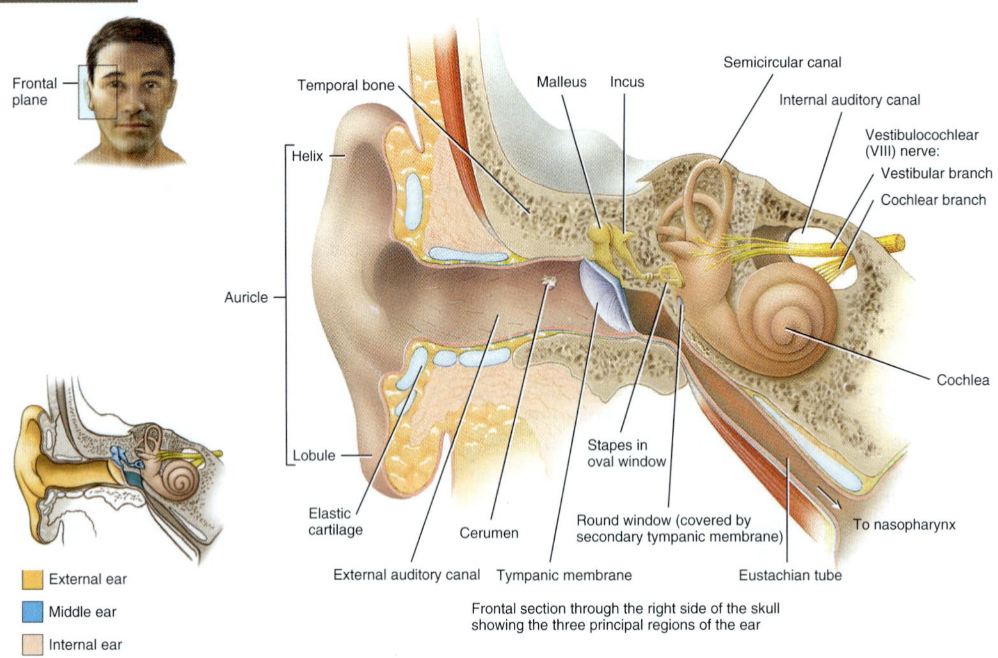

Source: Tortora and Derrickson (2009). Reproduced with permission of John Wiley & Sons.

The auricle is the shell-shaped projection surrounding the external auditory canal. It is made of elastic **cartilage** covered with skin. The auricle can be further broken down into the rim, known as the helix and the earlobe, which lacks supporting cartilage and so is soft. The function of the auricle is to direct soundwaves into the external auditory canal.

The external auditory canal (meatus) is a short, S-shaped, narrow passage about 2.5 cm long and 0.6 cm wide, which extends from the auricle to the tympanic membrane (figure 15.5). At the end closest to the auricle the external auditory ear canal is made of elastic cartilage; the rest of the canal is a channel through the temporal bone and thus needs no supporting cartilage. The entire canal is lined with skin with associated hairs, sebaceous (oil) glands and modified sweat glands called ceruminous glands. The ceruminous glands secrete a yellow-brown waxy cerumen (earwax). The purpose of the oils and the wax is to lubricate the ear canal, kill bacteria and, in conjunction with the hairs, keep the canal free of debris.

The end of the canal is sealed at the internal end by the tympanic membrane (eardrum). It is a cone-shaped structure which protrudes into the middle ear, made up of a thin translucent **connective tissue** membrane covered by skin on its external surface and internally by mucosa. This is the innermost structure of the external ear section. Soundwaves entering the external auditory canal travel along until they reach the tympanic membrane, making it vibrate, and this vibration is transmitted to the bones of the middle ear.

CLINICALLY REASONED EPISODE OF CARE

Ear care

Consider the patient situation

Stephen is a 21-year-old man with Down syndrome. He currently lives with his parents and attends college three days a week. He also attends a day centre two days a week.

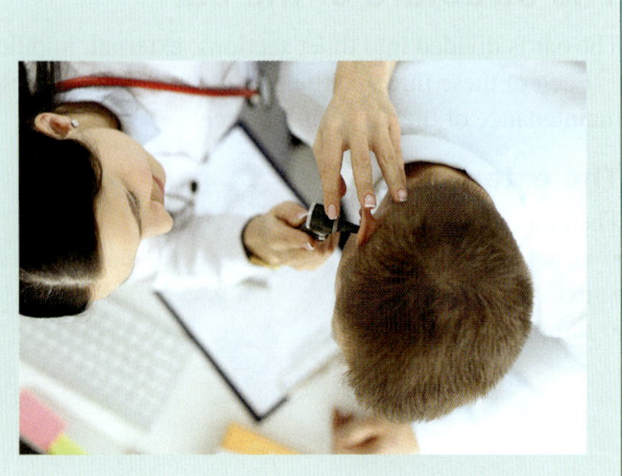

Collect cues and information

Stephen's peers notice that he has had a decreased attention span in class lately and has been speaking louder then usual. He has become withdrawn from his friends. His college instructors inform Stephen's parents that he needs to be given instructions several times and that he does not seem like himself.

Stephen's parents have taken him to the GP. On inspection, the GP finds wax in the ear canal and is concerned about a narrowed canal. The GP refers Stephen to an ear, nose and throat (ENT) specialist. Stephen and his family see the ENT nurse as part of the care team.

Process information

From birth, the person with Down syndrome will often have external ear canal stenosis (narrowing of the canal) which will usually resolve by the age of 3 years. However, even after this age a person with Down syndrome will be predisposed to chronic problems with the ear.

Upper respiratory tract infections are common in people with Down syndrome and thus predispose the patient to developing otitis media, potentially leading to 'glue ear' (otitis media with effusion), which is less likely to self-limit in those with Down syndrome. The reasons for this predisposition to respiratory and ear infections include anatomical differences in the structure of the mid face, a reduction in T and B lymphocytes which reduces the effectiveness of the immune system, differences in the shape and size of the Eustachian tube, and hypotonia of the muscles controlling the Eustachian tube leading to Eustachian tube collapse. Therefore, it is important that ear health is a priority for people living with Down syndrome.

Hearing has a significant role in the learning process. Hearing loss can cause issues with concentration and understanding and can lead to decreased participation and interest in schooling. In some cases, poor hearing can lead to behavioural issues and challenges.

Microsuction is one of the safest methods of earwax removal with few potential side effects. Patients may report feeling dizzy afterwards, but this usually passes quickly. Patients prone to the build-up of earwax should be advised of a few simple precautions to prevent the impaction of the wax in the ear canal (which makes the wax less likely to drain naturally).

Establish goals

1. Microsuctioning
2. Education for Stephen and family about good ear health
3. Coordination of follow-up appointments

Nursing actions

1. Prepare Stephen and family for microsuctioning procedure.
   Rationale:
   - Microsuctioning can be an unusual experience for any patient, especially for those with learning disabilities. It is therefore important that patients are prepared for how the procedure will be performed and what to expect.
   - Nurses will assist the care team in such procedures and work with patients and families before, during and after the procedure.
2. Provide education on long-term ear health strategies.
   Rationale:
   - Nurses are an important part of the care team who can educate patients and families on how to maintain ear health.
   - Education includes not putting anything in the ear canal, including cotton tips or anything to dry them, avoiding water in the ear and using a small amount of cotton wool in the ear when showering or bathing.
   - Due to the risk of perforation, consult with the practice nurse before using over-the-counter ear solutions.
3. Follow up appointment coordination.
   Rationale:
   - Due to the potential for ongoing issues, Stephen and his family will require follow-up appointments with the ENT specialist and team.
   - Nurses are well placed to check in with Stephen and his family on behalf of the care team.
   - Nurses can coordinate appointments and after-care as appropriate.

Evaluate outcomes

Following cleaning of the impacted earwax using microsuction, Stephen's hearing does improve but it is recommended that he is kept under review by the clinic as many of the otolaryngological features of Down syndrome predispose the patient to chronic otitis media.

As a result of the actions above, Stephen's college instructors and day centre peers report an improvement in his concentration and relationships.

Reflect on new processes and learning

What role does hearing play in the learning process?

Source: Based on the Clinical Reasoning Cycle, Levett-Jones (2013).

MEDICINES MANAGEMENT

Antibiotic ear drops

Infections of the external ear (otitis externa, or commonly known as swimmer's ear) are relatively common, especially in children aged 7–12 years. They are usually due to a bacterial infection and can be treated with antibiotic ear drops if necessary (Perth Children's Hospital 2021). The first-line treatment for any ear infection should be pain relief with simple analgesia, ear examinations, and placing a warm or cold flannel on the ear and removing any discharge by wiping the outside of the ear (never placing anything in the ear canal).

Outer ear infections usually present with the following symptoms:

- pain inside the ear
- a high temperature of 38 °C or above
- being sick
- a lack of energy
- difficulty hearing
- discharge running out of the ear
- a feeling of pressure or fullness inside the ear
- itching and irritation in and around the ear.

If the infection does not clear after 3 days, or the patient develops a very high temperature, a sore throat, or inflammation around the ear, then the patient should seek advice from a doctor or pharmacist.

If the infection is associated with significant inflammation, the GP may prescribe antibiotic ear drops with steroids to reduce the inflammation. In severe cases, oral antibiotics may be required. As with all antibiotics, it is important that they are used correctly and the entire course of treatment is taken.

Simple steps to prevent ear inflammation

Keeping the ear canals as dry as possible will minimise the risk of ear inflammation. Strategies include avoiding getting water into the ears by using earplugs, avoiding dirty water, removing the water that gets into the ear after a shower, and avoiding fingers or other objects from getting into the ear canal.

SKILLS IN PRACTICE

Instillation of ear drops

David is a 76-year-old gentleman who has been suffering with the build-up of earwax in his ear canals, leading to hearing loss. Prior to microsuction removal of the wax, he has been asked to instil olive oil into his ears to help soften the wax. He is to do this once a day for 7 days. You have been asked to teach David's partner how to put the olive oil into David's ears.

1. Gather the equipment. He will need a bottle of olive oil, an eye dropper with bulb (available from the local chemist — preferably with a small bottle to put the olive oil in) and some cotton wool.
2. He should wash his hands with soap and water.
3. If the olive oil is in the eye dropper bottle, hold it in your hands for a few minutes to warm it up — this prevents the shock of a cold fluid entering the ear canal.
4. David must lie on one side with the ear up and have 2–3 drops of olive oil dripped into the ear using the eye dropper (do not put the dropper into the ear). He then stays on his side for 5 minutes to allow the oil to seep down the canal. In the meantime, he can massage the ear just in front of the tragus (the small flap at the front of the ear) and pull the top of the ear upwards and backwards; this helps the olive oil work its way down the ear canal.
5. After 5 minutes, wipe any excess olive oil from the outside of the ear and be prepared to wipe away olive oil draining from the ear. Do not put anything in the ear canal.
6. Repeat on the other side.

Hearing aids and devices

Hearing aids work by converting speech and other sounds to acoustic signals; they then amplify these. There are some hearing aids that depress lower-frequency sounds and others that amplify higher frequency sounds. With advances in technology, increasingly smaller, more efficient hearing aids are now being produced. There are several different types, informally named by their placement in or around the ear: behind-the-ear, in-the-ear, or in-the-canal hearing aids. Although hearing aids can amplify sounds, they cannot make words clearer or speech any easier to understand, except by making thesounds louder.

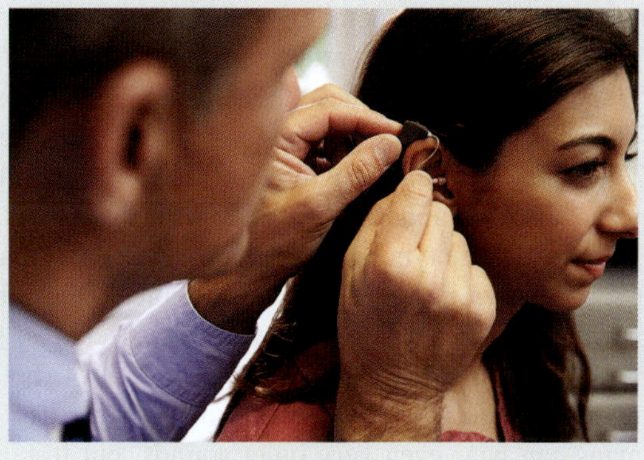

Hearing aids can pick up the sound that is entering the ear, process it to match the hearing loss and then release the signal back into the ear instantaneously. A digital hearing aid is much more advanced than an analogue aid. It contains a silicon chip made up of millions of electrical components, continuously processing incoming sound, converting it into clearer and more audible sounds and then releasing these at the appropriate sound level into the ear. This can help the user to distinguish between sounds that need to be amplified and unwanted noise that needs to be reduced. Moreover, digital hearing aids can be modified in order to work with an individual's personal degree of hearing loss and lifestyle needs.

The Australia-based medical device company Cochlear Limited is a world leader in the hearing implant market. Two types of hearing devices developed and sold by Cochlear are the bone-anchored hearing aid (BAHA®) and Cochlear™ implant. BAHA provides an alternative solution to achieving hearing through bone conduction, unlike hearing aids. A BAHA implant is suitable for people with mild to moderate hearing loss with external or middle ear problems since the sound bypasses these two areas, directing the sound towards the inner ear. This group of patients have partial or single-sided hearing loss with poor conduction and cannot use the standard in-the-ear or behind-the-ear hearing aids. Invasive surgery is required to implant the device, which carries direct localised sound via bone conduction directly into the inner ear, giving full directional sound awareness after filtering out external noise. However, this does not give true bilateral hearing. The BAHA device consists of a sound processor held in place by a titanium screw that is implanted into the skull behind the visual part of the external ear.

For patients with more severe hearing loss who are unable to successfully use traditional hearing aids or BAHA implants, a cochlear implant may be considered. Cochlear implants are specifically considered for those who have lost their inner ear function with poor conduction to the auditory nerve. While hearing aids amplify sounds to be detected by the damaged ears, cochlear implants generate signals bypassing damaged parts of the ear to stimulate the auditory nerve directly. These signals are then transmitted to the auditory centres in the brain.

See Happy Ears Hearing Center (2020).

Middle ear

Otherwise known as the tympanic cavity, this is a small, air-filled cavity lined with mucosa and contained within the temporal bone. It is enclosed at both ends, by the eardrum at the **lateral** end and medially by a bony wall with two openings:

- oval (vestibular) window
- round (cochlear) window.

The middle ear is connected to the **nasopharynx** by the Eustachian (auditory) tube, a 4 cm long tube that consists of two portions:

- the section near the connection to the middle ear, which is relatively narrow and is supported by elastic cartilage
- the section near the nasopharynx, which is relatively broad and funnel-shaped.

When open, the Eustachian tube allows the passage of air and thus ensures the equalisation of the pressures on both sides of the tympanic membrane so both are subject to the same atmospheric pressure. The Eustachian tube is normally closed at the end nearest the nasopharynx, but opens during yawning, chewing and swallowing (Jenkins & Tortora 2013). If equalisation of pressures does not happen, then the difference in pressures between the two sides can lead to reduced hearing as the tympanic membrane cannot move freely. Swellings caused by colds or infections can block the Eustachian tube and result in fluid build-up in the middle ear. If this leads to bacterial infection in the middle ear, then ear infection, known as otitis media, occurs.

Within the middle ear there are three bones known as the ossicles or ossicular chain. These three bones connect the tympanic membrane with the receptor complexes of the inner ear:

- The malleus (hammer) attaches at three points to the inner surface of the tympanic membrane.
- The incus (anvil) attaches the malleus to the stapes.
- The stapes (stirrup) — the edges of the base of the stapes are bound to the edge of the oval window.

The joints between these three bones are the smallest **synovial joints** in the body and each has its own tiny capsule and supporting extracapsular **ligaments**.

Vibration in the tympanic membrane is the first stage in the perception of sound; this vibration converts the soundwaves into mechanical movement (the vibration). The ossicles act as levers and conduct the vibrations to the inner ear. They are connected in such a way that the in–out movement of tympanic vibration is converted into a rocking motion of the stapes. The ossicles collect the force applied to the tympanic membrane, amplify it and transmit it to the oval window. This amplification explains why humans can hear even very quiet sounds, but it can also be a problem in very noisy environments. In order to protect the tympanic membrane and the ossicular chain from violent movement resulting from extreme noises, they are supported by two small muscles.

- The tensor tympani muscle is a short ribbon of muscle connected to the 'handle' of the malleus. When it contracts, the malleus is pulled medially (towards the inner ear), stiffening the tympanic membrane.
- The stapedius muscle is attached to the stapes and pulls it, reducing the movement against the oval window.

Inner ear

The senses of equilibrium (part of the sense of balance) and hearing are provided by the receptors in the inner ear.

The inner ear is also known as the labyrinth, owing to the complicated series of canals it contains. The inner ear is composed of two main, fluid-filled parts:

- bony labyrinth — a series of cavities within the temporal bone that contain the main organs of balance (the semicircular canals and the vestibule) and the main organ of hearing (the cochlea)
- membranous labyrinth — a series of fluid-filled sacs and tubes that are contained within the bony labyrinth.

Between the bony and membranous labyrinth flows **perilymph**, a liquid that is rather like cerebrospinal fluid; the fluid within the membranous labyrinth is known as **endolymph**.

As noted above, the bony labyrinth can be divided into three parts (figure 15.6).

- The vestibule consists of a pair of membranous sacs: the saccule and the utricle. Receptors in these two sacs provide the sensations of gravity and linear acceleration.
- The semicircular canals enclose slender semicircular ducts. Receptors in these ducts are stimulated by the rotation of the head. The combination of the vestibule and the semicircular canals is known as the vestibular complex.
- The cochlea is a spiral-shaped, bony chamber that contains the cochlear duct of the membranous labyrinth. Receptors within this duct give us the sense of hearing.

15.4 Equilibrium

LEARNING OBJECTIVE 15.4 Explain the way in which human beings maintain a sense of balance.

The sense of equilibrium is part of the sense of balance and is controlled by receptors in the semicircular ducts, the utricle and the saccule of the inner ear. The sensory receptors in the semicircular ducts are active during movement but inactive when the body is motionless. The sensory receptors in the ducts respond to rotational movements of the head. There are three of these ducts: lateral, posterior and anterior.

The ducts are continuous with the utricle. Each semicircular duct contains an **ampulla**, an expanded region that contains the majority of the receptors. The area in the wall of the ampulla that contains the receptors is known as the crista and each crista is bound to a cupula — a gelatinous structure that extends the full width of the ampulla. The hair cells (receptors) are surrounded by supporting cells and are monitored by the dendrites of sensory neurones.

The free surfaces of the hair cells are covered with stereocilia, which resemble very long microvilli. Along with the fine stereocilia, the hair cell will also have one kinocilium — a single, large and thick cilium. When an external force pushes against the cilia, the distortion of the plasma membrane of the hair cell alters the rate that the cell releases chemical transmitters. So, for instance, if a person moves their head to look to the left, the cilia of the lateral semicircular canal are subject to pressure and thus the cell membranes are distorted, leading to an altered release of neurotransmitters and the perception of rotational movement (figure 15.7). Any movement of the head can be perceived by varying combinations of stimulation of the three ducts and their receptors.

FIGURE 15.6 Inner ear

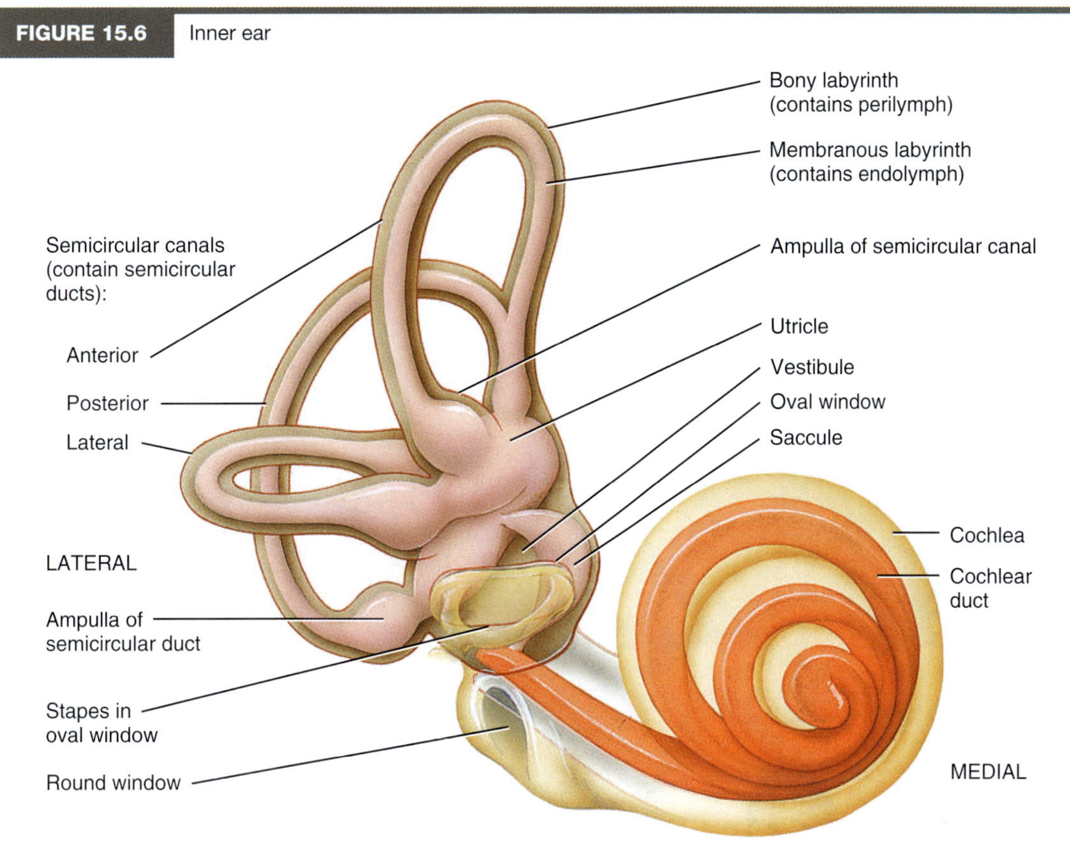

Components of the right internal ear

Source: Tortora and Derrickson (2009). Reproduced with permission of John Wiley & Sons.

A similar type of activity happens when the body is subject to linear acceleration; for example, as a car speeds up, the otolith lags behind due to inertia. The brain would normally differentiate between the action of gravity and the action of acceleration by integrating the information from the receptors with visual information.

In contrast to the semicircular canals, the utricle and the saccule provide equilibrium information whether the body is moving or stationary. The two chambers are connected by a narrow passageway that is also connected to the endolymphatic duct. The hair cells of the utricle and saccule are clustered in oval structures called maculae. As with the hair cells of the ampullae, the cilia of the hair cells in the utricle and saccule are embedded in a gelatine-like substance. However, the surface of this substance contains densely packed calcium carbonate crystals called statoconia. This combination of gelatine-like substance and calcium carbonate crystals is known as an otolith (figure 15.8).

When the head is in a neutral position, the statoconia sit on top of the macula. The pressure they generate is therefore downwards and the hair cell microvilli are pushed down. When the head is tilted, the pull of gravity on the statoconia shifts and the microvilli are moved to one side or the other. This distorts the cell membrane and triggers altered neurotransmitter release (figure 15.9).

FIGURE 15.7 (a, b) Ampulla at rest and in response to movement

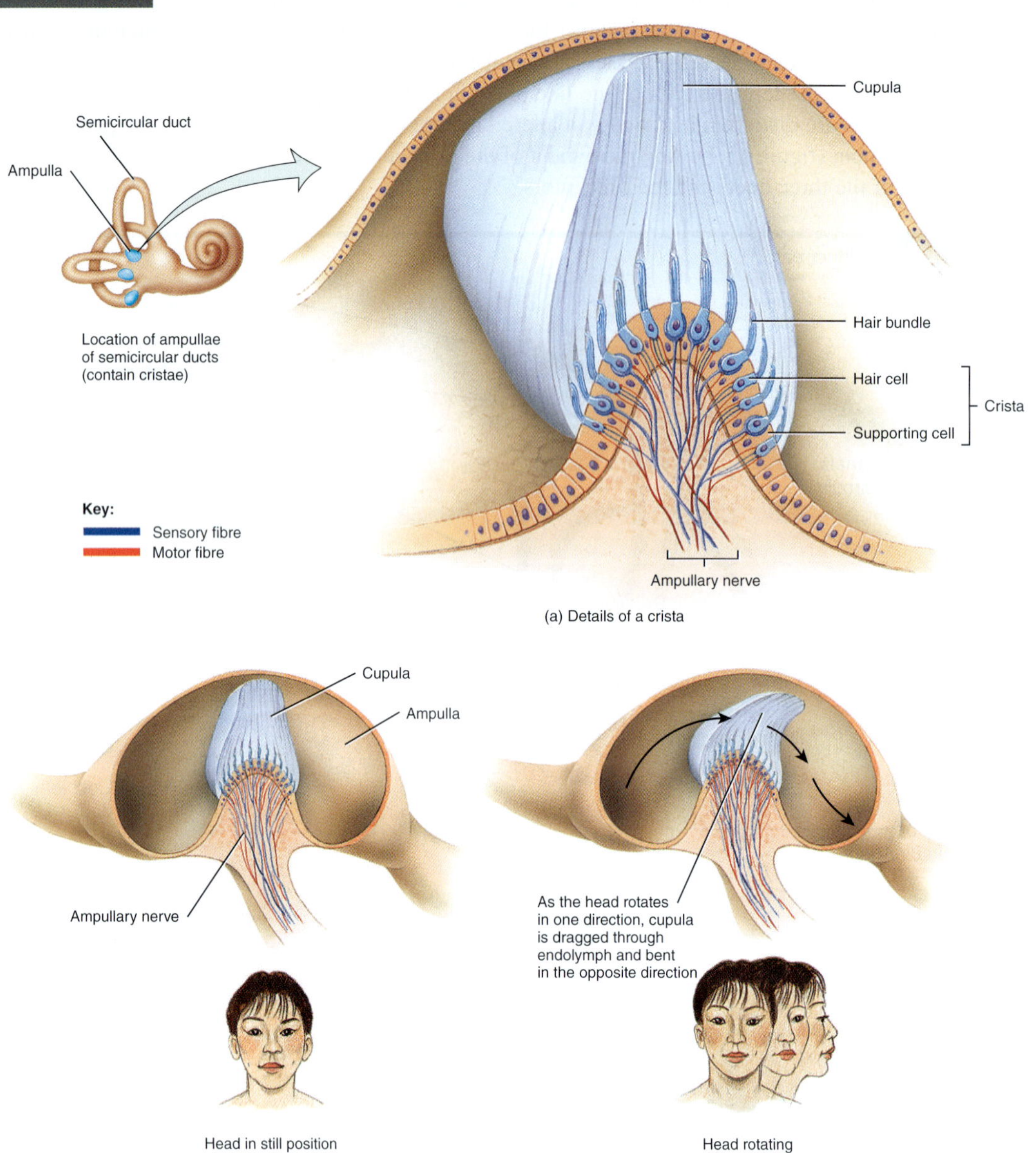

(a) Details of a crista

(b) Position of a cupula with the head in the still position (left) and when the head rotates (right)

Source: Tortora and Derrickson (2009). Reproduced with permission of John Wiley & Sons.

Pathways for the equilibrium sensations

The hair cells in the semicircular canals, the vestibule and the saccule are monitored by sensory neurones located in the vestibular ganglia. Sensory fibres from these ganglia form the vestibular branch of the vestibulocochlear nerve (cranial nerve VIII). These fibres feed into neurones within the vestibular nuclei at the boundary of the **pons** and the **medulla oblongata** in the brain.

The vestibular nuclei have four functions:

- integrating sensory information about equilibrium received from both sides of the head
- relaying information to the cerebellum
- relaying information to the cortex
- sending commands to motor nuclei in the brainstem and the spinal cord. The motor commands are reflex-type commands for eye, head and neck movements, such as the movement of the eyes that occurs in response to sensations of motion.

FIGURE 15.8 Hair cells and otolith

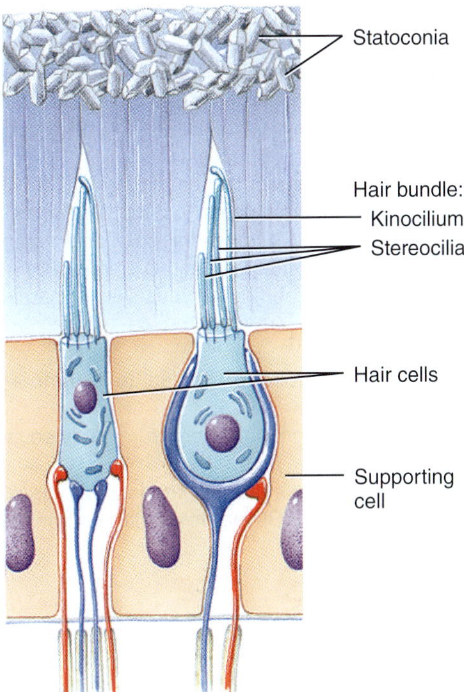

Details of two hair cells

Source: Tortora and Derrickson (2009). Reproduced with permission of John Wiley & Sons.

FIGURE 15.9 Action of gravity on the otolith

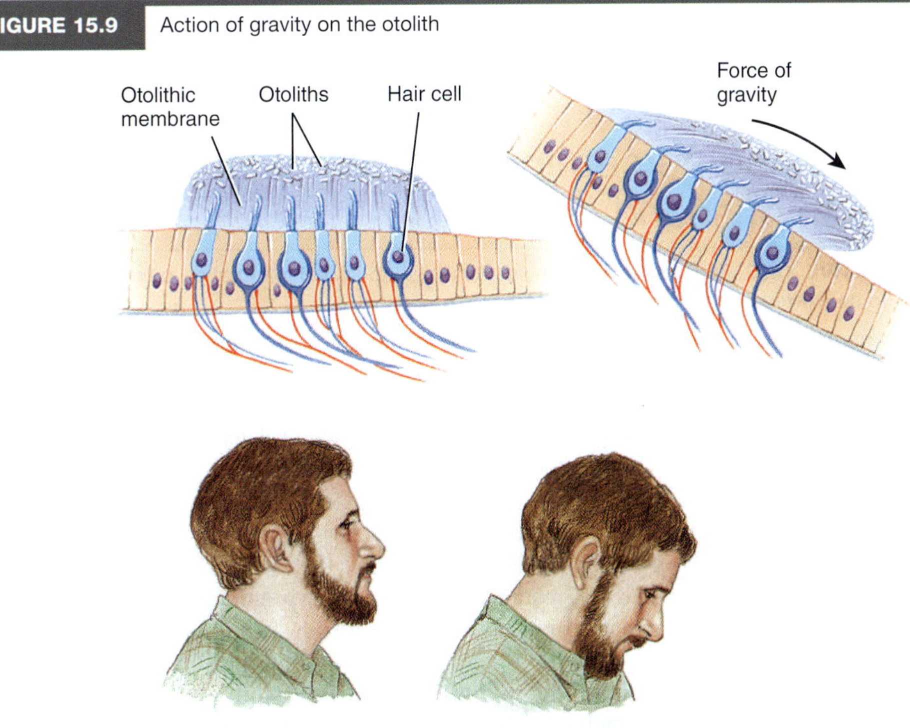

Position of macula with head upright (left) and tilted forward (right)

Source: Tortora and Derrickson (2009). Reproduced with permission of John Wiley & Sons.

MEDICINES MANAGEMENT

Vertigo

Vertigo is the sensation of spinning of self or surroundings, usually resulting in a combination of dizziness, disorientation, instability and nausea that affects the sense of balance. Vertigo occurs due to problems with equilibrioception when the visual system, vestibular system and proprioception do not act together to maintain balance with spatial awareness.

Vertigo may be classified as peripheral or central according to the clinical signs and symptoms. Peripheral conditions affecting the vestibular system include Ménière's disease, inner ear infection (labyrinthitis), vestibular neuronitis and benign paroxysmal positional vertigo (BPPV). BPPV is the most common cause of vertigo in clinical practice (Dommaraju & Perera 2016). Central causes include the dysfunction of the brainstem, cerebellum and central nervous system pathways such as strokes, lesions, drug toxicity and multiple sclerosis.

Clinical features:

- It may be sudden onset (e.g. BPPV or stroke) or gradual (e.g. tumour or demyelination in multiple sclerosis).
- BPPV, recent upper respiratory tract infection, stress or trauma may cause intermittent vertigo through changes to head position.
- Tinnitus and deafness may suggest Ménière's disease and labyrinthitis.
- Nystagmus or abnormal eye saccades in BPPV, vestibular neuronitis, labyrinthitis and Ménière's disease.
- It is associated with nausea and vomiting.
- Pain and fever may be bacterial labyrinthitis.

Physical examinations:

- An ear examination is required for infection and inflammation.
- A neurological examination, including speech assessment, is required to exclude central causes.
- Eye and visual examinations include nystagmus observation for types of conditions causing peripheral vertigo (see Emergency Care Institute 2021).
- Cardiovascular examination.

Clinical management:

- Administer ondansetron or prochlorperazine (antiemetic) for acute vertigo. Consider diazepam (anticholinergic) or betahistine (antihistamine) as second-line treatment.
- Administer IV fluids if patient is vomiting or dehydrated.
- If peripheral cause is not managed adequately, refer to an ENT specialist.

15.5 The hearing perception — discrimination and interpretation of sound energy

LEARNING OBJECTIVE 15.5 Explore the mechanisms that lead to sound information being converted into action potentials to be relayed to the brain.

Hearing is a perception of the energy from soundwaves, after the interpretation of the amplitude, frequency and duration of these waves, which are then discriminated by the auditory system as intensity (loudness or volume), pitch, and duration respectively. The interpretation of low-intensity sounds is influenced by sensitivity, which varies between individuals. The human ear is capable of detecting soundwaves with a wide range of frequencies ranging from 20 to 2000 Hz.

Initial sound processing for pitch, intensity and duration takes place in the cochlea of the ear, while location of sound involves sensory inputs from both ears together with additional higher function processing in the brain. The sense of hearing is provided by receptors in the cochlear duct; they are hair cells similar to those of the semicircular canals and vestibule. However, their positioning within the cochlear duct and the organisation of the surrounding structures protect them from stimuli generated by anything other than soundwaves.

The ossicular chains transmit and amplify pressure waves from the air into pressure waves in the perilymph of the cochlea. These waves stimulate the hair cells along the cochlear spiral.

- The *frequency* of the perceived sound is detected by the part of the cochlear duct that is stimulated.
- The *intensity* (volume) of the sound is detected by the number of hair cells that are stimulated at the particular point in the cochlea. The units for sound intensity are called decibels (dB).

Within the bony labyrinth of the cochlea there are three ducts (figure 15.10).

- The vestibular duct (scala vestibuli) connects to the oval window.
- The tympanic duct (scala tympani) connects to the round window.
- The cochlear duct (scala media) is separated from the tympanic duct by the basilar membrane.

FIGURE 15.10 Cross-section of the cochlea (highlighted section is shown in detail in figure 15.12)

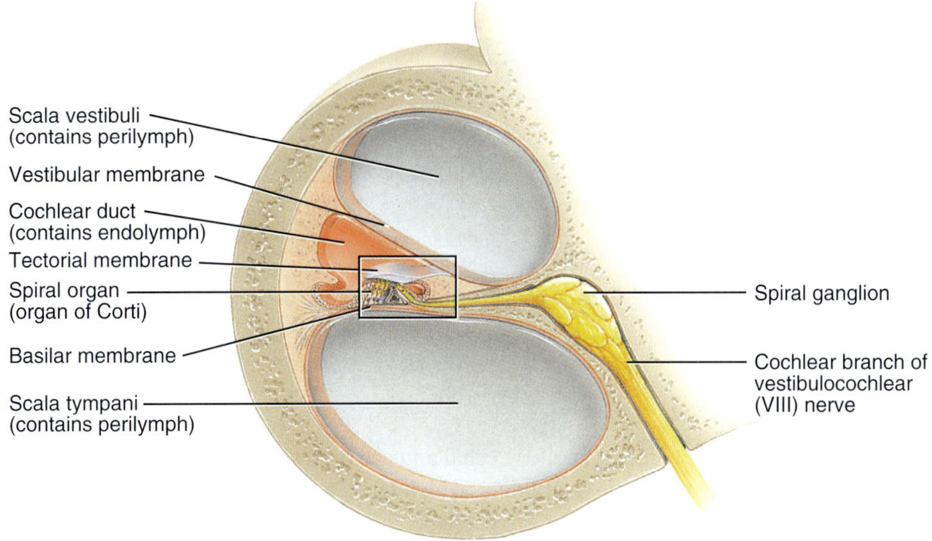

Section through one turn of the cochlea

Source: Tortora and Derrickson (2009). Reproduced with permission of John Wiley & Sons.

Both the vestibular and the tympanic duct are connected at the tip of the cochlear spiral and therefore make up one continuous perilymphatic chamber (figure 15.11).

FIGURE 15.11 Cochlea showing the continuous nature of the vestibular and tympanic ducts

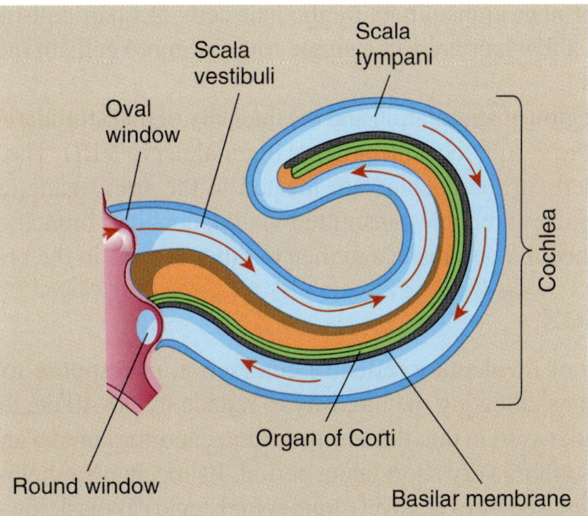

Between the vestibular and the tympanic ducts is the cochlear duct; the hair cells of this duct are located in a structure called the organ of Corti (figure 15.12). The organ of Corti sits on the basilar membrane and its hair cells are arranged in a series of longitudinal rows.

The hair cells of the organ of Corti do not have kinocilia and their stereocilia are in contact with the overlying tectorial membrane; this membrane is attached to the inner wall of the cochlear duct. When a portion of the basilar membrane bounces up and down in response to pressure waves in the perilymph, the stereocilia of the hair cells are pressed against the tectorial membrane and become distorted.

FIGURE 15.12 Organ of Corti

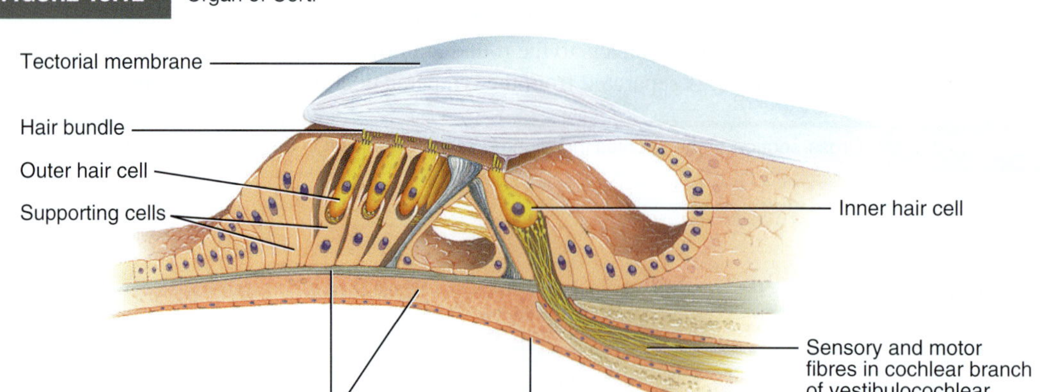

Source: Tortora and Derrickson (2009). Reproduced with permission of John Wiley & Sons.

The hearing process

1. Soundwaves travel down the external auditory canal and arrive at the tympanic membrane.
2. Movement is created in the tympanic membrane, which leads to the movement of the ossicles and the amplification of the movement.
3. Movement of the stapes at the oval window creates pressure waves in the perilymph of the vestibular duct.
4. The pressure waves distort the basilar membrane. The location of the maximum distortion depends on the frequency of the sound, as the basilar membrane varies in width and flexibility along its length. Higher pitch sounds create maximum distortion near to the oval window and lower pitch sounds further away from the window. The amount of distortion gives sensory information as to the volume of the sound.
5. Vibration in the basilar membrane leads to vibration of the hair cell cilia against the tectorial membrane, leading to the release of neurotransmitters by the hair cells. As hair cells are arranged in rows, a soft sound may only distort a few hair cells in a single row, but more cells in more rows will be stimulated as the volume increases.
6. Information about the region of stimulation and the intensity of that stimulation is relayed to the brain via the cochlear branch of the vestibulocochlear nerve (cranial nerve VIII). The cell bodies of the neurones that monitor the hair cells of the cochlea are located in the spiral ganglia at the centre of the bony cochlea. The nerve impulses are then transmitted via the cochlear branch of cranial nerve VIII to the cochlear nuclei of the medulla oblongata and then to other centres in the brain.

The hearing reflex

The middle ear is capable of involuntary reflexive contraction in response to a high intensity of lower-frequency sound stimulations, allowing the intensity to reduce by 30–40 decibels. When loud sounds are transmitted from the ossicular system into the auditory nerve, auditory nuclei and brainstem, a reflex called the **auditory reflex** occurs after a very short latent period. Its mechanism helps to: (1) protect the cochlea from damaging vibrations caused by excessively loud sounds; and (2) mask low-frequency sounds in a loud environment. For example, when a loud sound is presented, a reflex causes contraction to the stapedius muscle, and to a lesser extent, the tensor tympani muscle. This allows the tensor tympani muscle to pull the handle of the malleus inwards while the stapedius muscle pulls the stapes outwards. These opposing forces cause the entire ossicular system to become rigid, which in turn reduces the ossicular conductions of low-frequency sounds.

MEDICINES MANAGEMENT

Ototoxicity

Ototoxicity is the property of being toxic to the ear. There are over 200 drugs that can lead to ototoxicity, tinnitus and associated hearing loss. Ototoxicity effects can be short-term or long-term (i.e. temporary or permanent).

Many of the drugs are used in common practice, such as:

- furosemide
- gentamicin
- metropolol
- ramipril
- sodium valproate.

Patients should be informed that if they do experience any suspected tinnitus or hearing loss with a drug, it is important they do not stop taking the drug until they have talked to their doctor.

Avoiding ototoxicity

Many ototoxic drugs are excreted in the urine and thus it is best to avoid ototoxic drugs in patients with renal impairment and they should be used with caution in the elderly. Furthermore, the patient should be well hydrated to ensure good renal function.

Drugs such as gentamicin and vancomycin are normally given at set times and the nurse should avoid giving these drugs too early as it may cause an excessive blood level. Also, blood levels of these drugs are required at regular intervals and it is important to adhere to medical instructions regarding the administration before and after drug administration.

Furosemide toxicity is related to the speed of administration and, therefore, it is essential that the instructions for the speed of delivery of intravenous furosemide are followed.

CLINICAL CONSIDERATIONS

Noise exposure and ear damage

As noise levels increase, the chance of damage to the ear increases. The following table gives examples of the types of noise levels at certain decibel (dB) levels and the exposure time at which damage may occur.

dB level	Maximum exposure per day	Examples
10		Breathing
20		Rustling leaves
60		Conversation
75		Typical car interior on motorway
85	16 h	City traffic (inside car)
90	9 h	Power drill, food blender
97	3 h	French horn at 10 feet
100	2 h	Farm tractor, outboard motor, jet take-off at 1000 feet
110	0.5 h	Chainsaw, pneumatic drill, car horn at 3 feet
120	0 h	Typical rock concert, loud thunderclap
125	Hearing damage occurring	Pneumatic riveter at 4 feet
132–140	Permanent hearing damage	Gunshot, very loud rock concert 50 feet in front of speakers

dB level	Maximum exposure per day	Examples
150–160	Eardrum rupture	Jet take-off at 75 feet, gunshot at 1 foot
190	Immediate death of tissue	Jet engine at 1 foot
194		Loudest sound in air, air particle distortion (sonic boom)

15.6 The eye and the sense of sight

LEARNING OBJECTIVE 15.6 Describe the basic anatomical structures of the eye.

Vision is perhaps the sense that we value the most; we learn more about the world around us through sight than we do with any of the other senses. Vision is the process where light is reflected from external objects to the back of the eye and translated into a mental image involving various steps. Without sight many of our daily tasks and pleasures would be impossible and many others would become more difficult.

The structure of the eye

Accessory eye structures

The sense of sight is based on the eyes and around the eyes there are accessory structures that help to keep the eyes safe and working well (see figure 15.13):

- eyelids (palpebrae) — a continuation of the skin; continual blinking keeps the surface of the eye lubricated and removes dirt; the gap between them is known as the palpebral fissure
- eyelashes — robust hairs that help to keep foreign matter out of the eyes; they are associated with the tarsal glands which produce a lipid-rich secretion that helps to prevent the eyelids from sticking together
- **lacrimal** caruncle — a small collection of soft tissue that contains accessory glands
- commissure — the point where the eyelids meet; there are two: the lateral and the **medial**
- conjunctiva — the epithelial cell layer that lines the inside of the eyelids and the outer surface of the eye.

FIGURE 15.13 Accessory structures of the eye

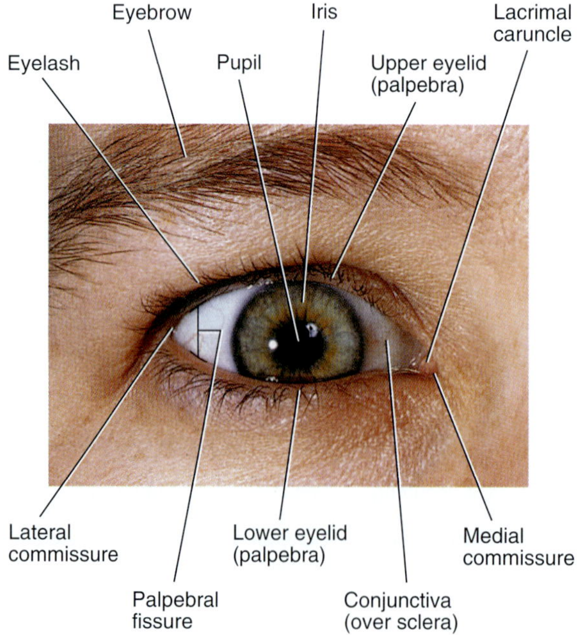

Source: Tortora and Derrickson (2009). Reproduced with permission of John Wiley & Sons.

MEDICINES MANAGEMENT

Conjunctivitis

Conjunctivitis is a condition where the conjunctiva, which covers the white part of the eye and the inside of the eyelid, is inflamed. Conjunctivitis causes the white part of the eye to appear pink or red with accompanying itchy and burning eyes. It is caused by either a bacterial or a viral infection and is highly contagious. Bacterial conjunctivitis is accompanied by gritty and copious yellowish discharge, making the eyelids stick together. Viral conjunctivitis leads to clear discharge with associated hayfever-like symptoms such as an itchy nose and sneezing. The patient generally experiences decreased **visual acuity** with discomfort in bright light settings.

When symptoms of conjunctivitis appear and do not disappear within a few hours, the individual is recommended to see a physician. Simple management includes constant cleaning of eye areas with warm moist towels once every hour, lubrication with eye drops and simple analgesics (paracetamol and ibuprofen) to manage the pain. The patient is usually prescribed broad-spectrum antibiotic drops (i.e. chloramphenicol (0.5%) or ciprofloxacin) once every few hours for a week (NSW Department of Health 2009). Whenever viral conjunctivitis is suspected, antihistamine drops such as Naphcon-A drops QID with nasal decongestants are prescribed and used for no longer than 14 days. The physician or nurse may also take a swab for culture and polymerase chain reaction. The patient should avoid wearing contact lenses until fully recovered, and additional care should be taken to avoid allergic triggers such as dust, mould and pollen in allergic conjunctivitis. It is also recommended to avoid workplace or school until the discharge from the eye has stopped.

Lacrimal apparatus

A constant flow of tears washes over the eyes to keep the conjunctiva moist and clean. Tears have several functions such as:

- reducing friction
- removing debris
- preventing bacterial infection
- providing nutrients and oxygen to parts of the conjunctiva.

The lacrimal apparatus produces, distributes and removes tears. It consists of:

- a lacrimal gland
- lacrimal canaliculi
- a lacrimal sac
- a nasolacrimal duct.

The lacrimal gland (tear gland) creates most of the content of tears (about 1 mL per day). Once the lacrimal secretions reach the eye they mix with the products of the accessory glands and the tarsal glands. This results in a mixture that lubricates the eye and reduces evaporation. The nutrient and oxygen demands of the corneal cells are supplied by diffusion from the lacrimal secretions. The secretions also contain antibacterial **enzymes** and **antibodies** to attack **pathogens** before they enter the body.

Blinking sweeps the tears across the ocular surface and they accumulate at the medial commissure from where they are drained by the lacrimal canaliculi into the lacrimal sac and from there into the nasal cavity through the nasolacrimal duct.

The main eye structures

The wall of the eye

The wall of the eye has three layers (figure 15.14):

- fibrous tunic
- vascular tunic
- neural tunic.

Fibrous tunic

The fibrous tunic is the outermost layer of the eye and consists of the sclera and the cornea; it has three main functions.

- It provides support and some protection.
- It is the attachment site for the **extrinsic** muscles.
- It contains structures that assist in the focusing process.

FIGURE 15.14 Anatomy of the eye

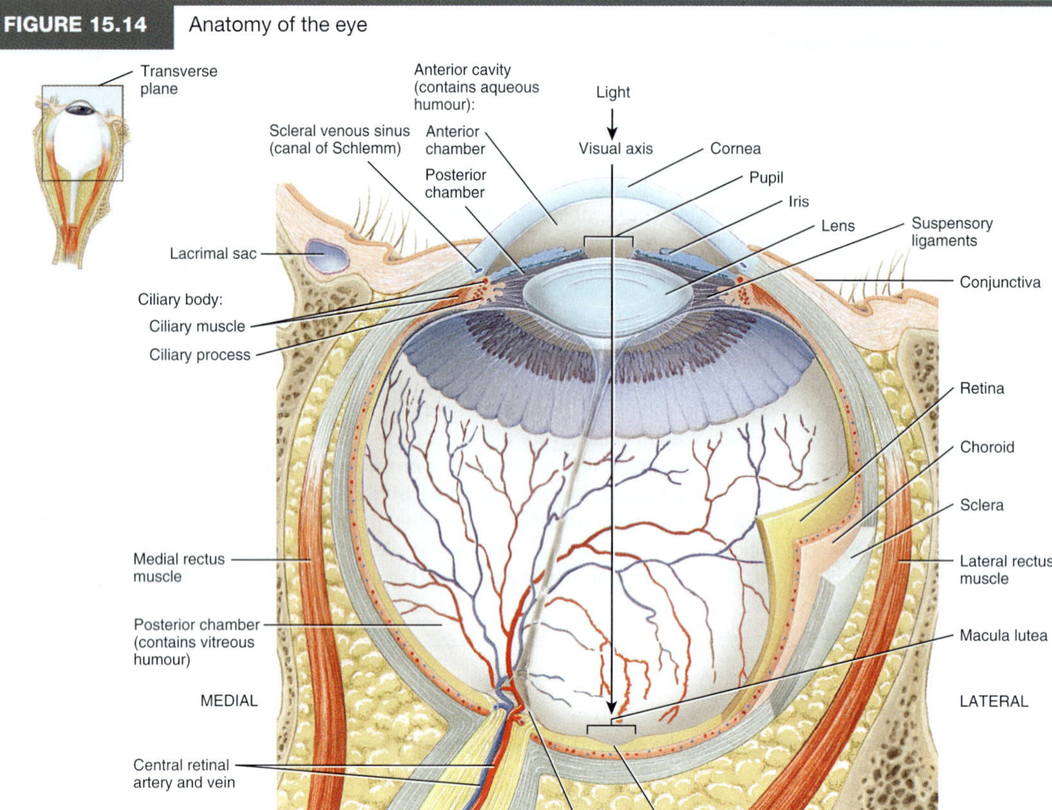

Source: Tortora and Derrickson (2009). Reproduced with permission of John Wiley & Sons.

Most of the ocular surface is covered by the sclera (the 'white' of the eye), which is made up of dense fibrous connective tissue containing collagen and elastic fibres. The surface of the sclera contains small blood vessels and nerves. The **transparent** cornea is continuous with the sclera and is made up of a dense matrix of fibres laid down in such a way that they do not interfere with the passage of light.

Vascular tunic (uvea)

The vascular tunic is the middle of the three layers of the eye and contains numerous blood vessels, lymph vessels and the smooth muscles involved in eye functioning. The functions of this layer include:

- providing a structure for the blood and lymph vessels that supply the tissues of the eye
- regulating the amount of light that enters the eye
- secreting and reabsorbing the aqueous humour
- controlling the shape of the lens.

The vascular tunic is made up of:

- the **iris**
- the ciliary body
- the choroid.

Iris

The iris is the central, coloured portion of the eye (figure 15.13) and regulates the amount of light entering the eye by adjusting the size or diameter of the central opening (the **pupil**). It is formed of two layers of pigmented cells and fibres and two layers of smooth muscle (the pupillary muscles):

- **pupillary constrictor muscles**
- **pupillary dilator muscles**.

Both sets of muscles are controlled by the **autonomic nervous system**; activation of the **parasympathetic nervous system** leads to constriction of the pupil in response to bright light. Activation of the **sympathetic nervous system** leads to the dilation of the pupil in response to dim light levels. Thus, the regulation of light entering the eye is controlled by the pupillary reflex. A standard part of a neurological examination is testing the pupillary reflex to check for damage in certain parts of the central nervous system. At its edge the iris attaches to the anterior part of the ciliary body.

Ciliary body

The greatest part of the ciliary body is made up of the ciliary muscle, a smooth muscular ring that projects into the interior of the eye. The epithelial covering of this muscle has many folds called ciliary processes. The suspensory ligaments of the lens attach to the tips of these processes.

Choroid

The choroid is a vascular layer that separates the fibrous and neural tunics. It is covered by the sclera and attached to the outermost layer of the retina. The choroid contains an extensive capillary network that delivers oxygen and nutrients to the retina.

Neural tunic (retina)

This is the innermost layer of the eye, consisting of a thin outer layer called the pigment epithelium and a thicker inner layer called the neural part.

- The retinal pigment epithelium absorbs the light that passes through the neural part; this prevents light bouncing back through the neural part and causing 'visual echoes'.
- The neural part of the retina contains light receptors and support cells and is responsible for the preliminary processing and integration of visual information.

The chambers of the eye

The eye is divided into two main cavities: a large posterior cavity and a smaller anterior cavity. The anterior cavity is further divided into the anterior chamber and the posterior chamber (figure 15.14).

- The anterior cavity is filled with a substance called aqueous humour that circulates between the anterior and posterior chambers by passing through the pupil and performing a vital role as a transport medium for nutrients and waste products. The fluid pressure created by the aqueous humour in the anterior cavity helps to maintain the shape of the eye. Aqueous humour is produced by the epithelial cells of the ciliary body and within a few hours is drained through the canal of Schlemm to the sclera to be recycled.
- The posterior cavity is the larger of the two cavities of the eye and is filled with a gelatinous mass known as vitreous humour. The vitreous humour helps to stabilise the shape of the eye as the activity of the extraocular muscles would otherwise distort the shape of the eye. Unlike aqueous humour, the vitreous humour is created during the development of the eye and is never replaced. A thin film of aqueous humour infiltrates the posterior chamber, bathing the retina, supplying nutrients and removing waste. The pressure it creates also helps to keep the neural part of the retina against the pigmented epithelium; though the two are close together, they are not fixed to each other and thus this external pressure is required.

CLINICAL CONSIDERATIONS

Glaucoma and tonometry

Globally, glaucoma is the most common cause of vision loss without any cure (Keel et al. 2017a). The incidence of glaucoma in non-Indigenous Australians over the age of 50 is approximately 3.5 per cent, while among similarly aged Indigenous Australians it is 1.6 per cent (Keel et al. 2017a). Glaucoma is a disease of the eye where the intraocular pressure (IOP) becomes abnormally high; the normal IOP is between about 10 and 21 mmHg. Even slight pressure changes (in the range of 21–30 mmHg) sustained for long time periods can lead to vision loss. When IOP rises, the axons of the optic nerve at the optic disc are compressed, leading to optic nerve fibres being damaged after being starved of nutrients and oxygen.

Measuring IOP is an important ophthalmic test and the correct term is tonometry. Tonometry is the objective measurement of IOP and is usually based on the assessment of resistance of the cornea to indent (usually a blast of air). This test has clinical relevance for glaucoma and aids in its early detection. There are several types of tonometer available; an applanation tonometer is a tool that measures the amount of force needed to temporarily flatten part of the cornea. The tonometer measures the degree of resistance provided by the cornea to gentle indentation, and converts this into a figure. A drop of fluorescein/anaesthetic provides a blue light filter. The procedure does not hurt; the patient has to keep their eyes wide open. While this test is completely painless, many patients find this test very difficult.

There are contraindications to this procedure, such as trauma or corneal ulcer. Measuring IOP is quick and simple and because of this it is routinely performed on all adults who require eye tests.

SKILLS IN PRACTICE

Using eye drops

Sarah is a 72-year-old woman who has been to see her optician for new glasses. During routine testing, the optician has detected the onset of glaucoma and referred Sarah to her GP. The treatment for early open-angle glaucoma is eye drops and the GP has prescribed prostaglandin eye drops to help the flow of aqueous humour from the eye and thus reduce the pressure. At present, glaucoma cannot be cured and the treatment is dependent on early recognition to avoid permanent damage. To use eye drops, the patient should be advised to carry out the following steps.

1. Wash their hands.
2. Ensure the eye drops are in date.
3. Put their head back.
4. Use their finger to pull down the lower eyelid.
5. Hold the bottle and allow a single drop to fall into the pocket made by pulling down the eyelid.
6. Close the eye and keep it closed for a few minutes.

Light rays enter the eye anteriorly via the transparent cornea, passing through the pupil and lens. The major optically refractive elements are the cornea and the lens. In a well-focused (emmetropic) eye, the optics form an image on the retina (figure 15.14). Although all parts of the eye are important for vision, the retina plays the critical role of absorbing visible light and converting it to neural signals which are propagated via the optic nerve to the higher-order processing centres in the brain.

15.7 Organisation of the retina

LEARNING OBJECTIVE 15.7 Describe the retina, and differences between rods and cones in the eye.

The retina, which is 250 μm thick, is the highly organised layer of the central nervous tissue. It is located at the back (posteriorly) of the eye, and forms the interior wall of the posterior part of the eyeball together with the choroid (figure 15.14). Figure 15.15 shows the two types of receptor cells contained within the outermost layer of the retina (closest to the retinal pigment epithelium part). These receptor cells are the cells that detect light (photoreceptors).

The photoreceptors are highly specialised neuronal cells that maintain high turnover of their components. In particular, a specialisation of each elongated outer segment photoreceptor plasma membrane is the ability to form a modified sensory cilium. The cilium then folds into thousands of flattened layers, called discs or folds (figure 15.15). In the rods the discs are separate and form the shape of a cylinder. In cones the discs are in fact folds of the plasma membrane and the outer segment tapers to a blunt point. The proteins in the photoreceptor discs or folds are able to capture light efficiently and convert the absorbed light into chemical and then electrical signals (a process called **phototransduction**), which are then sent to be processed by the visual centres of the brain.

- *Rods*. These photoreceptors do not discriminate between colours. They are very sensitive and enable us to see in very low or dim light levels. Rods are mostly concentrated in a band around the periphery of the retina and this density reduces towards the centre of the eye (**fovea**). There are about 92 million rods in the human retina. The rod photoreceptor protein is called **rhodopsin**.
- *Cones*. These photoreceptors provide colour vision and give sharper, clearer images than the rods do, but they require more intense light. Cones are mostly situated in the macula lutea and particularly at its centre in an area called the fovea (figure 15.14). The macula is the thinnest part of the retina caused by the radial migration of inner layers of retina away from central point during early development, where only the photoreceptors (mainly cones) are present. It then forms a small depression or pit in the retina to form the fovea (figure 15.14). In the mature human eye, the fovea is about 1.5 mm diameter, occupying the centre of the 5 mm wide macula lutea. The fovea contains the highest density of cone photoreceptor cells, necessary for colour acuity. As you move away from the fovea at either sides, the number of cone

photoreceptors falls with distance, while the number of rod photoreceptors increases. The human retina is made up of 4.5 million cones. The cone photoreceptor protein is called **opsin**.

FIGURE 15.15 Cross-section of the retina

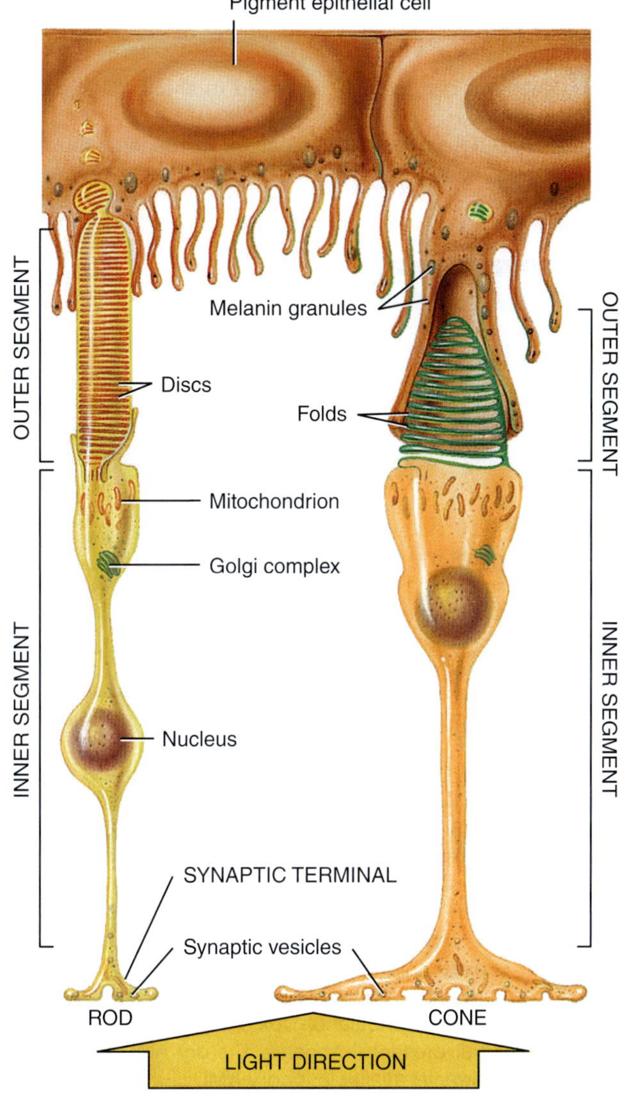

Source: Tortora and Derrickson (2009). Reproduced with permission of John Wiley & Sons.

HOMEOSTATIC IMBALANCE

Age-related macular degeneration

Age-related macular degeneration (AMD) is a disease that develops in middle to older age. It usually first affects people in their 50s and 60s. AMD is the most common cause of irreversible blindness among the global elderly (> 50 years) population. In Australia, late-stage AMD affects approximately 1 per cent (244 000) of non-Indigenous Australians and 0.2 per cent of Indigenous Australians (Keel et al. 2017b).

AMD is divided into two types.

- Dry AMD (or early AMD) is the slow degeneration of the cells in the retina; as the cells die they are not replaced, leading to a loss in visual acuity. It is a disease that is slow in progression (often months to years). There is no treatment for dry AMD.

- Wet AMD is a disease where new blood vessels grow in the retina and leak blood which leads to scarring. The protein vascular endothelial growth factor (VEGF) is mainly responsible for the leaky and abnormal growth of new blood vessels. Wet AMD is much quicker in onset but is treatable, so early diagnosis and referral is essential. Currently treatment involves either injections of anti-VEGF drugs into the eye to block the actions of VEGF protein or laser treatment for those patients who do not respond to the injections. Despite the eye injections sounding unpleasant they are hardly noticed by the patient as the eye is anaesthetised and the injection is into the corner of the eye so the patient does not see the needle.

The causes of AMD are unknown but seem to be linked to smoking, being overweight, high blood pressure and a family history of AMD.

It is important to note that AMD does not mean the patient will become totally blind as the peripheral vision is not affected.

CLINICALLY REASONED EPISODE OF CARE

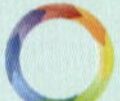

Macular degeneration

Consider the patient situation

Daphne is a 70-year-old lady who is reporting difficulty with her vision. She presents to the clinic for assessment and help.

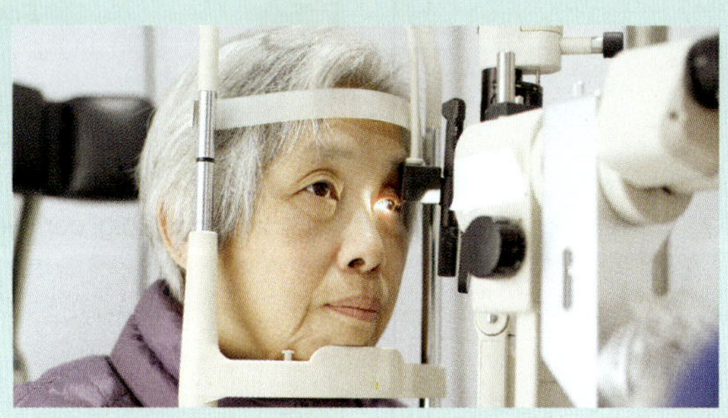

Collect cues and information

Vision assessment: Daphne states that her sense of colour is getting worse; she is finding it difficult to read and when she looks at straight lines, they look 'crooked'. When asked to view things out of the side of her eye, she states that these problems go away and they seem to only affect the centre of her vision.

Process information

Age-related macular degeneration (AMD) is the most common cause of sight loss, affecting approximately 1 in 7 Australians (1.29 million) over the age of 50 (Macular Disease Foundation Australia n.d.).

The macula lutea contains a very high concentration of photoreceptors and is crucial for detailed vision. Pathological changes result in the death of these photoreceptor cells.

The symptoms of AMD are blurred or 'fuzzy' vision; straight lines, such as sentences on a page, appearing wavy or distorted; blurry areas on a printed page; difficulty reading or seeing details in low light levels; and extra sensitivity to glare.

AMD is divided into two types: dry AMD and wet AMD. There is no treatment for dry AMD, and it can progress to wet AMD (see the homeostatic imbalance box on age-related macular degeneration).

Daphne is developing AMD, and at present it appears it is dry AMD. Beyond the recommendations given below there is no treatment currently available for dry AMD.

Nursing action

1. Provide support and education to Daphne, including referral to support networks. Education will include information on inhibiting progress of the disease by:
   - protecting the eyes from the sun by using good quality sunglasses
   - stopping smoking
   - having regular eye examinations (this especially helps if dry AMD develops into wet AMD)
   - eating a healthy diet rich in antioxidants, omega 3 and lutein (found in eggs and some fruits and vegetables) as there is some evidence that this may help prevent AMD and inhibit its progression
   - reassuring Daphne that AMD does not mean she will become totally blind as the peripheral vision is not affected.

   Rationale:
   - A person who is well informed about their condition is more likely to be concordant with suggested interventions, therapies and lifestyle changes, which may slow progress of a disease and thus improve health and life outcomes.

Evaluate outcomes
Daphne reports that she has been able to adopt the recommendations, which may inhibit progress of the disease. She reports that she is not overly anxious about living with dry AMD.
Source: Based on the Clinical Reasoning Cycle, Levett-Jones (2013).

There are three types of cones: blue, green and red, also known as short (S), medium (M) and long (L) wavelength cones respectively. They all have different types of cone opsins. Colour discrimination is based on the integration of information received from the three types of cones. For instance, yellow is shown by highly stimulated green cones, less strongly stimulated red cones and a relative lack of stimulation of the blue cones. Red-green colour blindness most commonly affects males. Since colour blindness is based on the X-linked inheritance, the inherited X-linked recessive allele expresses itself more readily in males, as described in the chapter on genetics.

A narrow connecting stalk links the outer segment to the inner segment, which is the part of the cell that contains all the usual cellular organelles. The inner segment is also the area where synapses with other cells are made and neurotransmitters are released.

The rods and cones synapse with neurones called bipolar cells, which in turn synapse within a layer of neurones called **ganglion** cells. At both these synapse areas there are associated cells that can stimulate or inhibit the communication between the two cells and therefore alter the sensitivity of the retina (e.g. in response to very bright, or dim, light levels).

Axons from approximately 1 million ganglion cells converge on the optic disc, at which point they turn and penetrate the wall of the eye and proceed to the diencephalon of the brain at the optic nerve. The central retinal artery and vein pass through the centre of the optic nerve. The optic disc contains no photoreceptors and thus this area is known as the blind spot (figure 15.14); however, we do not notice the blind spot in our vision as involuntary eye movements keep the visual image moving and the brain can thus supply the missing information.

15.8 Focusing images onto the retina

LEARNING OBJECTIVE 15.8 Explain how a visual image is focused on the retina.

In order for a visual image to be useful, it must be focused onto the retina; this is the purpose of the lens of the eye. First, the light entering the eye is subject to **refraction** and the lens provides the additional, adjustable refraction required to focus the image onto the retina.

Refraction

Light is refracted (bent) when it passes from one medium to another medium with a different density (figure 15.16).

FIGURE 15.16 Refraction of light passing from air (less dense) to water (dense)

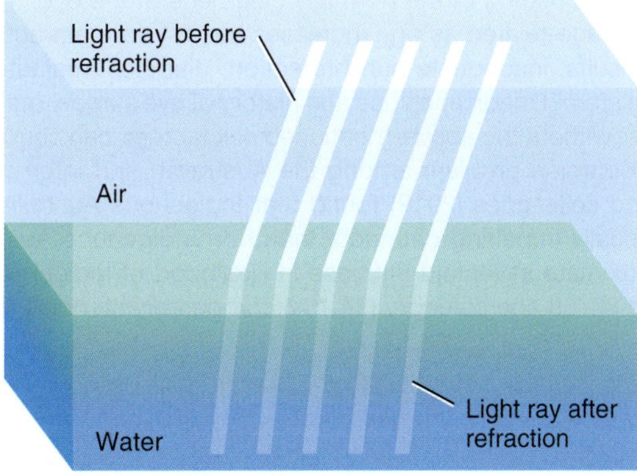

Refraction of light rays

Source: Tortora and Derrickson (2009). Reproduced with permission of John Wiley & Sons.

The majority of the refraction in the eye happens when light enters the cornea (80%) from the air; additional refraction occurs when light passes from the aqueous humour into the lens (20%). The lens provides the extra refraction to focus the light onto the retina and can adjust this refraction according to the **focal length**.

Focal length is the distance between the focal point (e.g. on the retina) and the centre of the lens (figure 15.17). It is dependent on:

- the distance from the object to the lens — the further away an object is, the shorter the focal length
- the shape of the lens — the rounder the lens, the more refraction occurs. A very round lens has a shorter focal length than a flatter lens.

FIGURE 15.17 Focal length

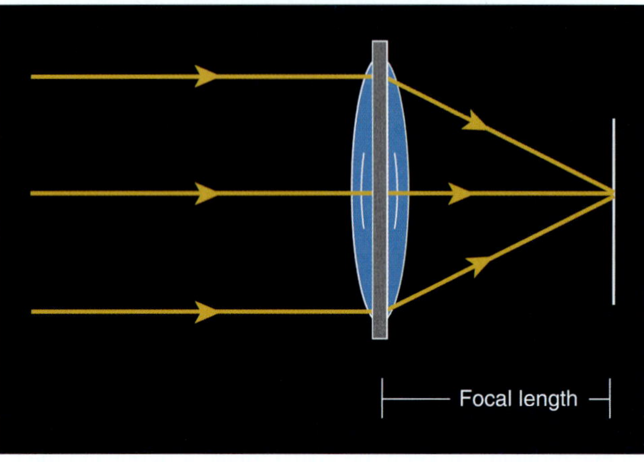

The lens lies behind the cornea and is held in place by ligaments that are attached to the ciliary body. The lens is made up of concentric layers of cells that are precisely organised and are covered by a fibrous capsule. Many of the capsule fibres are elastic and if it were not subject to external forces by the ligaments the lens would be spherical. Within the lens are lens fibres, specialised cells that have lost their nucleus and other organelles. They are filled with a protein called crystallin, which is responsible for the transparency and the focusing power of the lens.

HOMEOSTATIC IMBALANCE

Cataracts

The healthy adult lens in the eye is a biconvex and optically transparent intraocular structure that consists of a lens capsule, partial single-layered epithelium and lens fibres making up the cortex and nucleus (figure 15.18).

A cataract is the abnormal clouding of the normally clear lens of the eye. It mainly affects the elderly population, and is therefore age-related as age increases the risk for cataracts. Certain eye conditions, family history, traumatic insults, inadequate sun protection, diabetes, malnutrition and low antioxidant intake, smoking, long-term steroid medication use and history of eye surgery may increase the likelihood of developing a cataract. Age, without the above-mentioned risk factors, can cause the lens to lose flexibility and transparency. It is a common problem among the Australian and international populations. In the 50–59 age group, Keel and colleagues (2019) found that Indigenous Australians (3.2%) were threefold more likely to develop visually impairing cataracts than non-Indigenous Australians (0.9%). Strikingly, this increased to an approximate sevenfold increase in likelihood of Indigenous Australians developing significant cataracts in the 80–99 age category (34.1%) compared with non-Indigenous Australians (5%) (Keel et al. 2019).

FIGURE 15.18 The structure of the human lens

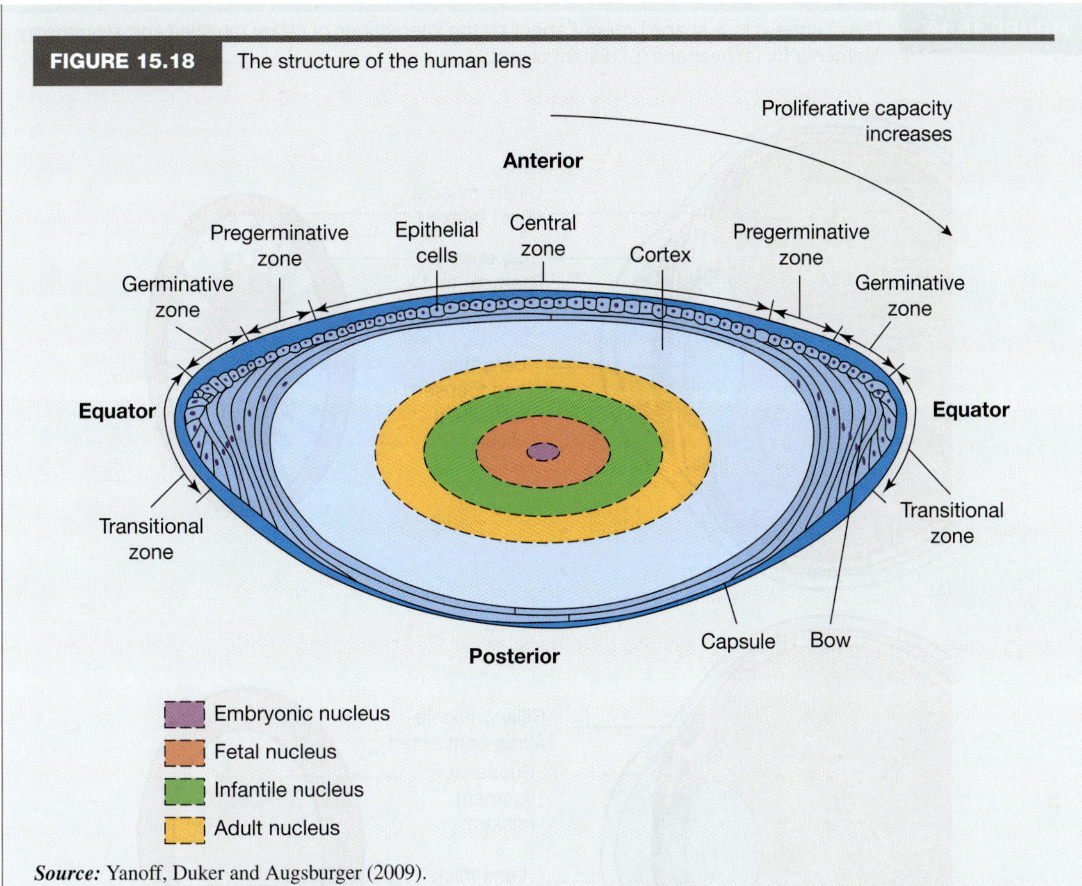

Source: Yanoff, Duker and Augsburger (2009).

The cataract process can occur in one or more areas of the lens and clinically be classified according to the anatomical location. For example, the lens capsule may undergo thinning or thickening, form plaques, rupture or wrinkle. The proteins in the lens fibres can start to denature and break down, eventually coagulating to form opaque areas in place of the normal transparent protein fibres. Sometimes, the nucleus fibres may start to yellow and harden. Cataracts usually develop in both eyes, but not uniformly. Lens with cataracts can significantly obscure light transmission towards the retina and seriously impair vision.

Symptoms, not entirely exclusive to cataracts, include:

- cloudy, blurred or dim vision
- increased light illumination needed for reading or other activities
- night vision difficulty
- being light sensitive and having a glare from bright lights
- presence of halos around light sources
- double vision
- colour fading or seeing objects with a yellowish or brownish tint
- increasing near-sightedness
- loss of contrast sensitivity.

Cataracts can be treated or corrected by laser and/or surgically replacing the entire lens, except for the lens capsule, with an artificial intraocular lens to retain the required refractive power for normal vision. The operation is a simple, quick and effective procedure that can restore vision. Although very rare, congenital cataracts may occur due to sporadic or familial causes (Ma et al. 2016). However, the pathological location within the lens differs in age-related cataracts versus congenital cataracts.

The process of changing the shape of the lens to focus an image onto the retina is known as accommodation. The shape of the lens is altered by tension being applied to or relaxed on the suspensory ligaments by smooth muscles within the ciliary body (figure 15.19). When the ciliary muscles relax, tension on the suspensory ligaments causes the lens to remain relatively flat for distance vision. Consequently, the contraction of either set of smooth muscles in the ciliary body relaxes the suspensory ligaments to the lens, which then assumes a more spherical shape required for near vision (figure 15.19).

FIGURE 15.19 The change in lens shape brought about by the interactions of ciliary muscles and suspensory ligaments for (a) near and (b) distant objects

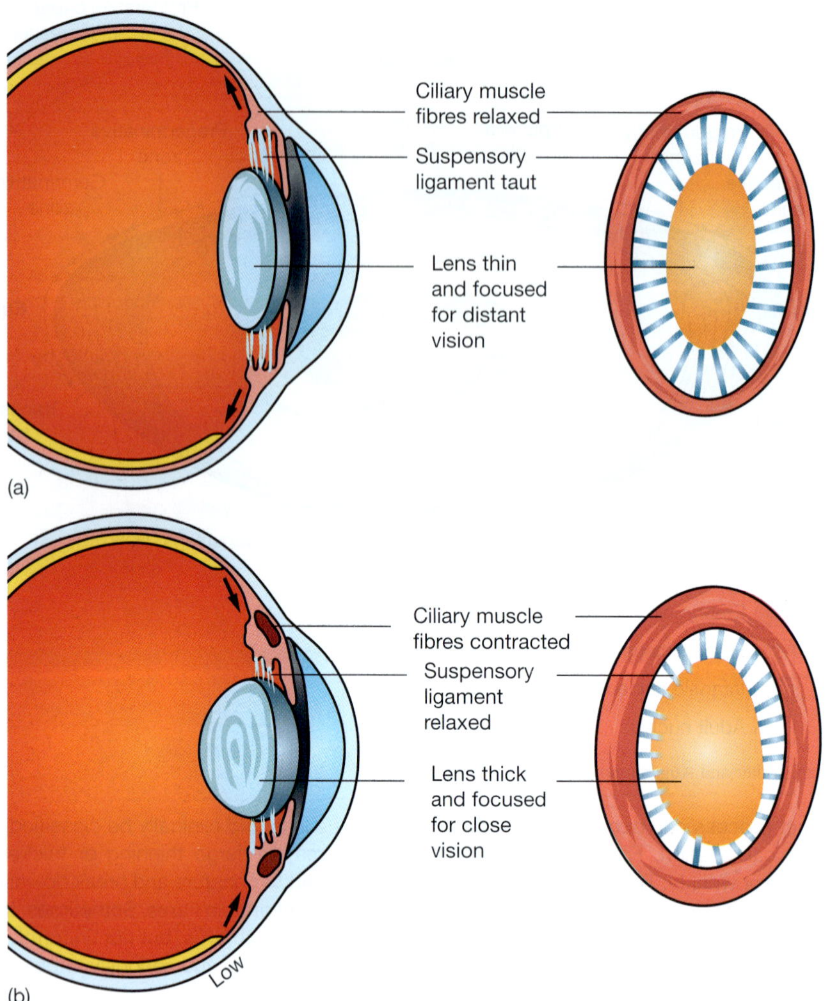

Source: 78 Steps Health (2020).

Myopia, hyperopia and presbyopia

In a person who has **myopia** (short-sightedness) the lens is unable to focus the image onto the retina and the focus of the image falls short (figure 15.20). With myopia, people can see objects close to them but those that are far away are blurred. Myopia is easily corrected for by the use of corrective lenses, either in the form of glasses or contact lenses.

FIGURE 15.20 (a) Myopic eye uncorrected, and (b) corrected by a concave lens

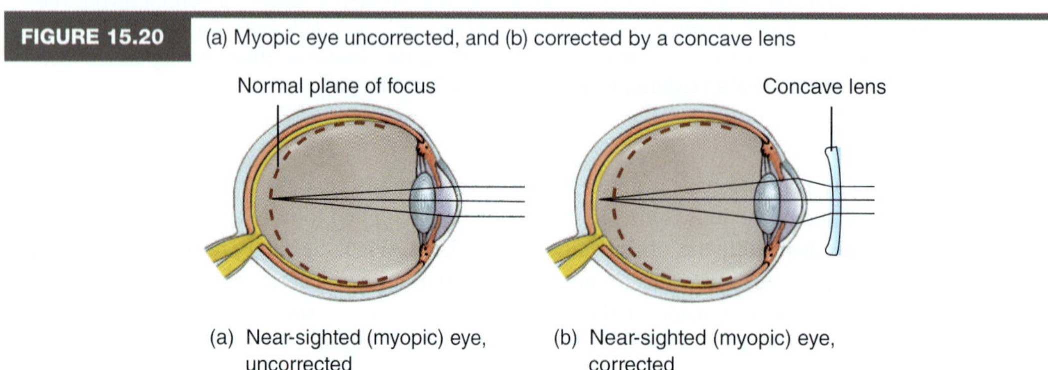

Source: Tortora and Derrickson (2009). Reproduced with permission of John Wiley & Sons.

In the person with **hyperopia** (long-sightedness) the image is focused onto a point behind the retina (figure 15.21); therefore, these people can see things at a distance but not near to them.

FIGURE 15.21 (a) Hyperopic eye uncorrected, and (b) corrected by a convex lens

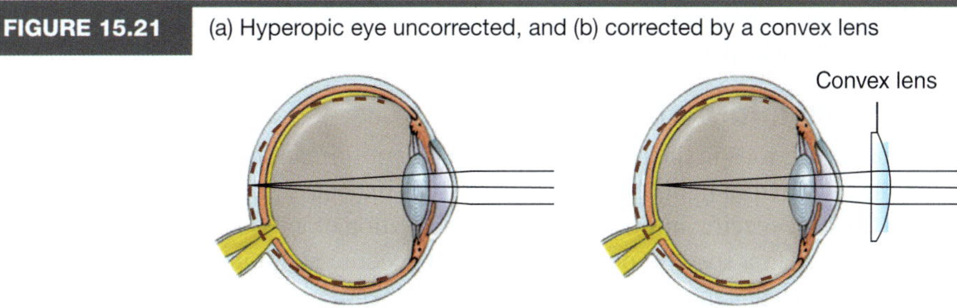

(a) Long-sighted (hyperopic) eye, uncorrected

(b) Long-sighted (hyperopic) eye, corrected

Source: Tortora and Derrickson (2009). Reproduced with permission of John Wiley & Sons.

CLINICAL CONSIDERATIONS

20/20 vision

The term '20/20 vision' refers to a measure of visual acuity. The meaning is that the person being tested can see the same detail from 20 feet away as a person with normal eyesight would see from 20 feet. In other words, 20/20 vision is normal vision. If a person has 20/40 vision they are only able to see detail at 20 feet that a person with normal vision can see at 40 feet. A person with a visual acuity of 20/70 can only see detail at 20 feet that a person with normal sight could see at 70 feet and so on. The visual acuity is not a direct correlation with the prescription for eyeglasses, but the prescribed glasses are intended to achieve 20/20 vision. Visual acuity is tested using a standard size **Snellen chart** at 20 feet and lit to a standard brightness (figure 15.22).

FIGURE 15.22 Snellen chart

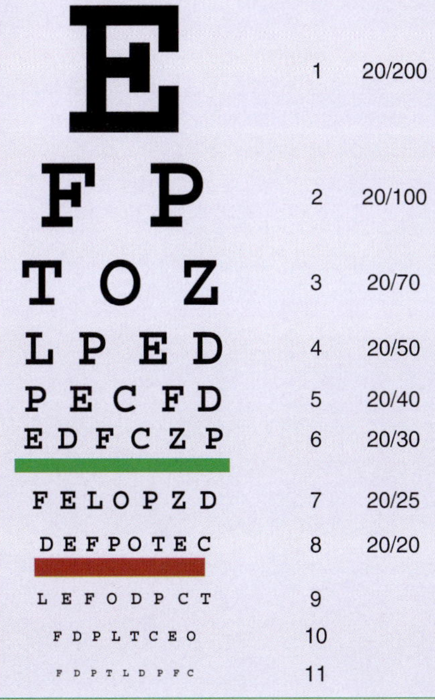

Presbyopia is the loss of the ability to focus on close objects as the person ages; the most common theory for this is the loss of elasticity in the lens. The loss of the ability to focus on near objects occurs in everyone, but at different rates and with different effects on vision. The onset of presbyopia is most commonly noticed at 40–50 years of age. Presbyopia is treatable with corrective glasses (usually known as reading glasses, though they are corrective for all tasks that require near vision).

The processing of visual information

The ganglion cells that monitor the rods in the retina (M cells) supply information about the general form of an object, motion and shadows in dim light. As many as 1000 rods may pass information to one M cell. This convergence leads to a loss of specific information and the activation of an M cell indicates that light has struck a general area rather than a specific point. This loss of specific location-based information is partially compensated for by the fact that the M cells' activity varies depending on the pattern of stimulation in their specific field (area of retina). So, for instance, an M cell would react differently to a stimulus at the edge of its receptive field than from one at its centre.

Cone cells show very little convergence; for instance, in the fovea the ratio of cones to ganglion is 1:1 (Martini & Nath 2009). The ganglion cells that monitor cones (P cells) are more numerous than M cells and because there is little convergence these cells provide location-specific information. As a result of this, cones supply more precise information about a visual image than do rods.

Central processing of visual information

Once axons from the ganglion cells have exited the eye through the optic disc they proceed to the diencephalon as the optic nerves (cranial nerve II). The two optic nerves (one for each eye) reach the diencephalon at the optic chiasm. From there, half the nerves go to the lateral geniculate nucleus on the same side of the brain and the other half cross over and proceed to the lateral geniculate nucleus on the opposite side. From each lateral geniculate nucleus, visual information also travels to the occipital cortex of the cerebral hemisphere on the same side. Involuntary eye control (such as pupillary reflexes) is processed in the diencephalon and the brainstem.

SUMMARY

In this chapter there has been a review of the senses:

- olfaction (smell), which is based in the olfactory receptors of the nose
- gustation (taste), which is partially based in the gustatory receptors on the tongue, but also has a large input from the olfactory receptors
- equilibrium, which is a part of the sense of balance and is based in the hair cells of the semicircular canals and the vestibule
- hearing, which is based in the hair cells in the organ of Corti in the cochlea of the inner ear
- sight, which is based in the photoreceptors of the eye.

With the exception of smell, all the information generated by the senses is processed in the thalamus before being transmitted on to the higher brain centres. Some of the senses (smell and taste) also have direct input into other centres of the limbic system, such as the hypothalamus, and this is an indication of both how ancient they are in evolutionary terms and the fact that certain smells and tastes can evoke subconscious responses, such as salivation and emotions.

KEY TERMS

afferent Heading towards a centre (e.g. the brain).
ampulla A sac-like enlargement of a canal or duct.
anterior Located at, or related to, the front of a structure.
antibodies Proteins in the blood that are used by the immune system to identify and destroy pathogens.
auditory reflex The auditory involuntary reflex system helps to reduce the intensity of lower-frequency sound transmission to protect the cochlea within the inner ear, and to mask sounds in a loud environment.
autonomic nervous system The part of the nervous system that controls involuntary functions, made up of the parasympathetic and sympathetic nervous systems.
axons Extension of a nerve cell that conducts impulses.
balance The ability to control equilibrium.
cartilage A supporting connective tissue made up of various cells and fibres.
cilia Small, hair-like processes on the outer surface of some cells.
connective tissue Tissue that supports and binds other body tissue.
convergence The movement of the eyes inwards to see an object close to the face.
efferent Heading away from a centre.
endolymph The fluid in the membranous labyrinth of the inner ear.
enzymes Proteins that increase the rate of a chemical reaction.
equilibrium Stability at rest or when moving.
ethmoid bone A bone in the skull that separates the nasal cavity from the brain.
extrinsic Not inherent to the process or object, external.
focal length The distance between the focal point (e.g. on the retina) and the centre of the lens of the eye.
fovea (fovea centralis) A small depression in the retina containing cones and where vision is the most acute.
ganglion A mass, or group, of nerve cells.
glomeruli (glomerulus — singular) In the olfactory pathway, a structure containing a mass of synapses.
gustatory Relating to the sense of taste.
hyperopia Long-sightedness.
iris The central, coloured portion of the eye.
lacrimal Relating to tears.
lateral Away from the midline of the body (to the left or right).
ligaments Fibrous tissue that binds joints together and connects bones and cartilage.
limbic system A group of structures/centres in the brain associated with various emotions and feelings, such as anger, fear, sadness and pleasure.
lipid A group of organic compounds, including the fats, oils, waxes, sterols and triglycerides.
medial Towards the midline of the body.
medulla oblongata A part of the brainstem that contains the cardiac and respiratory centres.
microvilli (microvillus – singular) Protrusions of the cell membrane that increase its surface area.

myopia Short-sightedness.
nasopharynx The part of the airway that begins in the nose and ends at the soft palate.
neurone Nerve cell.
olfaction The sense of smell.
olfactory Pertaining to the sense of smell.
olfactory bulb A structure of the brain involved in olfaction, the perception of odours.
opsin The proteins found in cone photoreceptor cells that are capable in converting absorbed light into chemical signals for phototransduction to start.
papillae (papilla — singular) Small, nipple-shaped projection.
parasympathetic nervous system Part of the autonomic nervous system.
pathogens Infectious agents that cause disease (e.g. bacteria or virus).
perilymph The clear fluid found between the bony labyrinth and the membranous labyrinth in the inner ear.
photoreceptors Light-sensing neurones.
phototransduction Process by which the absorbed light by photoreceptor rod or cone cells are converted to chemical and then electrical signals to be transmitted to the brain.
pons Part of the brainstem, the pons contains centres that deal with sleep, swallowing, hearing, equilibrium, taste, eye movement and many other functions.
posterior Located at, or related to, the rear of a structure.
presbyopia The loss of the ability to focus on close objects as the person ages.
pupil The opening in the centre of the iris of the eye that allows light to enter.
pupillary constrictor muscles Smooth muscles contained within the iris of the eye; when stimulated they lead to the constriction of the pupil.
pupillary dilator muscles Smooth muscles contained within the iris of the eye; when stimulated they lead to the dilation of the pupil.
reflexes Involuntary function or movement in response to a stimulus.
refraction The change of direction of light as it passes from one medium to another with a different density.
rhodopsin The proteins found in rod photoreceptor cells that are capable in converting absorbed light into chemical signals for phototransduction to occur.
Snellen chart Standardised chart for testing visual acuity.
sympathetic nervous system Part of the autonomic nervous system.
synapse A gap between two neurones or a neurone and an organ across which neurotransmitters diffuse to transmit a nerve impulse.
synovial joints A freely moving joint in which bony surfaces are covered with cartilage and connected by ligaments lined with a synovial membrane. The membrane secretes a lubricating fluid and keeps it around the joint.
thalamus A pair of structures in the brain that relay messages from most of the senses.
transparent Clear, can see through it.
umami The 'fifth taste', related to proteins found in meat and fish.
visual acuity Detailed central vision.

CONDITIONS

The following is a list of conditions that are associated with the senses. Take some time and write notes about each of the conditions. You may make the notes taken from textbooks or other resources (e.g. people you work with in a clinical area), or you may make the notes as a result of people you have cared for. If you are making notes about people you have cared for, you must ensure that you adhere to the rules of confidentiality.

Anosmia
Ageusia

Ménière's disease

Trauma and orbital cellulitis

Glaucoma

Uveitis

Retinopathy and retinitis pigmentosa

REFERENCES

78 Steps Health (2020) Accommodation. www.78stepshealth.us/human-physiology/accommodation.html (accessed May 2021).

Buitrago-Garcia, D., Egli-Gany, D., Counotte, M.J., Hossmann, S., Imeri, H., Ipekci, A.M., Salanti, G. and Low, N. (2020) Occurrence and transmission potential of asymptomatic and presymptomatic SARS-CoV-2 infections: a living systematic review and meta-analysis. *PLoS Medicine* 17(9): eCollection.doi: 10.1371/journal.pmed.1003346.

Dommaraju, S. and Perera, E. (2016) An approach to vertigo in general practice. *Australian Family Physician* 45(4): 190–194.

Emergency Care Institute (2021) Vertigo. https://aci.health.nsw.gov.au/networks/eci/clinical/clinical-resources/clinical-tools/neurology/vertigo (accessed March 2021).

Feng, P., Huang, L. and Wang, H. (2014) Taste bud homeostasis in health, disease and aging. *Chemical Senses* 39(1): 3–16.

Haehner, A., Tosch, C., Wolz, M., Klingelhoefer, L., Fauser, M., Storch, A., Reichman, H. and Hummel, T. (2013) Olfactory training in patients with Parkinson's disease. *PLoS ONE* 8(4): e61680.

Happy Ears Hearing Center (2020) Understanding the difference between BAHA and cochlear implants. https://aci.health.nsw.gov.au/networks/eci/clinical/clinical-resources/clinical-tools/neurology/vertigo (accessed March 2021).

Jenkins, G.W. and Tortora, G.J. (2013) *Anatomy and Physiology: From Science to Life*, 3rd edn. Hoboken, NJ: John Wiley & Sons. Inc.

Keel, S., McGuiness, M.B., Foreman, J. et al. (2019) The prevalence of visually significant cataract in the Australian National Eye Health Survey. *Eye* 33, 957–964. https://doi.org/10.1038/s41433-019-0354-x

Keel, S., Xie, X., Foreman, J., Lee, P.Y., Alwan, M., Fahy, E.T., van Wijngaarden, P., Gaskin, J.C.F., Ang, G.S., Crowston, J.G., Taylor, H.R. and Dirani, M. (2017a) Prevalence of glaucoma in the Australian National Eye Health Survey. *British Journal of Ophthalmology* 103: 191–195.

Keel, S., Xie, X., Foreman, J., van Wijngaarden, P., FRANZCO, Taylor, H.R. and Dirani, M. (2017b) Prevalence of age-related macular degeneration in Australia. *JAMA Ophthalmology* 135(11): 1242–1249.

Lechein, J.R., Chiesa-Estomba, C.M., Beckers, E., Mustin, V., Ducarme, M., Journe, F., Marchant, A., Jouffe, L., Barillari, M.R., Cammaroto, G., Circiu, M.P., Hans, S. and Saussez, S. (2021) Prevalence and 6-month recovery of olfactory dysfunction: a multicentre study of 1363 COVID-19 patients. *Journal of Internal Medicine*. https://doi.org/10.1111/joim.13209

Levett-Jones, T. (2013). *Clinical Reasoning: Learning to Think Like a Nurse.* Pearson Australia.

Li, J., Wang, X., Zhu, C., Lin, Z. and Xiong, N. (2020) Affected olfaction in COVID-19: re-defining 'asymptomatic'. *EClinicalMedicine* 100628: 29–30.

Ma, A.S., Grigg, J.R., Ho, G., Prokudin, I., Farnsworth, E., Holman, K., Cheng, A., Billson, F.A., Martin, F., Fraser, C., Mowat, D., Smith, J., Christodoulou, J., Flaherty, M., Bennetts, B. and Jamieson, R.V. (2016) Sporadic and familial congenital cataracts: mutational spectrum and new diagnoses using next-generation sequencing. *Human Mutation* 37(4): 371–384.

Macular Disease Foundation Australia (n.d.) Macular degeneration. www.mdfoundation.com.au/content/macular-degeneration-about (accessed 7 February 2021).

Martini, F.H. and Nath, J.L. (2009) *Fundamentals of Anatomy and Physiology*, 8th edn. San Francisco, CA: Pearson Benjamin Cummings.

Melbourne ENT Group (n.d.) Patient information on anosmia. https://melbentgroup.com.au/patient-information-on-anosmia (accessed 28 January 2021).

Meng, X., Deng, Y., Dai, Z. and Meng, Z. (2020) COVID-19 and anosmia: a review based on up-to-date knowledge. *American Journal of Otolaryngol* 41(5): 102581.

National Health Service (NHS) (2015) Lost or changed sense of smell. www.nhs.uk/conditions/lost-or-changed-sense-smell (accessed 7 August 2019).

National Institute for Health and Clinical Excellence (NICE) (2015) NG91 Otitis media (acute): antimicrobial prescribing. www.nice.org.uk/guidance/NG91 (accessed 7 August 2019).

Neuland, C., Bitter, T., Marschner, H., Gudziol, H. and Guntinas-Lichius, O. (2011) Health-related and specific olfaction-related quality of life in patients with chronic functional anosmia or severe hyposmia. *The Laryngoscope* 121(4): 867–872.

NSW Department of Health (2009) Eye emergency manual. www.aci.health.nsw.gov.au/__data/assets/pdf_file/0013/155011/eye_manual.pdf (accessed February 2021).

Osawa, Y. (2012) Glutamate perception, soup stock and the concept of umami: the ethnography, food ecology and history of dashi in Japan. *Ecology of Food and Nutrition* 51(4): 329–345.

Perth Children's Hospital (2021) Otitis externa. https://pch.health.wa.gov.au/For-health-professionals/Emergency-Department-Guidelines/Otitis-externa (accessed March 2021).

Tortora, G.J. and Derrickson, B.H. (2009) *Principles of Anatomy and Physiology*, 12th edn. Hoboken, NJ: John Wiley & Sons, Inc.

Tortora, G.J. and Derrickson, B.H. (2012) *Principles of Anatomy and Physiology*, 13th edn. Hoboken, NJ: John Wiley & Sons, Inc.

Yanoff, M., Duker J. S and Augsburger J. J (2009) *Opthalmology*, 3rd edn. Edinburgh: Mosby Elsevier.

FURTHER READING

Kikut-Ligaj, D. and Trzcielinska-Lorych, J. (2015) How taste works: cells, receptors and gustatory perception. *Cell Molecular Biology Letters* 20(5): 699–716.

ENT UK

https://entuk.org

The website of the British Association of Otorhinolaryngologists and the British Academic Conference in Otolaryngology. This group states its aims as including promoting care, professional education and information for the public. The site has useful information on a variety of conditions of the ear and the nose.

EXTERNAL EAR INFECTION HEALTH FACT SHEETS

www.betterhealth.vic.gov.au/health/ConditionsAndTreatments/swimmers-ear

www.health.qld.gov.au/__data/assets/pdf_file/0024/621267/ed-otitis_externa.pdf

Information on ear infections signs and symptoms, home care treatment options or remedies, and recommended preventative measures according to Australian state health departments.

ROYAL INSTITUTE FOR DEAF AND BLIND CHILDREN

https://ridbc.org.au

The Australian Royal Institute for Deaf and Blind Children provides specialist services towards detection, care and support for childhood vision and hearing developmental impairments. The website contains useful information for children and adults on current technologies and options.

EYESMART

www.geteyesmart.org/eyesmart/index.cfm

This is a website created and maintained by the American Association of Ophthalmology (eye doctors). It contains useful sections on eye conditions, symptoms and lifestyle advice related to eye health.

NATIONAL INSTITUTE ON DEAFNESS AND OTHER COMMUNICATION DISORDERS

www.nidcd.nih.gov/health/Pages/Default.aspx

A useful website maintained by the United States National Institutes of Health detailing various disorders of the ear and mouth, including taste disorders, balance disorders and disorders of the ear.

ROYAL NATIONAL INSTITUTE OF BLIND PEOPLE (RNIB)

www.rnib.org.uk

The RNIB is a UK-based charity offering information, support and advice to people experiencing sight loss. The website is a useful source of information, including sections on eye conditions, tests and coping with sight loss.

ACKNOWLEDGEMENTS

Photo: © Chinnapong / Shutterstock.com
Photo: © megaflopp / Shutterstock.com
Photo: © Monkey Business Images / Shutterstock.com
Photo: © goodluz / Shutterstock.com
Photo: © leungchopan / Shutterstock.com
Figure 15.19: © 78 Steps Health

The endocrine system

TEST YOUR PRIOR KNOWLEDGE

- How are hormones transported in the body?
- What is meant by the 'half-life' of a hormone?
- Name one hormone released by the pituitary gland.
- Where in the body is the thyroid gland found?
- What stimulates the release of insulin?

LEARNING OUTCOMES

After reading this chapter you will be able to:

16.1 name the endocrine glands in the body and the hormones they secrete

16.2 discuss the different forms of stimulus for the release of hormones and how those hormones have their effects

16.3 explain the control of hormone release by the hypothalamus

16.4 explain the role of insulin and glucagon in the control of blood glucose levels.

Body map

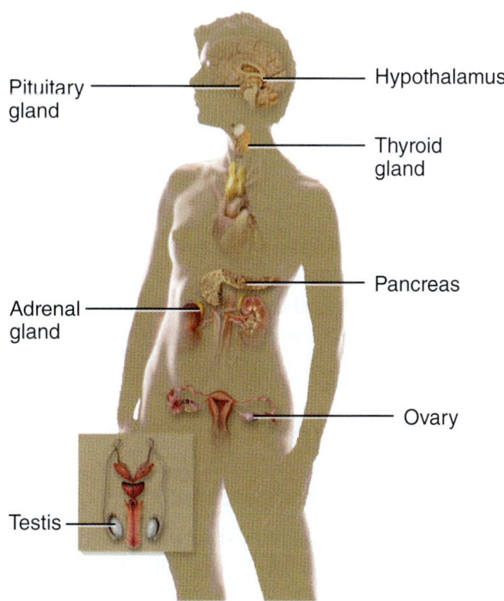

Introduction

Homeostasis (from the Greek *homoios*, 'similar'; and *histemi*, 'standing still') refers to the process of maintaining a stable internal environment. In other words, homeostasis refers to the maintenance of normal physiological balance and functioning within the body. There are two major systems in the body for maintaining homeostasis: the nervous system and the endocrine system. Table 16.1 shows the differences between these two systems.

TABLE 16.1 **Nervous system versus endocrine system**

	Nervous system	Endocrine system
Speed of action	Seconds	Minutes to hours (even days)
Duration of action	Seconds to minutes	Minutes to days
Method of transmitting messages	Electrical	Chemical
Transport method	Neurones	**Hormones**

The nervous system reacts rapidly to stimuli and affects its changes over a period of seconds or minutes; thus, it is involved in the immediate and short-term maintenance of homeostasis. Owing to its rapid onset of action, the nervous system is responsible for the control of rapid bodily processes such as breathing and movement. The endocrine system is often responsible for the regulation of longer-term processes. The major functions it coordinates are:

- homeostasis — maintains the internal body environment
- storage and utilisation of energy **substrates** (**carbohydrates**, proteins and fats)
- regulation of growth and reproduction
- control of the body's responses to external stimuli (particularly stress).

It should be noted, however, that though these two systems are separate, they often act together and complement each other in the maintenance of homeostasis.

The endocrine system is made up of a collection of small organs that are scattered throughout the body, each of which releases hormones into the blood supply ('endo' = within, 'crine' = to secrete). These hormone-releasing organs can be split into three main categories (Jenkins & Tortora 2013).

- Endocrine **glands** — organs whose only function is the production and release of hormones. These include:
  - pituitary gland
  - thyroid gland
  - parathyroid gland
  - adrenal gland
- Organs that are not pure glands (as they have other functions as well as the production of hormones) but contain relatively large areas of hormone-producing tissue. These include:
  - hypothalamus
  - pancreas
- Other tissues and organs that also produce hormones — areas of hormone-producing cells are found in the wall of the small intestine and the stomach.

There are no cell types, organs or processes that are not influenced by the endocrine system in some way, and while there are many hormones that we know of, there are probably many more that are yet to be discovered.

16.1 The endocrine organs

LEARNING OBJECTIVE 16.1 Name the endocrine glands in the body and the hormones they secrete.

Figure 16.1 shows the endocrine organs and their position within the body. Each of these organs will typically have a rich blood supply delivered by numerous blood vessels. The hormone-producing cells within the organ are arranged into branching networks around this supply. This arrangement of blood vessels and hormone-producing cells ensures that hormones enter the bloodstream rapidly and are then transported throughout the body to the target cells (see figure 16.2).

FIGURE 16.1 Location of the endocrine organs

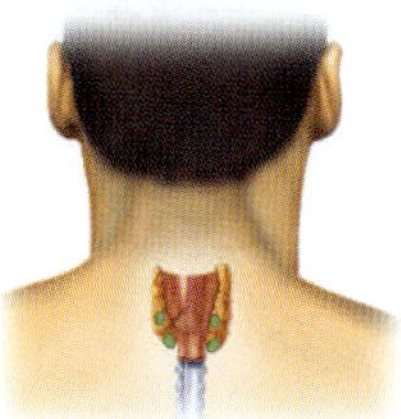

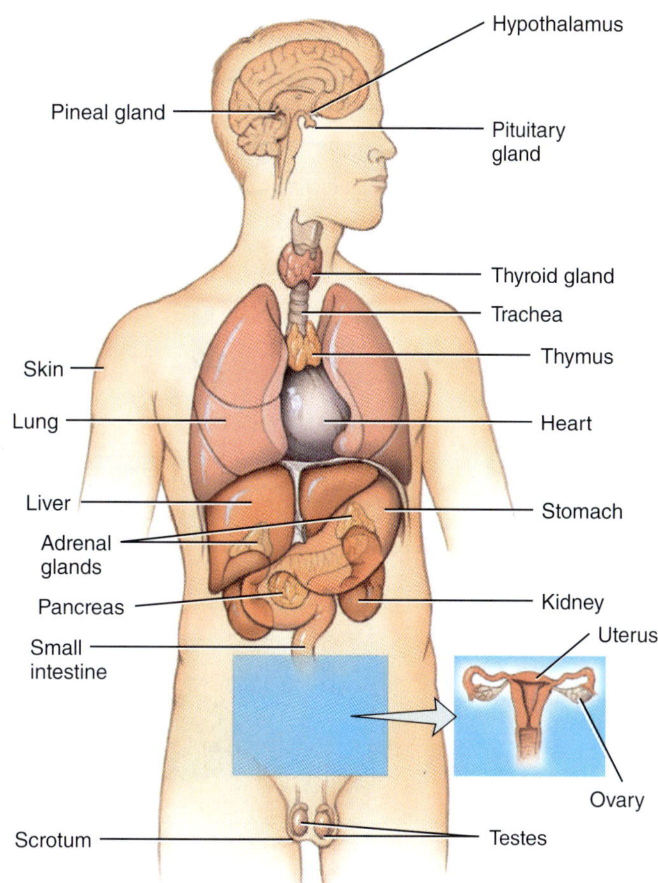

Source: Tortora and Derrickson (2009). Reproduced with permission of John Wiley & Sons.

FIGURE 16.2 Transportation of hormones in the blood

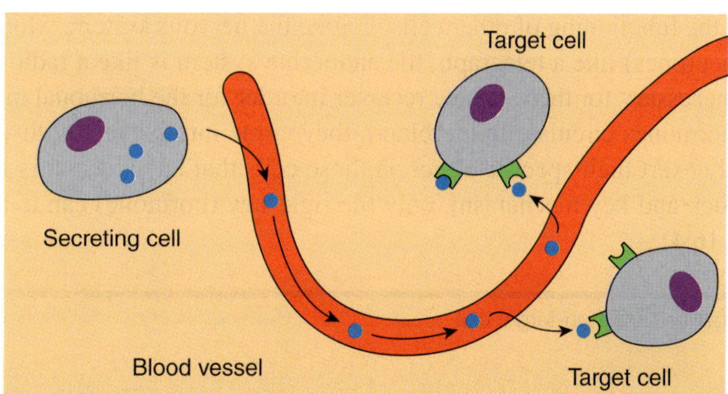

Endocrine, paracrine, exocrine and autocrine

Many words in anatomy and physiology have a similar ending to other words used about the same processes or areas of the body (figure 16.3). It is important to be aware of these as confusion can quickly take over.

Endocrine is usually used to refer to hormones that are secreted into the blood and have an effect on cells distant from those that released the hormone. However, many endocrine hormones are known to act locally and even on the cells that secrete them.

Paracrine refers to hormones that act locally and diffuse to the cells in the immediate neighbourhood to produce their action.

Autocrine refers to hormones that act on the cells that produce it.

Exocrine refers to glands/organs that secrete substances into ducts that eventually lead to the outside of the body (e.g. the sweat glands, the part of the pancreas that secretes digestive juices, the gallbladder).

FIGURE 16.3 Endocrine, paracrine and autocrine

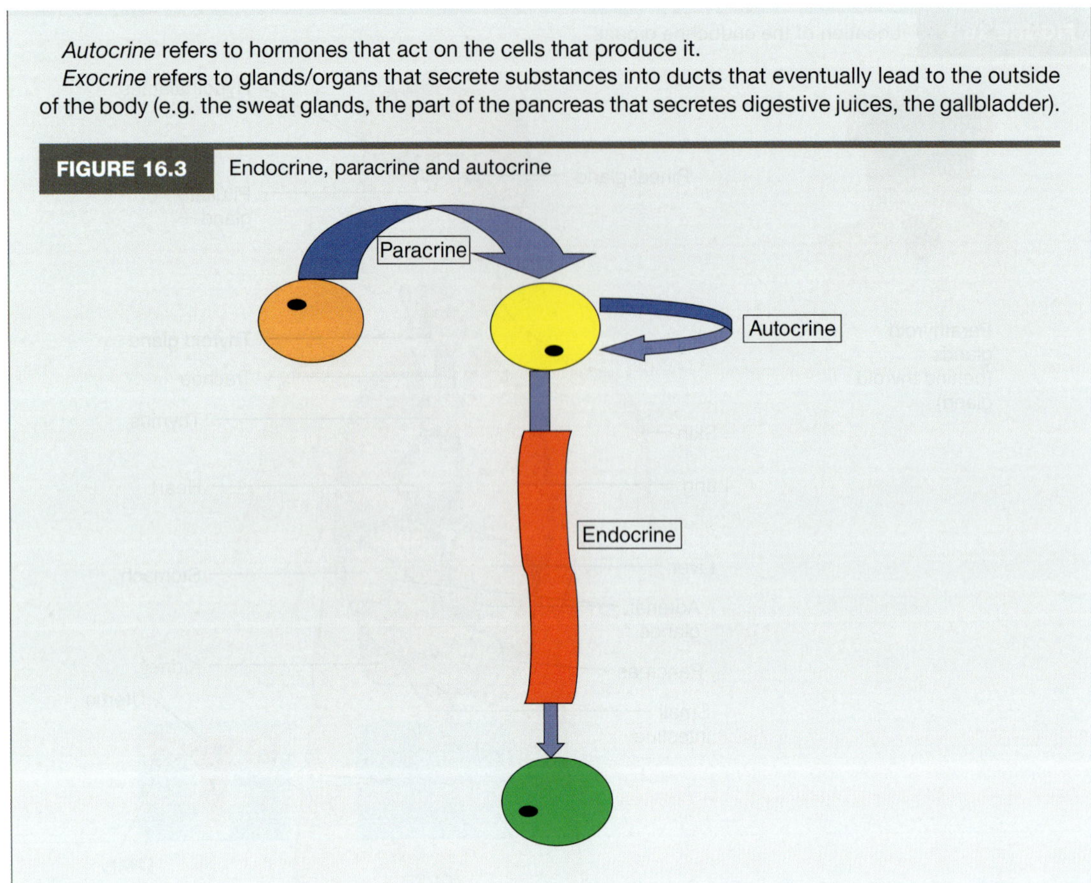

16.2 Hormones

LEARNING OBJECTIVE 16.2 Discuss the different forms of stimulus for the release of hormones and how those hormones have their effects.

Hormones are chemical messengers that are secreted into the blood or the extracellular fluid by one cell and have an effect on the functioning of other cells. Unlike the nervous system, which could be said to be based on wires (the neurones) like a telegraph, the endocrine system is like a radio broadcast. As with a radio broadcast, it is necessary for there to be a receiver in order for the hormonal message to be received and acted upon. As hormones circulate in the blood, they come into contact with virtually every cell in the body, but they only exert their specific effect on those cells that have receptors for that hormone (the target cells). Like a lock and key mechanism, only the right key (hormone) can unlock a particular lock (receptor) (see figure 16.4).

FIGURE 16.4 Target cell and non-target cell

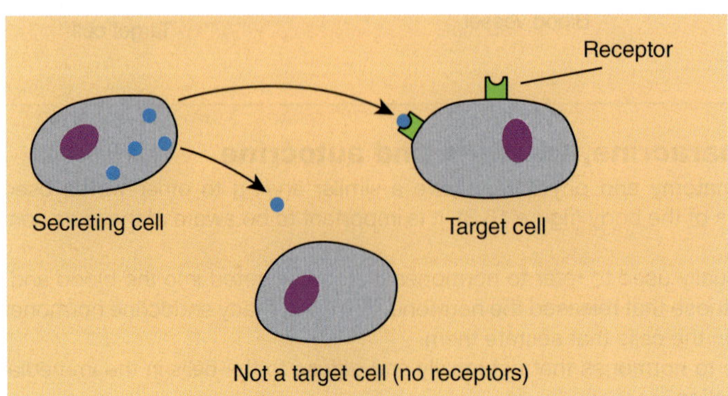

Hormone receptors are either found within the target cell or on its surface (as in figure 16.4). The site of the receptor is dependent on the type of hormone the receptor is for. Most hormones are made from **amino acids**, but some are made from cholesterol (the steroid hormones).

- Amino acid-based hormones cannot cross the cell membrane and thus their receptors are found on the cell wall. These hormones tend to exert their influence by activating enzymes and other molecules within the cell, which then affect the cell activity (secondary messengers). This is often through a cascade of changes, with the activation of the enzyme or molecule being the first step. The best understood example of this is cyclic adenosine monophosphate.
- The steroid hormones can cross the cell membrane because they are small and **lipid** soluble and thus their receptors are found within the cell itself. These hormones usually exert their effect by stimulating the production of genes within the target cell. The genes then stimulate the synthesis of new proteins.
- One exception is thyroid hormone, which is not a steroid hormone but is lipid soluble and very small and can diffuse easily across the cell membrane into the cell.

The activation of a target cell depends on the concentration of the hormone in the blood, the number of receptors on the cell and the affinity of the receptor for the hormone. Changes in these factors can happen quickly in response to a change in stimuli.

The most important factor influencing the effect of a hormone on its target cell is its concentration in the blood and/or extracellular fluid. This concentration of a hormone at the target cell is determined by three factors.

- *Rate of production of the hormone*. This is the most highly regulated aspect of the endocrine system.
- *Rate of delivery of the hormone.* An example of this is the blood flow to the organ or cell.
- *Rate of destruction and elimination of the hormone (half-life).* Hormones with a short half-life will rapidly drop in concentration once production decreases. If the half-life of the hormone is long, then the hormone will still be present in significant concentrations for some time after its production stops.

Changes in the concentration of hormones can be a rapid mechanism of control, especially the rate of production, but longer-term adjustments to target cell sensitivity to a hormone will almost certainly include changes in the numbers of receptors as well. Changes in the number of receptors are known as **upregulation** and **downregulation**.

- *Upregulation* is the creation of more receptors in response to low circulating levels of a hormone; the cell becomes more responsive to the presence of the hormone in the blood.
- *Downregulation* is the reduction in the number of receptors and is often the response of a cell to prolonged periods of high circulating levels of a hormone; the cell becomes less responsive (desensitised) to a hormone.

The transportation of hormones

Most hormones are secreted into the circulating blood, though there is the exception of hormones that are released into a local circulatory system known as a portal circulation. The two portal circulations in the human body are those connecting the hypothalamus and the anterior pituitary gland and the hepatic portal circulation that merges to form the portal vein entering the liver.

The steroid hormones are mostly conveyed within the circulation by being bound to transport proteins, with less than 10 per cent making up the 'free fraction' of the hormone (Jenkins & Tortora 2013). In clinical placements you may have noticed that some blood tests are specifically targeted at measuring both the bound and free elements of a hormone; the most common of these are the thyroid function tests, which measure both bound thyroxine (T_4) and **free T_4**. Water-soluble hormones are conveyed in their free form in the blood.

Effects of hormones

Hormones typically produce one of the following changes:

- changes in cell membrane permeability and/or the cell's electrical state (membrane potential) by opening or closing ion channels in the cell membrane
- synthesis of proteins or regulatory molecules (such as enzymes) within the cell
- enzyme activation or deactivation
- modulation of secretory activity
- stimulation of mitosis.

16.3 Control of hormone release

LEARNING OBJECTIVE 16.3 Explain the control of hormone release by the hypothalamus.

The creation and release of most hormones are preceded by a stimulus that can be internal or external; for instance, a rise in blood glucose levels or a cold environment. The further synthesis and release of hormones is then usually controlled by a negative feedback system. As can be seen in figure 16.5, the influence of a stimulus, from inside or outside the body (in this case a rise in blood glucose levels), leads to hormone release (insulin); following this, some aspect of the target organ function then inhibits further reaction to the stimulus and thus further release of the hormone by the organ.

FIGURE 16.5 The negative feedback system

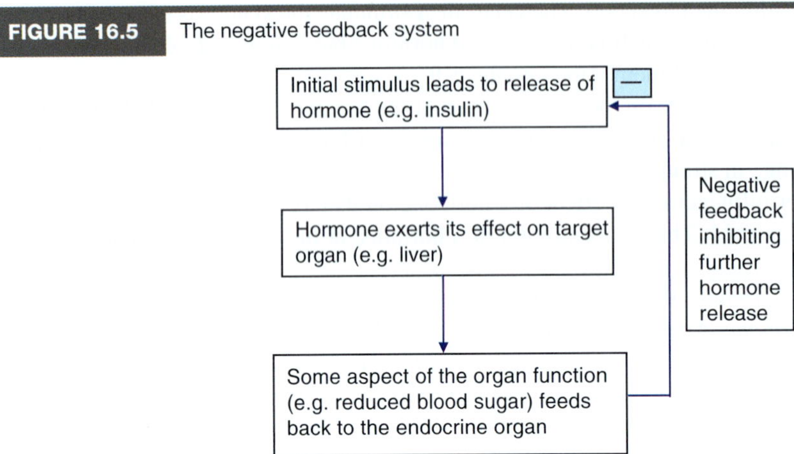

Source: Peate (2017). Reproduced with permission of John Wiley & Sons.

The initial stimulus for the release of a hormone is usually one of three types, though some organs respond to multiple stimuli.

- **Humoral stimulation** is a response to changing levels of certain **ions** and nutrients in the blood. For example, parathyroid hormone is stimulated by falling blood levels of calcium ions.
- **Neural stimulation** is a response to direct nervous stimulation. Very few endocrine organs are directly stimulated by the nervous system. An example is increased activity in the sympathetic nervous system that directly stimulates the release of **catecholamines** (adrenaline and noradrenaline) from the adrenal **medulla**.
- **Hormonal stimulation** is a response to hormones released by other organs. Hormones that are released in response to hormonal stimulation are usually rhythmical in their release (i.e. the levels rise and fall in a specific pattern). An example of hormonal control is the release of thyroid-stimulating hormone (TSH) from the anterior pituitary gland directly stimulating the production and release of T_4 from the thyroid gland.

Destruction and removal of hormones

Hormones are very powerful and can have a large effect at even low concentrations; therefore, it is essential that active hormones are efficiently removed from the blood. Some hormones are rapidly broken down within the target cells. Most are inactivated by enzyme systems in the liver and kidneys and then excreted mostly in the urine, but some are excreted in the faeces.

The physiology of the endocrine organs

The hypothalamus and the pituitary gland

The hypothalamus is a portion of the brain with a variety of functions. It is a small (about 4 g), cone-like structure that is directly connected to the pituitary gland by the pituitary stalk (or infundibulum). One of the most important functions of the hypothalamus is to link the nervous system to the endocrine system via the pituitary gland. Almost all hormone secretion by the pituitary gland is controlled by either hormonal or electrical signals from the hypothalamus (figure 16.6).

FIGURE 16.6 The hypothalamus and pituitary gland

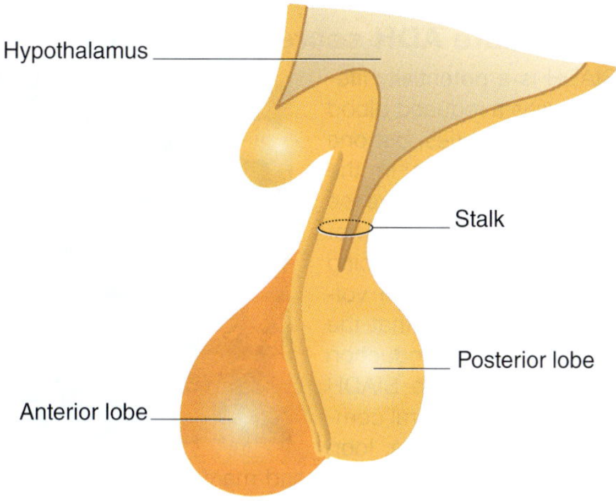

The hypothalamus receives signals from the nervous system but is also under negative feedback control by the hormones regulated by the pituitary gland. Thus, when there is a low level of a hormone in the blood supplying the hypothalamus, this leads to the release of the appropriate releasing hormone or factor that stimulates the release of the hormone by the pituitary, which in turn stimulates the release of the appropriate hormone. As the level of the target hormone rises in the blood, this is detected by receptors in the hypothalamus and the stimulus for the release of the stimulating factor is removed and thus release of this factor is reduced. A classic example of this system is the release of thyrotropin-releasing hormone (TRH) and the subsequent release of TSH by the anterior pituitary gland, which is described further on in this chapter.

The pituitary gland secretes at least nine major hormones and is the size and shape of a pea on a stalk. The pituitary gland is functionally and anatomically divided into two parts.

- The posterior lobe (neurohypophysis) is made up mostly of nerve fibres that originate in the hypothalamus and terminate on the surface of capillaries in the posterior lobe. The posterior lobe releases two hormones that it receives directly from the hypothalamus. In this sense it is in fact a storage area rather than a gland in the true sense of the term. The hypothalamus and the posterior pituitary are linked by a nerve bundle called the hypothalamic-hypophyseal tract.
- The anterior lobe (adenohypophysis) is much larger than the posterior lobe and partly surrounds the posterior lobe and the infundibulum. It is made up of glandular tissue and produces and releases several hormones. The hypothalamus and the anterior pituitary have no direct nerve connections but do have a vascular (blood vessel) connection known as the hypothalamo-hypophyseal portal system, whereby venous blood from the hypothalamus flows to the anterior lobe. Thus, control of the anterior pituitary is by releasing and inhibiting factors (or hormones) released by the hypothalamus.

Hormones that are secreted by the posterior pituitary are the following.

- *Oxytocin.* Oxytocin has an effect on uterine contraction in childbirth and is responsible for the 'let down' response in breastfeeding mothers (the release of milk in response to suckling). In men and non-pregnant women it appears to play a role in sexual arousal and orgasm (Jenkins & Tortora 2013).
- *Antidiuretic hormone (ADH).* Under resting conditions, large quantities of ADH accumulate in the posterior pituitary; excitation by nervous impulses leads to the release of the ADH from where it is stored into the adjacent blood vessels. The effects of ADH are that it increases water retention by the kidneys by increasing the permeability of the collecting ducts in the kidneys. The secretion of ADH is stimulated:
  - by increased plasma **osmolality** — increased levels of certain substances in the plasma, such as sodium
  - by decreased extracellular fluid volume
  - by pain and other stressed states
  - in response to certain drugs.

CLINICAL CONSIDERATIONS

Syndrome of inappropriate ADH secretion (SIADH)

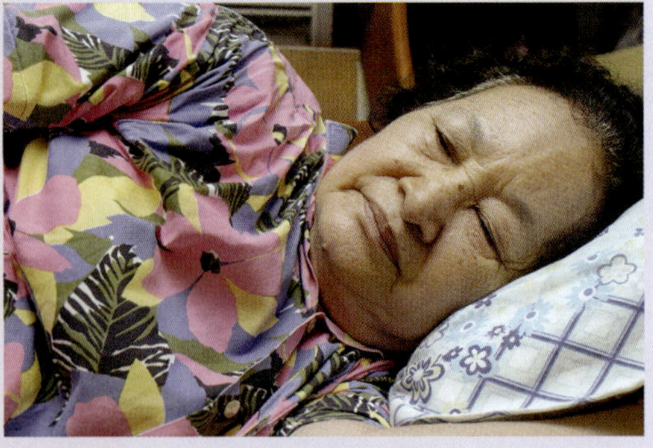

Though relatively rare, SIADH is a potentially life-threatening condition that causes a reduced blood sodium level. The pathophysiology varies, but one type is thought to be due to changes in the ability of the hypothalamus to detect a decrease in blood osmolality and thus ADH release is not reduced and the blood volume increases, reducing the concentration of sodium relative to the volume of blood. In the elderly it is thought that the cells of the hypothalamus increase ADH production with increasing age. Clinically detectable SIADH has many potential causes, including several commonly used medications (such as morphine, loop diuretics, angiotensin-converting enzyme inhibitors and many antidepressants), some neurological disorders, several types of cancer and hypothyroidism. It is the most common cause of hyponatraemia in critical care patients (Friedman & Cirulli 2013) and is also common in the elderly.

The symptoms of SIADH include loss of appetite, nausea, weakness, confusion and delirium. In the elderly, the diagnosis of SIADH can be late as one of the common presenting factors is altered mental states (including confusion) which can be mistakenly ascribed to many other factors or conditions such as dementia, infection and cerebrovascular events (Nelson & Robinson 2012).

The diagnosis of SIADH includes the detection of a low blood sodium concentration with a normal blood volume (euvolaemia).

The treatment of SIADH involves fluid restriction, thus increasing relative sodium levels in the blood by reducing blood volume and where possible treating the cause. In cases requiring urgent treatment, hypertonic saline (3% saline) can be infused to temporarily increase the blood sodium level (Gross 2012).

Hormones released by the anterior pituitary gland

Table 16.2 summarises the range of hormones released by the anterior pituitary gland and the releasing or inhibiting hormones (or factors) from the hypothalamus that influence this release.

TABLE 16.2 Hormones released by the hypothalamus and the anterior pituitary gland

Hypothalamus	Anterior pituitary gland	Target organ or tissues	Action
Growth-hormone-releasing factor	Growth hormone	Many (especially bones)	Stimulates growth of body cells
Growth-hormone-release-inhibiting factor	Growth hormone (inhibits release)	Many	
Thyrotropin-releasing hormone (TRH)	Thyroid-stimulating hormone (TSH)	Thyroid gland	Stimulates thyroid hormone release
Corticotropin-releasing hormone (CRH)	Adrenocorticotropic hormone (ACTH)	Adrenal **cortex**	Stimulates **corticosteroid** release
Prolactin-releasing hormone	Prolactin	Breasts	Stimulates milk production
Prolactin-inhibiting hormone	Prolactin (inhibits release)	Breasts	
Gonadotropin-releasing hormone	Follicle-stimulating hormone Luteinising hormone	Gonads	Various reproductive functions

Source: Peate (2017). Reproduced with permission of John Wiley & Sons.

There are five types of pituitary cell in the anterior lobe:

- somatotropes, which secrete growth hormones
- lactotropes, which secrete prolactin
- thyrotropes, which secrete TSH
- gonadotropes, which secrete luteinising hormone (LH) and follicle-stimulating hormone (FSH)
- corticotropes, which secrete adrenocorticotropic hormone (ACTH).

Growth hormone

Effects

As its name suggests, growth hormone promotes the growth of bone, cartilage and soft tissue by stimulating the production and release of insulin-like growth factor (IGF-1).

Regulation

Growth hormone release from the anterior pituitary is regulated by the release of growth-hormone-releasing hormone and growth-hormone-release-inhibiting hormone (somatostatin) by the hypothalamus. Both growth hormone and IGF-1 produce a negative feedback effect on the hypothalamus.

HOMEOSTATIC IMBALANCE

Gigantism and acromegaly

Gigantism and acromegaly are two disorders associated with excessive secretion of growth hormone (GH), usually due to a GH-secreting benign pituitary adenoma (Vilar et al. 2017). The difference between gigantism and acromegaly is largely due to the time of onset. Gigantism typically occurs in early childhood and results in increased height and rapid growth, while acromegaly occurs in adults after epiphyseal plate closure and results in enlarged bones in the hands, feet, skull and jaw (Better Health Channel 2021). In addition to these symptoms, these conditions also cause joint pains, headaches, cardiomegaly, enlarged tongue and lips, excessive sweat production and coarse-looking facial features (Better Health Channel 2021; Health Direct 2021a). Comparatively, gigantism and acromegaly are very rare, with only 1000 sufferers identified within Australia.

Prolactin

Effects

Prolactin stimulates the secretion of milk in the breast.

Regulation

Secretion is inhibited by the release of dopamine from the hypothalamus. Secretion can be intermittently increased by the release of prolactin-releasing hormone from the hypothalamus in response to the baby suckling at the breast.

Follicle-stimulating hormone and luteinising hormone (gonadotrophins)

Effects

In males, FSH stimulates sperm production. In females, it leads to the early maturation of ovarian follicles and oestrogen secretion.

LH is responsible for the final maturation of the ovarian follicles and oestrogen secretion in females, and stimulates testosterone secretion in males.

Regulation

In males and females, LH and FSH production are regulated by the release of gonadotrophin-releasing hormone (GnRH). Testosterone and oestrogen exert a negative feedback effect on the release of GnRH from the hypothalamus.

Thyroid-stimulating hormone

Effects

TSH stimulates the activity of the cells of the thyroid gland leading to an increased production and secretion of thyroxine (T_4) and triiodothyronine (T_3).

Regulation

TSH is produced and released in response to the release of TRH from the hypothalamus. The hypothalamus can also inhibit the release of TSH through the action of somatostatin.

Free T_3 and T_4 in the blood have a direct negative feedback effect on the hypothalamus and the anterior pituitary gland.

Adrenocorticotrophic hormone

Effects

ACTH stimulates the production of **cortisol** and androgens from the cortex of the adrenal gland. It also leads to the production of aldosterone in response to increased concentrations of potassium ions, increased angiotensin levels or decreased total body sodium.

Regulation

ACTH is secreted from the anterior pituitary in response to the secretion of corticotropin-releasing hormone (CRH) from the hypothalamus. Excitation of the hypothalamus by any form of stress leads to the release of CRH and the subsequent release of ACTH and then cortisol. Cortisol exerts a direct negative feedback on the hypothalamus and the anterior pituitary gland.

CLINICALLY REASONED EPISODE OF CARE

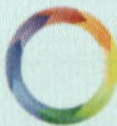

Cushing's disease

Consider the patient situation

Mary is a 50-year-old woman who has reported significant depression for which she has been prescribed antidepressants. Mary returns to the GP after one month for a review and while she feels somewhat better, the depression remains and she reports increasing weight gain and excess hair growth.

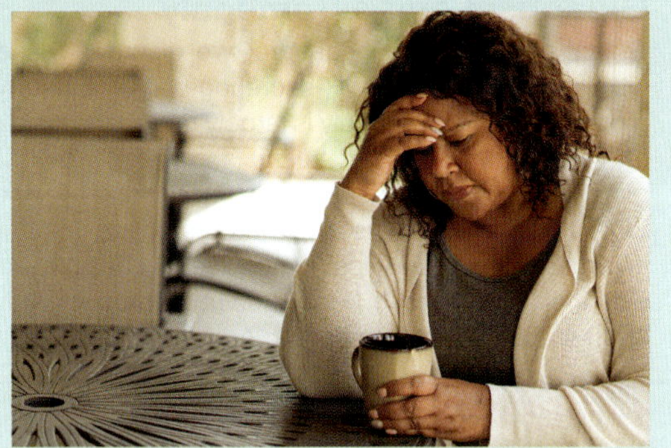

Collect cues and information

On further questioning, Mary reports increasing weight gain, especially in the face and on the back of the neck. She also reports that her skin is bruising easily, and she is constantly tired.

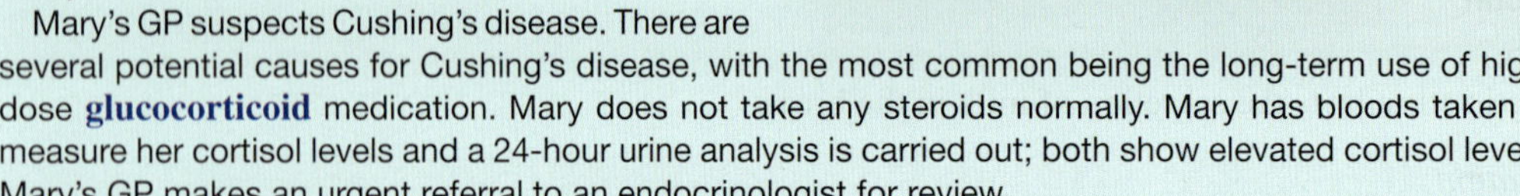

Mary's GP suspects Cushing's disease. There are several potential causes for Cushing's disease, with the most common being the long-term use of high-dose **glucocorticoid** medication. Mary does not take any steroids normally. Mary has bloods taken to measure her cortisol levels and a 24-hour urine analysis is carried out; both show elevated cortisol levels. Mary's GP makes an urgent referral to an endocrinologist for review.

Process information

Cushing's disease occurs in response to a long-term overproduction of the hormone cortisol in the body. Signs and symptoms of Cushing's include a fatty hump on the back between the shoulder blade and neck, weight gain around the face (known as moon face), purple stretchmarks and fragile skin.

Along with long-term steroid use, Cushing's syndrome can also be caused by several intrinsic causes including a pituitary gland tumour. A pituitary gland tumour is a noncancerous (benign) tumour of the pituitary gland, located at the base of the brain. The pituitary gland produces an excess amount of adrenocorticotropic hormone (ACTH), which in turn stimulates the adrenal glands to make more cortisol. When this form of the syndrome develops, it is called Cushing's disease. It occurs more often in women and is the most common form of endogenous Cushing's syndrome.

After an MRI, Mary is diagnosed with a pituitary tumour and Cushing's disease. Mary is quickly passed on to the care of a neurosurgeon for an operation known as transsphenoidal hypophysectomy (the removal of the pituitary gland via the nasal cavity). The procedure can involve removing part or all of the pituitary gland. In Mary's case it was necessary to remove the whole gland.

Following this procedure, Mary will no longer have a pituitary gland and will no longer produce any of the pituitary hormones, including thyrotropin-releasing hormone (TRH) and ACTH. The loss of TRH and ACTH production will mean there will be no stimulus for the thyroid gland and the adrenal glands to produce hormones; thus, hormone replacement therapy for hypothyroidism (thyroxine) and hypoadrenalism (hydrocortisone and fludrocortisone) will be required.

In Cushing's disease, a major depressive syndrome is seen in 50–70 per cent of patients, which often improves once the condition is treated. Psychiatric disorders, especially depression, are a common finding in most patients with an endocrine disorder, with anxiety being the second most common finding. Traditionally, depression and anxiety have been considered a consequence of diagnosis, but increasingly it is being recognised that the endocrine disorders themselves may be the cause of psychiatric disturbances, and treatment of the endocrine disorder will often improve any psychiatric symptoms.

Having completed her surgery, Mary returns to the general practice where she sees the GP and practice nurse.

Establish goals

1. Cessation of antidepressants
2. Commencement of hormone therapy
3. Ongoing support and postoperative care

Nursing actions

1. Organise for medication management.
   Rationale:
   - Post surgery, Mary's depression symptoms have resolved, and her antidepressant medication is ceased. Antidepressants should be ceased under the guidance of the care team and weaned over a period of weeks. Nurses are well placed to liaise with both patient and GP during this process.
   - After the removal of the whole pituitary gland, Mary will need to be on hormone replacement therapy (HRT) for the remainder of her life.
   - There can be side effects with starting HRT (e.g. sweating, mood swings, trouble sleeping) and nurses should provide education, information and support with the management of HRT.
2. Provide ongoing support and postoperative care.
   Rationale:
   - Recovery from surgery typically occurs within two weeks; however, symptoms associated with surgery via the nasal cavity, such as headache, congestion, numbness and fatigue, are common.
   - Nurses are well placed to provide ongoing support and assessment postoperatively, and in conjunction with the GP to organise for review and medication as required.

Evaluate outcomes

Mary commences HRT with minimal symptoms, and she is feeling well post surgery.

Reflect on new processes and learning

How can nurses support patients taking hormone replacement therapy? What changes are patients likely to see and how can nurses make this transition easier for individuals?

Source: Based on the Clinical Reasoning Cycle, Levett-Jones (2013).

SKILLS IN PRACTICE

Twenty-four-hour urine collection

Twenty-four-hour urine collections are undertaken for many reasons. For instance, in suspected Cushing's disease, a 24-hour collection of urine is undertaken to assess the excretion of cortisol in the urine. While a simple test from the patient's point of view, it is important that the test is carried out correctly.

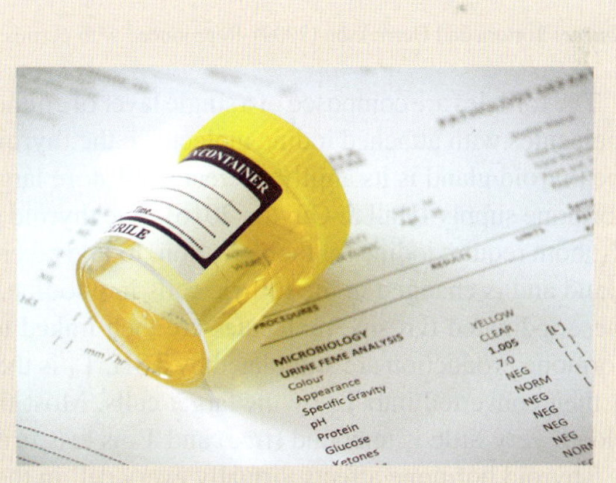

- Record all medications that the patient is taking; some medications can affect the test results (e.g. if the patient is taking oestrogen or corticosteroids).
- The urine will be collected in a large container that may contain preservatives; it is therefore essential that the patient is informed not to pass urine directly into the container or touch the inside of the container as this may lead to skin contact with the preservative.
- Patients must use a clean receptacle every time they pass urine and to avoid contaminating the sample with faeces, menstrual blood, toilet paper or pubic hair.
- When the patient passes the first urine of the day (first thing in the morning), this urine is discarded and the time recorded (this is the time of the start of the test).
- All urine passed for the next 24 hours is then collected in the receptacle and the receptacle is normally kept in a cool area.

- Not collecting all the urine passed over 24 hours may affect the outcome of the test.
- At the point the 24 hours are up (or just before), the patient should empty their bladder and add this to the collection. The final time should be noted, and the collection returned to the hospital laboratory.

The thyroid gland

The thyroid gland is a butterfly-shaped gland located in the front of the neck on the trachea just below the larynx (figure 16.7). It is made up of two lobes joined by an isthmus (a narrow strip; isthmus = neck). The upper extremities of the lobes are known as the upper poles and the lower extremities the lower poles. Each lobe is made up of hollow, spherical follicles surrounded by capillaries. This leads to an abundant blood supply; although the thyroid gland accounts for 0.4 per cent of the total body weight, it receives 2 per cent of the circulating blood supply.

FIGURE 16.7 (a, b) Position of the thyroid gland and parathyroid glands

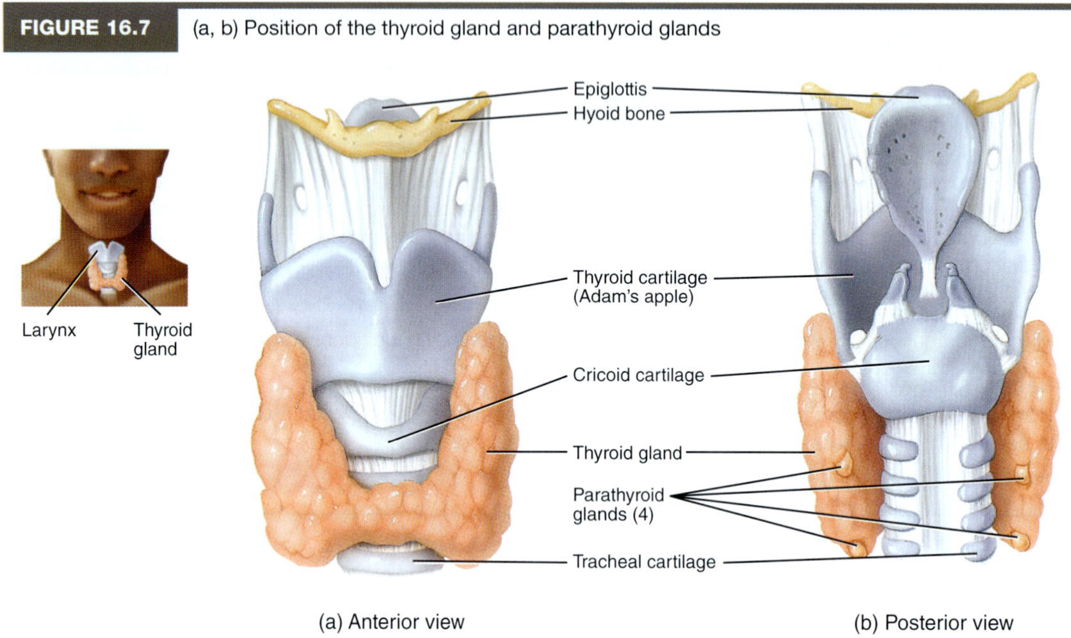

Source: Tortora and Derrickson (2009). Reproduced with permission of John Wiley & Sons.

The follicles are composed of a single layer of epithelial cells that form a cavity that contains thyroglobulin molecules with attached iodine molecules; the thyroid hormone is created from this. One unique factor of the thyroid gland is its ability to create and store large amounts of hormone; this can be up to 100 days of hormone supply (Hall & Guyton 2016). The thyroid gland releases two forms of thyroid hormone: T_4 and T_3; both require iodine for their creation. Iodide taken in with the normal diet is concentrated by the thyroid gland and is changed in the follicle cells into iodine. This iodine is then linked to tyrosine molecules and these iodinated tyrosine molecules are then linked together to create T_3 and T_4. All the steps in thyroid hormone production are stimulated by TSH. T_4 is the primary hormone released by the thyroid gland; this is then converted into T_3 by the target cells. Most thyroid hormone is bound to transport proteins in the blood; very little is unbound (free) and T_3 is less firmly bound to transport proteins than is T_4.

Thyroid hormone affects virtually every cell in the body, except:

- the adult brain
- spleen
- testes
- uterus
- thyroid gland.

Both T_4 and T_3 easily cross the cell membrane and interact with receptors inside the cell. In the target cells, thyroid hormone stimulates enzymes that are involved with glucose oxidation. This is known as the calorigenic effect and its overall effects are:

- an increase in the basal metabolic rate
- an increase in oxygen consumption by the cell
- an increase in the production of body heat.

Basal metabolic rate is the amount of energy expended while at rest in a temperate environment (not hot or cold). The release of energy in this state is enough for the functioning of the vital organs. As basal metabolic rate is increased, oxygen consumption is increased, as oxygen is required in the production of energy.

Thyroid hormone also has an important role in the maintenance of blood pressure as it stimulates an increase in the number of receptors in the walls of the blood vessels.

The control of the release of thyroid hormone is mediated by a negative feedback system that involves the hypothalamus and cascades through the pituitary gland (figure 16.8).

FIGURE 16.8 Negative feedback control of thyroid hormone production

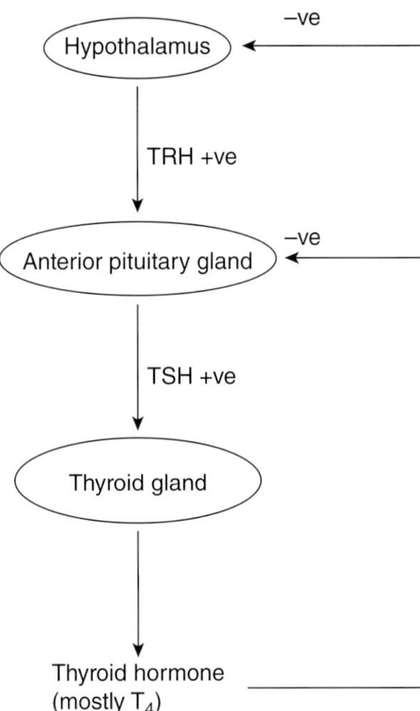

Plasma levels of thyroid hormone are monitored in the hypothalamus and by cells in the anterior lobe of the pituitary gland. Increased levels of T_4 in the blood inhibit the release of TRH from the hypothalamus, thus reducing the stimulation for the release of TSH from the anterior pituitary gland. Thyroid hormones also have a direct negative feedback effect on the anterior pituitary gland. The effect of TSH on the thyroid gland is to promote the release of thyroid hormone into the blood; therefore, a reduction in TSH reduces the release of T_3 and T_4. A reduced level of T_4 in the blood reduces the negative feedback and thus there is an increase in the release of TRH, which leads to an increase in thyroid gland function. Conditions that increase the energy requirements of the body (such as pregnancy or prolonged cold) also stimulate the release of TRH from the hypothalamus and therefore lead to an increase in blood levels of thyroid hormone. In these situations, the stimulating conditions override the normal negative feedback system (Jenkins & Tortora 2013). The negative feedback control of thyroid hormone can be likened to a central heating system. The hypothalamus and pituitary gland are the thermostat and the thyroid gland is the boiler. As the room temperature increases, the thermostat turns off the central heating boiler; when the temperature decreases, the thermostat turns the boiler on to increase the temperature.

The half-life of T_4 is approximately 7 days and the half-life of T_3 is 1 day. Thyroid hormones are broken down in the liver and the skeletal muscle and while much of the iodine is recycled, some is lost in the urine and the faeces. Therefore, there is a need for daily replacement of iodine in the diet.

HOMEOSTATIC IMBALANCE

Goitre

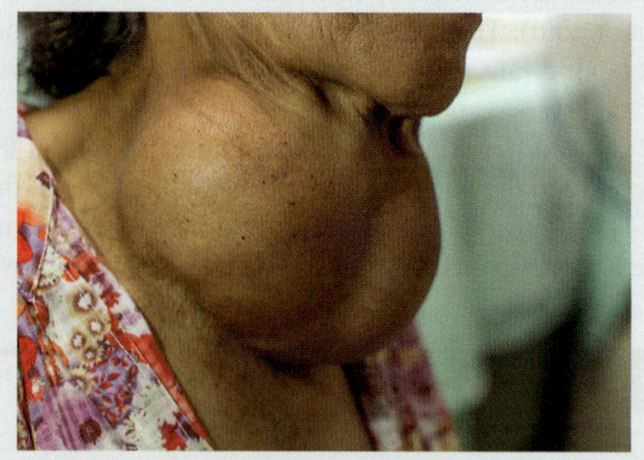

Goitre is a benign enlargement of the thyroid gland caused predominantly by a lack of dietary iodine. Goitre can also be caused by autoimmune conditions, injury, infection and cancers of the thyroid gland (Health Direct 2021b). Goitre due to lack of iodine is very rare in Australia as there is iodine supplementation in both salt and bread products.

While generally benign, goitre can cause difficulties in speaking, swallowing and breathing, but it is usually easily treated through supplementation of iodine or the prescription of synthetic thyroid hormone (levothyroxine). In cancer and severe enlargement of the thyroid, partial or total thyroidectomy is also a potential treatment option alongside radioactive iodine therapy to diminish the size of the goitre (Health Direct 2021b).

CLINICAL CONSIDERATIONS

Hypothyroidism and hyperthyroidism

A patient's blood level of thyroid hormone can be measured. Depending on whether the thyroid gland is overactive or underactive, different levels of hormones will be shown by the test. Generally, the patient would have their free T_4 and TSH levels assessed.

	TSH	Free T_4
Hyperthyroidism	Reduced	Elevated
Hypothyroidism	Elevated	Reduced

In the case of a patient with an overactive thyroid gland (hyperthyroidism), free T_4 will often be elevated but TSH levels will be reduced as the levels of thyroid hormone will be exerting a negative feedback effect on the hypothalamus and the pituitary gland. Despite the reduced TSH levels and the negative feedback effect on the pituitary gland as well, hormone levels will remain elevated.

A patient with hypothyroidism (an underactive thyroid gland) will often present with a reduced free T_4 and an elevated TSH as the reduced hormone levels remove the negative feedback on the hypothalamus and the pituitary and thus TSH levels rise. The patient with a test result within normal ranges is called 'euthyroid'.

Sick euthyroid syndrome

During severe illness or starvation, the metabolic drive on the human body by the thyroid is reduced. The term 'sick euthyroid' is used in this condition since it represents a state of thyroid function appropriate for a sick individual; and it returns to normal with the return of good health.

T_3 is largely produced by target cell conversion of T_4. In the typical sick euthyroid patient, circulating T_3 is usually low but the total T_4 may be normal or even raised since there is reduced conversion to T_3. Conversely, T_4 may be low since the majority is carried on serum-binding proteins and their synthesis may be suppressed by severe illness. In these cases, the absence of a raised TSH excludes a diagnosis of primary hypothyroidism (McDermott 2013).

Critically ill patients with sick euthyroid syndrome are known to have increased rates of mortality, but at present the routine testing of thyroid function in the critically ill is not recommended and should only be carried out when there is clinical suspicion of hypothyroidism (Economidou et al. 2011).

In addition to the thyroid epithelial cells there are C cells, which are found between the follicles and secrete calcitonin. Calcitonin is involved in the metabolism of calcium and phosphorus within the body. It decreases calcium levels in the blood by reducing the activity of **osteoclasts** (cells that 'digest' bone and thus release calcium and phosphorus into the blood); due to this action, calcitonin is used as a treatment for osteoporosis and may also have a future role in the treatment of osteoarthritis (Mero et al. 2014). Calcitonin also inhibits the reabsorption of calcium from urine in the kidneys.

CLINICALLY REASONED EPISODE OF CARE

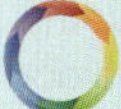

Hypothyroidism in Down syndrome

Consider the patient situation

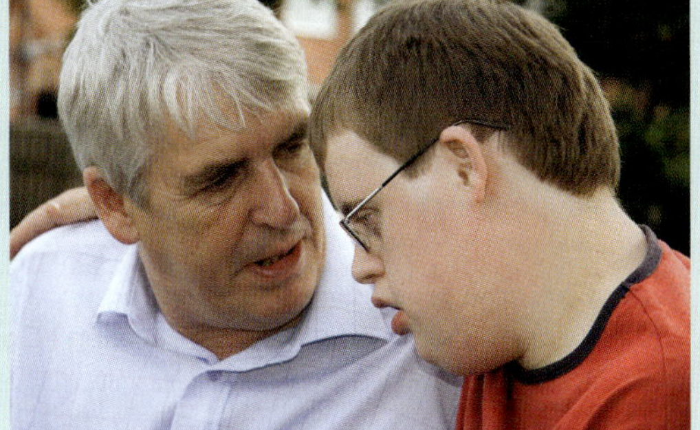

Daniel is a 28-year-old man with Down syndrome. Daniel lives at home with his mother, father and sister in a semi-detached house. He attends a day centre from Monday to Friday and enjoys a wide range of activities. Recently, his parents have noted that Daniel has become less interested in activities other than watching television and is reluctant to get out of bed in the morning.

He attends the GP with his family as they are concerned about his weight gain and constipation.

Collect cues and information

On review, the GP considers his symptoms in the context of Down syndrome. Lethargy, constipation and weight gain are common in patients with Down syndrome. The GP counsels Daniel and his family on getting exercise to lose weight and eating fibre.

The GP also recognises these changes as possible signs of hypothyroidism and sends Daniel for a thyroid function test. Daniel is found to have hypothyroidism. The GP prescribes Daniel levothyroxine but warns that it will be several weeks before he feels completely better; in the meantime, repeated blood tests are required to monitor his blood levels of T_4 to ensure that he is receiving the correct dose.

Process information

The thyroid gland is located at the anterior of the neck below the larynx. The thyroid gland produces several different hormones including thyroxine (T_4) and triiodothyronine (T_3). These hormones help to regulate energy levels and they play an important part in physical and mental development. Thyroid cells combine iodine and the amino acid tyrosine to make T_3 and T_4, which are then released into the bloodstream and transported throughout the body where they control the conversion of oxygen and calories to energy, controlling the metabolism.

People with Down syndrome are more likely to experience hypothyroidism than those without. The symptoms of hypothyroidism include weight gain, slow pulse, constipation, tiredness, rough skin, hair loss and mental deterioration.

Hypothyroidism is usually treated with a medication such as levothyroxine. It is recommended that patients with Down syndrome are screened for hypothyroidism at birth and then every two years thereafter.

Establish goals

1. Education on thyroid medication
2. Management of constipation
3. Follow-up blood test for thyroid levels

Nursing actions

1. Provide education on medication for hypothyroidism.
   Rationale:
   - Daniel and his family will require education on how and when to take levothyroxine.
   - Levothyroxine should be taken on an empty stomach at least 30–60 minutes before breakfast. Levothyroxine should not be taken within four hours of ingesting products containing iron or calcium, nor should it be taken with antacids or proton pump inhibitors.
   - Adverse events are rare but may include tachycardia, palpitations, arrhythmias, dyspnoea, anxiety, fatigue, headache, heat intolerance, insomnia, irritability, skin rash, alopecia, goitre, weight loss, abdominal cramps or diarrhoea.
2. Provide education on management of constipation.
   Rationale:
   - The commencement of levothyroxine should ease the symptoms of constipation; however, there are additional steps that Daniel and his family can be educated on to address constipation.
   - Management includes drinking plenty of water, eating 30 g of fibre per day, defecating as soon as one feels the urge and exercising regularly.
   - Medications such as laxatives can help; however, patients should be discouraged from regular use of laxatives as a dependence can occur.

3. Follow up post medication commencement.
   Rationale:
   - Thyroid levels will need to be monitored approximately 6–8 weeks post commencement of levothyroxine. Once the therapeutic dose is achieved, thyroid levels will need to be monitored via a blood test 6 months after commencement and then every 12 months thereafter.
   - Nurses are well placed to liaise with Daniel and his family and the GP, ensuring that regular follow-up occurs.

Evaluate outcomes

As a result of the actions above, Daniel reports that he is feeling much better. He has more energy at the day centre and is engaging with activities. His parents report that he is sleeping well and his bowel habits have greatly improved. The family are now taking regular walks to ensure that Daniel maintains a healthy weight.

Reflect on new processes and learning

What role does the thyroid play in constipation? Consider the pathophysiology of hormones T_3 and T_4.

Source: Based on the Clinical Reasoning Cycle, Levett-Jones (2013).

MEDICINES MANAGEMENT

Levothyroxine

Holly is a 24-year-old woman who has been experiencing symptoms of lethargy, a loss of appetite, weight gain and mild depression. Initially her GP decided her symptoms were due to Holly's lifestyle and advised Holly to get sufficient rest and exercise. As the months went by, the symptoms did not improve and Holly began to lose her hair. Holly's GP took blood and sent it to the local hospital for thyroid function testing. The results showed an increase in TSH and a decrease in free T_4, suggestive of hypothyroid disease.

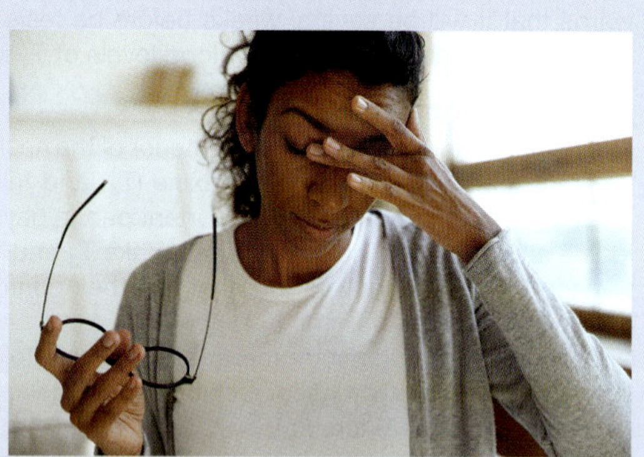

The GP prescribed Holly levothyroxine but warned her that it would be several weeks (if not months) before she felt completely better and in the meantime there would be a need for repeated blood tests to monitor her blood levels of T_4 to ensure that she is receiving the correct dose.

Levothyroxine is a synthetic version of the hormone T_4 and is generally free from side effects at the correct dose. Levothyroxine should be taken at the same time every day, preferably on an empty stomach. Where possible, patients are advised to take their levothyroxine an hour before breakfast.

Holly should also be counselled that before she intends to become pregnant she should discuss this with her endocrinologist. Pre-conception measurement of thyroid replacement levels is advised as low levels of maternal T_4 in the first trimester are associated with intellectual impairment in the baby. Levothyroxine requirements increase by about 50 per cent in pregnancy and the patient should be advised to increase their dose as soon as they are aware that they are pregnant (Weetman 2013).

The parathyroid glands

The parathyroid glands (figure 16.7) are small glands located on the back (posterior) of the thyroid gland. There are usually two pairs of glands, but the precise number varies and some patients have been reported to have up to four pairs. The cells that create and secrete parathyroid hormone (parathyroid chief cells) are arranged in cords or nests around a dense capillary network. Parathyroid hormone is the single most important hormone for the control of the calcium balance in the body. Its major target cells are in the bones and the kidneys.

- It increases intestinal calcium absorption.
- It stimulates renal calcium absorption.
- It stimulates osteoclast activity and therefore reabsorption of calcium from the bones.

Physiologically, calcium is important in the transmission of nerve impulses, is involved in muscle contraction and is also required in the creation of clotting factors in the blood. The regulation of parathyroid hormone synthesis and secretion is in response to the levels of calcium in the blood, which is monitored by cells in the gland. A reduced blood calcium level leads to an increase in the synthesis and secretion of parathyroid hormone.

Calcitriol is a hormone released by the kidneys in response to a decrease in calcium ions in the blood; it is known to have some effect on parathyroid hormone secretion and inhibits the release of calcitonin. It also promotes the absorption of calcium from the gut and the reabsorption of calcium from the renal tubules. Parathyroid hormone is a known stimulus for the release of calcitriol, but when calcitriol levels achieve a high enough level, its effect changes to that of inhibiting the release of parathyroid hormone. This prevents an uncontrollable increase in calcium in the blood.

The adrenal glands

The adrenal glands are complex, multifunctional organs whose secretions are essential for the maintenance of homeostasis. The two adrenal glands are found on the top of each of the two kidneys (figure 16.9). The right gland is roughly triangular in shape and the left, which is commonly the larger of the two, is crescent-shaped. Both glands are encased in a connective tissue capsule and embedded in an area of fat. Adrenal glands are very vascular (have a rich blood supply from many blood vessels).

FIGURE 16.9 Position of the adrenal glands

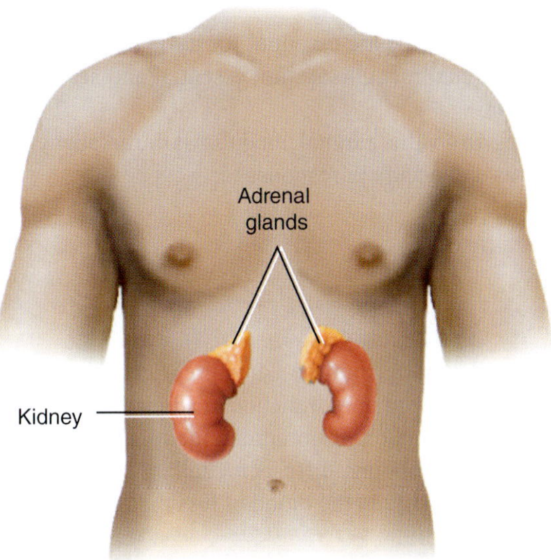

Source: Tortora and Derrickson (2009). Reproduced with permission of John Wiley & Sons.

Functionally, each adrenal gland is actually two glands and is composed of two major regions (figure 16.10):
- adrenal medulla
- adrenal cortex.

Adrenal medulla

The adrenal medulla is the inner part of the adrenal gland; it makes up about 30 per cent of the total mass of the adrenal gland. The function of the adrenal medulla is the secretion of catecholamines:
- adrenaline
- noradrenaline
- dopamine.

The adrenal medulla is mostly a modified, densely innervated, sympathetic **ganglion** made up of granule-containing cells. Within the adrenal medulla approximately 90 per cent of the cells secrete adrenaline, and the remaining 10 per cent secrete noradrenaline. It is unclear which cells secrete dopamine at this time. The effects of the catecholamines are many and varied.
- They stimulate the nervous system.
- They have metabolic effects — for instance, **glycogenolysis** in the liver and skeletal muscle.
- They increase metabolic rate.
- They increase heart rate.

- They increase alertness — though adrenaline frequently evokes anxiety and fear.
- Noradrenaline causes significant, widespread vasoconstriction.
- Adrenaline causes vasoconstriction in the skin and viscera but vasodilatation in skeletal muscles.

FIGURE 16.10 Cross-section of an adrenal gland

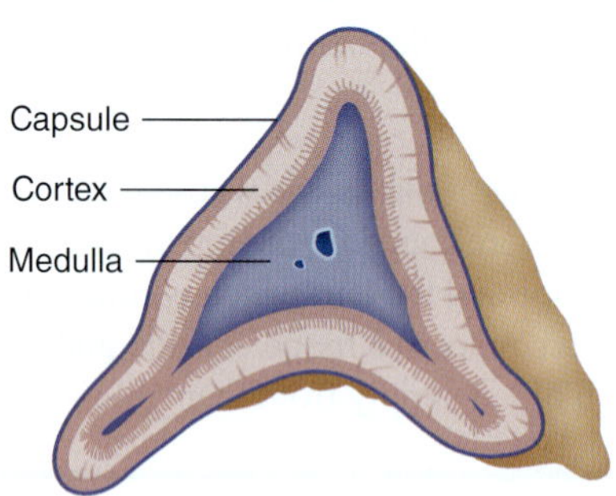

Source: Peate (2017). Reproduced with permission of John Wiley & Sons.

Although adrenaline and noradrenaline are essential for normal bodily functioning, adrenaline and the noradrenaline secreted by the adrenal medulla are not essential and serve only to intensify the effects of sympathetic nervous stimulation.

Secretion of catecholamines from the adrenal medulla is initiated by sympathetic nervous activity controlled by the hypothalamus and occurs in response to:

- pain
- anxiety
- excitement
- **hypovolaemia**
- **hypoglycaemia**.

The medulla receives its blood supply from the adrenal cortex rich in corticosteroids. These regulate the production of the enzymes that convert noradrenaline to adrenaline. Thus, an increase in corticosteroid production leads to an increased conversion of noradrenaline to adrenaline. With emergency stimulation of the hypothalamus there is a responding diffuse medullary activity preparing for fight or flight. Catecholamines have a very short half-life in the blood of less than 2 minutes as they are rapidly degraded by blood-borne enzymes.

Adrenal cortex

The outer part of each adrenal gland is made up of three distinct functional layers (figure 16.11). Each layer is involved in the production of steroid-based hormones (known collectively as the corticosteroids):

- zona glomerulosa — produces the **mineralocorticoids**
- zona fasciculata — produces the glucocorticoids
- zona reticularis — this zone is also involved in the production of glucocorticoids but also produces small amounts of adrenal sex hormones (the gonadocorticoids).

Mineralocorticoids

Mineralocorticoids are the group of hormones whose main function is the regulation of the concentration of the **electrolytes** in the blood. There are several known mineralocorticoids, but the most common is aldosterone, which accounts for 95 per cent of all the mineralocorticoids synthesised and is also the most potent.

The effect of aldosterone is to reduce the excretion of sodium in the urine by regulating the reabsorption of sodium from the urine in the distal portion of the renal tubules. Sodium is in effect exchanged for potassium and hydrogen, which results in the renal excretion of potassium and acidic urine. Aldosterone also has an effect on the levels of water in the body and several other ions (including potassium, bicarbonate and chloride) due to the fact that their regulation is coupled to the regulation of sodium in the body. The control of aldosterone secretion is primarily related to the blood concentrations of sodium (Na^+) and potassium (K^+), the mean arterial blood pressure and blood volume. Increased concentrations of potassium, reduced blood concentrations of sodium and a reduction in blood pressure and/or blood volume all stimulate the release of aldosterone, while the opposite inhibits release (figure 16.12). High blood levels of potassium are also known to have a direct effect on the adrenal cortex in the stimulation of aldosterone production and secretion.

FIGURE 16.11 Cross-section of the adrenal cortex

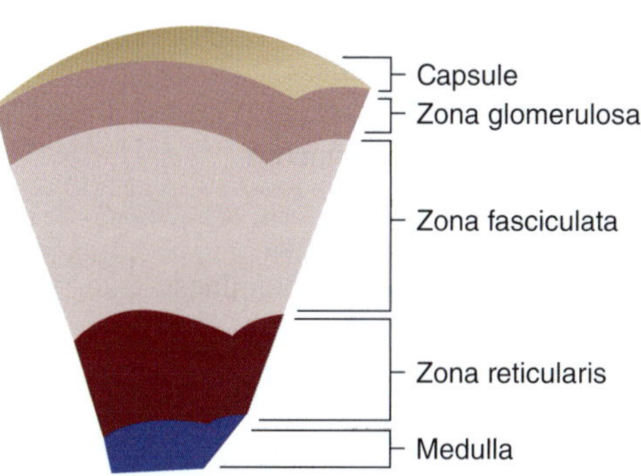

Source: Peate (2017). Reproduced with permission of John Wiley & Sons.

FIGURE 16.12 Control of aldosterone secretion

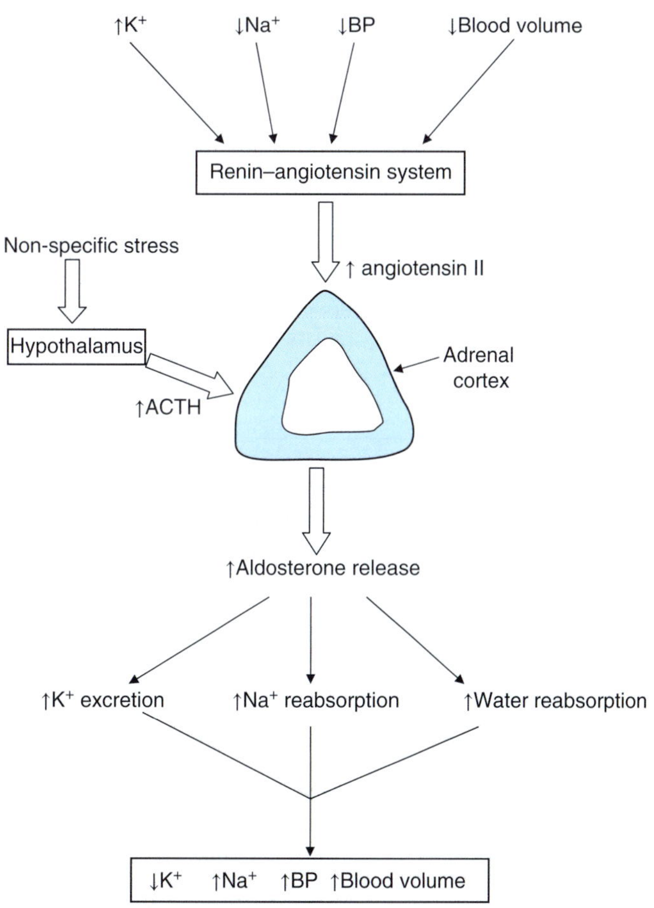

Source: Peate (2017). Reproduced with permission of John Wiley & Sons.

There are several mechanisms that regulate the release of aldosterone. The primary control mechanism is the production of angiotensin II by the renin-angiotensin system in response to reduced blood pressure in the kidneys or reduced sodium delivery to the distal tubules of the kidneys. Raised levels of potassium and reduced levels of sodium in the blood are also known to have a direct effect on the adrenal cortex and stimulate the release of mineralocorticoids. However, in response to a severe, non-specific stressor, hypothalamic release of CRH stimulates the increased release of ACTH. This increase in ACTH stimulates a slight increase in the release of aldosterone, leading to a slight increase in blood volume and pressure, which will help to maintain delivery of oxygen and nutrients to the tissues.

Glucocorticoids

There appears to be no cell within the body that does not have receptors for the glucocorticoid hormones. The glucocorticoid hormones have several effects.

- They influence the metabolism of most body cells.
- They promote **glycogen** storage in the liver.
- During fasting they stimulate the generation of glucose.
- They increase blood glucose levels.
- They are involved in providing resistance to stressors.
- They potentiate the vasoconstrictor effect of catecholamines.
- They decrease the permeability of vascular endothelium.
- They promote the repair of damaged tissues by promoting the breakdown of stored protein to create amino acids.
- They suppress the immune system.
- They suppress inflammatory processes.

The glucocorticoid hormones include:

- cortisol (hydrocortisone)
- cortisone
- corticosterone.

Only cortisol is secreted in any significant amounts. Cortisol is normally released in a rhythmical pattern, with most being released shortly after the person gets up from sleep and the lowest amount being released just before, and shortly after, sleep commences.

Cortisol release is stimulated by ACTH from the anterior pituitary gland. ACTH releases cholesterol from the **cytoplasm** in the cells, which is then converted and modified to create the steroid hormones. ACTH secretion is regulated by the release of CRH from the hypothalamus. Increasing levels of cortisol have a negative feedback effect on both the hypothalamus and the pituitary gland, inhibiting further release of both CRH and ACTH. However, this negative feedback system can be overridden by acute physiological stress (e.g. trauma, infection or haemorrhage) and mental stress. The increase in sympathetic nervous system activity in response to an acute stress triggers greater CRH release and thus there is a significant increase in subsequent cortisol production (figure 16.13).

CLINICAL CONSIDERATIONS

Glucocorticoid steroids and inflammatory diseases

Synthetic glucocorticoid steroid hormones are used widely in healthcare for the suppression of inflammation in diseases such as arthritis, ulcerative colitis and acute severe asthma. However, after taking glucocorticoid steroids such as prednisolone for a significant length of time (except in asthma inhalers), steroid treatment should be gradually reduced, not stopped suddenly. Trials have shown that a short-term (5 days) course of high-dose prednisolone (60 mg) led to some suppression of ACTH production in children, but this did not require a tapering dose of steroids to prevent hypoadrenalism. However, it is felt that these patients should be counselled as to the potential symptoms of hypoadrenalism and to seek medical aid if these symptoms did appear (Crowley et al. 2014).

The constant intake of synthetic steroids for long-term treatment of inflammatory disease leads to a reduction in the production of steroids by the adrenal cortex (probably due to reduced CRH and ACTH secretion because of negative feedback to the hypothalamus and pituitary gland) and suddenly stopping steroid treatment may leave the patient with reduced levels of glucocorticoid steroids in their blood and may lead to a life-threatening hypoadrenal crisis. Thus, the patient will be advised to take a gradually reducing dose of steroids to allow the hypothalamus, pituitary gland and adrenal glands to respond to the reducing blood levels of steroids.

The need for adherence to the prescribed regimen of any course of steroid medication and advice on what to do in the event of gastrointestinal disease preventing the patient taking their steroids must be impressed on the patient. The patient should also carry a blue 'steroid card' at all times detailing the dose and type of steroid taken so that healthcare professionals can respond appropriately, even when the patient is unconscious.

FIGURE 16.13 Response of the endocrine system to stress

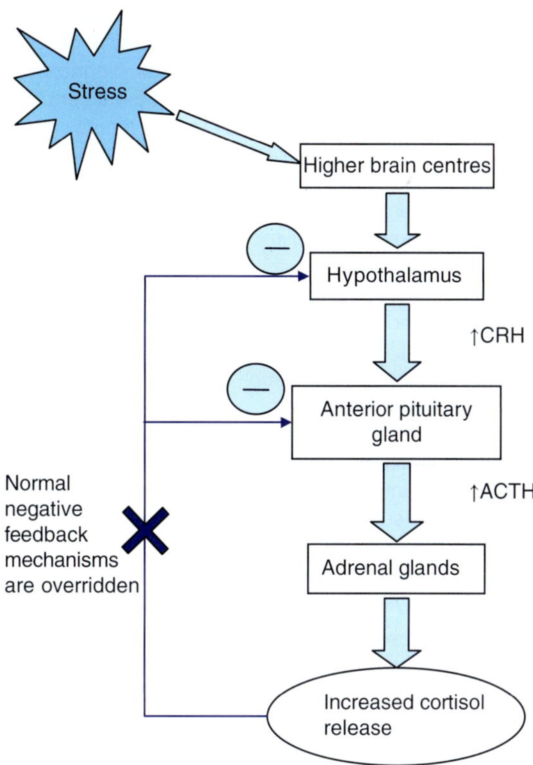

Source: Peate (2017). Reproduced with permission of John Wiley & Sons.

Pancreas

The pancreas is an elongated organ and is found next to the first part of the small intestine. The pancreas is composed of two different types of tissues. The majority of the pancreas is made up of exocrine tissue and the associated ducts. This tissue produces and secretes a fluid rich with digestive enzymes into the small intestine. Scattered throughout the exocrine tissue are many small clusters of cells called islets of Langerhans (islets). These islets are the site of the endocrine cells of the pancreas. Each islet has three major cell types, each of which produces a different hormone:

- alpha cells, which secrete glucagon
- beta cells, the most abundant of the three cell types and which secrete insulin
- delta cells, which secrete somatostatin.

The different cell types within each islet are distributed in a set pattern, with the beta cells being the central portion of the islet, surrounded by alpha and delta cells. The islets are highly vascularised, ensuring rapid transit of the hormones into the bloodstream. Although the islets only account for 1–2 per cent of the mass of the pancreas, they receive about 10–15 per cent of the pancreatic blood flow. The pancreas is innervated by the parasympathetic and sympathetic nervous systems and it is clear that nervous stimulation influences the secretion of insulin and glucagon.

HOMEOSTATIC IMBALANCE

Diabetes mellitus

Diabetes mellitus is a term used to describe a number of conditions, of differing aetiology, that lead to **hyperglycaemia** and impaired glucose tolerance. Type 1 diabetes is an autoimmune disease caused by the destruction of the beta islet cells by the immune system, with onset typically occurring during childhood or adolescence. Type 2 diabetes, on the other hand, is a progressive illness that develops due to a combination of lifestyle and genetic factors affecting the body's ability to respond to normal insulin signalling (insulin resistance) and typically occurs later in life. Over time this insulin resistance leads to an inability to produce sufficient insulin to maintain homeostasis, resulting in hyperglycaemia. If uncontrolled, diabetes mellitus can lead to serious complications such as neurological damage (neuropathy), eye damage (retinopathy), cardiovascular damage, renal damage (nephropathy), impaired healing, increased risk of Alzheimer's disease and damage to blood vessels (angiopathy) (Forbes & Cooper 2013).

Type 1 diabetes occurs in about 10–15 per cent of diabetes diagnoses in Australia and requires treatment using supplemental insulin. Type 2 diabetes occurs in 85–90 per cent of diagnoses in Australia and is an emerging health concern as rates of type 2 diabetes are increasing globally. Type 2 diabetes is largely preventable as the insulin resistance is linked to modifiable lifestyle factors such as a high-fat diet, lack of physical activity and excess body weight. Treatment and prevention of type 2 diabetes is largely centred on lifestyle modifications and improving the quality of the patient's diet. In more severe cases it can also be treated by using supplemental insulin or hypoglycaemic medications such as metformin hydrochloride (Diabetes Australia 2021).

Roughly one million Australians (~4.9%) are currently living with type 2 diabetes, with the highest prevalence appearing in low socioeconomic and remote communities when compared with those living in major cities (Diabetes Australia 2021). This prevalence coupled with the costs associated with treating type 2 diabetes and its associated comorbidities (such as obesity) has made the prevention of type 2 diabetes one of Australia's national health priorities.

Gestational diabetes is the third form of diabetes mellitus and occurs in roughly 7 per cent of pregnancies (American Diabetes Association 2004). Gestational diabetes is caused by insulin resistance arising as a consequence of hormonal interference from the placenta. This insulin resistance requires the mother's pancreas to produce more insulin to try and compensate. As the foetus develops, the insulin demand increases two to threefold mid-pregnancy, and this compensatory insulin production begins to fail, leading to hyperglycaemia (Better Health Channel 2021). In mild cases gestational diabetes is usually treated using dietary and lifestyle changes (e.g. increased physical activity) but can be treated using supplementary insulin if blood glucose levels become too high. Typically, gestational diabetes will disappear rapidly once the baby is born; however, both the mother and baby will have an increased risk of developing type 2 diabetes later in life (Better Health Channel 2021).

CLINICAL CONSIDERATIONS

Type 2 diabetes in Indigenous communities

An area of concern in Australia is the high rate of type 2 diabetes within Indigenous communities. The prevalence is 7.9 per cent in urban centres and 12 per cent in rural and remote communities (Davey 2021). This is further exacerbated by the dietary and lifestyle changes that these communities have experienced since European settlement, including decreased physical activity and increased access to high-fat and calorie-dense foods.

MEDICINES MANAGEMENT

Type 2 diabetes

George is a 56-year-old gentleman who has recently been diagnosed with type 2 diabetes. For the past few months he has noticed that he feels increasingly thirsty and is also constantly tired. George has been reluctant to go to the GP as he does not feel that there is anything really wrong with him and he does not like to bother the doctor anyway. During a routine health screening the practice nurse carries out a dipstick test on George's urine and it is found that there is a significant level of glucose in it. The diagnosis is made of type 2 diabetes; in addition to being educated about lifestyle and dietary changes, George is prescribed metformin.

Metformin is an oral antidiabetic drug that is normally used as the first-line drug in the treatment of type 2 diabetes. It works by reducing the amount of glucose produced by the liver. To try to prevent the development of gastrointestinal side effects the GP has decided to start George on a relatively low dose of metformin and then to slowly increase the dose. If George is unable to tolerate metformin due to gastrointestinal side effects, current guidelines suggest a trial of extended absorption metformin (Health Direct 2021c).

16.4 Insulin

LEARNING OBJECTIVE 16.4 Explain the role of insulin and glucagon in the control of blood glucose levels.

Insulin is well known for its effect in reducing the blood glucose levels. It does this by:

- facilitating the entry of glucose into muscle, adipose tissue and several other tissues; note that the brain and the liver do not require insulin to facilitate the uptake of glucose
- stimulating the liver to store glucose in the form of glycogen.

However, as well as its effects on glucose, insulin is known to have an effect on protein and mineral metabolism. Finally, insulin has an effect on lipid metabolism. As has been noted, insulin promotes the synthesis of glycogen in the liver. As glycogen accumulation in the liver rises to higher levels (5% of the total liver mass), further glycogen synthesis is suppressed. Further uptake of glucose is then diverted by insulin into the production of **fatty acids** and insulin inhibits the breakdown of fat in adipose tissue and facilitates the production of **triglycerides** from glucose for further storage in these tissues.

From a whole-body perspective, insulin has a fat-sparing effect in that it promotes the use of glucose instead of fatty acids and stimulates the storage of fat in the adipose tissue.

The stimulation of insulin synthesis and secretion is primarily a response to a rise in blood glucose levels, but rises in blood levels of amino acids and fatty acids also have a stimulating effect. Some neural stimuli (e.g. the sight and smell of food) also increase insulin secretion. The pancreas is innervated by the sympathetic and parasympathetic nervous systems and nervous stimulation clearly influences the secretion of insulin (and glucagon).

As blood glucose levels fall, there is a corresponding fall in the production and secretion of insulin. When insulin levels in the blood fall, glycogen synthesis in the liver reduces and enzymes that break down glycogen become active. The half-life of insulin is approximately 5 minutes and it is destroyed in the liver.

SKILLS IN PRACTICE

Injecting insulin with a pen

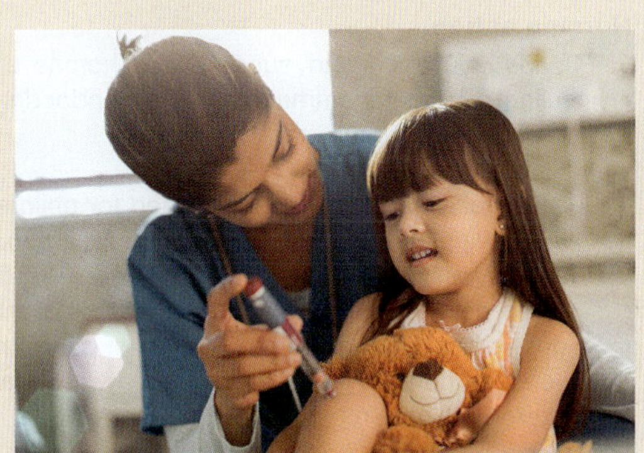

- Follow local policy on medicine administration (right patient, right time and so forth).
- Put a new needle on the pen (reusing needles causes more pain and bruising).
- Remove the cap from the needle.
- Hold the pen upright (needle uppermost) and dial 2–3 units of insulin and press the plunger. Watch for a steady stream of insulin — if a steady stream is not seen then repeat (carrying out an 'air shot' removes bubbles fromthe needle).
- Dial the correct (prescribed) dose.
- Pick an area of soft 'fatty' skin (top of the thigh, stomach, buttock) — in thinner people it may be necessary to pinch a fold of skin to inject into.
- Hold the pen straight and push the needle into the skin.
- Push down the plunger slowly (pushing the plunger too fast can cause pain).
- Hold the pen in place for 10 seconds to ensure the whole dose is delivered.
- Dispose of the needle according to local policy.
- Return the insulin pen to safe storage.

CLINICALLY REASONED EPISODE OF CARE

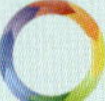

Type 1 diabetes

Consider the patient situation

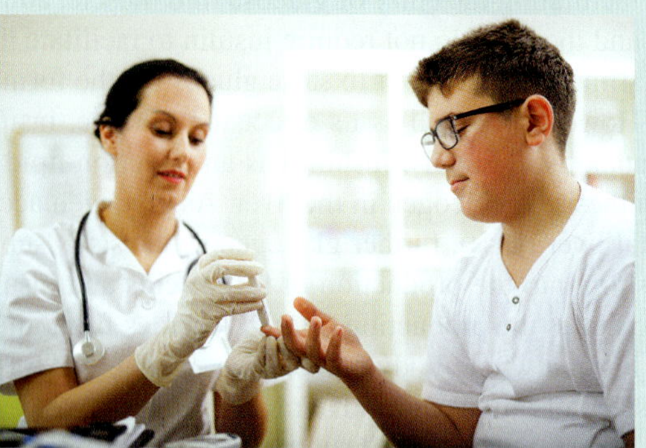

Thomas is a 14-year-old boy who was diagnosed with type 1 diabetes mellitus at the age of 8. Since the onset of puberty, Thomas and his family have found that glucose control has become difficult with repeated episodes of hypoglycaemia and hyperglycaemia.

Collect cues and information

HbA1c: consistently $> 8\%$ — the target is $\leq 7.5\%$ (Phelan et al. 2017).

Process information

Diabetes mellitus is a chronic condition in which glucose is present in the bloodstream in higher levels than is normal. Type 1 diabetes occurs when there is a failure of the cells in the pancreas which produce insulin. The reasons why this happens are complex. These cells never recover, and the person will require insulin injections for the rest of their life. They will also need to monitor their blood glucose levels several times a day.

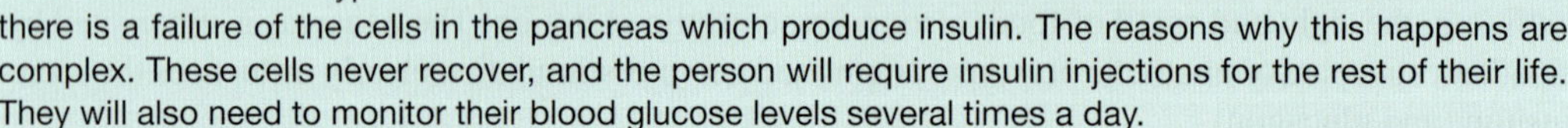

Puberty includes a marked increase in the release of growth hormone, causing the body mass to increase significantly. However, growth hormone also causes cellular resistance to insulin and the liver to release more glucose. This can make the control of blood glucose during this time very difficult.

A person with type 1 diabetes will self-test their blood glucose levels several times a day. They will also have bloods taken every 2–3 months to check the average blood glucose over that time. This is an accurate assessment on which management can be based. An HbA1c result $> 8\%$ indicates that Thomas had a blood glucose average greater than 10.2 mmol/L. The normal blood glucose range is 4–6 mmol/L.

The use of a continuous subcutaneous insulin infusion (CSII) can mitigate some of these issues.

Nursing action

1. Provide education and support for Thomas and his family in the establishment and use of an insulin pump as recommended by the endocrine specialist. This education will include management and troubleshooting.

   Rationale:

   - CSII management is recommended for children and adolescents with type 1 diabetes in Australia (Australian Living Evidence Consortium 2020). The device is a pump unit with a reservoir of short-acting insulin attached to a subcutaneous needle via a thin tube. The use of the pump allows for both timed delivery of insulin at different times of the day and allows the wearer to modify the immediate dose of insulin at any time. The use of pump therapy in children has been associated with a greater sense of control, greater satisfaction with treatment and a greater sense of freedom over diet and exercise (Hussein et al. 2017).

Evaluate outcomes

Thomas and his family report satisfaction with management of the insulin pump. Thomas has an HbA1c result < 7.5 per cent and reports fewer hypoglycaemic episodes.

Source: Based on the Clinical Reasoning Cycle, Levett-Jones (2013).

MEDICINES MANAGEMENT

Insulin

There are more than 20 types of insulin available in four basic forms. Insulin types have three important factors to be considered when prescribing and using them:

1. how soon they start working (onset)
2. when they work the hardest (peak time)
3. how long they last in the body (duration).

The decision as to which insulin to prescribe a patient is based on multiple factors, including the patient's lifestyle and blood glucose levels.

On the ward, insulin is usually stored in the fridge, but cold insulin increases the pain of the injection and slows down the insulin absorption, so for better injection comfort and insulin efficiency it is advisable to take the insulin out of the refrigerator a minimum of 1 hour prior to injection.

Insulin pens

Patients should be advised not to store opened insulin pens in the fridge (especially with the needle attached). Refrigerating a fluid leads to it contracting and warming it up causes it to expand. This is especially dangerous with cloudy insulins. Taking cloudy insulin from the fridge and allowing it to warm in a pen with needle attached can lead to the leakage of either the insulin or the inert carrier fluid, thus changing the strength of the insulin preparation. Leakage into the needle also leads to the formation of insulin crystals, which can block the needle and change the injection pressure or the amount injected.

Taking a pen (and needle) from the warm and putting it into the fridge leads to the contraction of the fluid and the development of air bubbles. Air bubbles are compressible and lengthen injection time. Even after the standard 10 seconds count, insulin can still be leaking from the needle when it is withdrawn.

Unopened pen cartridges are stored in a fridge, but once inserted into an insulin pen the pen should be kept out of the fridge. The insulin can be stored at room temperature for 28 days (NDSS 2020).

Premixed insulins

When a patient (or nurse) is going to administer a cloudy, or premixed, insulin it is important that the pen or vial is rotated end over end 20 times (not shaken), otherwise the insulin may not be mixed correctly (Frid et al. 2010). Research has shown that patients are often confused about this technique and the actual mixing of insulin by patients has a large variation that may be affecting glycaemic control (Frid et al. 2010).

CLINICAL CONSIDERATIONS

Hypoglycaemia

Hypoglycaemia is a constant worry in the patient with diabetes and as many hypoglycaemic episodes are associated with exercise, the fear of hypoglycaemia prevents many patients with diabetes from undertaking regular exercise (Kennedy et al. 2018). This is unfortunate, as exercise is one of the cornerstones in the prevention of diabetes-related complications and aids in the control of diabetes by assisting with weight loss and promoting vascular health (reducing heart attack and stroke risk).

Current guidelines suggest that the promotion of exercise in patients with both type 1 and type 2 diabetes should be associated with guidance on the management of blood glucose level changes linked with exercise. The patient should take their blood glucose before and after exercise and again several hours later. Patients with either very high or very low blood glucose should avoid exercising until the blood glucose has normalised (Kourtoglou 2011). Patients using insulin therapy are advised to either omit the insulin dose prior to exercise or consume a carbohydrate load (such as a carbohydrate drink) before exercise; patients on medication regimens other than insulin are at a much lower risk of exercise hypoglycaemia and do not need to take this precaution (American Diabetes Association 2019).

Any patient with diabetes who is considering exercise as part of their diabetes management should be encouraged, but they should always be advised to consult with their endocrinologist first for advice on the intensity and timing of exercise.

Glucagon

Glucagon has an important role in maintaining normal blood glucose levels, especially as the brain and neurones can only use glucose as a fuel.

Glucagon has the opposite effect on blood glucose levels to insulin (figure 16.14).

- It stimulates the breakdown of glycogen stored in the liver.
- It activates hepatic **gluconeogenesis** (the creation of glucose from substrates such as amino acids).
- It has a minor effect enhancing triglyceride breakdown in adipose tissue — providing fatty acid fuel for most cells and thus conserving glucose for the brain and neurones.

The production and secretion of glucagon are stimulated in response to a reduction in blood glucose concentrations and elevated blood levels of amino acids (e.g. after a protein-rich meal). It has also been found that glucagon levels in the blood rise in response to exercise, but it is unclear whether this is a response to the exercise itself or a response to the reduced blood glucose levels that exercise creates.

FIGURE 16.14 Effects of insulin and glucagon on blood glucose concentrations

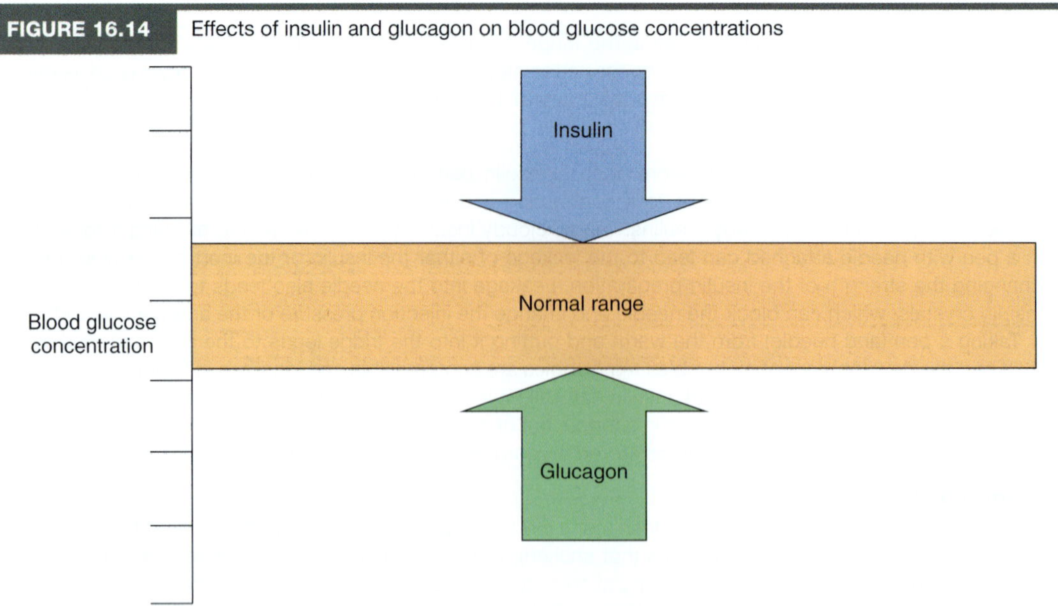

Glucagon production and secretion are inhibited when there are increased glucose levels in the blood; however, it is unknown whether this is a direct effect of the glucose levels or a response to rising levels of insulin, as insulin is known to inhibit the release of glucagon.

Somatostatin

Somatostatin is actually released by a broad range of tissues. Its physiological effect in the pancreas is to inhibit the release of insulin and glucagon; it does this in a paracrine fashion; that is, the hormone is released and has its effect locally. The exact mechanism of control of this hormone is unknown.

SUMMARY

This chapter has introduced the reader to the endocrine system, a diverse system that is one of the two bodily systems necessary for the maintenance of homeostasis. While often working in close conjunction with the nervous system, the endocrine system is often responsible for the control of longer-term processes. The major functions of the endocrine system are based on four main areas:

- the maintenance of homeostasis (especially electrolyte levels and fluid balance)
- metabolism
- growth and development
- responses to stress.

The secretion of hormones can be stimulated by nervous impulses, hormones or changes in the body levels of ions and nutrients; and further regulation of hormone release is then often controlled by negative feedback loops. Hormones can only have an effect on a cell if that cell has a receptor for the hormone; however, there appears to be virtually no cell within the body that is not affected by the endocrine system.

KEY TERMS

amino acids Chemical compound that is the basic building block of proteins and enzymes.
carbohydrates A group of compounds (including starches and sugars) that are a major food source.
catecholamines A collective term for adrenaline, noradrenaline and dopamine.
cortex The outermost layer of an organ.
corticosteroid A steroid hormone released by the adrenal cortex, further divided into glucocorticoids and mineralocorticoids.
cortisol The major glucocorticoid steroid released by the adrenal gland.
cytoplasm The part of the cell enclosed within the cell membrane.
downregulation The reduction in the number of hormone receptors of a cell, often the response of a cell to prolonged periods of high circulating levels of a hormone.
electrolytes A group of chemical elements or compounds that includes sodium, potassium, calcium, chloride and bicarbonate.
fatty acids Dietary fats that have broken down into elements that can be absorbed into the blood.
free T_4 Thyroxine in the blood that is not bound to proteins.
ganglion A mass, or group, of nerve cells.
glands Any organ in the body that secretes substances not related to its own, internal, functioning.
glucocorticoid A group of hormones that exert their major effect on the metabolism of carbohydrates.
gluconeogenesis Creation of new glucose from non-carbohydrate substrates.
glycogen A carbohydrate (complex sugar) made from glucose.
glycogenolysis Breakdown of glycogen to create glucose.
hormonal stimulation Stimulation of a gland that produces a change in the activity of that gland in response to hormones released by other organs.
hormones Chemical substances that are released into the blood by the endocrine system and have a physiological control over the function of cells or organs other than those that created them.
humoral stimulation Stimulation of a gland that produces a change in the activity of that gland in response to changing levels of certain ions and nutrients in the blood.
hyperglycaemia High blood levels of glucose.
hypoglycaemia Low blood levels of glucose.
hypovolaemia Low levels of fluid in the circulation.
ions An atom or group of atoms that carry an electrical charge.
lipid A group of organic compounds, including the fats, oils, waxes, sterols and triglycerides.
medulla The most internal part of an organ.
mineralocorticoids A group of hormones released by the adrenal glands that exert their effect on the electrolytes and water balance in the body.
neural stimulation Stimulation of a gland that produces a change in the activity of that gland in response to direct nervous activity.
osmolality A measure of how much of a substance has dissolved in a solvent.
osteoclasts A type of cell that breaks down bone tissue and thus releases the calcium used to create bones.

substrates Molecules on which an enzyme acts.
triglycerides A form of fatty acid having three fatty acid components.
upregulation The increase of hormone receptors of a cell, usually in response to low circulating levels of a hormone.

CONDITIONS

The following is a list of conditions that are associated with the endocrine system. Take some time and write notes about each of the conditions. You may make the notes taken from textbooks or other resources (e.g. people you work with in a clinical area), or you may make the notes as a result of people you have cared for. If you are making notes about people you have cared for, you must ensure that you adhere to the rules of confidentiality.

Addison's disease
Cushing's disease
Diabetes insipidus
Diabetes mellitus
Graves' disease

REFERENCES

American Diabetes Association (2004) Gestational diabetes mellitus. *Diabetes Care* 27(supplement 1): S88–S90.

American Diabetes Association (2019) Standards of medical care in diabetes — 2019. *Diabetes Care* 42 (supplement 1): S11–S61.

Australian Living Evidence Consortium (2020) Living guidelines for diabetes. https://livingevidence.org.au/new-index-3#Living-Guidelines-for-Diabetes (accessed 6 February 2021).

Better Health Channel (2021) Acromegaly. www.betterhealth.vic.gov.au/health/conditionsandtreatments/acromegaly (accessed 10 January 2021).

Better Health Channel (2021) Diabetes — gestational. www.betterhealth.vic.gov.au/health/conditionsandtreatments/diabetes-gestational (accessed 10 January 2021).

Crowley, R.K., Argese, N., Tomlinson, J.W. and Stewart, P.M. (2014) Central hypoadrenalism. *Journal of Clinical Endocrinology and Metabolism* 99(11): 4027–4036.

Davey, R.X. (2021) Health disparities among Australia's remote-dwelling Aboriginal people: a report from 2020. *JALM* 126: 125–141.

Diabetes Australia (2021) Type 2 diabetes. www.diabetesaustralia.com.au/about-diabetes/type-2-diabetes (accessed 10 February 2021).

Economidou, F., Douka, E., Tzanela, M., Nanas, S. and Kotanidou, A. (2011) Thyroid function during critical illness. *Hormones* 10(2): 117–124.

Forbes, J. M. and Cooper, M. E. (2013) Mechanisms of diabetic complications. *Physiological reviews* 93(1): 137–188.

Frid, A., Hirsch, L., Gaspar, R., Hicks, D., Kreugel, G., Liersch, J. and Strauss, K. (2010) New injection recommendations for patients with diabetes. *Diabetes and Metabolism* 36: S3–S18.

Friedman, B. and Cirulli, J. (2013) Hyponatremia in critical care patients: frequency, outcome, characteristics and treatment with the vasopressin V2 receptor antagonist tolvaptan. *Journal of Critical Care* 28(2): 219.e1–219.e12.

Gross, P. (2012) Clinical management of SIADH. *Therapeutic Advances in Endocrinology and Metabolism* 3(2): 61–73. doi: 10.1177/2042018812437561.

Hall, J.E. and Guyton, A.C. (2016) *Guyton and Hall, Textbook of Medical Physiology,* 13th edn. Philadelphia, PA: Elsevier Saunders.

Health Direct (2021a) Gigantism. www.healthdirect.gov.au/gigantism (accessed 10 January 2021).

Health Direct (2021b) Goitre. www.healthdirect.gov.au/goitre (accessed 10 January 2021).
Health Direct (2021c) Metformin. www.healthdirect.gov.au/metformin (accessed 25 February 2021).
Hussain, T., Akle, M., Nagelkerke, N. and Deeb, A. (2017) Comparative study on treatment satisfaction and health perception in children and adolescents with type 1 diabetes mellitus on multiple daily injection of insulin, insulin pump and sensor-augmented pump therapy. *SAGE Open Medicine.* https://doi.org/10.1177/2050312117694938
Jenkins, G. and Tortora, G.J. (2013) *Anatomy and Physiology: From Science to Life,* 3rd edn. Singapore: John Wiley & Sons.
Kennedy, A., Narendran, P., Andrews, R.C. for the EXTOD Group, et al. (2018) Attitudes and barriers to exercise in adults with a recent diagnosis of type 1 diabetes: a qualitative study of participants in the Exercise for Type 1 Diabetes (EXTOD) study. *BMJ Open* 8: e017813. doi: 10.1136/bmjopen-2017-017813.
Kourtoglou, G.I. (2011) Insulin therapy and exercise. *Diabetes Research and Clinical Practice* 93: S73–S77.
Levett-Jones, T. (2013). *Clinical Reasoning: Learning to Think Like a Nurse.* Pearson Australia.
McDermott, M.T. (2013) *Endocrine Secrets,* 6th edn. Philadelphia, PA. Elsevier Health Sciences.
Mero, A., Campisi, M., Favero, M., Barbera, C., Secchieri, C., Dayer, J.M. and Pasut, G. (2014) A hyaluronic acid-salmon calcitonin conjugate for the local treatment of osteoarthritis: chondro-protective effect in a rabbit model of early OA. *Journal of Controlled Release* 187: 30–38.
Peate, I. (2017) *Fundamentals of Applied Pathophysiology: An Essential Guide for Nursing Students*, 3rd edn. Oxford: John Wiley & Sons, Ltd.
National Diabetes Services Scheme (2020) Insulin. www.ndss.com.au/about-diabetes/resources/find-a-resource/insulin-fact-sheet (accessed 10 February 2021).
Nelson, J.M. and Robinson, M.V. (2012) Hyponatremia in older adults presenting to the emergency department. *International Emergency Nursing* 20(4): 251–254.
Phelan, H., Clapin, H., Bruns, L. et al. (2017) The Australasian Diabetes Data Network: first national audit of children and adolescents with type 1 diabetes. *MJA* 206(3): 121–125.
Tortora, G.J. and Derrickson, B.H. (2009) *Principles of Anatomy and Physiology,* 12th edn. Hoboken, NJ: John Wiley & Sons, Inc.
Vilar, L., Vilar, C.F., Lyra, R., Lyra, R. and Naves, L.A. (2017) Acromegaly: clinical features at diagnosis. *Pituitary* 20(1): 22–32.
Weetman, A. (2013) Current choice of treatment for hypo-and hyperthyroidism. *Prescriber* 24(13–16): 23–33.

FURTHER READING

AUSTRALIAN ADDISON'S DISEASE ASSOCIATION INC.

https://addisons.org.au

The Australian Addison's Disease Association Inc. is a charity that aims to provide information about Addison's disease to patients, families and professionals. There are many publications on the site.

AUSTRALIAN THYROID FOUNDATION

https://thyroidfoundation.org.au

The Australian Thyroid Foundation is a charity dedicated to helping people with thyroid disorders and their families.

DIABETES AUSTRALIA

www.diabetesaustralia.com.au

Diabetes Australia is the country's leading charity for people with diabetes. As well as providing information for patients and their families, it is also a pressure group, campaigning both for better diabetes care and funding diabetes research.

ACKNOWLEDGEMENTS

Photo: © SrsPvl Witch / Shutterstock.com
Photo: © pixelheadphoto digitalskillet / Shutterstock.com
Photo: © JCREATION / Shutterstock.com
Photo: © Karan Bunjean / Shutterstock.com
Photo: © Science Photo Library / Shutterstock.com
Photo: © fizkes / Shutterstock.com
Photo: © Hoxton / Getty Images

CHAPTER 17

The immune system

TEST YOUR PRIOR KNOWLEDGE

- How do the T-helper and T-suppressor cells work together in helping to control the immune system?
- Which cells are involved in humoral immunity?
- Discuss the role of immunoglobulin E (IgE) in fighting infections.
- Identify the organs of the lymphatic system.
- What is meant by phagocytosis?

LEARNING OUTCOMES

After reading this chapter you will be able to:

17.1 describe and discuss the development of white blood cells and their roles in immunity

17.2 explain how the immune system works to protect us from infections, listing the various barriers used to prevent infectious organisms from entering the body

17.3 explain the process of phagocytosis and explain how inflammation works to protect the body

17.4 describe and discuss cellular and humoral immunity

17.5 explain the body's response to infection and the rationale for immunisations.

Body map

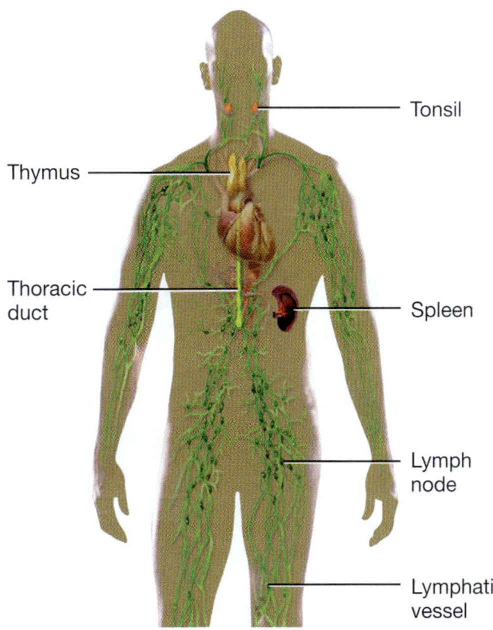

Introduction

Our bodies are continuously under attack from organisms that are out to destroy it. This may sound dramatic, but it is true. Infectious microorganisms, toxins and pollutants are some of the harmful substances from which it needs to defend itself. Fortunately, the body has evolved and developed many defences to repel and destroy these harmful substances — this is what we call the immune system.

The immune system is a complicated and wonderful system that underpins so much of our understanding of disease and disease processes. This applies not only to those diseases caused by infectious microorganisms, but also many others, including cancer, arthritis, stress, and so on.

This chapter will show what the body's immunological defences consist of and how they work together to give the body an opportunity of surviving the continuous assaults by microorganisms, toxins and other pollutants.

17.1 Blood cell development

LEARNING OBJECTIVE 17.1 Describe and discuss the development of white blood cells and their roles in immunity.

All our blood cells are descended from multipotent **stem cells**, which have the ability to switch to different types of cells. In terms of the immune system, the blood cells that form a substantial part of the immune system are the white blood cells, of which there are two major branches. One branch develops into the myeloid family of cells, which include the **neutrophils** and **monocytes**, and the other branch develops into the lymphoid family of cells, made up of **lymphocytes**. Figure 17.1 shows the development of the white blood cells from the initial multipotent stem cell.

FIGURE 17.1 The development of blood cells

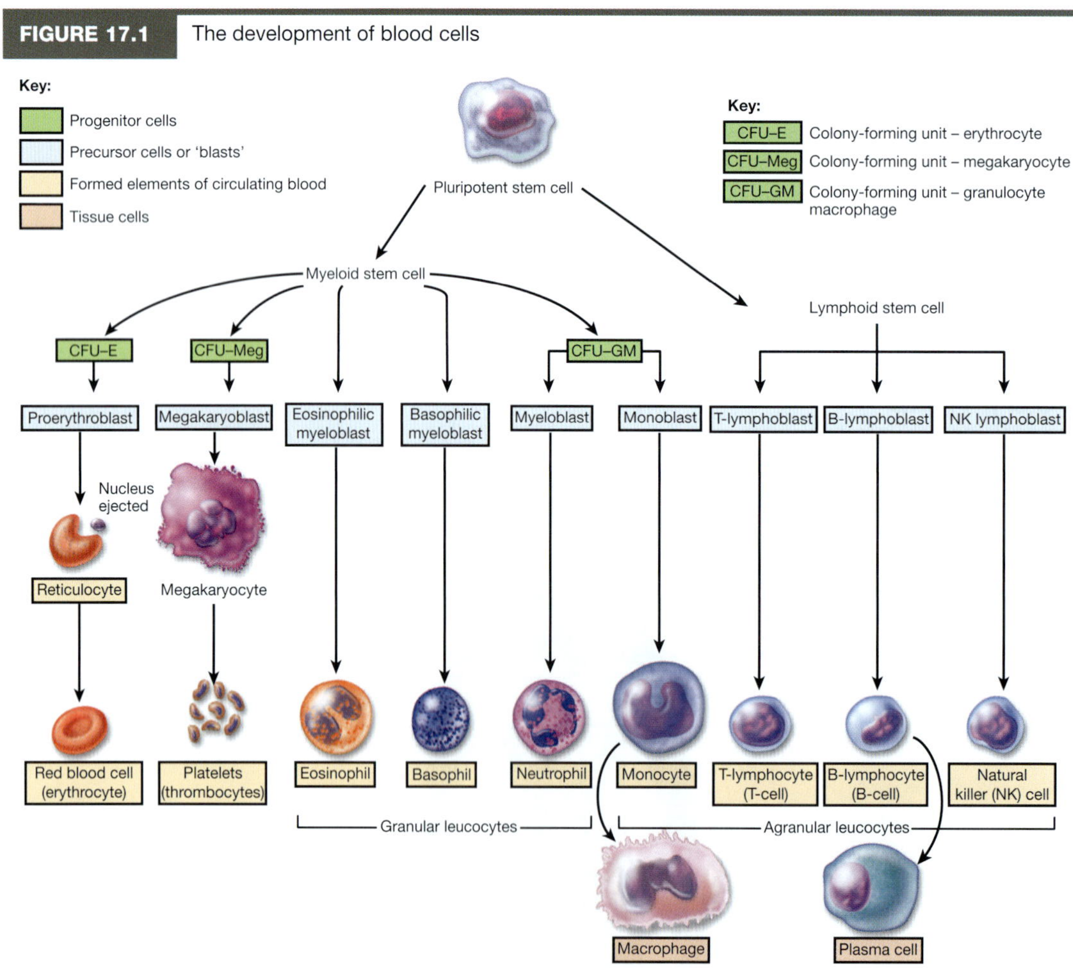

Source: Tortora and Derrickson (2009). Reproduced with permission of John Wiley & Sons.

It can be seen from the family tree of blood cells that the myeloid family includes the **macrophages** (monocytes and tissue macrophages) and **granulocytes** (neutrophils, **eosinophils** and **basophils**). The lymphoid branch of white blood cells gives us T-lymphocytes and B-lymphocytes (with many of the B-lymphocytes developing into **plasma cells**). The myeloid branch also provides us with megakaryocytes (leading to **platelets**) and erythroid cells, which develop into erythrocytes (i.e. **red blood cells**). Red blood cells and platelets are discussed in the chapter on the circulatory system.

All the white blood cells arise initially in the **bone marrow** as stem cells, but, as they slowly mature through their various stages, they are found in different places around the body, including:

- the blood and **lymph** circulation
- the **thymus**
- the **spleen**
- the **tonsils** and other **lymph nodes**.

They are also found in all the mucosal membranes, such as the lining of the mouth and the gastro intestinal tract.

17.2 Organs of the immune system

LEARNING OBJECTIVE 17.2 Explain how the immune system works to protect us from infections, listing the various barriers used to prevent infectious organisms from entering the body.

The main organs of the immune system are all part of the **lymphatic system** consisting of:

- the thymus
- the spleen
- the lymph nodes
- the lymphoid tissues scattered throughout the gastrointestinal, respiratory and urinary tracts.

The thymus

The thymus is located in the chest (figure 17.2), and in babies it is a large organ (relative to size) playing a major role in the development of competent immunological cells. It shrinks (atrophies) with age.

FIGURE 17.2 Position of the thymus within the body

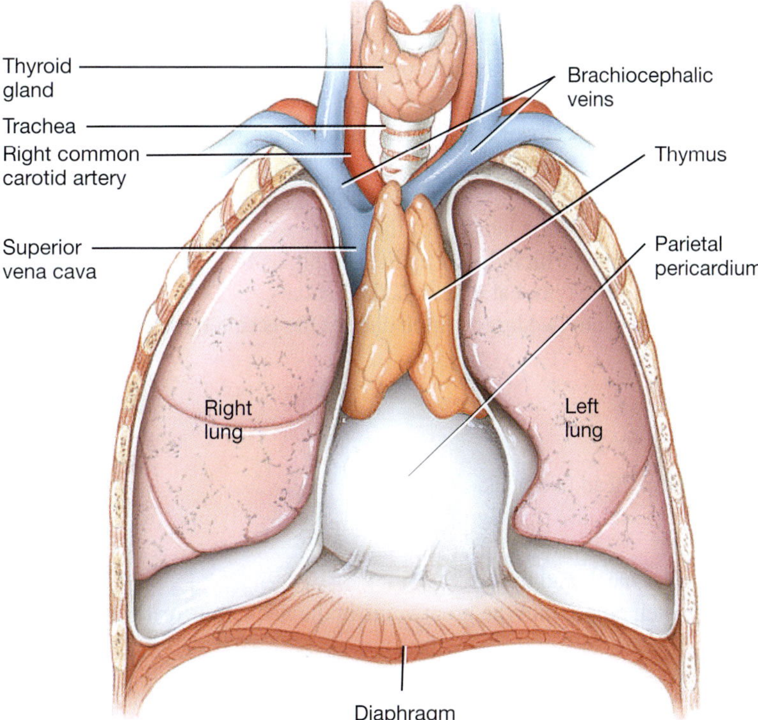

Source: Tortora and Derrickson (2009). Reproduced with permission of John Wiley & Sons.

Within the thymus, certain blood stem cells mature and differentiate into various **T-cell lymphocyte** subclasses. In addition, they also acquire the ability to recognise and differentiate 'self' cells from 'non-self' cells — an important role in cell-mediated responses to an **antigen**, the continued production of T-cells throughout life and the development of an immunological memory.

'Self' cells originate and belong to the individual with that thymus, while 'non-self' cells come from outside of the individual such as from contact with viruses and bacteria. T-cells that recognise self-antigens are destroyed.

The lymphatic system

The lymphatic system is a specialised system of **lymph vessels** (similar to blood vessels) and lymph nodes. The lymphatic vessels contain lymph, a fluid formed from the plasma that leaks from blood capillaries into the interstitial space. This fluid is then collected by the lymph capillaries from where it drains into the larger lymphatic vessels and the organs of the lymphatic system.

Lymphocytes migrate from the blood system by passing through the walls of the smallest capillaries in the lymph nodes. Lymphocytes spend only a few minutes in the bloodstream during each circuit of the body, but, in contrast, spend several hours in the lymphoid system.

The lymphatic system can be thought of as a parallel system to the circulatory system, except that it does not have a pump like the heart. Instead, the lymph is moved around the body by a combination of the smooth muscle contraction (in the walls of the lymph vessels) and the contraction and relaxation of skeletal muscle during both movement and breathing in combination, which is facilitated by the presence of valves in the larger lymphatic vessels. This occurs in a similar way to blood movement through the venous system.

The peripheral lymphatic system (figure 17.3) is made up of lymphatic vessels and lymphatic capillaries, as well as encapsulated organs (i.e. organs that are situated within their own 'capsule').

These include:

- spleen
- tonsils
- lymph nodes.

The lymphatic system also includes unencapsulated (not bound by a capsule, but more diffuse) lymphoid tissue in the gastrointestinal tract (Peyer's patches), the urogenital tract and the lungs.

The lymph vessels and capillaries form a network throughout the body and connect the tissues of the body to the lymphoid organs, such as the spleen, and the lymph nodes.

Lymphatic capillaries have some anatomical similarities to blood capillaries in that their walls consist of a layer of endothelial cells. However, lymphatic capillary walls do not have a basement membrane. This lack of a basement membrane allows relatively large molecules, such as plasma proteins, to enter the lymphatic capillaries between the cells of the capillary walls.

Lymph flows through the vessels by means of:

- muscle contraction in the limbs
- the pulsing of arteries (caused by the beating of the heart)
- negative intrathoracic pressure (which draws up the lymph, as from a vacuum)
- the rhythmic contraction of the lymphatic vessels themselves.

The lymph eventually flows into two large lymph ducts. One is called the thoracic duct, and this receives lymph from:

- the lower limbs
- the digestive tract
- the left arm
- the left side of the thorax, head and neck.

The other large lymph vessel, the right lymphatic duct, receives lymph from:

- the right arm
- the right side of the head, neck and thorax.

The two lymph ducts then empty into the great veins in the neck, thus restoring fluid and proteins to the venous circulation.

FIGURE 17.3 Principal components of the lymphatic system

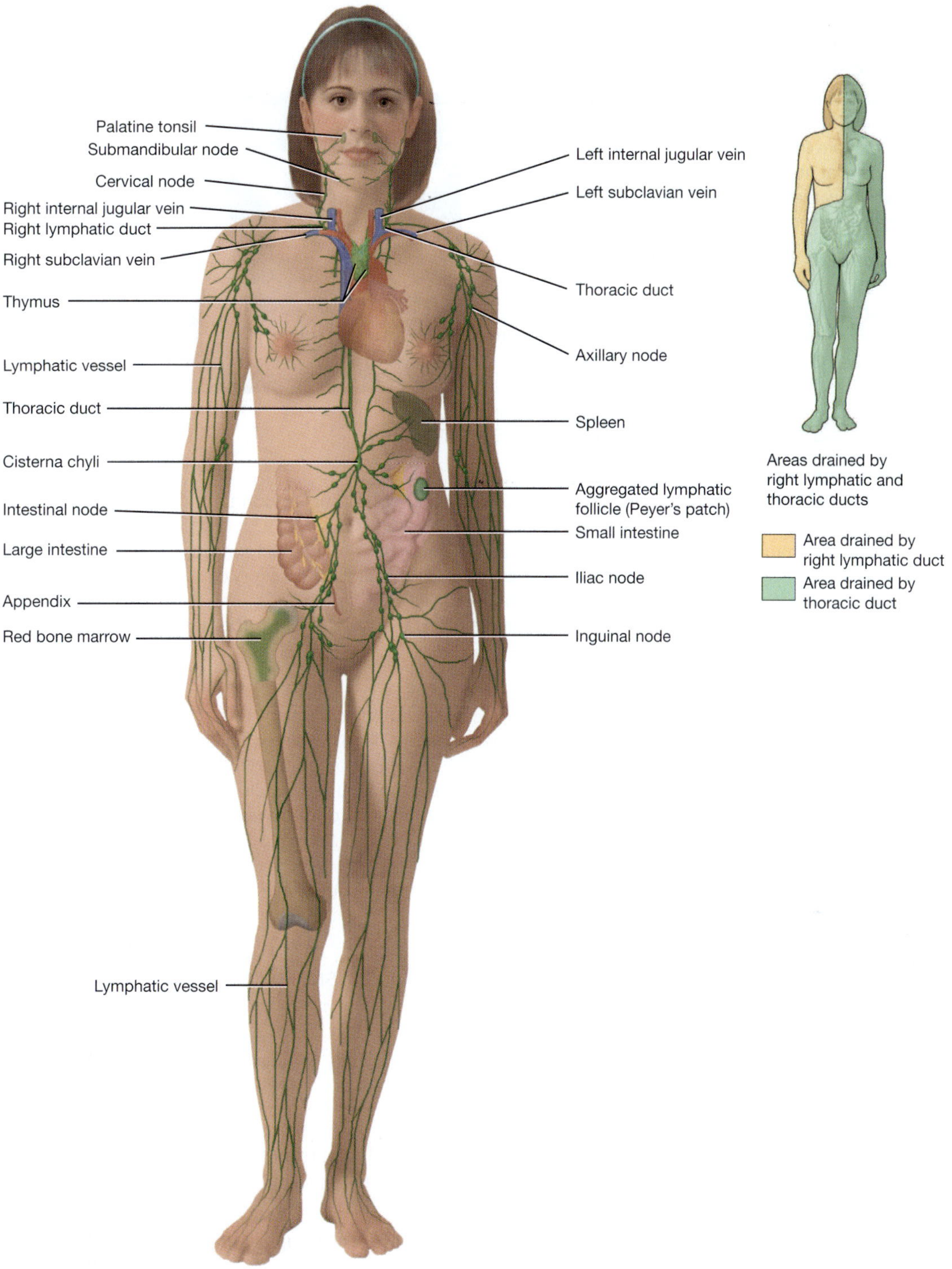

Palatine tonsil
Submandibular node
Cervical node
Right internal jugular vein
Right lymphatic duct
Right subclavian vein
Thymus
Lymphatic vessel
Thoracic duct
Cisterna chyli
Intestinal node
Large intestine
Appendix
Red bone marrow
Lymphatic vessel
Left internal jugular vein
Left subclavian vein
Thoracic duct
Axillary node
Spleen
Aggregated lymphatic follicle (Peyer's patch)
Small intestine
Iliac node
Inguinal node

Areas drained by right lymphatic and thoracic ducts
Area drained by right lymphatic duct
Area drained by thoracic duct

Source: Tortora and Derrickson (2009). Reproduced with permission of John Wiley & Sons.

CLINICALLY REASONED EPISODE OF CARE

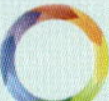

Epstein–Barr virus (EBV)

Consider the patient situation

Sally, a 14-year-old schoolgirl, has been sent home from school as she is feeling unwell and complaining of a sore throat and headache. Despite resting for 2 days at home and taking regular paracetamol, Sally is now feeling worse. Sally's mother takes her to the clinic and sees the nurse practitioner.

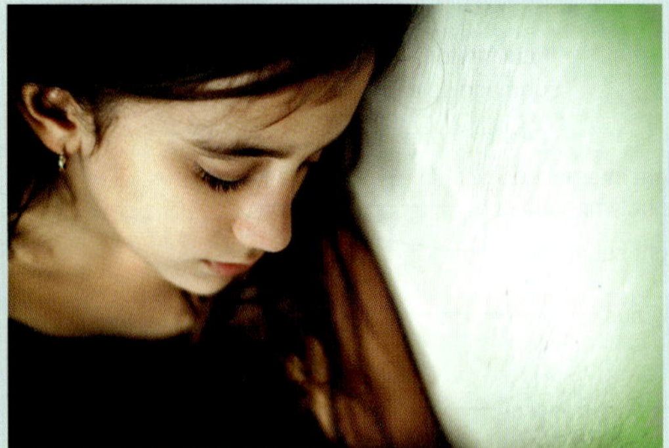

Collect cues and information

Physical examination: Sally's cervical glands are swollen, and she is finding it difficult to move her neck from side to side. She has a high temperature and is feeling tired and listless.

Sally has bloods taken to confirm or rule out a provisional diagnosis of glandular fever (infectious mononucleosis) due to contact with the Epstein–Barr virus (EBV).

Process information

EBV belongs to the herpes group of viruses; once acquired, it remains dormant in the body for the individual's lifetime.

EBV is a common illness that is easily contracted through close contact with saliva of an infected individual (hence it is also known as kissing disease) or using the utensils/crockery of an infected individual. In individuals with no other underlying disease, the illness is self-limiting.

Confirmation of the virus is made by undertaking a blood test to look for **antibodies** to EBV. If positive, this indicates a current, recent or past exposure to EBV.

Nursing action

1. Provide education and support to Sally and her family about her condition. This education will include:
   - minimising transmission risk (NSW Health 2012) — careful handwashing with soap and running water, especially after sneezing and coughing and before touching other people; avoiding saliva contact (e.g. kissing) with people who are sick with infectious mononucleosis; cleaning soiled objects with soap and water, such as toys of sick children; and not sharing drink containers
   - symptom management — rest, drinking adequate fluids, fever and pain management with simple analgaesia
   - advice on avoiding high contact sports for at least 6 months due to risk of spleen rupture as virally induced spleen enlargement is a possibility.

Evaluate outcomes

As a result of the nursing actions above, Sally recovers from EBV. She is careful to avoid high contact sports during her recovery period.

Source: Based on the Clinical Reasoning Cycle, Levett-Jones (2013).

Lymph nodes

Lymph enters the lymph nodes from the afferent lymphatic vessels and from there it goes to the **trabeculae**. Afferent means 'leading towards'; therefore, in the case of lymph nodes, afferent vessels are those vessels that lead towards the lymph node.

The lymph node is made up of a mesh of cells — just like a net. The lymph at this stage contains antigens from infected cells and tissues. This lymph passes through this mesh in the lymph node and the antigens are trapped (figure 17.4).

Antigens entering the body at any point are rapidly swept along the lymph vessels towards a lymphoid organ or lymph node.

Within the lymph node, **B-cell lymphocytes** are located in the primary lymphoid follicles as well as the secondary lymphoid follicles (which contain the germinal centres), and it is inside these germinal centres that the B-cells proliferate after encountering their specific antigen and its cooperating T-helper cell. The B-cells at the centre of the secondary lymphoid follicles are actively dividing, while those at the periphery are antibody forming.

FIGURE 17.4 Structure of a lymph node

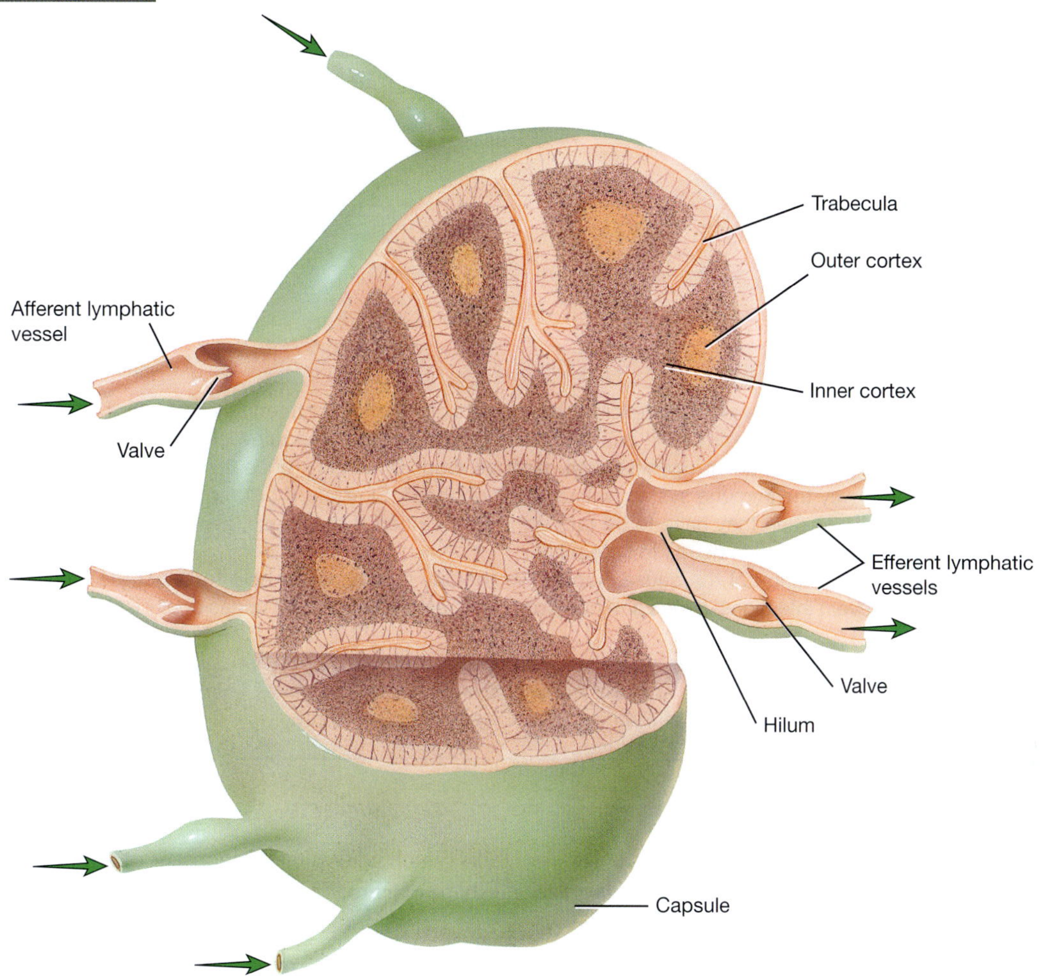

Source: Nair and Peate (2009). Reproduced with permission of John Wiley & Sons.

In addition, large numbers of phagocytic macrophages and plasma cells producing antibodies are found in the **medulla** of the gland. Macrophages and other antigen-presenting cells spend most of their lives migrating through the tissues until they encounter antigens. These are then phagocytosed (engulfed by **phagocytes** and 'eaten') and transported to the nearest lymph node.

Macrophages in the lymph node also encounter trapped antigens within the meshwork of reticular cells, and they phagocytose the dead cells and bacteria and present the antigens from these on their cell surface for recognition by lymphocytes. The lymph that has passed through the lymph nodes then leaves through the efferent lymphatic vessel. Efferent means 'to lead away from'.

CLINICAL CONSIDERATIONS

Secondary immunodeficiencies

Secondary immunodeficiencies are disorders that result in an increased susceptibility to infection due to another illness, age, injury, environmental poisons or treatment. Almost all serious illnesses are associated with some impairment of one or more components of the immune system.

One of the major causes of immunodeficiency globally is protein deficiency due to malnutrition or to such disorders as Kwashiorkor disease. In developed countries, the major causes of secondary immunodeficiencies are iatrogenic (apart from HIV); that is, they are caused by medical personnel/treatment. These particularly include immunodeficiencies that occur following steroid or cytotoxic drug therapy for various diseases.

Someone with a secondary immunodeficiency will have a susceptibility to opportunistic infections, anorexia, diarrhoea and an increased risk of cancer.

Secondary immunodeficiencies are associated with a multitude of factors including:

- infections — for example, HIV, hepatitis, measles, mumps, TB, congenital rubella, cytomegalovirus and infectious mononucleosis (glandular fever)
- medications — for example, steroids, cytotoxic drugs and immunosuppressive drugs, and even antibiotics, as well as alcohol, cocaine and heroin
- stress — psychological and physical stress
- malnutrition
- cancers
- autoimmune diseases
- ageing
- environmental chemicals
- burns and other traumas
- pregnancy
- anaesthesia and surgery
- radiation.

The treatment of secondary immunodeficiencies consists of removing or treating the cause (if possible) and supportive therapy. For example, if an infection is the cause, then the relevant antimicrobial drugs need to be given. If there is an iatrogenic cause, such as drugs or surgery, once these are stopped and recovery is under way the immune system will usually right itself. Similarly, if other diseases are causing the immunodeficiency, then they have to be tackled. If malnutrition is the cause, then the solving of the problem leading to malnutrition needs to take place.

Along with the elimination of the cause, supportive therapy is required to help to boost the immune system and to prevent infections. Drugs and nutrition, changes of lifestyle, and occasionally isolation may be necessary.

Secondary immunodeficiencies are often transient, and supportive therapy is usually only necessary until the cause has been dealt with and the immune system starts to recover. Unfortunately, however, there are some secondary immunodeficiencies to which this does not apply.

Lymphoid tissue

As well as lymphatic vessels, the lymphatic system contains lymphoid tissue. This consists of lymph glands (i.e. lymph nodes), which are approximately the size and shape of a broad bean, and lymphoid tissue, found in specific organs, particularly:

- the spleen
- the bone marrow
- the lungs
- the liver
- other lymphoid tissue.

The spleen

The spleen is situated just behind the stomach and is about the size of a fist. It collects antigens from the blood for presentation to phagocytes and lymphocytes, and also collects, and disposes of, dead red blood cells.

In summary, the lymphoid systems play a key role in the immune system by enabling lymphocytes to protect the tissues and vessels of the body from infectious microorganisms. It achieves this by holding microorganisms in antigen 'traps' in the lymph nodes and other lymphoid organs, and it brings them into close proximity with other immune cells. This allows for the cell-to-cell communication required to recruit, direct and regulate a coordinated immune response. Lymph glands are the major centres for lymphocyte proliferation and antibody production, as well as for filtering the lymph.

Types of immunity

There are two major types of **immunity**: the innate and the acquired.

Innate immunity is the immunity we possess at birth, so it is innate in all of us. On the other hand, **acquired immunity** is not present at birth; instead, it is something acquired as we go through life.

Innate immunity is the oldest type of immunity and is present in all creatures, whereas the second type of immunity, acquired immunity, is only found in more developed organisms, such as humans.

Another name for innate immunity is non-specific immunity. This means that these defences come into action no matter what infectious or non-self antigen is present or trying to attack us; therefore, they are non-specific. Similarly, acquired immunity is also known as specific immunity because it responds to known specific antigens or organisms.

The innate immune system

Many parts of the body, as well as the white blood cells, combine to make up the innate immune system.

It is possible to categorise the innate immune system into four groups, although some parts may use more than one class of defence:

- physical barriers
- mechanical barriers
- chemical barriers
- blood cells.

Physical barriers

These include the skin and mucosal membranes. The skin acts as a physical barrier to prevent infectious organisms and other substances from gaining access to the more 'at risk' and undefended organs within our body. However, not only is skin a physical barrier, but it is also a chemical barrier, in that sweat produced from the skin is **bactericidal** (dangerous for bacteria). However, skin also has weak spots, namely the various orifices that connect the internal body to the outside, such as the mouth, nose, external urethral opening and anus.

Mechanical barriers

In this category are included cilia, coughing, sneezing and tears.

- Cilia are the tiny hairs found in the nose. They are constantly beating and moving dirt, microorganisms and mucus away to the adenoids (made of lymphatic tissue) where they can be dealt with.
- Sneezing and coughing work by expelling any microorganisms or irritants out of the body and into the external atmosphere. So, if someone has a cold or a cough and sneezes or coughs, millions of viruses are expelled into the atmosphere, which means that there are fewer viruses in that person's body to cause even worse problems. This is very effective for the infected person, but means that there are many viruses in the tiny droplets suspended in the air, just waiting for someone else to come along and breathe them in, thereby becoming infected themselves.
- Tears are also a mechanical barrier. Tears wash any dirt particles or microorganisms away from the eyes (like a windscreen washer in a car). Tears are also a chemical barrier because they contain a bactericidal enzyme known as lysozyme. Lysozyme will crop up quite a lot in the section on the innate immune system.

Chemical barriers

Chemical barriers include tears, breastmilk, sweat, saliva, acidic secretions including stomach acid, and semen.

Most of these secretions contain either bactericidal enzymes, such as lysozyme, or antibodies. In addition, bacteria cannot survive in acidic secretions.

Blood cells

As well as the previously mentioned defences, the innate system includes certain blood cells, namely **leucocytes** (white cells) and **thrombocytes** (platelets).

The white cells involved in the innate immune system are:

- neutrophils (making up 60 per cent of the leucocytes in the body)
- monocytes and tissue macrophages (making up a total of 3 per cent of leucocytes)
- eosinophils (making up only 1 per cent of leucocytes)
- basophils (also making up only 1 per cent of leucocytes).

The neutrophils, eosinophils and basophils are also known as granulocytes, because when seen through a powerful microscope they appear to be full of little granules (or grains). In fact, these granules are vacuoles, or empty spaces, within the cells, and are very important when looking at one particular function of these white cells, namely **phagocytosis**.

Blood cells of the immune system

These, as mentioned previously, are the white blood cells. There are three main activities of the white blood cells.

- *Phagocytosis*. This is the destruction of infectious organisms/non-self matter by engulfing and then ingesting them/it. This will be explained a little later in this chapter.

- ***Cytotoxicity***. Cyto means 'cell' and toxicity means 'poisonous' or, in immunological terms, 'lethal to'. So, cytotoxicity is the action that some types of white cells take in killing infected cells or infectious organisms by damaging their cell membranes (see also complement system).
- ***Inflammation***. White cells are very much involved in the response of body tissue to infection and injury.

There are many other roles that white cells play within the immune system, and these will be discussed throughout this chapter. Table 17.1 provides a summary of the blood cells and their role in the immune system.

The three main functions of the immune cells are as follows.

TABLE 17.1 Summary of blood cells and their roles within the immune system

Cells involved in the innate immune system	
Natural killer cells	Kill (apoptosis) of virally infected cells
Neutrophils	Phagocytosis
Macrophages	Phagocytosis
Tissue **mast cells**	Release histamine and other inflammatory mediators
Cells involved in the adaptive immune system	
B-lymphocytes	Produce plasma cells which secrete **immunoglobulins** (antibodies)
T-lymphocytes	Release **cytokines** when activated, kill (apoptosis) virally infected cells

17.3 Phagocytosis

LEARNING OBJECTIVE 17.3 Explain the process of phagocytosis and explain how inflammation works to protect the body.

The cells that make up our innate immunity have two major functions: they are either phagocytes or mediator cells.

The phagocytes are cells that devour infectious organisms that have managed to get through the other innate immune defences previously mentioned.

There are two types of phagocytes: mononuclear phagocytes and polymorphonuclear phagocytes.

Mononuclear phagocytes include monocytes and macrophages. They are called mononuclear because the nuclei of the cells are single round blobs (or spheres) when looked at through a microscope; in other words, they have a clearly defined single nucleus; neutrophils, on the other hand, make up the polymorphonuclear phagocytes.

When looked at through a microscope, the nuclei of neutrophils are seen as a blob which can take many shapes, hence poly (many) morpho (shape) nucleocyte (cell nucleus) — in other words, polymorphonucleocyte.

CLINICALLY REASONED EPISODE OF CARE

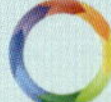

Neutropenia

Consider the patient situation

Jerome is a 33-year-old man living with paranoid schizophrenia. He presents to the hospital with a fever and productive cough.

Collect cues and information

Jerome was recently diagnosed with paranoid schizophrenia and has been taking clozapine for approximately four months. Jerome has recently complained of feeling feverish, unwell and having a productive cough. A recent blood test has indicated that Jerome's white blood cells (neutrophils) are low at 0.8 x 10^9/L.

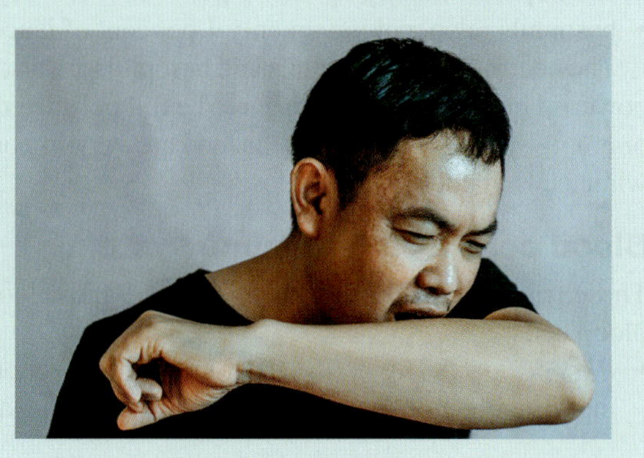

Jerome is diagnosed with a chest infection, secondary to a reduced immune system due to his clozapine. He is admitted to the medical ward for treatment.

Process information

Clozapine is a form of antipsychotic medication used to treat schizophrenia, and in particular treatment-resistant schizophrenia. In some circumstances, patients taking clozapine can develop neutropenia — this occurs in approximately 0.9–3.8 per cent of patients, with the peak incidence occurring at one month post commencement.

Neutrophils are a type of white blood cell which make up the majority of circulating white blood cells and serve as the primary defence against infections by destroying bacteria, bacterial fragments and immunoglobulin-bound viruses in the blood. Neutropenia is characterised by neutrophil levels falling below 1500/mm^3.

Neutropenia can occur for many reasons including exposure to certain toxins and using certain medications. Jerome has no other history of causative factors; therefore it is assumed that he has become neutropenic due to the medication he is taking, as psychotropic drugs (of which clozapine is one) can cause bone marrow suppression, consequently affecting the production of blood cells and leaving the person vulnerable to opportunistic infection. Other medications that can cause neutropenia include cancer treatments, antibiotics and cardiovascular agents.

Neutropenia treatment is dependent on the cause and will usually include cessation of the contributing medications and commencement of antibiotics to treat infection.

Establish goals

1. Commencement of antibiotic treatment
2. Cessation of clozapine and commencement of alternative antipsychotic
3. Monitoring of treatment and condition

Nursing actions

1. Commence antibiotic treatment.
   Rationale:
   - Given Jerome's neutropenia and reduced immunity, antibiotic treatment is a priority and should be administered within 60 minutes.
   - Antibiotic treatment will be administered intravenously at regular intervals on the ward. Standard infection control precautions, such as hand hygiene, gloves and mask, are required when caring for Jerome.
   - Nurses will need to monitor intravenous therapy closely for reaction, efficacy and clinical deterioration as the risk of deterioration with febrile neutropenia is high.
   - Patients should be in a single room with their own ensuite to limit the risk of contamination and infection.
2. Monitor the cessation of clozapine and commencement of olanzapine.
   Rationale:
   - A decision has been made to cease Jerome's clozapine due to his neutrophil count. Usually, clozapine is decreased slowly; however, Jerome's neutrophils are too low to continue.
   - In abrupt cessation, the patient should be monitored for rebound psychosis and cholinergic rebound including headache, nausea, vomiting and diarrhoea.
   - Nurses can monitor this via regular observation and assessment including vital signs, pain scale, Glasgow coma scale and other assessment tools.
   - The introduction of an alternative antipsychotic is clinically indicated.
   - Commencement of a new medication, olanzapine, will require monitoring by the nurse. Side effects of this medication include feeling lightheaded and dizzy; therefore there is an increased risk of falls.
3. Regularly monitor and assess condition.
   Rationale:
   - Jerome is unwell with an acute chest infection, lowered immune system and adjustment of medications for his paranoid schizophrenia; therefore he is at risk of clinical deterioration.
   - Regular monitoring of medical and psychological issues is required by the nursing team.
   - Jerome will require frequent and timely observations and treatments, including regular blood tests to ensure that he recovers from his chest infection and does not relapse into psychosis or have any other clinical deterioration.

Evaluate outcomes

As a result of the interventions above, Jerome recovers from his chest infection and adjusts to olanzapine. After one week of treatment, he is discharged from hospital under the care of his GP.

Reflect on new processes and learning

Reflect on the role of the biopsychosocial model of care. How would such a model support nurses in caring for Jerome and his family?

Source: Based on the Clinical Reasoning Cycle, Levett-Jones (2013).

The role of a phagocytic cell is to phagocytose, or consume, any infectious organism or non-self matter that overcomes the external barriers. This process is known as phagocytosis, and it works as follows.

- *Stage 1*. A bacterium approaches a phagocyte — in this case a neutrophil (figure 17.5). It is held in place by **opsonins** — **complement factors** or antibodies (immunoglobulins). Opsonins prepare the bacterium for being digested by the phagocyte by firmly holding the bacterium to the phagocyte so that it cannot escape.
- *Stage 2*. As the bacterium binds to the neutrophil, the neutrophil recognises that it is 'non-self' matter and it sends out **pseudopodia** (false arms) and starts to surround the bacterium (figure 17.6).
- *Stage 3*. Once surrounded by the phagocyte, the bacterium comes into contact with the vacuoles (as mentioned above). A vesicle completely surrounds the bacterium and kills it, and then breaks it up by means of bactericidal enzymes such as lysozyme. The phagocyte then uses what it can from the bacterium for its own functions (e.g. growth, nutrition) and ejects the parts that it cannot use and presents any foreign antigens to the cells of the adaptive immune system. This is the process of phagocytosis (figure 17.7).

As well as bacteria, phagocytes also remove pus and other infected matter, as well as any other non-self matter that has found its way into the body.

FIGURE 17.5 Phagocytosis (stage 1)

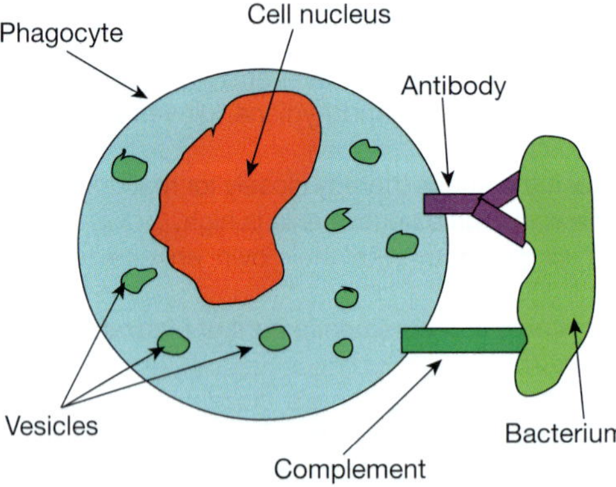

FIGURE 17.6 Phagocytosis (stage 2)

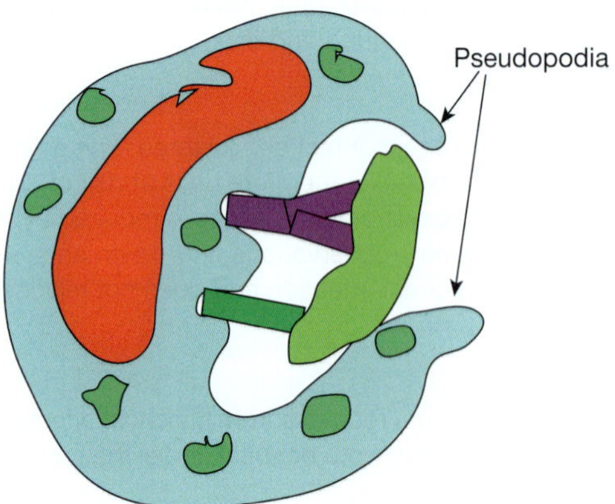

FIGURE 17.7 Phagocytosis (stage 3)

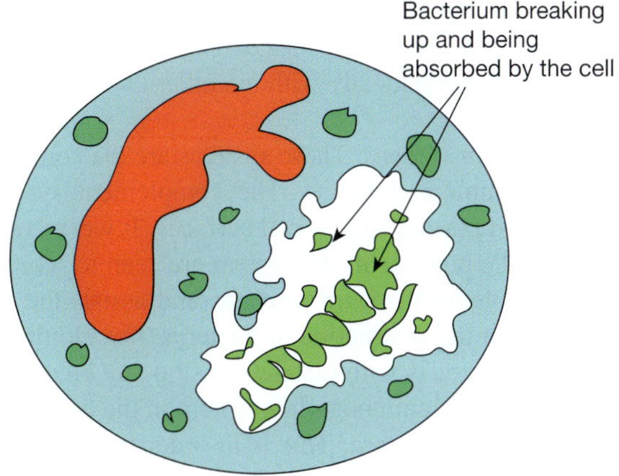

Cytotoxicity

Cytotoxicity is the process of damaging or killing cells. Many substances are toxic to cells, including certain chemicals, components of the immune system, viruses and bacteria, and some types of venom (e.g. from certain snakes).

Within the immune system, T-cells that can kill other cells are known as cytotoxic T-cells, and produce proteins that play a role in the destruction of target cells. Cytotoxic T-cells (Tc cells) work by programming their target cells (often cells that have been infected by viruses, or even cancerous/pre-cancerous cells) to undergo apoptosis — otherwise known as programmed cell death.

Inflammation

Inflammation is the body's immediate reaction to tissue injury or damage. This can be caused by:

- physical trauma
- intense heat
- irritating chemicals
- infection by viruses, fungi or bacteria.

The inflammatory process involves the movement of white cells, complement and other plasma proteins into a site of infection or injury (Delves et al. 2017).

There are four cardinal signs and symptoms of inflammation at the site of the injury:

- swelling (also known as **oedema**)
- pain
- heat
- redness.

There may also be:

- nausea
- loss of function at joints
- sweating
- raised pulse
- lowered blood pressure
- possibly loss of consciousness.

These last symptoms and signs are the body's response to pain and shock, but in terms of immunology, the first four signs and symptoms are the important ones, hence this is why they are known as the 'four cardinal signs of inflammation'.

According to Helbert (2016), inflammation can be defined clinically as the presence of swelling, redness and pain. Although inflammation does cause pain and other problems, it actually has beneficial properties and effects. These are:

- containment of infectious microorganisms and other damaging agents to prevent their spread to nearby tissues
- the disposal of killed pathogens and cell debris
- preparation for repair of the damage.

Following injury or other damage to the body, three processes occur at the same time.

- *Mast cell degranulation*. Mast cells are tissue cells that contain granules in their cytoplasm. These granules contain, among other substances, serotonin and histamine, which are released into the tissues during the process of degranulation. These substances cause some of the signs and symptoms of inflammation, but they also work synergistically with the other two processes to provide the complete inflammatory signs and symptoms.
- *The activation of four plasma protein systems*. These systems are the complement system, the **clotting system**, the **kinin** system and immunoglobulins. The complement system consists of more than 30 proteins that are found in blood plasma and on cell surfaces. It works very closely with antibodies, and indeed is so called because the proteins in the system are seen to 'complement' antibodies in the destruction of bacteria. The complement system activates and assists the inflammatory and immune processes and plays a major role in the destruction of bacteria. The clotting system traps bacteria that have entered the wound and also interacts with platelets to stop any bleeding. The **kinin system** helps to control vascular permeability, while immunoglobulins help in the destruction of bacteria.
- *The movement of phagocytic cells to the area*. This is in order to phagocytose bacteria or any other non-self debris in the wound (figure 17.8).

FIGURE 17.8 Phagocytes migrate from blood to the site of tissue injury

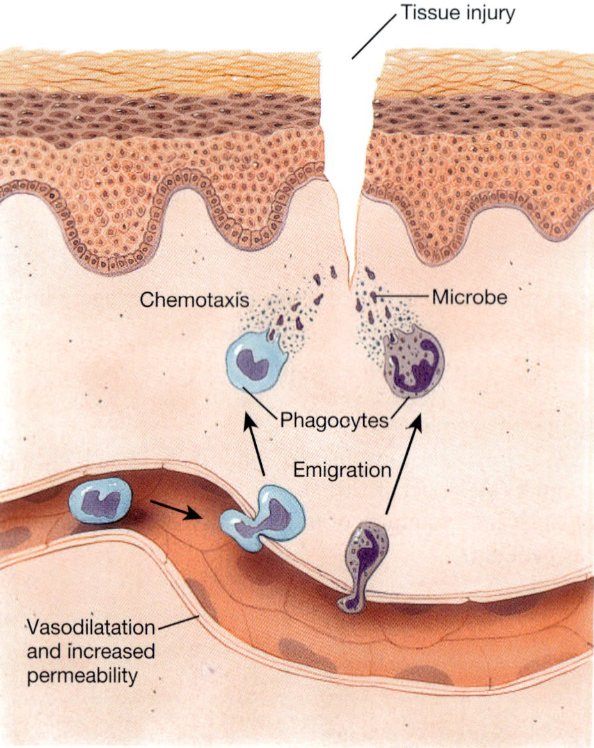

Source: Tortora and Derrickson (2014). Reproduced with permission of John Wiley & Sons.

Complement factors stimulate the mast cells to release histamine and other chemicals, which in turn can increase the permeability of blood vessels (Tortora et al. 2015).

Other factors involved in vascular permeability are:

- cytokines (cell messengers), which promote inflammation and also attract white blood cells to the affected area
- kinins and **prostaglandins**, which are chemical messengers released from damaged and stressed tissue cells, phagocytes and lymphocytes.

All of these factors (histamine, complement, cytokines and kinins), as well as having their own specific individual inflammatory roles, cause the small blood vessels in the area that has been damaged to dilate so that more blood is able to flow into the region surrounding the damaged area. This causes the redness and heat associated with inflammation.

HOMEOSTATIC IMBALANCE

Sepsis

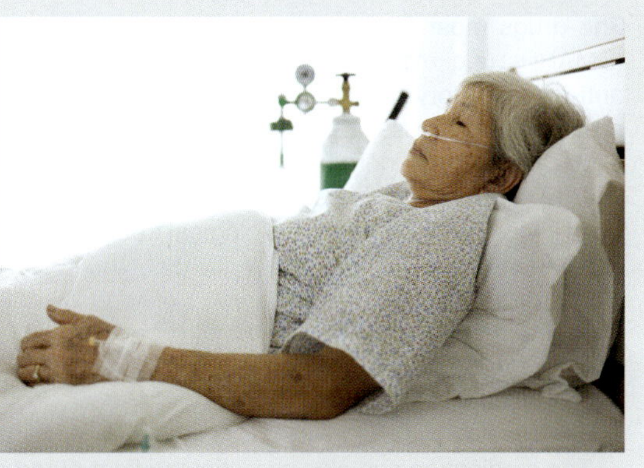

Sepsis is a serious, life-threatening condition caused by bacteria and bacterial toxins in the blood. Sepsis causes a range of symptoms including increased heart rate, increased respiratory rate, headache, fever, nausea/vomiting and chest pain (Health Direct 2020). Additionally, immune intervention (particularly in the form of neutrophil degranulation) can cause the progression to septic shock. Septic shock results in multiple organ dysfunction and a sudden drop in systemic blood pressure due to increased endothelial permeability (circulatory shock) which rapidly progresses to death in the absence of medical intervention (Martin-Fernandez et al. 2020). Sepsis is a major cause of morbidity and mortality worldwide, with the largest burden of disease (~85%) occurring in low- to medium-income countries such as sub-Saharan Africa and South-East Asia, with 49 million cases of sepsis worldwide in 2017 and 11 million deaths (Rudd et al. 2020).

Sepsis requires emergency treatment, particularly as it can progress quickly to shock and organ failure, with delays in treatment resulting in a greater risk of death. Treatment usually involves a combination of IV fluids and antibacterial therapies, but can also involve other therapies to support the respiratory and renal systems (Health Direct 2020).

CLINICAL CONSIDERATIONS

Australian focus: sepsis

While Australia has a much lower rate of both sepsis and sepsis-related mortality when compared with less wealthy nations, the most recent evidence suggests that annually there are approximately 55 000 cases and approximately 8700 deaths (ASN 2020). In 2019, the Australian government allocated $1.5 million to the development of treatment and public awareness programs in an attempt to reduce the burden of disease, particularly with respect to the elderly, the very young and Indigenous Australians who are disproportionately affected by sepsis (ASN 2020).

CLINICAL CONSIDERATIONS

Rheumatoid disease

Rheumatoid disease is caused by an autoimmune reaction (this is the body's immune system attacking the body's own cells); it is one of the most common chronic inflammatory conditions. Some inflammatory cytokines have a key role to play in the pathogenesis of this disease. Rheumatoid arthritis is a common cause of disability, with one-third of patients likely to be severely disabled. The joint changes, which almost certainly represent an autoimmune reaction, consist of:

- inflammation
- erosion of cartilage and bone.

Autoimmune diseases

Specific examples of autoimmune diseases include such diverse conditions as rheumatoid arthritis, type 1 diabetes mellitus, multiple sclerosis and systemic lupus erythromatosus (lupus). Autoimmune diseases affect 3 per cent of the Western population and are found to be more common in people living in the more northerly latitudes. Almost all autoimmune diseases are more common in women with onset usually occurring between puberty and retirement. In addition, there tend to be clusters in families — not necessarily of the same disease, but of a tendency to an autoimmune disease.

MEDICINES MANAGEMENT

Autoimmune diseases

The drugs most frequently used in rheumatoid disease are disease-modifying anti-rheumatoid drugs (DMARDs) (e.g. methotrexate, leflunomide, hydroxychloroquine and sulfasalazine) as well as non-steroidal anti-inflammatory drugs (NSAIDs). These drugs reduce the symptoms of rheumatoid disease, but do not prevent the progression of the disease.

Methotrexate is normally the first medicine given for rheumatoid arthritis, often alongside another DMARD and a short course of corticosteroids to relieve any pain (Lee & Pile 2003). The drug may also be used in combination with the biological treatments. The common side effects of methotrexate can include:

- nausea
- loss of appetite
- a sore mouth
- diarrhoea
- headache
- hair loss.

The medication can also sometimes affect blood cell counts and liver function.

Other drugs that are used with this disease include:

- some immunosuppressants (drugs that suppress the immune system to try to prevent it from attacking the body's own cells)
- steroids
- anticytokine drugs — these are newer drugs and they have more specific action against the disease processes of rheumatoid disease.

Included within the category of DMARDs are a variety of drugs with different chemical structures and mechanisms of action. They can improve symptoms and reduce disease activity in rheumatoid arthritis. This can be measured by a reduction in:

- the number of swollen and tender joints
- the pain score
- the disability score.

However, there are doubts as to their efficacy in halting the long-term progress of the disease.

SKILLS IN PRACTICE

The nurse's role(s) in assessing the needs of a patient with multiple sclerosis

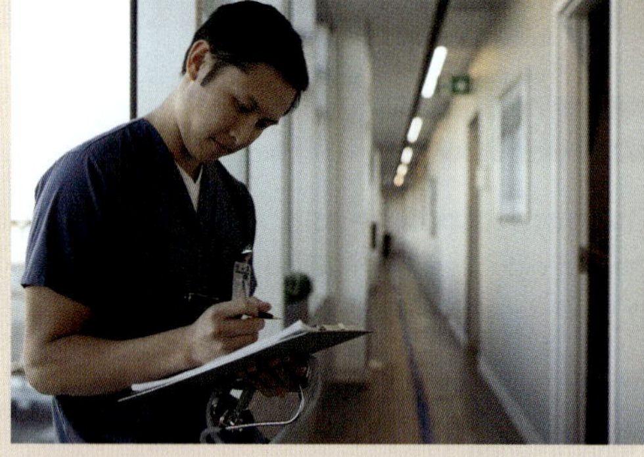

Multiple sclerosis (MS) is an autoimmune disorder in which the myelin sheath surrounding and protecting the nerve fibres is damaged by the body's own immune system. This, in turn, leads to the damage of the underlying nerve fibres.

The signs and symptoms of MS are many and varied and depend upon which part of the central nervous system is affected. Potential symptoms can include problems with vision and balance, dizziness, fatigue, bladder and bowel problems, speech and swallowing difficulties, stiffness and/or spasms, and tremors, as well as memory, cognitive and emotional problems. It is also important for the nurse to know that there are different types of MS: new, relapsing, progressive and advanced forms.

Consequently, the role of the nurse is to ensure that they have a sufficient knowledge of the signs, symptoms, cause and effects of MS, as well as knowledge of the patient. This knowledge will allow the nurse to provide explanations, initiate education of patients and families regarding MS, its treatment and prognosis, and to take part in (or provide referrals for) counselling for patients and their families.

To assist in this role of guiding the patients and family affected by this condition, nurses first of all must undertake a comprehensive assessment of the individual patient, looking at such areas as physical, cognitive, emotional, sensory effects and coping strategies, along with any problems concerning bowel and bladder functioning (and any sexual issues that may arise). These assessments must continually be updated throughout the course of the patient's life in order to ensure that the best physical, psychological, emotional and social support is always available and relevant for that patient and family. To that end, nurses need to have a knowledge and understanding of how various MS drugs work, and, with the medical team, ensure that the drug regimen is the most suitable for that patient in order to minimise the patient's MS symptoms and to ensure the best quality of life possible. This will help to enhance patient compliance with the drug and other therapeutic regimens. Within this category, nurses must be aware of how the individual patient's condition responds to the therapies, as well as any side effects that may arise.

The nurse must also become an advocate for patient follow-up within the appropriate interdisciplinary health and social/psychological teams that may be involved.

Above all, the nurse needs to know the individual requirements of the patient (and family) to aid them in retaining as much autonomy as possible while managing this disease, its effects and therapies; while keeping in mind that this is a lifelong condition for which, at the moment, there is no cure, and that the patient and their family will always be aware of this fact.

These chemicals also increase the permeability of the capillary walls, which allows blood cells and protein-rich fluid to seep into the surrounding tissues, leading to oedema — the third of the classic signs of inflammation. Oedema performs three functions that are important to the healing of damaged tissue:

- the dilution of harmful substances in the area to make them less concentrated
- the movement of large quantities of oxygen and the nutrients necessary for the repair of any damage into the area
- the entry of clotting proteins to help seal off the damage.

That leaves pain as the remaining classic sign of inflammation. Pain is caused partly by the pressure on the nerve endings as a result of the oedema in the tissues and partly by the release of bacterial toxins.

Summary of inflammation

Irrespective of cause, the timetable of a typical inflammatory response to tissue in injury is the following.

- Arterioles near the injury site constrict briefly.
- This vasoconstriction is followed by vasodilatation, increasing blood flow to the site of the injury (redness and heat).
- Dilatation of the arterioles at the injury site increases the pressure in the circulation.
- This increases the exudation of both plasma proteins and blood cells into the affected tissues.
- Exudation causes oedema and swelling.
- The nerve endings in the area are stimulated, partly by pressure (pain).
- The clotting and kinin systems, along with platelets, move into the area and block any tissue damage by commencing the clotting process.
- White blood cells — phagocytes and lymphocytes — move into the area and start to destroy any infectious organisms in the vicinity of the trauma.
- These phagocytes, along with the substances they produce, kill any bacteria or other microorganisms in the vicinity and remove the debris that results from the battle between the microorganisms and the immune system — this includes exudates and dead cells (pus).
- All of these components of the immune and blood systems remain in the area until tissue regeneration (repair) takes place — this is known as resolution.

MEDICINES MANAGEMENT

New therapies: adalimumab

Adalimumab is a synthetic drug and is fundamentally a fully human anti-tumour necrosis factor alpha monoclonal antibody. It is derived from synthetic antibodies that are programmed to target tumour necrosis factor alpha (TNFa) (Australian Prescriber 2004). TNFa is a normal part of the human immune system, which, following an infection, allows for an increasing inflammatory reaction within the body as well as helping to mobilise the various cells of the immune system (e.g. lymphocytes) to fight the invading infectious microorganism.

Adalimumab is used as a component of the drug therapy for people with autoimmune diseases such as rheumatoid arthritis. In an autoimmune condition, the body's own immune system attacks the body cells and tissues. Because circulating levels of TNFa remain constantly high whether or not there is an infection, these high levels of TNFa cause the immune cells to malfunction and attack the body's own cells. Adalimumab blocks this TNFa production and consequently reduces the physical effects of rheumatoid arthritis, psoriasis and other autoimmune disorders (Australian Prescriber 2004).

17.4 The acquired immune system

LEARNING OBJECTIVE 17.4 Describe and discuss cellular and humoral immunity.

Acquired or adaptive immunity is the immunity that we acquire as we go through life — the acquired immune system is barely functioning when we are born and is reliant upon the mother's own acquired immune system giving protection in utero — some of which (mainly certain immunoglobulins) are retained by the infant for a short time postnatally. Another name for the acquired immune system is the specific immune system, as it is aimed at specific infectious organisms and antigens. It is very much based upon the class of white blood cells known as lymphocytes.

There are two types of acquired immunity: **cell-mediated immunity** and **humoral immunity**.

Cell-mediated immunity (T-cell lymphocytes)

This type of immunity is known as cell-mediated immunity because the cells themselves destroy any invading antigens.

T-lymphocytes originate in the bone marrow, but, at a certain stage in their development, leave the bone marrow as immature lymphocytes. These immature lymphocytes find their way to the thymus, where they fully develop. In addition, they learn to recognise our own cells, and so, do not destroy these, but only destroy or target invading cells; for example, bacteria and viruses (see figure 17.11). The thymus is situated in the chest. In babies it is a large organ (relative to size), but atrophies with age.

T-lymphocytes have different functions to perform within the acquired immune system, and the functions that they perform are dependent upon the differentiation they undergo within the thymus (figure 17.9). Different types of T-cells carry different receptors on their surfaces, and these are known as clusters of definition (CDs) — so called because the way in which these receptors are organised on the cell surface defines their role and function.

FIGURE 17.9 Development and types of T-lymphocytes

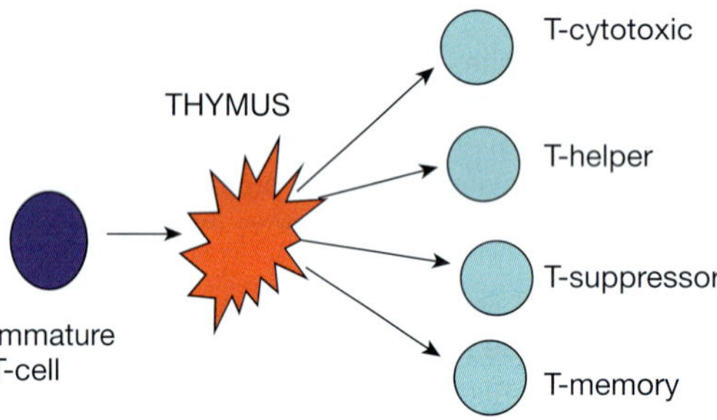

There are four classes of T-lymphocytes:

- T-cytotoxic lymphocytes
- T-helper lymphocytes
- T-suppressor lymphocytes
- T-memory lymphocytes.

The major functions performed by the T-lymphocytes are:

- cytotoxicity (cell destruction)
- control of the immune system
- memory.

HOMEOSTATIC IMBALANCE

HIV/AIDS

Human immunodeficiency virus is a transmissible infection that infects and destroys T-helper cells (reduced CD4 cell count) or impairs their function. The destruction of T-helper cells reduces the adaptive immune response and increases the risk of opportunistic infection by a large number of pathogenic and normally harmless organisms, as well as other diseases and some cancers (e.g. lymphoma & Kaposi's sarcoma) (WHO 2020). HIV is most commonly spread through body fluid exchanges such as sexual contact, sharing needles and needlestick injuries (WHO 2020). Globally, there are currently

38 million people living with HIV and, with advances in anti-retroviral therapy, it is becoming a manageable chronic health condition rather than the 'death sentence' it once was. Despite this, the costs associated with the lifelong treatment required place a great deal of strain on the healthcare systems of heavily affected countries.

While it is becoming increasingly rare, untreated HIV infection inevitably progresses to AIDS or acquired immunodeficiency syndrome. This typically occurs within 10 years due to the severe damage inflicted on the immune system over time, rendering it unable to respond to infections and cancerous cells (WHO 2020). Because of the damage inflicted on the immune system and the opportunistic infections associated with AIDS, the life expectancy of AIDS suffers is only 1–3 years (HIV.gov 2020).

CLINICAL CONSIDERATIONS

Australian focus: HIV

As previously mentioned, Aboriginal and Torres Strait Islander peoples suffer from a large number of socioeconomic, geographical and educational disadvantages that complicate the provision of timely and effective healthcare (Davey 2021). This is concerning given the higher rates of HIV infection in Indigenous communities when compared with non-Indigenous Australians (Ward et al. 2018). Australia has committed to eliminating HIV, which will require greater integration of Indigenous Australians in the planning and implementation of prevention strategies and better healthcare for remote communities.

Cytotoxicity (cell destruction)

This function is performed by the T-cytotoxic lymphocytes that possess the CD8 glycoprotein on their membrane. These cells mediate the direct cellular killing of target cells (Rote & Crippes Trask 2018). The target cells may be virally infected cells, tumours or 'non-self' grafts, such as kidney transplants.

The T-cytotoxic lymphocytes bind to the target cell and release toxic substances into the target cell, which are capable of destroying it. If the target cell is a virally infected cell, that cell is destroyed, as are the viruses that have infected it. In this way the viruses are unable to go on to invade other cells.

Control of the immune system

This is a task undertaken by the T-helper and T-suppressor lymphocytes working together.

T-helper cells are coated with CD4 proteins and they stimulate the immune system — both the acquired immune system and many parts of the innate immune system — to proliferate in response to infectious organisms (or other antigens) present in the body. There are two types of T-helper cell: type 1 T-helper cells and type 2 T-helper cells based on their individual cytokine profiles.

The body is usually very efficient at stimulating immune activity in response to an invasion by antigens, but there is a need for balances and checks to prevent the overstimulation of immunological activity, and this function is performed by the T-suppressor cells.

While many studies have identified T-suppressor cells, there appears to be no unique receptor marker for T-suppressor cells, and so immune suppression may actually be a task performed by a combination of T-helper and T-cytotoxic cells by means of a negative feedback mechanism (Male 2013).

Memory

A special quality that the acquired immune system possesses is the ability to remember antigens — or, more specifically, the antigen receptors that have been previously detected by the immune system, and so produce a group of lymphocytes which can stimulate the parts of the immune system that are able to counter these antigens immediately if that antigen is detected in future infections. T-memory lymphocytes are responsible for a rapid response to further attacks by specific infectious microorganisms (Rote & McCance 2018). This process is known as the secondary immune response and will be explained towards the end of this chapter (figures 17.10 and 17.11).

Memory cells are long-lived and there is always a constant number of T-memory cells for a given antigen in circulation (Murphy & Weaver 2016).

FIGURE 17.10 Cellular and humoral immune responses

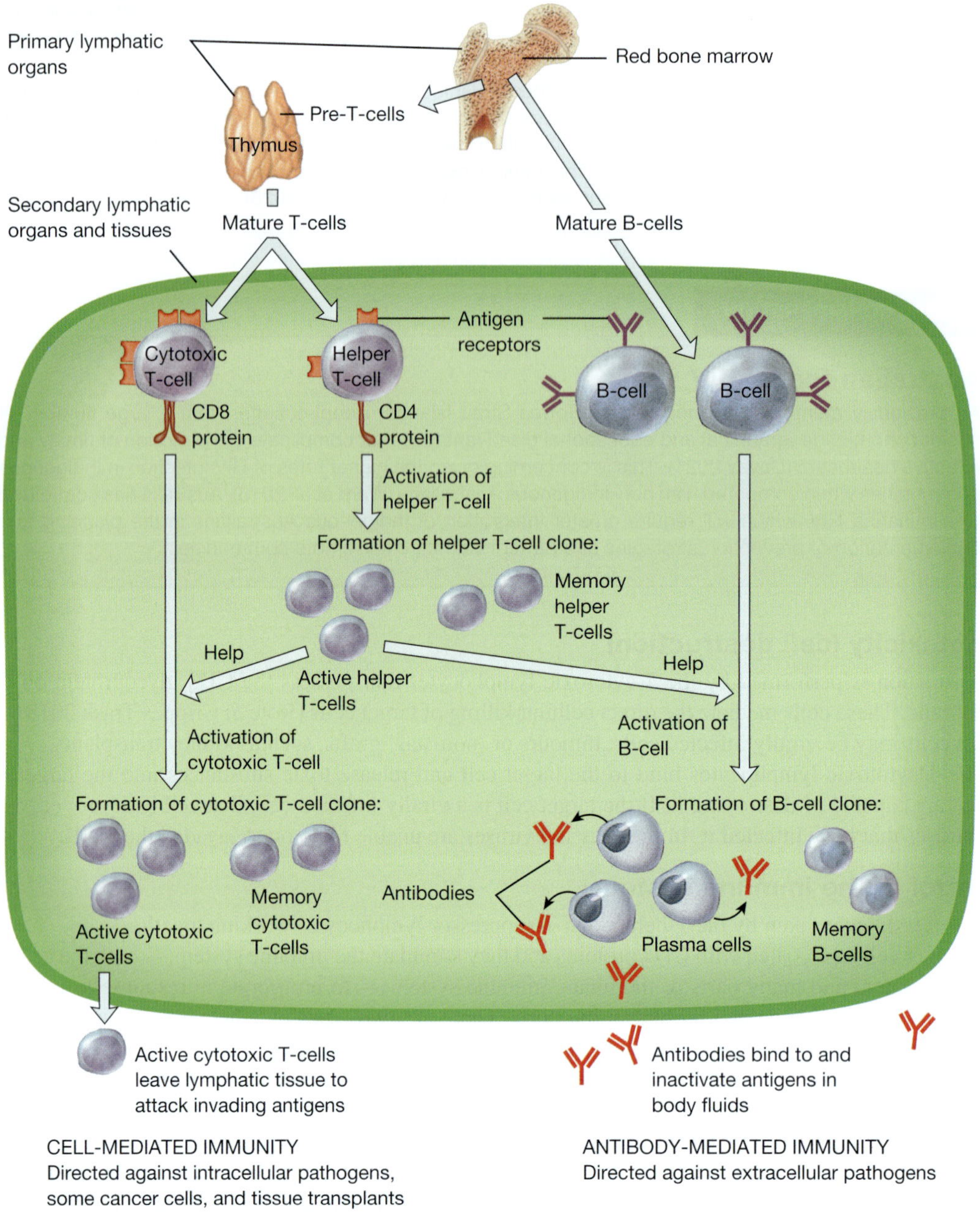

Primary lymphatic organs
Red bone marrow
Pre-T-cells
Thymus
Secondary lymphatic organs and tissues
Mature T-cells
Mature B-cells
Antigen receptors
Cytotoxic T-cell
Helper T-cell
B-cell
B-cell
CD8 protein
CD4 protein
Activation of helper T-cell
Formation of helper T-cell clone:
Memory helper T-cells
Help
Active helper T-cells
Help
Activation of cytotoxic T-cell
Activation of B-cell
Formation of cytotoxic T-cell clone:
Formation of B-cell clone:
Antibodies
Active cytotoxic T-cells
Memory cytotoxic T-cells
Plasma cells
Memory B-cells
Active cytotoxic T-cells leave lymphatic tissue to attack invading antigens
Antibodies bind to and inactivate antigens in body fluids
CELL-MEDIATED IMMUNITY
Directed against intracellular pathogens, some cancer cells, and tissue transplants
ANTIBODY-MEDIATED IMMUNITY
Directed against extracellular pathogens

Source: Tortora and Derrickson (2009). Reproduced with permission of John Wiley & Sons.

Humoral immunity (B-cell lymphocytes)

This second type of acquired immunity (which involves B-cell lymphocytes) is known as humoral immunity because the components effective in the immune system are soluble in fluids (and so is called humoral immunity).

B-cell lymphocytes originate and mature within the bone marrow.

As with the T-cell lymphocytes, the B-cells need to undergo a maturation process in which they have to survive a negative selection process. This is an attempt to ensure that the antigen receptors on their surface membrane do not display self-reactivity (i.e. do not react against our own cells) (Helbert 2016).

During this process, those B-cell lymphocytes that are autoreactive to the host cells and tissues are destroyed, leaving only non-autoreactive naive lymphocytes behind, which will then be able to go on to the next stage of maturation and selection (figure 17.10). This is a very important process, because if there should be any self-reactivity of the B-cells, as with T-cell self-reactivity, then autoimmunity may be the result.

FIGURE 17.11 (a–c) Process of teaching T-cells and B-cells to recognise pathogens (infectious organisms)

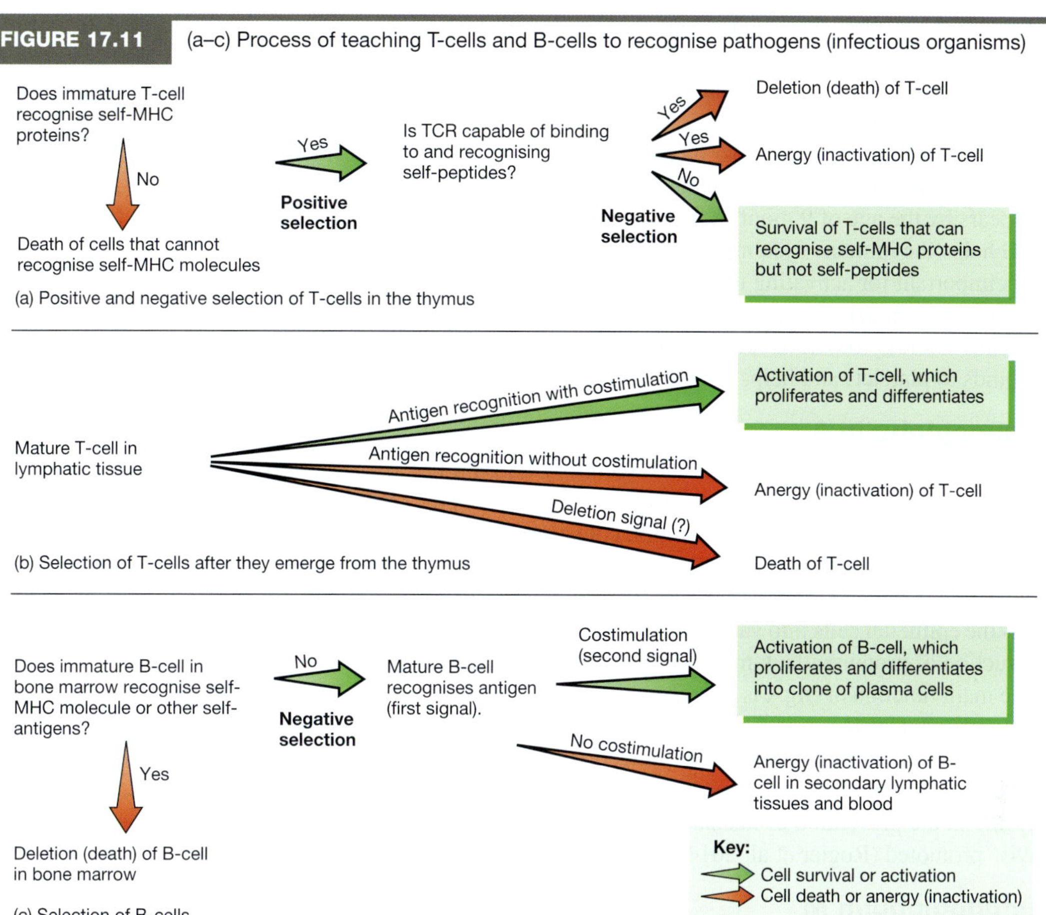

Source: Tortora and Derrickson (2009). Reproduced with permission of John Wiley & Sons.

The actual mechanism of the B-cell negative selection process within the bone marrow is similar to that process which is undergone by T-cells during their maturation and differentiation within the thymus (figure 17.11). However, in addition, B-cells undergo a positive selection process in which those lymphocytes that are able to respond to non-self antigens are preserved, while those that are not are left to die. The B-cells that have survived this negative selection find their way to the peripheral lymphoid organs, where they may encounter actual non-self antigens for which they have specificity. It is thought that more than 100 000 000 different antigens may be recognised by the B-cell lymphocytes.

Mature B-cells are of two types: B-memory cells (with a similar role to play as the T-memory cells) and antibody-secreting plasma cells.

Immunoglobulins (antibodies)

The antibodies secreted by the plasma cells are also known as immunoglobulins, and their role is to act as mediators in the destruction of non-self antigens. These immunoglobulins are not responsible for the actual killing. Instead, they assist other components of the immune system in destroying non-self antigens.

There are five classes of immunoglobulin:

- IgG
- IgA
- IgM
- IgE
- IgD.

Immunoglobulin G

This is the most important class of immunoglobulins involved in the secondary immune response. It makes up about 75 per cent of total serum immunoglobulin (Helbert 2016), and is divided into four subclasses: IgG1, IgG2, IgG3 and IgG4.

Because it has a low molecular weight (i.e. it is very small), IgG is found within both the intravascular and extravascular areas of the body. This means that it can reach all parts of the body, and therefore its effects are far-reaching. In particular, it plays a major role against blood-borne infective organisms as well as those invading the tissues.

The low molecular weight also means that IgG can cross the placental barrier to give a high degree of temporary **passive immunity** to the newborn child. This is important, because although maternal IgG disappears by the age of 9 months, by then the infant is usually producing its own IgG.

IgG helps the immune system in several ways (Helbert 2016).

- It is important for activating the complement system.
- It can bind to macrophages, and so enhance phagocytosis.
- It binds to the cytotoxic T-cells and helps them in destroying infected cells.
- It binds to platelets and helps with the inflammatory response.

Immunoglobulin A

There are two types of IgA: 'serum' and 'secretory'. Serum IgA has similar roles to IgG.

Secretory IgA (SIgA) is the most important because it is the major immunoglobulin found in external body secretions, such as saliva, breastmilk, colostrum, tears, nasal secretions, sweat, and the secretions of the respiratory tract and gastrointestinal tract.

As its name suggests, SIgA has a secretory component, which allows for the easy transfer of SIgA across the epithelial cells into various bodily secretions. It also helps to protect the IgA from the proteolytic (destruction of protein) attack mounted by enzymes that are themselves secreted by bacteria.

The main function of SIgA is to prevent antigens crossing the epithelium. In addition, SIgA can activate the complement system.

SIgA plays an important role in the protection of the host's body against respiratory, urinary and bowel infections. Also, because it is present in such large quantities in colostrum and breastmilk, it performs a vital role in the prevention of neonatal gut infections — this is one of the reasons why breastfeeding is so heavily promoted (Rogier et al. 2014).

Immunoglobulin M

IgM is the predominant antibody involved in the primary immune response (see the section on primary immune response), as well as being involved in the early stages of the secondary immune response.

It is very effective in activating the classic pathway of the complement system.

Because of its large size, IgM is restricted almost entirely to the intravascular (within blood vessels) spaces, and it is also often involved with any response by the immune system to complex, blood-borne infectious microorganisms (Helbert 2016).

Immunoglobulin E

Only very small amounts of IgE are found in the body — in normal circumstances it makes up less than 0.01 per cent of the total serum immunoglobulins, but is also found on the surfaces of mast cells and basophils because it has a very high avidity (binding potential) to tissue mast cells and circulatory basophils, and it is the binding of IgE to receptors on these cells in the presence of antigen that can trigger an allergic reaction.

This allergic reaction consists of:

- the activation of the mast cell
- the degranulation of the cell
- the release of mediators such as histamine.

Degranulation of the mast cell and release of histamine helps to cause an acute inflammatory response, which leads to the classic signs of allergic reactions, such as those seen in hayfever and asthma. IgE is also responsible for sensitising cells on mucosal surfaces, such as the conjunctival, nasal and bronchial mucosa. This gives rise to other symptoms of an allergy, including rhinitis and conjunctivitis (Helbert 2016).

The main role of IgE in helping to maintain good health is that it can bind onto helminths and other intestinal worms and so lead to their destruction. Allergic reactions and autoimmune diseases are less common in areas where worm and parasitic infestation is rife. In societies where helminth infestation is rare, it is thought that the IgE then turns its attention to the cells of the body, and allergy/autoimmunity is a response to this.

MEDICINES MANAGEMENT

New therapies: nematode therapy

As discussed, IgE is a major factor in allergic reactions. However, it is known that allergic reactions (e.g. eczema, food allergies) are not as prevalent in countries where there is a high parasitic infestation, particularly in terms of intestinal nematodes and helminths, and particularly hookworm or ascaris. At the same time, in more developed countries with high levels of hygiene and general cleanliness, allergies are very much on the increase. It is this dichotomy that has persuaded researchers to think about helminth therapy to alleviate allergies (Wu et al. 2017; Alvarado et al. 2015). Indeed, there have been trials where patients with allergies have swallowed hookworm larvae (the maximum tolerated number being 10) and have reported improvements — although not enough to significantly improve allergic symptoms. However, because the treatment made some subjects 'feel better', they opted to remain in the treatment once the trial had ended. Although not proven as such, further trials may well take place in the future, and hookworm therapy may become one of the standard therapies for allergies.

Immunoglobulin D

There is little known about the functions of IgD. However, we do know that it is chiefly found on B-cell surface membranes and that it acts as a receptor molecule. Work is ongoing in trying to decipher and understand this particular immunoglobulin.

Role of immunoglobulins

The primary function of an antibody is to bind to foreign antigens and facilitate phagocytosis and other functions of the immune system by attaching to **epitopes** (sites of immune recognition) on the surface of the antigen (figures 17.12 and 17.13); thus, the main functions of antibodies are to protect the host by (Rote & McCance 2018):

- neutralising bacterial toxins
- neutralising viruses
- opsonising bacteria — opsonins are molecules that bind to non-self matter and to receptors on phagocytes, and in this way acting as a bridge between the two and holding the non-self matter bound to the phagocytes (Male 2013)
- activating components of the inflammatory response.

Antibodies rarely act in isolation. Instead, they cooperate with other components of the immune system to destroy infecting organisms.

A second role of the immunoglobulin is the neutralisation of bacterial toxins. These toxins are produced by the bacteria and make them more pathogenic (harmful), thus causing more harm to the host. When this happens, the immunoglobulins function as antitoxins.

Similarly, the immunoglobulins neutralise viruses by binding to the viral surface receptors, preventing them from binding to the host's cells and allowing the viruses then to be phagocytosed, thus preventing the viruses from infecting cells of the body.

Immunoglobulins also activate components of the inflammatory response.

FIGURE 17.12 (a, b) Model of an antibody (IgG)

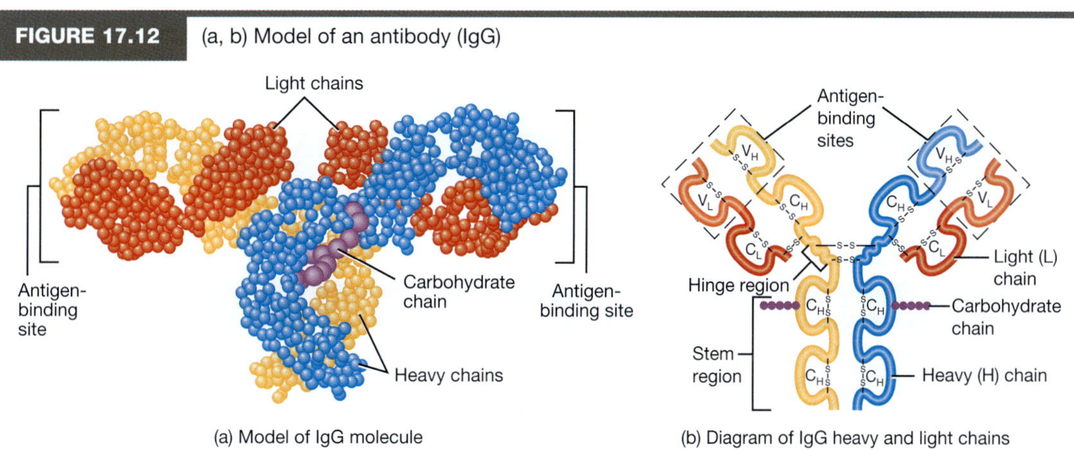

Source: Tortora and Derrickson (2014). Reproduced with permission of John Wiley & Sons.

FIGURE 17.13 Model of an antigen showing the epitopes (receptors)

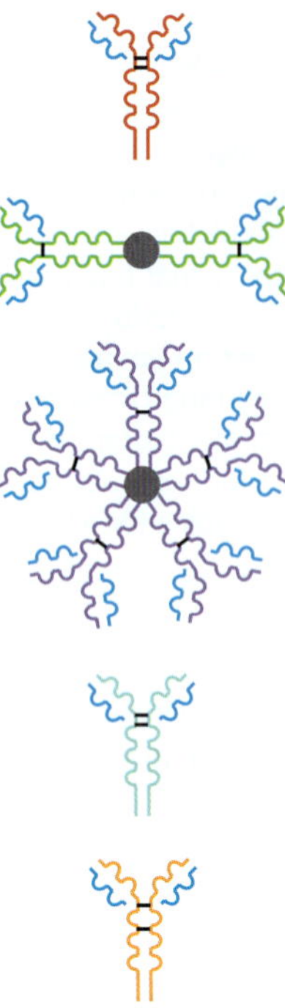

Source: Tortora and Derrickson (2014). Reproduced with permission of John Wiley & Sons.

MEDICINES MANAGEMENT

New therapies: immunoglobulin therapy

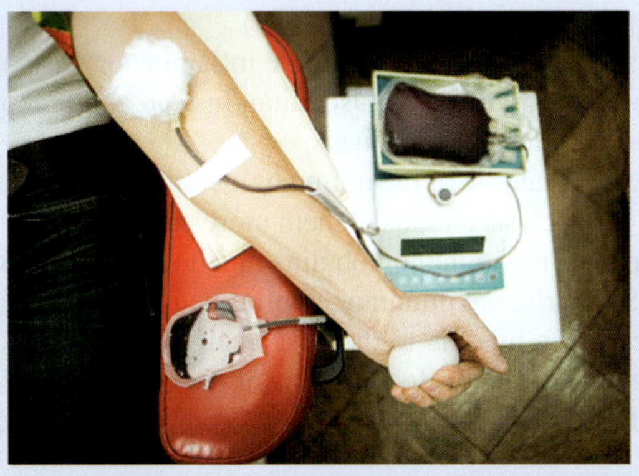

Immunoglobulin therapy uses purified immunoglobulins (antibodies) taken from the blood of volunteer donors. It can be administered intramuscularly, intravenously or subcutaneously. It is particularly important for people with antibody or combined immunodeficiencies and has become essential for the management of these conditions. Immunoglobulin therapy has been available for patients with immunodeficiencies for many years, but in recent years these therapies have been found to be important for many other medical conditions, so that, no matter in what ward, clinic or home therapy situation that a nurse is working, you will likely encounter this therapy at some time.

What is new about this therapy is that it can also be used for a huge number of medical conditions — and the list is continuously growing. The following are just a few of the conditions for which immunoglobulin therapy may be useful, or which are under review.

Immunological conditions	
Antibody deficiency Combined immunodeficiency (T-and B-cells) Complement deficiencies	HIV
Haematological/oncological conditions	
Various types of leukaemia Haemophagocytic syndrome Idiopathic thrombocytopaenia purpura	Aplastic anaemia

Infectious conditions	
Rheumatic fevers Recurrent otitis media	Lyme disease Chronic sinusitis
Neurologic conditions	
Alzheimer's disease Epilepsy Myeloma	Encephalopathy Multiple sclerosis
Rheumatological diseases	
Rheumatoid arthritis Kawasaki disease	Scleroderma Systemic lupus erythematosus
Other conditions	
Asthma Cystic fibrosis Sepsis and septic shock Recurrent pregnancy loss or miscarriage	Atopic dermatitis Diabetes mellitus Transplant rejection

SKILLS IN PRACTICE

Education of patients with hypogammaglobulinaemia to self-administer subcutaneous immunoglobulin therapy at home

For chronic conditions, such as hypogammaglobulinaemia (low or absent B-lymphocytes leading to a lack of antibodies), the ability to self-treat at home leads to a better quality of life for the patient and family, because the patient is taking control of their condition and there is also less disruption to the patient's (and family's) lifestyle. Additionally, it is more cost-effective in terms of the healthcare professional's time. This then allows for more new patients or patients with complex conditions to be seen and monitored in a clinical setting. However, for this to happen, some form of home therapy management needs to be put into place, and the first and most important is the ability of the nurse to teach the methods of subcutaneous treatment as well as monitoring of the ongoing treatment at home along with support of the patient and family. This requires the nurse to set up a teaching/training course once the patient has been deemed to be coping well with hospital/clinic-based treatment and after being assured that the patient (and/or a family member) has the desire, cognitive ability and manual dexterity to carry out this procedure at home. This is a new skill for many nurses and will require time and expertise to accomplish.

Protocols will have to be written and then agreed to by the hospital/clinic before training can begin for this procedure to be undertaken by the patient/family at home.

First, there is the home visit to ensure that the home environment and facilities available are suitable for this procedure to be carried out at home.

For training in self-administration of subcutaneous immunoglobulins, there are three steps during the training sessions for each patient, which may also include the family of the patient.

1. Nurse demonstration of the procedure.
2. The procedure carried out by the patient with the help of the nurse.
3. The patient carrying out self-administration on their own — validated by the nurse observing.

The whole training period can last for several weeks until the nurse is assured that the patient can safely cope at home.

Arrangements will need to be made for regular monitoring by the nurse to ensure that no problems occur, such as regular monitoring of the ongoing ability of the patient/family to carry out this procedure safely, as well as setting up a system of being able to be contacted to deal with questions or emergencies if/as they arise at home.

CLINICAL CONSIDERATIONS

Snake antivenom

A constant risk for rural communities and those enjoying nature in Australia is an encounter with a venomous animal such as a snake, stonefish or spider. Of particular concern is the large array of highly venomous endemic snake species including the inland taipan, coastal taipan, tiger snake and the eastern brown snake.

Antivenom is produced by injecting animals (typically horses for Australian snakes) with venom or venom components and then harvesting and purifying the antibodies from the blood of these animals. Antibody preparations can either be monovalent and neutralise the venom of a single species, or polyvalent and able to neutralise the venom of multiple species. If the species of snake is known, a monovalent preparation is used due to the very large dose size required when using polyvalent preparations and the increased risk of side effects. When administered, the antibodies will bind to the venom, neutralising it and allowing it to be removed by the immune system. Prior to the development of antivenoms in the twentieth century, tiger snake envenomation resulted in death 45 per cent of the time and taipan bites 90 per cent of the time (University of Melbourne 2020).

In Australia there are roughly 3000 snakebites per year which account for roughly 550 hospitalisations and 2 deaths annually. Not surprisingly, nearly 60 per cent of these incidents occur in rural and remote areas (RFDS 2018). Because most fatalities from snakebites occur due to delays in receiving antivenom, the Royal Flying Doctor Service carries a selection of antivenoms on their aircraft.

Natural killer cells

There is a further type of lymphocyte, which appears to express only the earliest markers of T-cell differentiation. These are known as **null cells** or NK (natural killer) cells. The **NK cells** do not bind antigens, nor are they induced to proliferate by contact with an antigen. Rather, they bind to chemical changes on the surfaces of virally infected cells or malignant cells, rather than antigen receptors (Rote & McCance 2018).

Although they are lymphocytes, these cells are usually classified within the innate immune system.

17.5 Primary and secondary response to infection

LEARNING OBJECTIVE 17.5 Explain the body's response to infection and the rationale for immunisations.

Finally, we will examine the immune system's response to infections. The one thing that really marks out the acquired immune system as special is its ability to 'remember' previous encounters with an antigen. Without this ability, each time an individual comes into contact with a particular antigen there would be a risk of a serious, and possibly fatal, illness. This immune memory is crucial because it allows the body to mount an immediate immune response to an antigen without waiting for the immune system to work out a way of destroying that antigen each time it infects us.

How does the immune system gain this memory of a specific antigen? There are two immune responses: the **primary response** and **secondary response**. The primary response occurs when the immune system first comes into contact with a new antigen (such as an infectious organism), and the secondary response occurs with all subsequent encounters with that same antigen.

Primary immune response

With the primary immune response, there is always a long time period before a response can be made. This is known as the 'lag' phase because the response lags some way behind the encounter with the antigen (figure 17.14). During this time there are no detectable antibodies produced by the mature B-cell lymphocytes, but the immune system is working out how to destroy the antigen.

In the case of the primary immune response, the lag phase can take anything from 5 to 10 days before there has been sufficient production of antibodies to have an effect. During this period, the host can become very sick and may even die.

The major immunoglobulin class produced at this stage is IgM, and only small amounts of IgG are produced, but hopefully enough to destroy the antigen.

FIGURE 17.14 Antibody responses to an infection

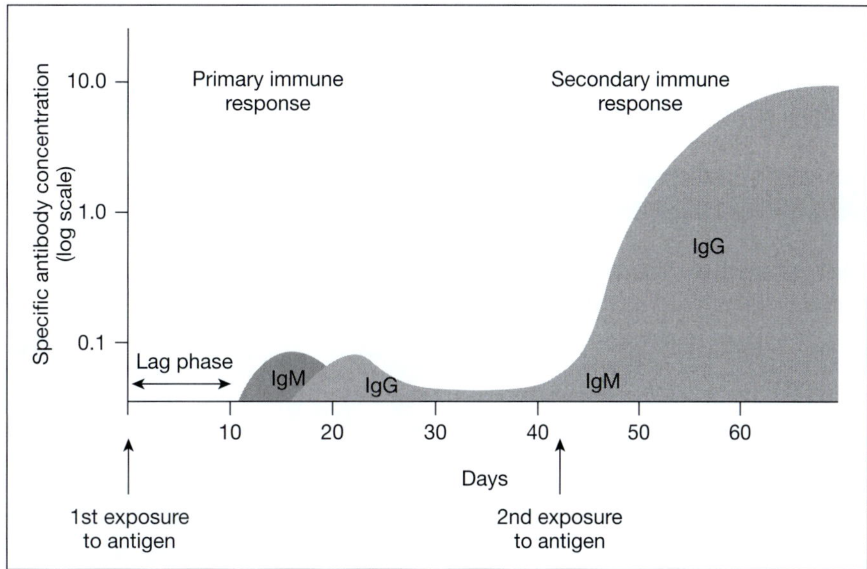

At the same time as the antigen is being destroyed, the memory cells are being produced to retain a memory of this specific antigen and how to defeat it. This memory will stay with the host for a long time. Each time the host is infected by that same antigen, the memory cells are reinforced.

CLINICAL CONSIDERATIONS

Handwashing

Handwashing is the single most important measure in preventing cross-infection. The technique employed involves thoroughly cleaning, rinsing and drying both hands. Hands are the principal route by which cross-infection occurs.

Effective handwashing remains an essential public health initiative. Handwashing is an essential aspect of any caregiver's repertoire of skills, and these skills must be mastered in order to provide all people with a safe environment. Those people with immunological deficiencies are at a particular risk of infection; and, as such, attention to scrupulous handwashing techniques must be carried out at all times.

All healthcare providers should strive to make handwashing an automatic behaviour that is performed by all in homes, schools and other environments. Families and carers who come into contact with those people with an immunological deficiency must adhere to effective handwashing. The key aim of effective handwashing is to prevent the spread of microorganisms between people or between other living things and people. Inanimate objects and surfaces, such as contaminated cutlery or clinical equipment, may put the health and wellbeing of an immunologically compromised person at risk.

Using the correct handwashing technique not only saves lives but can also save money. Poor handwashing practices can lead to urinary tract infections, bloodstream infections, respiratory infections and infection of incisional wounds. These infections are caused by the transfer of microorganisms from staff and families to vulnerable people, which could be prevented by using the correct handwashing procedures.

In all healthcare environments, handwashing is mandatory and must be carried out using established policies and procedures. There are a number of practices associated with hand hygiene — for example, using alcohol hand rubs and the act of physically washing the hands. The consequences of failing to use the correct procedure are many; the impact this can have on the health and wellbeing of the person you are caring for can be devastating.

Secondary immune response

If, at a later date, the same antigen infects the body again, because of the memory T-cell lymphocytes, the body is capable of mounting a secondary immune response that is much quicker. Because the memory cells are carrying their memory of this antigen, production of antibodies can take place very quickly, so that there is a very short lag phase.

In a secondary immune response, the major antibody class produced is IgG, although occasionally IgA or IgE may be produced depending upon the nature of the antigen and its route of entry (Helbert 2016). IgG is produced in huge quantities very quickly, and therefore the response is very rapid and effective — often, the antigen is destroyed before any signs and symptoms appear.

CLINICALLY REASONED EPISODE OF CARE

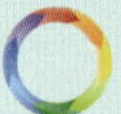

Allergy and asthma

Consider the patient situation

Nathan is a 24-year-old man with a learning disability who has asthma. He has attended the emergency department with shortnessof breath.

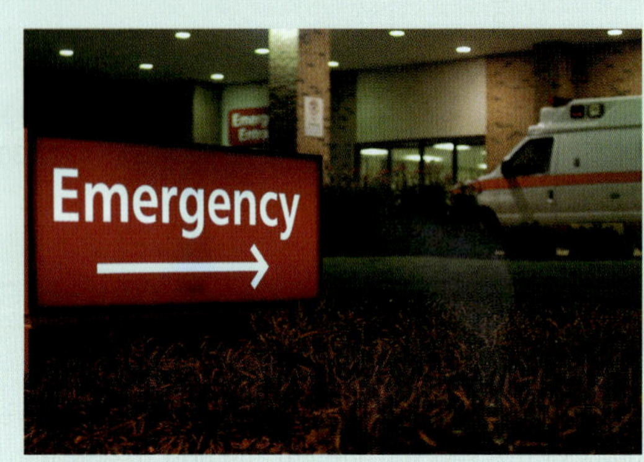

Collect cues and information

Nathan lives independently with the help of a local support provider. His parents live nearby and visit him daily. Nathan has recently started working part-time in a garden centre and in his spare time enjoys playing football and attending a local social club. Nathan suffers from asthma, which is normally well controlled with medication. However, as of late, Nathan has had repeated asthma attacks, with his most recent requiring hospitalisation and treatment.

Nathan sees the nurse as part of the emergency department team.

Process information

Asthma is a chronic inflammatory condition in which the airways and lungs narrow and swell with an increased production of mucus. Asthma can be mild to severe and can be present throughout the entire lifespan. Some people will only require symptom relief such as an inhaler, while others, such as Nathan, will require long-term inhalers and medication to prevent the onset. In its most extreme form, asthma attacks can be a life-threatening situation where the airway can close.

Allergies occur as an immune response to antigens. The immune response is dependent on the body's T-helper cells TH1 and TH2. In individuals with allergies, TH2 cells encourage the immune system to recognise allergens as invaders and create a response against the allergen. Once these antigen-presenting cells identify the allergen, it is absorbed and processed. This cell then migrates to the T-cell, which encourages the B-cells to produce antibodies to the allergen. This stimulates an IgE response. When the allergen is identified in the body again, the immune response recognises it and releases IgE to attack the allergen. Allergy symptoms can include skin rashes, itching, nausea, vomiting, breathlessness, swelling and pain.

Allergies and asthma can occur separately or together. The same substances that initiate an immune response, such as pollen or dust, can also cause asthma to flare. This is called allergic asthma. In Nathan's case, it was noted that his asthma symptoms had become worse since he had started working at the garden centre and his doctor considered it highly likely that increased exposure to plants and grasses at the garden centre was the trigger for his asthma.

Establish goals

1. Asthma management
2. Allergy management
3. Education and information on prophylactic treatment

Nursing actions

1. Asthma management

   Rationale:
   - Asthma is a potentially life-threatening situation involving the airway and is therefore a priority for emergency nurses.
   - Asthma should be immediately treated:
     - assess Airway Breathing Circulation and Disability (ABCD)
     - in consultation with a prescribing doctor, administer bronchodilator with a spacer and puffer, or if severe, a nebuliser

- administer corticosteroids such as prednisone or hydrocortisone within the first hour
- administer bronchodilators every 20 minutes
- Patients should be continuously monitored for treatment efficacy and clinical deterioration.

2. Allergy management
   Rationale:
   - Corticosteroids will likely have some benefit to allergies; however, additional treatments such as antihistamines may also be prescribed.
   - This should be administered only after initial treatment for asthma is initiated.
3. Provide education and information.
   Rationale:
   - Once initial asthma treatment is effective and Nathan is in a clinically stable condition, asthma and allergy education and information can be delivered to him and his family.
   - Prophylactic antihistamines have been shown to reduce symptoms and severity of allergies and will be helpful for Nathan in his work life.
   - Nathan and his family should also be educated on when to seek care should his symptoms worsen, even with prophylactic treatment.
   - Nurses are well placed to provide education and information to patients and families being discharged from the emergency department. This information should include the how and when to take antihistamines and when to seek help.

Evaluate outcomes

As a result of the interventions above, Nathan's asthma settles within the hour. He is observed in the department for a further two hours and his symptoms resolve.

It is noted that his emergency presentations decrease, and he reports to his GP that his symptoms are less frequent and severe.

Reflect on new processes and learning

Reflect on the diverse role of the emergency nurse. Consider how nurses can move from critical care management to education and support in their role.

Source: Based on the Clinical Reasoning Cycle, Levett-Jones (2013).

Hypersensitivity

While it is evident that the immune system provides protection for the individual, at times this ability may become compromised and an excessive or inappropriate immune response (or **hypersensitivity** reaction) can occur and may prove life-threatening. Types of hypersensitivity reactions are summarised in table 17.2.

TABLE 17.2 Types of hypersensitivity disorders

Hypersensitivity type	Antibodies/cells involved	Effector cells	Mediators	Associated disorders
I — immediate	IgE	Mast cells Basophils	Histamine	Anaphylaxis Allergic rhinitis Extrinsic asthma
II — cytotoxic	IgG IgM	**Polymorphonuclear leukocytes**	Complement K cells	Transfusion reactions Myasthenia gravis Graft rejection Haemolytic disease of the newborn
III — immune complex	IgG IgM	Polymorphonuclear leukocytes	Complement	Rheumatoid arthritis Systemic lupus erythematosus
IV — cell mediated	T-cells	Mononuclear leukocytes	Lymphokines	Tuberculosis Contact dermatitis Protozoal or fungal infections Sarcoidosis

SKILLS IN PRACTICE

Patient assessment

Assessing and planning the care of patients is a fundamental aspect of a healthcare professional's role. As part of this process it is imperative that any known allergies are documented. Where the patient is unsure as to whether they have an allergy or not, it is safer to document it as an allergy just in case.

Anaphylaxis

Anaphylaxis is the most severe form of allergic reaction and requires prompt action. Anaphylaxis is a severe allergic response that can be triggered in sensitive individuals by substances such as penicillin, peanuts or latex rubber. Onset is usually sudden and in severe cases death may ensue in a matter of minutes if untreated. Anaphylaxis is classified as type I anaphylactic hypersensitivity. This occurs in those people with very high levels of IgE. When these people have been exposed to an allergen — for example, peanuts or penicillin — these high levels of antibody will activate mast cells and basophils that will then degranulate. Histamine is released and this constricts some smooth muscle, such as airway smooth muscle, vasodilation occurs and this increases vascular permeability. A type I reaction includes anaphylaxis where there is profound bronchoconstriction and shock due to the widespread vasodilation.

Immunisations

Immunisation, or vaccination, is either the process of transferring antibodies to an individual who is lacking them (passive immunisation) or the process of inducing an immune reaction in an individual (active immunisation). Immunisations induce the primary response by exposing the immune system to a vaccine that includes an infectious organism which is either inactivated (killed) or attenuated (weakened) so that it is no longer infectious but still possesses the receptors that can stimulate the immune system.

Passive immunisation

In passive immunisation, the individual is actually injected with the antibodies. There are two types of passive immunisation, which are natural and very common.

- The mother transfers IgG antibodies across the placenta to the foetus. Whatever organisms the mother is immune to, the newborn baby will also be immune to them.
- During breastfeeding, when the mother passes IgA antibodies to the baby in her colostrum and milk.

Passive immunisation is also short-lived and lasts only as long as it takes for these antibodies to be cleared from the body. This type of immunisation will not normally provoke an immune response in the recipient; therefore, there will be no immunological cover for subsequent exposure to that particular antigen.

Active immunity

Active immunity is the process of presenting antigen to the immune system to induce an immune response to it. This is the type of immunity that takes advantage of the primary and secondary responses to immunity and is the basis for all the immunisations/vaccinations that we have throughout our lives.

A vaccine has to be able to stimulate both T-and B-cell lymphocytes to provide an immune response. If a vaccine is effective, it provides common immunity to a population.

SUMMARY

This completes the chapter on the immune system. As you have learned, it is a very complex system, with each of the many components interacting with others to provide us with the protection that we need to survive in this very dangerous world. But, above all, hopefully you will be amazed and awestruck at its ability to fulfil its major role: that of keeping us safe from infections and other potential harm that could befall us.

What you must remember is that immunology is a dynamic subject. Research in the specialty is continually bringing us new knowledge, not only of the anatomy and physiology of the immune system but also of disorders affected by it and of new therapies.

There is now so much progress being made in immunology that it is impossible to predict the future. But then, this is what makes immunology so exciting!

KEY TERMS

acquired immunity Immunity that is acquired throughout life by coming into contact with many different infectious agents.

active immunity Immunity developed inside the body as a result of encountering infectious agents.

antibodies Also known as immunoglobulins, antibodies can recognise and attach to infectious agents and so provoke an immune response to these infectious agents. They are also opsonins.

antigen Anything that provokes an antibody response.

bactericidal The ability to kill bacteria.

basophils White blood cells that take part in the process of phagocytosis. Also involved in allergic/atopic reactions.

B-cell lymphocytes Blood cells from which antibodies (immunoglobulins) develop. Part of the humoral immune system.

bone marrow The site in the body where most of the cells of the immune system are produced as immature stem cells.

cell-mediated immunity The type of acquired immunity generated by the T-cell lymphocytes.

clotting system The clotting of blood to reduce blood loss. Also involving thrombocytes (platelets).

complement factors A group of proteins that are involved in many of the immune processes (e.g. phagocytosis and inflammation). They are also opsonins.

cytokines Chemical messengers that affect the behaviour of other cells, including cells of the immune system.

cytotoxicity The process by which infectious microorganisms are killed or damaged (cyto = cell, toxicity = dangerous to).

eosinophils White blood cells involved in the destruction of parasitic worms, but also linked to hypersensitivity.

epitopes The parts of a cell that can bind to other cells (i.e. cell receptors).

granulocytes White blood cells that take part in the process of phagocytosis.

humoral immunity Another name for antibody immunity. This is the part of the acquired immune system that relies upon antibodies to help in the destruction of infectious agents.

hypersensitivity A heightened immune response that can cause allergies and atopic diseases.

immunisation The process of either transferring antibodies to someone (i.e. passive immunisation) or inducing an immune reaction naturally but safely (i.e. active immunity).

immunity The body's response to infection, damage or other diseases.

immunoglobulins Also known as antibodies, they are highly specialised protein molecules that hold onto foreign antigens to enable their destruction by other cells of the immune system.

inflammation The body's immediate reaction to tissue injury or damage.

innate immunity The immunity with which we are born.

kinin A specialist group of plasma proteins (i.e. proteins that circulate within blood plasma) and have a role to play in the process of inflammation.

kinin system The system in which kinins operate in order to activate and help inflammatory cells, such as neutrophils, to function properly as well as being involved in making the blood vessels more permeable to allow cells of the immune system to get to the area of inflammation or damage.

leucocytes Another term for a white blood cell (leuco = white, cyte = cell).

lymph A colourless liquid derived from blood.

lymphatic system This shadows the blood system, but is very much involved in immunity. It consists of lymph vessels that contain lymph (which transports antigens and antibodies) and also lymph nodes and other lymphatic tissues (such as the tonsils and the spleen).

lymph nodes Nodules within the lymphatic system that contain mesh traps which are able to trap antigens in order for them to be destroyed by antibodies and other components of the immune system.

lymphocytes The major white blood cell of the acquired immune system.

lymph vessels These are similar to blood vessels, but they carry lymph, antigens (e.g. bacteria), antibodies and other components of the immune system, from the site of infection towards lymph nodes.

macrophages Also known as a tissue macrophage, it is a white blood cell that takes part in the process of phagocytosis within the tissues as opposed to within the blood circulation.

mast cells Cells of connective tissue that are involved in the activation of the inflammatory response (inflammation).

medulla The central part of an organ.

monocytes A type of phagocytic white blood cell (known as a tissue macrophage once it migrates into the tissues).

neutrophils White blood cells that take part in the process of phagocytosis.

NK cells Natural killer cells are a class of lymphocytes that are not specific to certain infectious agents and so are often classed with innate immunity as opposed to acquired immunity.

null cells Another name for the NK cells.

oedema A scientific term for swelling.

opsonins Substances that bind antigens to phagocytic cells, and so enhance the process of phagocytosis (e.g. complement factors and antibodies).

passive immunity The process of transferring antibodies to someone who is vulnerable to infections and cannot make their own active immunity.

phagocytes White blood cells that are able to ingest and destroy infectious microorganisms and other non-self matter, and include, among others, neutrophils and macrophages.

phagocytosis The ingestion and destruction of infectious microorganisms and other non-self matter by specialised cells (phagocytes).

plasma cells Cells that develop from B-cell lymphocytes and that produce antibodies.

platelets See thrombocyte.

polymorphonuclear leucocytes Also known as phagocytes, these are found in the blood.

primary response The immune response that occurs when we first come into contact with a new infectious agent.

prostaglandins Fatty acids that function as part of the inflammatory process (inflammation).

pseudopodia (Literal meaning = 'false arms'). These are finger-like projections that emerge from cells and, within immunity, they are very important in the process of phagocytosis.

red blood cells These cells carry oxygen from the lungs to the tissues.

secondary response The immune response that, following a successful primary immune response to a specific infectious agent, occurs every time we encounter that same specific infectious agent.

spleen Part of the lymphatic system, it functions to fight infections and to filter and clean blood. In addition, it serves as a blood reservoir.

stem cells Cells that have the potential to differentiate and mature into the different cells of the immune system.

T-cell lymphocyte White blood cells that have many functions, including control of the acquired immune system and killing viruses. The major component of the cell-mediated immune system.

thrombocytes Another name for a platelet; it is important in the clotting process.

thymus The organ of the body where T-cell lymphocytes mature, distinguish between self and non-self cells and differentiate into various types of T-cells that each have different functions within the acquired immune system.

tonsils Lymph tissue that is situated within the oral region (the mouth) and helps to protect the respiratory and gastrointestinal tracts from infections.

trabeculae Connective tissue strands that help to form part of the framework of organs, so giving them rigidity.

ACTIVITIES

TRUE OR FALSE

1. Phagocytes are red blood cells.
2. The thymus is where immature T-cells mature.
3. Another name for an antibody is an immunoglobulin.
4. White blood cells are descended from omnipotent stem cells.
5. Macrophages include monocytes and granulocytes.
6. One branch of T-cells develops into plasma cells.
7. The spleen is a lymphatic organ.
8. The right lymphatic duct receives lymph from the right arm.
9. The lymphoid system enables lymphocytes to protect tissues from infections.
10. Sneezing is a physical barrier within the immune system.

FIND OUT MORE

1. What are the immunisation schedules for your country?
2. Find out the differences, in terms of cause, symptoms and treatment, between rheumatoid arthritis and osteoarthritis.
3. Explore the different methods of immunoglobulin therapy for people with primary immunodeficiency disorders.
4. Look at what medical conditions are treated by immunoglobulin therapy, other than primary immunodeficiencies.
5. What is anaphylaxis and how is it treated?
6. What are the differences between bacteria and viruses, and what are the differences between how these infectious conditions are treated?
7. What is the normal treatment for a patient diagnosed with pulmonary tuberculosis (TB)?
8. Find out about and discuss the isolation policy for the hospital/healthcare centre, etc., that you are working in or have worked in as part of your nurse education.
9. How can nurses prevent infectious disease in hospitals and other healthcare institutions, as well as the home?
10. Find more out about the link between stress (physical, social, and psychological) and the immune system.

CONDITIONS

The following is a list of conditions that are associated with the immune system. Take some time and write notes about each of the conditions. You may make the notes taken from textbooks or other resources (e.g. people you work with in a clinical area), or you may make the notes as a result of people you have cared for. If you are making notes about people you have cared for, you must ensure that you adhere to the rules of confidentiality.

Septicaemia
Myasthenia gravis
Pernicious anaemia

(continued)

Skin allergy
Hayfever
Coeliac disease
Multiple sclerosis
Tuberculosis

REFERENCES

Alvarado R., O'Brien B., Tanaka A., Dalton J.P. and Donnelly S. (2015). A parasitic helminth-derived peptide that targets the macrophage lysosome is a novel therapeutic option for autoimmune disease. *Immunobiology* 220: 262–269.

Australian Prescriber (2004). Adalimumab. *Australian Prescriber* 27: 101–105.

Australian Sepsis Network (2020) Sepsis epidemiology. www.australiansepsisnetwork.net.au/healthcare-providers/sepsis-epidemiology (accessed 10 February 2021).

Davey, R.X. (2021) Health disparities among Australia's remote-dwelling Aboriginal people: a report from 2020. *JALM* 126: 125–141.

Delves, P.J., Martin, S.J., Burton, D.R. and Roitt, I.M. (2017) *Roitt's Essential Immunology*, 13th edn. Oxford: Blackwell Science.

Health Direct (2020) Sepsis (septicaemia, or blood poisoning). www.healthdirect.gov.au/sepsis-septicaemia (accessed 10 February 2021).

Helbert, M. (2016) *Immunology for Medical Students*, 3rd edn. St Louis, MO: Mosby.

HIV.gov (2020) What are HIV and AIDS? www.hiv.gov/hiv-basics/overview/about-hiv-and-aids/what-are-hiv-and-aids (accessed 10 February 2021).

Lee, A.T. and Pile, K. (2003) Disease modifying drugs in adult rheumatoid arthritis. *Australian Prescriber* 26: 36–40.

Levett-Jones, T. (2013). *Clinical Reasoning: Learning to Think Like a Nurse*. Pearson Australia.

Male, D. (2013) *Immunology: An Illustrated Outline*, 5th edn. London; Garland Science Publishing.

Martin-Fernandez, M., Vaquero-Roncero, L.M., Almansa, R., Gómez-Sánchez, E., Martín, S., Tamayo, E., Esteban-Velasco, M.C., Ruiz-Granado, P., Aragón, M., Calvo, D., Rico-Feijoo, J., Ortega, A., Gómez-Pesquera, E., Lorenzo-López, M., López, J., Doncel, C., González-Sanchez, C., Álvarez, D., Zarca, E., Ríos-Llorente, A., … Heredia-Rodríguez, M. (2020) Endothelial dysfunction is an early indicator of sepsis and neutrophil degranulation of septic shock in surgical patients. *BJS Open* 4(3): 524–534.

Murphy, K. and Weaver C. (2016) *Janeway's Immunobiology*, 9th edn. New York: Garland Publishing.

Nair, M. and Peate, I. (2009) *Fundamentals of Applied Pathophysiology: An Essential Guide for Nursing Students*. Oxford: John Wiley & Sons, Ltd.

Nair, M. and Peate, I. (2017) *Fundamentals of Applied Pathophysiology: An Essential Guide for Nursing Students*, 3rd edn. Oxford: John Wiley & Sons, Ltd.

NSW Health (2012) Glandular fever (infectious mononucleosis) factsheet. www.health.nsw.gov.au/Infectious/factsheets/Pages/mononucleosis.aspx (accessed February 2021).

Rogier, E.W., Aubrey, L., Frantz, M.E., Bruno, C., Wedlund, L., Cohen, D.A., Stromberg, A.J. and Kaetzel. C.S. (2014) Breast milk SLgA promotes intestinal homeostasis. *Proceedings of the National Academy of Sciences* 111(8): 3074–3079. doi: 10.1073/pnas.1315792111

Rote, N.S. and Crippes Trask, B. (2018) Adaptive immunity. In McCance, K.L. and Huether, S.E. (eds), *Pathophysiology: The Biologic Basis for Disease in Adults and Children*, 8th edn. St Louis: Mosby.

Royal Flying Doctor Service (RFDS) (2018) Outback survival: snakes and snakebites. www.flyingdoctor.org.au/qld/news/outback-survival-snakes-and-snakebites (accessed 10 February 2021).

Rudd, K.E., Johnson, S.C., Agesa, K.M., Shackelford, K.A., Tsoi, D., Kievlan, D.R., Colombara, D.V., Ikuta, K.S., Kissoon, N., Finfer, S., Fleischmann-Struzek, C., Machado, F.R., Reinhart, K.K., Rowan, K., Seymour, C.W., Watson, R.S., West, T.E., Marinho, F., Hay, S.I., Lozano, R., … Naghavi, M. (2020) Global, regional, and national sepsis incidence and mortality, 1990–2017: analysis for the Global Burden of Disease Study. *Lancet* 395(10219): 200–211.

Tortora, G.J. and Derrickson, B.H. (2009) *Principles of Anatomy and Physiology*, 12th edn. Hoboken, NJ: John Wiley & Sons, Inc.

Tortora, G.J. and Derrickson, B.H. (2014) *Principles of Anatomy and Physiology*, 14th edn. Hoboken, NJ: John Wiley & Sons.

Tortora, G.J., Funke, B.R. and Case, C.L. (2015) *Microbiology: An Introduction*, 12th edn. San Francisco, CA: Pearson.

University of Melbourne (2020) What is antivenom? https://biomedicalsciences.unimelb.edu.au/departments/department-of-biochemistry-and-pharmacology/engage/avru/discover/what-is-antivenom (accessed 10 February 2021).
Ward, J., McManus, H., McGregor, S., Hawke, K., Giele, C., Su, J.Y., McDonald, A., Guy, R., Donovan, B. and Kaldor, J.M. (2018) HIV incidence in Indigenous and non-Indigenous populations in Australia: a population-level observational study. *Lancet HIV* 5(9): e506–e514.
World Health Organization (2020) HIV/AIDS. www.who.int/news-room/fact-sheets/detail/hiv-aids (accessed 10 February 2021).
Wu, Z., Wang, L., Tang, Y. and Suyn, S. (2017) Parasite-derived proteins for the treatment of allergies and autoimmune diseases. *Frontiers in Microbiology* 8: 2164. doi: 10.3389/fmicb.2017.02164. eCollection 2017.

FURTHER READING

THE AUSTRALASIAN SOCIETY OF CLINICAL IMMUNOLOGY AND ALLERGY (ASCIA)

www.allergy.org.au

ASCIA offers support and advice to adults and children on all allergies and intolerances, including allergic conditions such as eczema, dermatitis, asthma, and so on.

IMMUNE DEFICIENCIES FOUNDATION AUSTRALIA (IDFA)

www.idfa.org.au

IDFA is an Australian immune deficiency organisation offering education, advocacy and awareness for Australians living with immune deficiencies.

EUROPEAN FEDERATION OF IMMUNOLOGICAL SOCIETIES (EFIS)

www.efis.org

An umbrella organisation for all European immunology societies.

INGID (INTERNATIONAL NURSING GROUP FOR IMMUNODEFICIENCIES)

www.ingid.org

This website contains excellent learning/teaching materials and information on immunologyand immunodeficiencies.

ACKNOWLEDGEMENTS

Photo: © Kamira / Shutterstock.com
Photo: © joloei / Shutterstock.com
Photo: © Akkalak Aiempradit / Shutterstock.om
Photo: © Hero Images / Getty Images
Photo: © Vesnaandjic / Getty Images
Photo: © sshepard / Getty Images

CHAPTER 18

The skin

TEST YOUR PRIOR KNOWLEDGE

- List the layers of the skin.
- What is the role of the skin in health?
- Describe three key functions of the skin.
- Discuss how the skin provides or helps to provide the body with various defence mechanisms.
- Ultraviolet light is said to be sometimes harmful to the skin. Why is this?

LEARNING OUTCOMES

After reading this chapter you will be able to:

18.1 discuss the anatomy and physiology related to the skin and outline the factors that determine skin colour

18.2 discuss the structure and growth of the appendages

18.3 describe the various functions associated with the skin, including how the skin functions as a homeostatic mechanism.

Body map

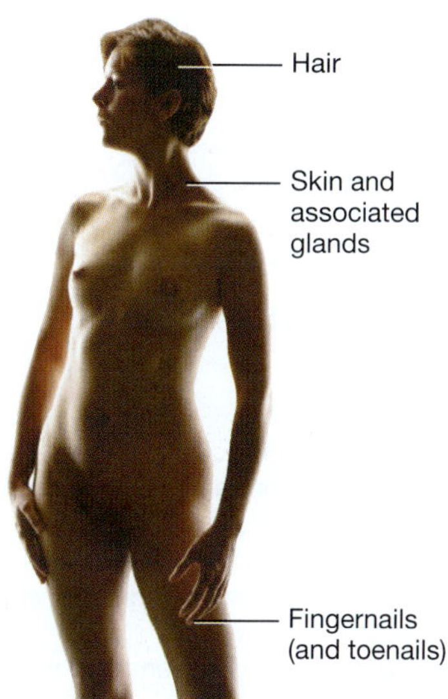

Introduction

The skin and associated structures (sometimes known as the **integumentary** system) protect the body in a number of ways; the simple fact is that without skin and its protective mechanisms we would not survive. The skin is often the only **organ** of the body that is on show all of the time, and because of this the skin can reveal how we feel emotionally; for example, we may blush. Importantly for healthcare professionals, it can also reveal how we are from a physiological perspective; for example, skin can appear cyanosed (a bluish tint), indicating low blood-oxygen levels. As a barrier to the outside world, the skin is the organ that is the most commonly exposed to disease or infection, and is almost entirely waterproof.

This system has a number of homeostatic elements; for example, it can regulate body temperature with the help of a variety of appendages (accessory structures of the skin). Waugh and Grant (2018) suggest that the average adult has 1.5–2 m^2 of skin and it weighs approximately 4.1 kg, making it twice as heavy as the brain! There are about 4.5 m blood vessels, 3.6 m nerves, 2.6 million sweat glands, 1500 sensory receptors and over 3 million cells that are continuously dying and being replaced. The skin receives nearly one-third of all blood that flows through the body, acting as a reservoir for up to 5 per cent of your blood at any one time (McLaughlin 2018).

The skin plays an essential role in health and wellbeing. Any disturbance in skin can lead to physical and/or psychological problems, and this in turn has the ability to impact on a person's quality of life. Just as a house needs bricks and mortar to act as a framework, the house would be of little value if it were not waterproof; using this analogy, the house also needs shelter from the environment, and in humans this job is carried out by the skin. The skin provides a defensive barrier, protecting the body from the elements as well as offering a defence against **pathogens**. It also has a number of other functions. The skin is made up of a superficial epidermis and a deeper structure called the dermis. Prior to discussing the functions of the skin, we will first outline the structure of the skin.

CLINICALLY REASONED EPISODE OF CARE

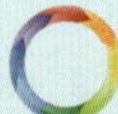

Acne

Consider the patient situation

Karl is 15 years of age and has acne vulgaris; he also has moderate learning disabilities and struggles with anxiety and depression. The acne has impacted his self-confidence.

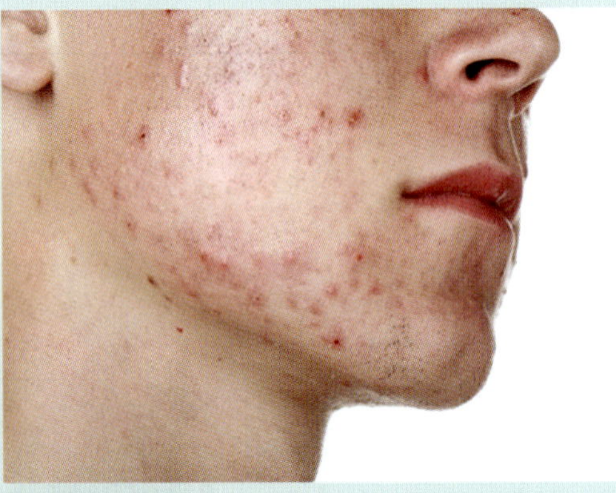

Collect cues and information

Karl's father reports that Karl has become so withdrawn that he dreads going to school as his classmates not only tease him about his learning disability but also his acne.

Karl's teachers have reported that he is displaying a number of challenging behaviours that they have not seen in him before; he is angry and has occasional aggressive outbursts. He is often seen rubbing and scratching the skin lesions.

Karl is referred to a dermatologist.

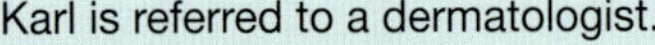

Process information

Acne vulgaris is a disorder of the pilosebaceous follicles located in the face and upper trunk. At puberty, androgens increase the production of **sebum** from enlarged sebaceous glands; these become blocked and infected, causing an inflammatory reaction.

Follicles that are impacted and distended by incompletely desquamated keratinocytes and sebum are known as comedones. These can be open (blackheads) or closed (whiteheads). The inflammation causes **papules**, **pustules** and nodules to appear.

Acne is a mild and self-limiting condition; however, teenagers like Karl can be very sensitive about it. Acne can cause severe psychological problems, undermining the person's self-assurance and self-esteem at a vulnerable time in their life.

Nursing actions

1. Support Karl and his family with empathetic, sensitive education on the prescribed treatment and management which includes:

- topical and systemic treatment, including an oral antibiotic and a cream (eTG complete 2020a)
- avoiding over-cleaning of the skin — twice daily washing with soap and fragrance-free cleanser is adequate for skin cleaning (acne is not caused by poor hygiene)
- avoiding picking and squeezing spots as this can increase the risk of scarring
- following instructions carefully when applying topical medication to reduce the risk of irritation
- engaging in sunsmart behaviours as the topical medication can cause sun sensitivity
- understanding the spots will not disappear overnight and that it may take some time for treatment to work; even after successful treatment, the spots are likely to reappear and Karl should follow up with the GP for consideration of maintenance treatment.

Rationale:

- It is very important to take antibiotics as prescribed for effective treatment and to reduce the risk of antimicrobial drug resistance. Advice and reassurance will promote treatment concordance and improve the chance of positive health outcomes for Karl.

Evaluate outcomes

After 8 weeks, Karl reports that his face is clearing up. His father reports that Karl feels much better about his appearance and his confidence has increased.

Source: Based on the Clinical Reasoning Cycle, Levett-Jones (2013).

18.1 The structure of skin

LEARNING OBJECTIVE 18.1 Discuss the anatomy and physiology related to the skin and outline the factors that determine skin colour.

According to Shier et al. (2016), the skin is one of the more versatile organs of the body. The skin is composed of two distinct regions: the dermis and the epidermis. The subcutaneous facia (often referred to as the hypodermis) lies under the dermis (Colbert et al. 2012); these masses of loose connective and adipose tissue attach to the skin and organs beneath; they are not part of the skin.

The epidermis

The superficial and thinnest aspect of the skin, the epidermis, is the area of skin that can most commonly be seen. While the skin covers the whole of the body, there are several regional distinctions, and these are associated with flexibility, distribution and type of **hair**, density and types of gland, pigmentation, vascularity, **innervations** and thickness (Jenkins et al. 2013). The thinnest part of the skin can be found on the eyelids; here, it is just 0.5 mm in thickness, whereas at sites of abrasion, such as the heel, it is 4.0 mm thick.

The epidermis is made up of specific epithelial tissue called keratinised stratified squamous epithelium; this means that it predominantly contains **keratin** (a protein), in addition to layers (stratified) of squashed (squamous) epithelial cells. There are four key cell types within the epidermis (figure 18.1):

- keratinocytes
- melanocytes
- Langerhans cells
- Merkel cells.

Keratinocytes

These cells are organised in four layers and are responsible for producing a protein called keratin. Keratin is a tough, fibrous protein that aids in the protection of the skin and tissues below from the heat, microorganisms and chemicals. In response to rubbing, pressure and local irritation, skin can thicken by producing excess keratin (**hyperkeratosis**); this is often visible in the form of calluses and corns on the hands and feet. Keratinocytes are also responsible for the production of the water-resistant properties of the skin, and act as a type of sealant that reduces water entry as well as water loss; they also prevent the entry of foreign matter.

Melanocytes

The developing embryo produces the pigment **melanin** from the melanocytes. Melanocytes are most profuse in the epidermis of the penis, nipples, the areola, face and limbs. Melanocytes have long, slender projections that extend between the keratinocytes and have the ability to transfer melanin granules. Melanin is responsible for the natural colour of a person's skin, and it helps to defend it from the damaging effects of the sun.

FIGURE 18.1 (a–d) The types of cells in the epidermis

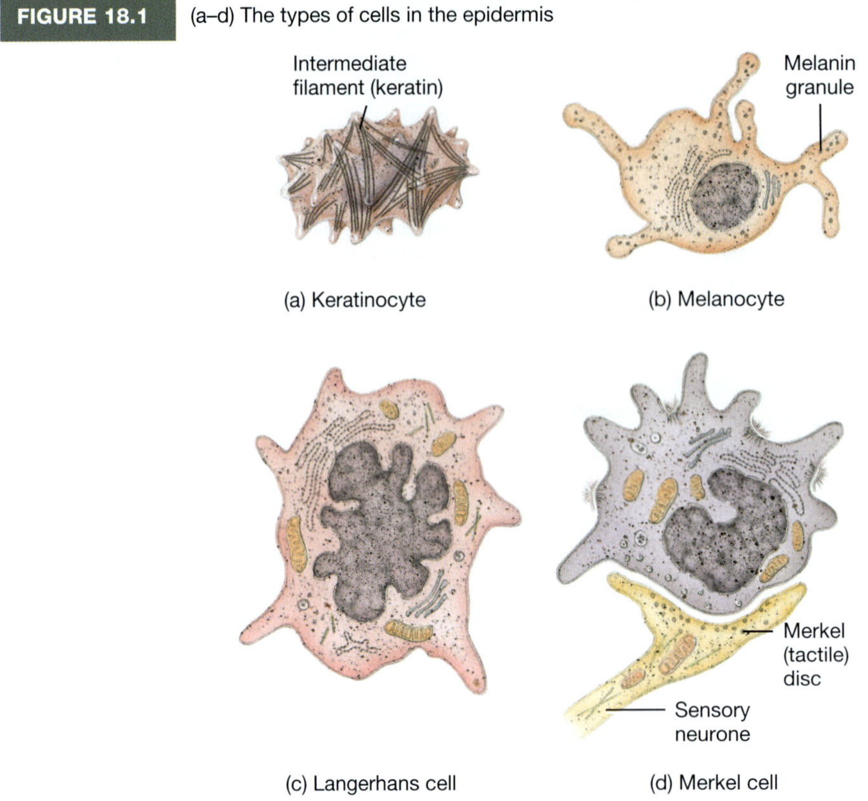

Source: Tortora and Derrickson (2009). Reproduced with permission of John Wiley & Sons.

When skin has been exposed to a great deal of sun, the melanocytes multiply the quantity of melanin in order to absorb more ultraviolet rays. This activity makes the skin darker, giving it a suntanned appearance. A suntan indicates that the skin has been harmed and is attempting to defend itself.

All people have about the same number of melanocytes; people with brown or black skin have the same number of melanocytes but they make more of the pigment melanin. It is the amount of melanin produced and how it is distributed that results in a variation of skin colour. Brown or black skinned people have more natural protection from the harmful ultraviolet rays of the sun. Moles (sometimes called naevi) are a group or a cluster of melanocytes that lie close together. The majority of people with white skin have approximately 10–50 moles on their skin.

CLINICAL CONSIDERATIONS

Skin cancer

The protection afforded by melanin is particularly important in Australia and New Zealand for the prevention of skin cancer. Many people migrate to these countries from less sunnier climates (e.g. Europeans migrating to Oceania), and so lack the requisite level of protection, or melanin production, for the level of sun exposure (as shown by their fair-skinned appearance). As a result, the skin cells of these individuals are vulnerable to the DNA-damaging rays of the sun, leaving Australia and New Zealand with skin cancer rates that are the highest in the world. Skin cancer is more common in older adults, and in males than in females, and it is estimated that around two in three Australians will be diagnosed with some form of skin cancer before the age of 70 years old (see figure 18.2). It is important to note that although the skin of Indigenous populations is well adapted to the local environment, melanoma still occurs in these populations, albeit at a far lower rate.

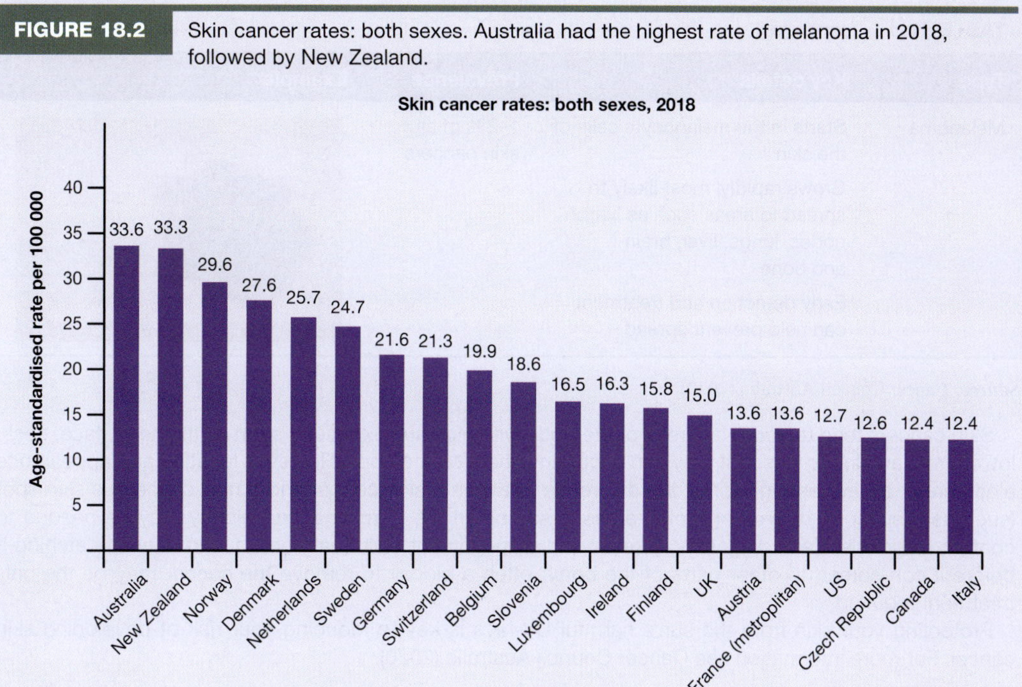

FIGURE 18.2 Skin cancer rates: both sexes. Australia had the highest rate of melanoma in 2018, followed by New Zealand.

Source: Data from World Cancer Research Fund (n.d.).

Skin cancer can occur when the sun's ultraviolet rays damage the DNA of cells, impacting on their ability to function, replicate or even carry out programmed cell death (**apoptosis**). As a result, damaged cells become abnormal and keep growing uncontrollably; in skin cancer, these form a lump of cells called a tumour. Some skin cancers can spread to other parts of the body, while others increase the risk of further occurrences. The three main types of skin cancer most commonly diagnosed in Australia are detailed in table 18.1.

TABLE 18.1 **The three main types of skin cancer most commonly diagnosed in Australia**

Type	Key details	Prevalence	Example
Basal cell carcinoma (BCC)	Occurs in the basal cells of the epidermis Grows slowly, rarely spreads to other parts of the body Increases the chance of further BCC	Approximately 70% of non-melanoma skin cancer	
Squamous cell carcinoma (SCC)	Forms in the squamous cells of the epidermis Grows rapidly, can spread across the body — particularly if on the lips and ears	Approximately 30% of non-melanoma skin cancer	

TABLE 18.1 *(continued)*

Type	Key details	Prevalence	Example
Melanoma	Starts in the melanocyte cells of the skin Grows rapidly, most likely to spread to areas such as lymph nodes, lungs, liver, brain and bone Early detection and treatment can help prevent spread	1–2% of all skin cancers	

Source: Cancer Council Australia (2020).

Skin cancers tend to occur on areas of the body with high sun exposure, such as the head, face, neck, lower arms and lower legs, but they can occur anywhere on the body. However, location and appearance alone aren't always enough to tell the difference between a skin cancer and a non-cancerous skin spot (such as a sunspot, naevus or mole); a tissue sample in the form of a skin biopsy may be needed to confirm diagnosis. Early diagnosis is key in the management and treatment of skin cancer, catching it before it can spread to other parts of the body; often a biopsy to remove the cancer may be the only treatment required.

Protecting your skin from the sun's harmful UV-rays is key to reducing your risk of developing skin cancer. For more information see Cancer Council Australia (2020).

SKILLS IN PRACTICE

Skin biopsy

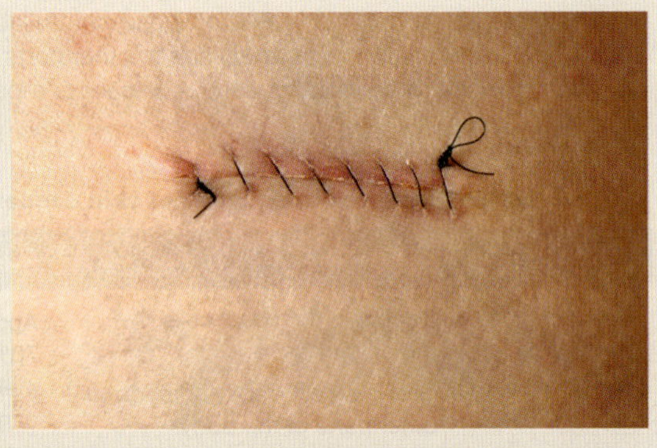

A skin biopsy is a procedure in which a sample of skin tissue is removed and this is then processed and examined under a microscope; it is usually undertaken to diagnose skin cancer or other skin conditions, and may be carried out by a GP or specialised skin cancer nurse. There are several methods that may be used to obtain a skin sample; the method selected depends on the size and location of the abnormal area of skin (the skin lesion). When the specimen has been obtained, it is placed in a solution (such as formaldehyde) and sent to the laboratory where it is processed and examined.

An assessment of the patient is carried out prior to a skin biopsy being performed. There is no special preparation required before having the biopsy. The procedure must be explained and a consent form will need to be signed.

The skin is cleaned and a marker may be used to outline the edges of the skin sample. The procedure is undertaken using a sterile approach. A local anaesthetic is injected and the procedure is performed; sutures will not be needed in some cases (e.g. a shave biopsy). The biopsy site is then covered with a sterile dressing. In a punch biopsy there may be a need for sutures, and this will depend on the size of biopsy. In excision biopsy, pressure may be applied to the site until the bleeding stops; sutures are needed to close the wound.

After the procedure, specific instructions are given to the patient on how to care for the biopsy site. The biopsy site should be kept clean and dry until it has healed completely. The clinic or hospital where the biopsy took place should be contacted if the patient experiences excessive bleeding or drainage through the dressing. If there is increased tenderness, pain, redness or swelling at the biopsy site, then the dermatology nurse or doctor should be contacted.

Langerhans cells

These cells are part of the immune system and arise from the red bone marrow (see the chapter on the skeletal system for a discussion on red bone marrow), they migrate from the bone marrow to the epidermis and make up a small part of the epidermal cells. The Langerhans cells regulate immune reactions in the skin as a defence against microorganisms that invade it (Waugh & Grant 2018); when the Langerhan cells are exposed to the sun they become very fragile and this impacts on their function.

The Langerhans cells are responsible for the processing of microbial antigens (helping to stimulate lymphocytes); their role is to assist other cells of the immune system in recognition of and response to microorganisms and destroy/remove the invading microbes via **phagocytosis**.

Merkel cells

A Merkel cell has the ability to have contact with a flattened process of a sensory neuron (a synaptic contact); this is a structure called a **tactile** disc (sometimes called a Merkel disc). The Merkel cells and the tactile discs (the least numerous of cells on the epidermis) are capable of detecting touch sensations; the greater the number of these, the more sensitive an area is (Tortora & Derrickson 2014).

Layers of the epidermis

Just as there are two distinct layers of skin — the dermis and epidermis — there are also a number of distinct layers of keratinocytes within the epidermis. These layers are developed over time and form the epidermis. These layers are called strata and are microscopically visible (see figure 18.3).

FIGURE 18.3 A microscopic perspective of the skin with the various strata

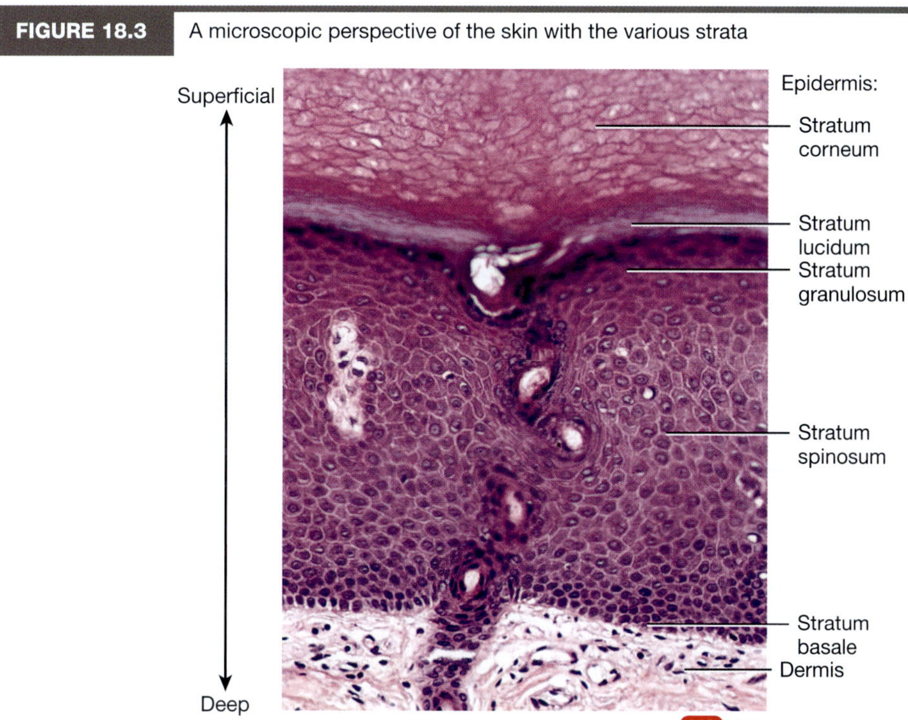

Source: Tortora and Derrickson (2009). Reproduced with permission of John Wiley & Sons.

The superficial and deeper levels of the epidermis are:

- the **stratum** corneum
- the stratum lucidum
- the stratum granulosum
- the stratum spinosum
- the stratum basale.

Table 18.2 provides an overview of the layers of the epidermis, and these are discussed in detail in the chapter.

TABLE 18.2 **The layers of the epidermis**

Layer	Location	Description
Stratum corneum	The most superficial of layers	Several layers of keratinised, dead epithelial cells These cells are flattened and have no nucleus
Stratum lucidum	When present, situated between the stratum corneum and the stratum granulosum	These cells are not present on the soles and palms The cells have no nucleus and are tightly packed
Stratum granulosum	Under the stratum corneum	Flattened cells arranged in approximately three to five layers Protect the body from losing fluid and also protect from harm Compact brittle cells as they lose their nucleus
Stratum spinosum	Above the stratum basale and below the stratum granulosum	These keratinocytes are tightly packed, flat and have spine-like projections
Stratum basale (sometimes called the basal cell layer)	The deepest layer	Cuboidal cells that are arranged as a single row; these divide and grow Also contains melanocytes

CLINICAL CONSIDERATIONS

Assisting with personal hygiene

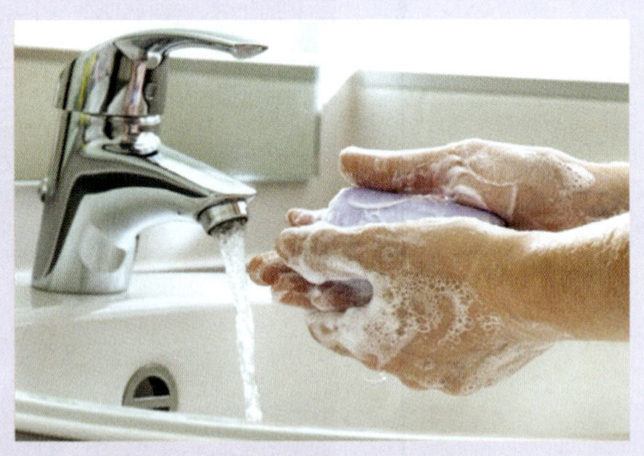

Healthcare professionals are required to demonstrate the knowledge, skills and an ability to meet people's needs related to personal and skin integrity and they must do this competently, with compassion and with due regard to dignity. One of the most important aspects of the role and function of the nurse and healthcare professional is to help people to attend to their personal hygiene when they are unable to do this. Washing a patient may be regarded a basic task that can be delegated to others; however, this important activity is a skilled activity that requires much thought as well as an assessment of the person being cared for. When assisting people with their hygiene needs, observe, assess and enhance skin and hygiene status and establish if there is any need for further support and intervention.

Understanding the anatomy and physiology of the skin and the complexities associated with this body system can help you offer high-quality care to those people you care for. When helping a person to maintain personal hygiene, take care and ensure that you use soaps and other toiletries that will not damage or potentially damage skin integrity. This will include ensuring that the person is not allergic to any of the products that have been chosen to wash and cleanse the skin. As far as is possible you should always ask the person if they are allergic to any toiletries or other skin products, as there are some people who are allergic to the chemicals found in soaps and cleansing products. This element of care provision requires you to be able to assess an individual's needs holistically.

You should bear in mind that when using some kinds of soap, this can have the same effect on the skin as swimming in the sea; the lather worked up by the soap when it is on the person's skin has a higher concentration of glycerine and as a result of this it can then draw out water from the epidermis. The product that has been chosen to clean the skin may have a harmful effect on the person's skin and this may potentially lead to the development of some skin conditions; for example, **dermatitis** and eczema.

Stratum corneum

The stratum corneum is the outer layer of the epidermis and it is made up of a number (about 25) of scale-like layers that are non-dividing (i.e. dead) and overlap with each other; the chief component of these cells is keratin; most of the fluid within these cells has been lost. The cells of the lower layers are composed of approximately 70 per cent water, whereas this layer is made up of 20 per cent fluid (Rizzo 2006). These cells are very tough and horny. The surface is covered in lipids, which provide a protective barrier; this layer provides structural strength. Constant friction means that this layer is being continuously rubbed off (sloughed off). The thickness of this specific layer will vary depending on the abrasion it is exposed to; the soles of your feet have a much thicker layer than your eyelids, for example.

There are other important functions associated with this layer, and these are in relation to a physical barrier to light and heat waves, microorganisms, chemicals and injury. The stratum corneum becomes thicker when it is exposed to strong sunlight, providing a barrier to ultraviolet rays. If the ultraviolet rays do reach through to the dermis, they will destroy the protein content of the skin, and this can lead to cancer of the skin (as explored earlier).

Stratum lucidum

Lying below the stratum corneum is the stratum lucidum, also known as the clear layer. There are five layers of flat dead cells here; this layer is not found on all aspects of the body, but rather only on areas of thick skin; for example, the heels. The cells have no nucleus and are tightly packed, providing a barrier to fluid loss.

Stratum granulosum

As the layers move towards the deeper level, the next layer is the stratum granulosum. There are between three and five layers of flattened keratinocytes in this aspect of the skin. These cells contain granules (hence the name stratum granulosum) that form a water-resistant lipid (lamellar granules), protecting the body from losing excess fluid and at the same time guarding against the entry of microbes. The flattening of the cells occurs as a result of pressure from below. The cells here undergo apoptosis; they lose their nucleus prior to dying, becoming compact and brittle as they move slowly up towards the surface; this process is known as **keratinisation**. The skin is now becoming tougher and stronger, getting ready to perform its protective function. This layer lies below the stratum lucidum.

Stratum spinosum

Below the stratum granulosum lies the stratum spinosum. The keratinocytes in this layer have spine-like projections (spinosum means thorn-like or prickly). The keratinocytes are tightly packed here. This tightly packed arrangement provides strength and flexibility to the skin.

Stratum basale

The stratum basale rests on the basement membrane and is the deepest layer of the epidermis; this layer provides a definite border between the dermis and epidermis. This is made up of a single row of columnar keratinocytes. The cells (stem cells or mother cells) of the epidermis originate from this deep layer. New cells are being constantly produced; they are continually dividing (the constant regeneration of the skin), slowly pushing older cells (called daughter cells) up through the other layers of the epidermis until they reach the surface. As we age, our ability to produce new epidermal cells reduces, contributing towards epidermal atrophy and resultant thinning of the skin (Nigam & Knight 2017).

CLINICALLY REASONED EPISODE OF CARE

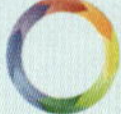

Antipsychotics and sun exposure

Consider the patient situation

Kylma is a 65-year-old woman who is currently taking clozapine for treatment-resistant bipolar disorder. Kylma was recently invited to attend a fishing trip; and while she wore a hat and protective clothing, she was exposed to the sun for approximately 40 minutes. She subsequently experienced sunburn to her shoulders and arms.

Kylma is experiencing pain and discomfort and is feeling unwell with nausea and cramps. She attends the emergency department later that evening as she is unable to sleep.

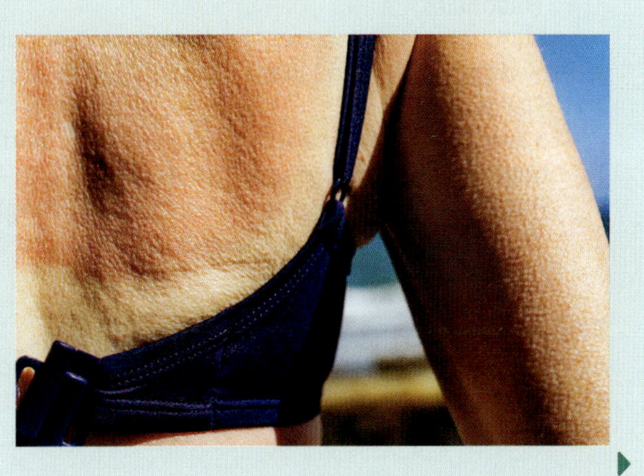

Collect cues and information

On arrival to the emergency department, Kylma has some visible **erythema** to her shoulders and arms with a small amount of blistering on her shoulders.

Observations: temperature 37 °C, heart rate 105 beats per minutes, respiratory rate 20 breaths per minute, oxygen saturation 98% on room air, and her pain is 2/10 due to intermittent cramping.

Kylma is diagnosed with heat stress and commences treatment in the emergency department.

Process information

Kylma has bipolar disorder and is taking psychotropic medications. This means that she is at a higher risk for heatstroke and heat-related illnesses. Antipsychotic medications can interfere with Kylma's ability to regulate heat and her awareness that her body temperature is rising.

Heat stress or exhaustion occurs after exposure to heat. Symptoms can be mild to extreme, including sweating, dizziness, fatigue, muscle cramps, nausea, vomiting and headache. Certain risk factors can exacerbate heat stress, such as being over the age of 65, being overweight and certain medications including antipsychotics.

Photosensitivity is a side effect of several medications, including psychiatric drugs. Most psychiatric medications will increase the body's sensitivity to the heat or sun. Photosensitivity is due to medications combining with proteins in the skin to form substances that react with direct light. The most common type of drug-induced photosensitivity is phototoxic reaction. In a phototoxic reaction, ultraviolet radiation converts drugs within the skin to a toxic metabolite. This produces an immediate exaggerated sunburn, often with oedema and a burning sensation. Being in the sun for as little as 30 to 60 minutes can cause a variety of symptoms.

This increased reaction to the sun can lead to heat stress and exhaustion; therefore, patients must be adequately educated on how to protect themselves when outdoors.

Establish goals

1. Commencement of treatment for heat exhaustion
2. Treatment of sunburn
3. Education on safe sun exposure

Nursing actions

1. Commence treatment for heat stress. Treatment should include:
   - removing excess clothing
   - commencing intravenous normal saline 0.9% solution
   - managing urine output at above 1–2 mL/kg/hr
   - administering analgesia and antiemetics
   - encouraging the oral intake of cool fluids and rest
   - commencing passive cooling such as sponging or spraying; icepacks may be used in extreme heat exhaustion
   - performing urinalysis for assessment of myoglobin and rhabdomyolysis
   - performing electrocardiogram (ECG) for assessment of tachycardia and electrolyte disturbance
   - performing blood tests.

   Rationale:
   - If left untreated, heat stress can lead to heat exhaustion, which is a medical emergency.
   - Assessment and reassessment should occur regularly for efficacy of treatment and to check for exacerbation of condition.
2. Commence treatment for sunburn. Treatment should include:
   - actively cooling the skin by sponging the area
   - applying water-based emollient or cream
   - encouraging oral water intake.

   Rationale:
   - Sunburn can exacerbate heat stress and should be managed.
3. Provide education and information on sun exposure.

   Rationale:
   - It is important that people taking high-risk medications are aware of the effects of sun exposure and how to limit the risk of adverse events.
   - Patients on medications which react to sunlight should avoid long periods of sun exposure, drink plenty of fluids, wear loose and light-coloured clothing, apply sunscreen and try to stay in the shade or indoors.

Evaluate outcomes

As a result of the intervention above, Kylma's condition stabilises and she can go home the next day. Having now experienced a phototoxic reaction and heat stress, she reports that she will take particular care when in the sun.

Reflect on new processes and learning
Consider the scenario. What clinical markers will nurses assess and reassess in the context of heat exhaustion?
Source: Based on the Clinical Reasoning Cycle, Levett-Jones (2013).

The dermis

The deepest part of the skin is called the dermis and lies directly below the epidermis; it is predominantly composed of dense connective tissue that contains **collagen** and elastic fibres. Embedded within the dermis are various structures which help the integumentary system carry out its vast range of functions:

- blood vessels
- nerves
- lymph vessels
- smooth muscles
- sweat glands
- hair follicles
- sebaceous glands.

The elastic system associated with the dermis supports the components above, as well as allowing the skin to flex with movement and to return to its normal shape when at rest. The dermis can be divided into two layers:

- the papillary aspect
- the reticular aspect.

The surface area of the dermis is much increased as a result of the finger-like papillary layers; the papillary layers connect the dermis to the epidermis (providing nutrients and waste removal to this avascularised layer). The fingerprints arise from this layer. The deeper aspect of the dermis is attached to the subcutaneous layer. Figure 18.4 shows the epidermis, the dermis and the subcutaneous layer.

FIGURE 18.4 Three layers of skin: the epidermis, the dermis and subcutaneous layer

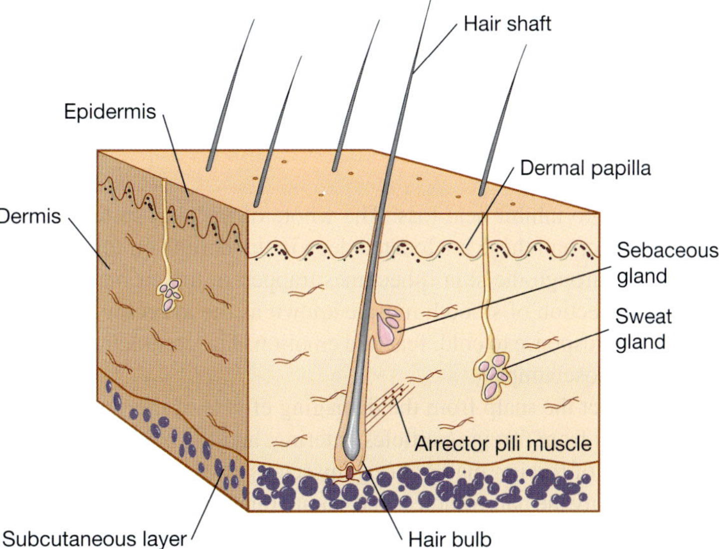

Source: Nair and Peate (2009). Reproduced with permission of John Wiley & Sons.

The papillary and reticular aspects

These aspects of the dermis, according to Tortora and Derrickson (2014), account for one-fifth of the total dermal layer, the superficial layer. The ridges caused by the papillary aspect are also known as friction ridges. These friction ridges can help the hand or foot grasp by increasing friction.

There is a capillary network within the papillary aspect. The dermal papillae also contain Meissner's corpuscles, and these are tactile receptors or touch receptors. The nerve endings here are sensitive to touch, as well as to sensations associated with warmth, coolness, pain and itching (**pruritus**).

Attached to the subcutaneous layer are irregular, dense connective tissues containing fibroblasts and collagen bundles, and coarse elastic fibre forms the reticular aspect. Other sensory receptors are found in this layer; for example, the Pacinian receptors for deep sensory pressure. This layer also contains sweat glands, lymph vessels, smooth muscle and hair follicles; these are called the accessory structures and are discussed next.

Tattoos inject ink deep into the dermal layer of the skin — if the ink were only injected into the epidermis, your tattoo would fade as epidermal layers are shed.

18.2 The accessory skin structures

LEARNING OBJECTIVE 18.2 Discuss the structure and growth of the appendages.

The accessory structures of skin are also known as the appendages. The following accessory structures of the skin will be outlined in this section of the chapter:

- hair
- sweat glands
- **nails**.

The hair

Hair can be found on most surfaces of the body apart from the palms, soles and lips; the amount, distribution, colour and texture differ depending on location, gender, age and ethnic group. There are different types of hair, and the earliest type is distinctive at approximately the fifth month of foetal development. Known as **lanugo**, it is a very fine, downy, non-pigmented hair and covers the body of the foetus. Just prior to birth, the lanugo of the eyelashes, eyebrows and scalp is shed and replaced by coarse hair, longer in length and heavily pigmented.

The hair can play a part in a person's distinctive appearance. The colour of the hair is influenced by the melanocytes that are found within the hair bulb. A progressive decline in melanin results in hair that is grey in colour. Hair growth is determined by genetic and hormonal factors.

Hairs are growths of dead keratin; each hair is a thread of keratin and is formed from cells at the base of a single follicle (Timby 2016). There are a number of functions associated with hair:

- sexual
- social
- **thermoregulation**
- protection.

The primary role of hair is to inhibit heat loss. The whole of the skin surface has hair follicles; every pore is an opening to a follicle, and these are located deep in the dermis on top of the subcutaneous layer. When heat leaves the body through the skin it becomes trapped in the air between the hairs. Each gland has attached to it a small collection of smooth muscle known as the **arrector pili** muscle. These muscles contract and become erect in response to cold, fear and emotion. The contraction of the muscle can be seen on the skin in the form of 'goosebumps'.

Hair on the head can protect the scalp from the damaging effects of the sun. The hair on the eyelashes and eyebrows guards the eyes from foreign particles entering, and the hair situated in the nostrils helps to protect against the inhalation of foreign material (e.g. insects).

Sebaceous glands accompany the hair follicles, and sebum (an oily substance) is exuded by these glands, supplying lubrication to the skin and at the same time ensuring that the skin and hair are waterproof as well as removing waste (e.g. old dead cells). Sebum is a slightly acidic substance and has antibacterial and antifungal properties (Boore et al. 2016). The distribution of the sebaceous glands differs. They are foremost on the scalp, face, upper torso and anogenital region, and these glands are at their most active during puberty; the manufacture of sebum is influenced by sex hormone levels. Figure 18.5 shows a pilosebaceous unit; this is made up of the follicle, the hair shaft, the sebaceous gland and the arrector pili.

The base of the onion-shaped bulb — the follicle — contains blood vessels, providing nourishment for the developing hair.

FIGURE 18.5 A pilosebaceous unit

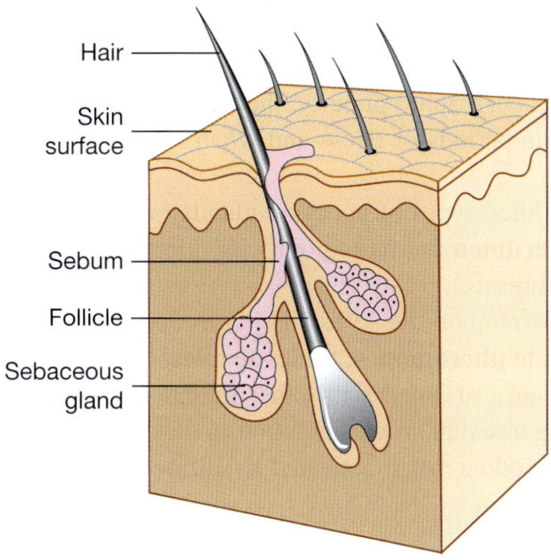

Source: Nair and Peate (2009). Reproduced with permission of John Wiley & Sons.

Sweat glands

There are a number of glands located within the skin; these can be thought of as mini-organs of the skin, which have a number of functions to fulfil. Sweat glands, also known as sudoriferous glands (from the Latin word *sudor*, meaning sweat), are coiled tubes composed of epithelial tissue and open out to pores that excrete onto the skin surface (see figure 18.6). All of the glands have separate nerve and blood supplies; each secretes a slightly acidic fluid made up of water and salts.

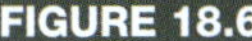
FIGURE 18.6 A sweat gland

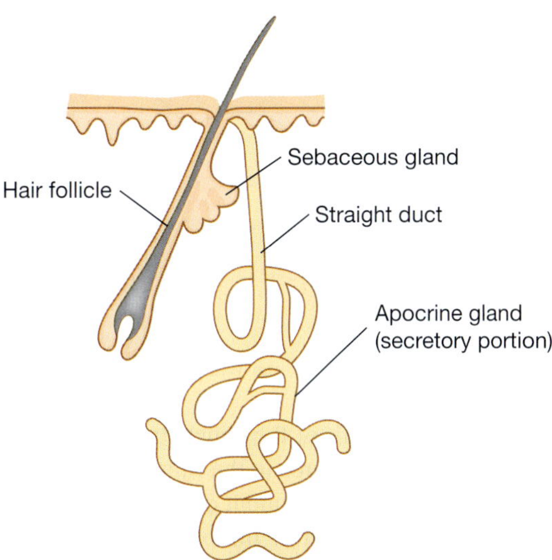

Source: Nair and Peate (2009). Reproduced with permission of John Wiley & Sons.

There are two kinds of sweat gland: eccrine and **apocrine**.

Eccrine glands

Reaction to heat and fear and the production of secretions by the eccrine glands occur in response to activity of the sympathetic nervous system. These types of gland are located all over the body. There are, however, sites on the body where they are more numerous; for example, the forehead, axillae, soles and palms.

The primary function of the eccrine glands is associated with thermoregulation. This is accomplished through the cooling effect of the evaporation of sweat on the surface of the skin. During hot weather, stress, exercise and pyrexia these glands produce more sweat.

Apocrine glands

Similar in structure, apocrine glands are also coiled; there are not as many of these in comparison with the eccrine glands, and they are found in more localised sites; for example, the pubic and axillary areas, the nipples and perineum. The exact function of the apocrine glands is not fully understood. These glands are not fully active until the person reaches puberty; they are larger, deeper and produce thicker secretions than the eccrine glands. During periods of stress and when in a heightened emotional state these glands produce more sweat.

There are a number of modified types of apocrine glands (specialised types); for example, those that are seen on the eyelids, the **cerumen**-producing (earwax) glands of the external auditory canal, and the milk-producing glands of the breasts.

The apocrine glands first develop on the soles and palms and then gradually appear all over the body. It is understood that they secrete **pheromones**; these are released into the external environment, enabling communication through the sense of smell with other members of the species, and this can provoke a number of reactions, including a sexual arousal reaction (a 'sexy sweat', if you like!). A viscous material is excreted that results in body odour when activated by surface bacteria — this is what we recognise as the **malodorous** properties of sweat.

Nails

The nails provide a protective covering for the ends of the fingers and the toes. Nails are tightly packed, dead, hard, keratinised epidermal cells that form a clean, solid covering over the digits (see figure 18.7).

FIGURE 18.7 The nail

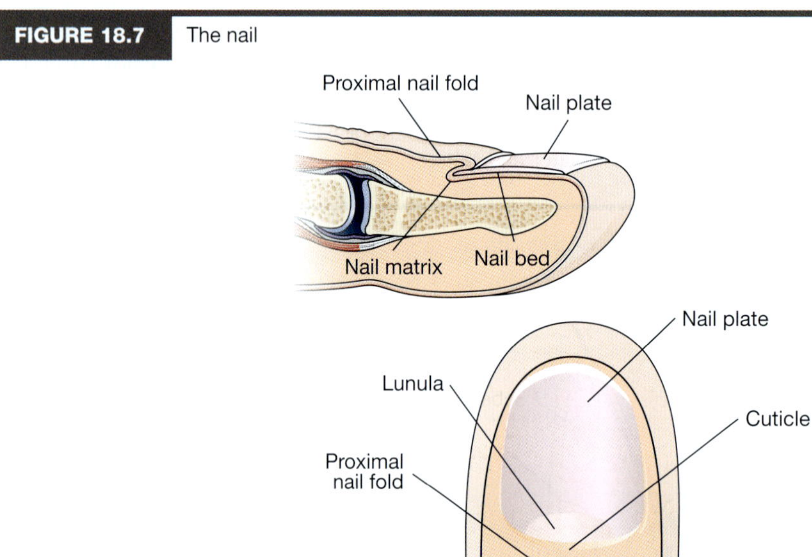

Source: Nair and Peate (2009). Reproduced with permission of John Wiley & Sons.

The horn-like structure of the nails is a result of the concentrated amount of keratin present; there are no nerve endings in nails. Nails act as a counterforce to the fingertips, the fingertips have numerous nerve endings, permitting a person to receive information about objects that are touched.

The majority of the nail body is pink, a result of the blood capillaries lying underneath. The white crescent present at the proximal ends of the nail is known as the **lunula** and is formed by air mixed with keratin matrix. The size of the lunula varies with individuals. The cuticle (also called the eponychium) is stratum corneum extending over the proximal end of the nail body.

Fingernails grow faster than toenails; as a person ages, the growth of nails slows. Nail growth varies, and on average they grow at a rate of 0.01 cm per day (1 cm per 100 days). Four to six months is required for fingernails to regrow completely; it takes toenails between 12 and 18 months for total regrowth. There are a number of factors that will influence the growth; for example, the age of the individual, diet, genetics, the time of year and the amount of exercise/activity undertaken (nails grow faster during the day, when you are more active). The growth of nails can be delayed by trauma and inflammation; changes in the integrity of the nails can be caused by injury or infection. In some cases, evidence of systemic diseases can be identified by the condition of the nails; for example, chronic cardiopulmonary disease or fungal infection (Fickertt-Wilson & Foret-Giddens 2017; Timby 2016).

CLINICALLY REASONED EPISODE OF CARE

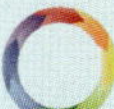

Tinea

Consider the patient situation

Maya is a 12-year-old who has been selected to represent her school in the national basketball championships; the competitions take her all over the country. Ever since Maya returned from a match in Queensland six weeks ago she has been experiencing a problem with her feet itching. During a visit to the school nurse for booster vaccinations, the nurse asks Maya how the basketball is going, and Maya tells the nurse that she is enjoying it but says her itchy feet are driving her crazy. The nurse assesses Maya.

Collect cues and information

Maya says that the area in between the toes of her left foot itches like crazy. The bottom of her right foot is red and itchy and some of the skin is even peeling off.

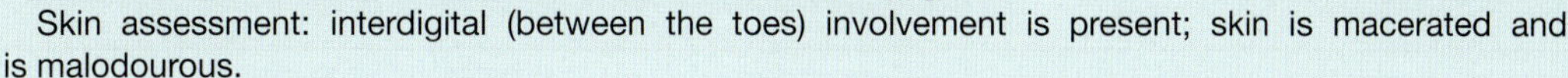

Skin assessment: interdigital (between the toes) involvement is present; skin is macerated and is malodourous.

A diagnosis of tinea pedis is made.

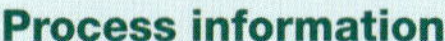

Process information

Tinea pedis is also known as athlete's foot. This condition is a common fungal condition and is caused by a dermatophyte (a type of fungus). Dermatophytosis infections are caused by a group of fungi that invade and grow in dead keratin. These infections can also appear on the body (tinea corporis), the groin (tinea cruris), the hands (tinea manuum), the scalp (tinea capitis), the nails (tinea unguium) and the face (tinea faciei).

Most infections are passed on from person to person (anthropophilic), but the infection can also be passed on by animals (zoophilic).

Nursing action

1. Support Maya and her family with education on the prescribed treatment for tinea pedis which includes:
   - a topical treatment applied to both feet including the soles and the interdigital spaces. Terbinafine 1% cream is prescribed for application 2–3 times a day for at least 4 weeks (AMH 2021; eTG complete 2020b)
   - advising Maya to keep her feet well aerated by wearing breathable footwear and leaving shoes off around the home; she should ensure her feet (particularly in between the toes) are dried thoroughly when wet as dry skin discourages fungal growth
   - dabbing, as opposed to rubbing, when drying the affected area, to help reduce the risk of local spreading of the infection
   - using a separate towel for the feet which should be washed regularly, and if possible dried in the sun (the sun will help to destroy the fungus), to reduce the risk of the infection spreading to other parts of the body (cross-infection)
   - prophylactic treatment with topical antifungals, which can be used once to twice a week on non-infected feet areas, to reduce the risk of the infection spreading
   - washing socks frequently and airing shoes and runners (not wearing the same pair of shoes for more than 2 days in a row), to ensure that the fungus will have died before reusing the socks or shoes and reduce the risk of reinfection
   - avoiding scratching the affected skin as doing so can cause cross-infection
   - not walking barefoot in places such as changing rooms and showers, and not sharing towels, socks or shoes with others, to reduce the risk of spreading the infection to other people
   - continuing the treatment for 4 weeks even if symptoms are reducing, to ensure that the infection is completely controlled
   - using an antifungal powder on feet and in shoes after finishing treatment, to prevent reinfection.

   Rationale:
   - Advice and reassurance will promote treatment concordance and improve the chance of positive health outcomes for Maya.

Evaluate outcomes

Maya reports that her feet are no longer red and itchy.

Source: Based on the Clinical Reasoning Cycle, Levett-Jones (2013).

SKILLS IN PRACTICE

Capillary nail bed refill

Also known as the nail blanch test, this is a simple and non-invasive test that can be used to assess cardiovascular status and is performed on the nail bed. It is often underused but can easily be carried out in hospital or in the field by healthcare practitioners to provide a good indication of peripheral tissue perfusion. When carrying out this test, it is important that the ambient environment should be warm and the following guidelines adhered to.

An explanation of the test is given to the patient; it should be explained that there will be minor pressure to the bed of the nail and this should not cause discomfort. If the person is using nail polish, this must be removed prior to taking the test. It will not be possible to perform this activity if the person is wearing false or acrylic nails.

Gently apply pressure to the nail bed until it turns white, indicating that the blood has been forced from the tissue (blanching). Once the tissue has blanched, pressure is removed. While the patient holds their hand at the level of their heart for 5 seconds, the healthcare practitioner measures the time it takes for blood to return to the tissue. Return of blood is indicated by the nail turning back to a pink colour. If there is a good blood flow to the nail bed, a pink colour should return in less than 2 seconds after pressure is removed.

Any abnormalities must be reported to the person in charge. The outcome of the test should be documented in the person's notes, and local policy and procedure must be adhered to at all times.

18.3 The functions of the skin

LEARNING OBJECTIVE 18.3 Describe the various functions associated with the skin, including how the skin functions as a homeostatic mechanism.

A fundamental understanding of the structure of the skin allows the reader to begin to understand the numerous functions of the skin. These functions include:

- sensation
- thermoregulation
- protection
- **excretion** and **absorption**
- synthesis of vitamin D.

Sensation

There are several receptor sites on the skin that have the ability to sense change in the external environment with respect to temperature and pressure; these receptors throughout the skin are made up of a wide and varied range of nerve endings. The messages picked up in the skin are then usually transferred to the brain. The chapter on the senses considers the senses in more detail.

Sensations that arise in the skin are known as **cutaneous** sensations; other sensations are those associated with vibration, tickling and irritations. There are some areas of the body that have more sensory receptors than others; for example, the lips, genitalia and tips of the fingers. The sensation of pain can signify actual or potential tissue injury.

MEDICINES MANAGEMENT

Administration of medicines

There are some medications that you may be asked to administer via the skin. These include ointments, lotions, creams, gels and patches (see the medicines management boxes on transdermal patches and use of topical steroids). The application of medicines via the skin through an adhesive patch is also used in a number of care areas. All of these medicines are subject to the same rules and regulations associated with the administration of any medicine. Medicines applied to skin are often needed to treat skin conditions, and they are known as topical medications; they are administered externally onto the body as opposed to being ingested or injected.

Lotions are used to protect, soften and soothe and can provide relief from itching. Ointments are oil-based, and body heat causes them to melt after application; often, these medications are used to fight infection or relieve inflamed tissue. Gloves must be used when applying these medicines; they must be applied in thin, even layers unless the prescription states otherwise (Gawthorpe 2018).

Most skin medications are provided for use in tubes; one tube must only be used for one person in order to prevent cross-infection. There are some skin medicines that must be sterile for use; when this is the case, after application, the leftover medication must be discarded.

When you are applying the medication, you must take care that you do not increase discomfort by using too much pressure or rubbing areas that are inflamed or causing the person pain.

HOMEOSTATIC IMBALANCE

Thermoregulation

The skin has a role to play in **homeostasis** through thermoregulation, helping to keep the temperature of the body within narrow ranges, adapting and adjusting as a person engages in a number of different activities. Effective thermoregulation is essential for survival; temperature changes can alter **enzyme** function and, as such, can impact on the chemical makeup of cells and their functions. The skin acts as a temperature regulator through a range of complex and integrated activities.

Changes in the size of blood vessels in the skin can help to regulate temperature. As body temperature rises, so the blood vessels dilate — this is known as **vasodilatation**; this is a multifaceted bodily defence mechanism that is attempting to get hot blood from the deeper tissues beneath to the surface of the skin for cooling down: the surface of the skin is cooler as heat radiates away from the body (this is why you might find yourself 'glowing bright red' after a session at the gym!). As this is happening, the sweat glands secrete water onto the surface of the skin. Evaporation occurs and, as a result of this, so too does cooling. (To help cool you, sweat has to evaporate off — the sweat dripping from you doesn't have the same effect.)

The opposite will occur when the person is in a cold environment. The blood vessels constrict — **vasoconstriction** — and blood stays closer to the core of the body, preserving heat. This contributes towards the pale appearance associated with being cold (think of your fingers and toes getting paler or losing colouration when you spend too long in the sea).

The hair (as previously described) plays an important part in thermoregulation. Pockets of air are trapped in the hair when the arrector pili muscles are stimulated to contract, making the hairs stand up. The trapped air causes insulation to occur, insulating the surrounding environment on the skin from the cooler atmosphere.

MEDICINES MANAGEMENT

Transdermal patches

Transdermal drug administration (skin patch) provides consistent, continuous drug delivery through the skin into the bloodstream. When applying the medication, the nurse should follow the manufacturer's instructions, adhere to local policy and procedure, and carry out the following instructions.

- Follow the 'five rights' of drug administration.
- Provide privacy, perform hand hygiene and explain the procedure to the patient.
- Use gloves.
- If applicable, remove the old patch and dispose of it.
- Select a new site for the patch on a flat surface, such as the chest, back, flank or upper arm. Rotate sites throughout therapy.
- Ensure the skin is intact, non-irritated and non-irradiated.
- Avoid hairy areas if possible, or shave/cut excessive hair.
- If the site needs to be cleaned prior to application, use only clear water; let the skin dry completely.
- Open the packing carefully and remove the patch from its pouch and peel half of its protective liner. If the patch is damaged during opening, then throw it away and start again.
- Take care not to touch the sticky side of the patch. Place the adhesive side on the skin and then peel off the other half of the liner. Press the skin patch firmly with the palm of your hand for at least 30 seconds, making sure it adheres to the skin, particularly at the edges.
- Remove gloves and perform hand hygiene.
- Document the medication administration.

The patient can shower as usual and get the patch wet. However, the patch should not be kept under water for long periods of time as this can cause it to loosen or fall off.

Advise the person not to use a heating pad on the body where wearing a patch. The heat can cause the patch to release its drug faster, and this could result in overdose.

Patches should be stored as per the manufacturer's instructions and they should be kept away from children.

Source: Pullen (2008).

Protection

There are many ways in which the skin protects the body, and a number of these have already been discussed; for example, the skin's ability to protect by the production of melanin against the harmful effects of ultraviolet light. Through its ability to intensify normal cell replacement when needed and the ability to shed dead skin and cause the migration of cells, the skin maintains the integrity of the body.

CLINICAL CONSIDERATIONS

Wound healing

Wound healing is an example of the skin's protective mechanism; this process consists of four distinct, sequential phases (Han & Ceilley 2017).

1. *Haemostasis*. The process of vascular constriction and clotting to prevent blood loss and temporarily seal the wound (see the chapter on the circulatory system).
2. *Inflammation*. White blood cells (neutrophils, macrophages and lymphocytes) infiltrate the wound site, in accordance with an increase in blood flow to the site. This process helps 'tidy' the site of foreign pathogens and waste products; the white 'pus' you see at an inflamed wound/pustule is the collection of dead white blood cells and their debris.
3. *Proliferation*. Generally overlapping the late inflammatory phase, epithelial tissue proliferates (replicates/grows) in tandem with the formation of new capillaries, collagen and granulation tissue (in the dermis).
4. *Remodelling*. New tissue remodels and matures over time to either: 1) regain original function; or 2) become scar tissue.

Wounds generally heal in approximately 6 weeks, depending on the depth and severity of the wound. However, multiple factors can lead to impaired wound healing; these are categorised into local (to the wound itself) or systemic factors (relating to the overall health of the individual). Local factors include tissue oxygenation, infection, the presence of a foreign body and poor vascular flow (either through conditions such as peripheral vascular disease or due to sustained pressure, such as during bed rest). Systemic factors include age (older adults experience impaired wound healing), comorbidities (such as diabetes, jaundice, hereditary healing disorders), suppressed immunity, obesity, medications (particularly non-steroidal anti-inflammatory drugs and corticosteroids), alcoholism, smoking and poor nutrition. It is important to note that these factors are not mutually exclusive, with many interacting to significantly impede the wound-healing process.

Sebum (an oily substance) secreted by the skin contains bacterial chemicals that have the ability to destroy surface bacteria. When sweat is produced, the acidic pH has the potential to hamper the proliferation of bacteria. Phagocytic macrophages present in the dermis have the ability to ingest and destroy viruses and bacteria that have penetrated the surface of the skin. By eliminating waste products through the pores on the skin (and there are over 2 million of these), the skin can help to protect the body from a build-up of poisonous substances. The skin also has the ability to prevent body fluids from escaping, preventing dehydration and helping to regulate the amount of fluid through the content and volume of sweat produced. As a waterproof barrier, the skin can also ensure that harmful fluids in the environment are prevented from entering the body.

CLINICAL CONSIDERATIONS

Occupational dermatitis

The use of vinyl gloves (these are considered 'hypoallergenic') has increased and is believed to be safer than latex gloves. However, contact allergy to vinyl gloves is not rare and vinyl can also be responsible for dermatitis. Dermatitis can occur on any part of the body; however, the skin on the hands is the most commonly affected area. Wearing gloves for long periods — during clinical practice, for example — increases the risk of the healthcare worker developing occupational dermatitis; using the wrong type of glove for a particular task has the potential to cause the condition to develop and can exacerbate an existing condition.

If the healthcare worker is concerned about occupational dermatitis, they should contact their occupational health services as soon as possible to seek advice. If the dermatitis does not resolve with treatment and modifications at work have been instigated, then a referral to a dermatologist for patch testing to identify or exclude sensitisers that may be causing the problem will be required.

CLINICAL CONSIDERATIONS

Dehydration

Many people in a number of care environments are prone to dehydration. The older person is particularly at risk, and your role is to prevent and identify dehydration and to take actions to remedy any deficits; you will be required to assess, plan, implement and evaluate care.

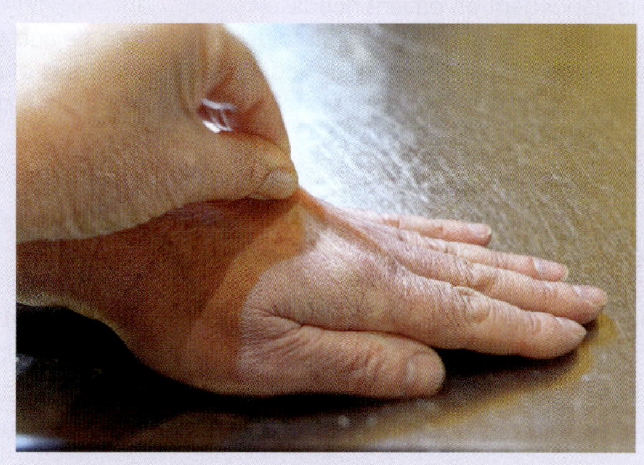

Undertaking a safe and effective assessment of needs requires a variety of skills: you will be required to observe, measure and ask questions (Lapin 2018). The skin can tell you much about the people you care for. You can make a diagnosis of dehydration by observing the skin of those in your care, although this is not and should not be used as the sole diagnostic tool. The classic signs of dehydration in older people include loss of skin recoil (also described as loss of skin turgor), increased thirst, reduced urinary output, tachycardia and hypotension; the person may also be confused. However, these signs are late signs of dehydration.

The skin may lack its normal elasticity and revert to its usual position slowly when gently pinched up into a fold if lack of skin turgor is present. Normally, the skin springs right back into position in a hydrated person. Care must be taken not to harm the person when trying to make an assessment and diagnosis.

Excretion and absorption

Some elements of secretion and absorption have already been mentioned with respect to the skin's function in protecting the person. The skin has the ability to excrete substances from the body; sweat is composed of water, sodium, carbon dioxide, ammonia and urea. Jenkins et al. (2013) point out that the body (despite its almost waterproof nature) can excrete approximately 400 mL of water daily; those who lead a less active lifestyle will lose less, and a more active person will lose more.

The skin also has the ability to absorb substances from the environment. Materials are absorbed from the external environment into the body cells, and some of these substances when absorbed are toxic; for example, heavy metals such as lead and mercury. There are some therapeutic and non-therapeutic medications that can be absorbed through the skin. A number of fat-soluble vitamins — A, D, E and K — oxygen and carbon dioxide are also absorbed.

MEDICINES MANAGEMENT

Use of topical steroids

Topical steroids are used in addition to emollients (moisturisers) for treating skin conditions such as eczema. Topical steroids reduce skin inflammation and they are available as creams, ointments, gels, mousses and lotions; they work by reducing inflammation in the skin (inflamed skin is easily infected). Steroid medicines that reduce inflammation are also known as corticosteroids (cortisone creams).

They are generally grouped into four categories, depending on their strength: mild, moderate, potent and very potent. There are various brands and types in each category. Some mild corticosteroids can be bought over the counter at a pharmacy; however, stronger corticosteroids are prescription only. Hydrocortisone cream 1%, for example, is a commonly used steroid cream and is classified as a mild topical steroid. The greater the strength, the more effect it has on reducing inflammation, but with this comes the greater risk of side effects with continued use. Creams are usually best to treat moist or weeping areas of skin. Ointments are usually best to treat areas of skin that are dry or thickened. Lotions may be useful to treat hairy areas, such as the scalp.

It is usual to use the lowest strength topical steroid first. If there is no improvement after 3–7 days, a stronger topical steroid may be prescribed. For severe cases a stronger topical steroid may be prescribed from the outset. Occasionally, two or more preparations of different strengths are used at the same time; for example, a mild steroid for the face and a moderately strong steroid for patches of eczema on the thicker skin of the arms or legs. A very strong topical steroid is often needed for eczema on the palms and soles of the feet of adults as these areas have thick skin.

In most cases, a course of treatment for 7–14 days is enough to clear a flare-up of eczema. In some cases, a longer course is needed. Many people with eczema may require a course of topical steroids to clear a flare-up. The frequency of flare-ups and the number of times a course of topical steroids is needed is dependent on patient needs.

Short courses of topical steroids are usually safe and cause no problems. Problems may arise if topical steroids are used for long periods, or if short courses of stronger steroids are often repeated. Side effects associated with mild topical steroids are uncommon. Side effects from topical steroids can either be local or systemic.

Synthesis of vitamin D

The skin is actively involved in the production and synthesis of vitamin D. For vitamin D to synthesise effectively, activation of a precursor molecule in the skin by ultraviolet rays in the sunlight (ultraviolet radiation) is required. Enzymes present in the kidneys and liver alter the molecules, producing calcitriol. Calcitriol (a hormone) assists in the absorption of calcium present in food in the intestines into the blood.

SUMMARY

The skin is an exceptional organ and is also known as the integumentary system. There are a variety of diseases or injuries that can easily be observed on the surface of the skin; for example, a skin rash, the presence of jaundice or **cyanosis**. It is the largest organ in the body in weight and surface area (Hubert & VanMeter 2018). The skin has the ability to reveal how we feel and what emotional state we may be in: humans blush, sweat and tremble. No other organ in the body is as easily looked over or palpated as the skin; the skin is also more easily exposed to injury such as infection and trauma.

This organ is the interface between the external and internal environments. The skin contributes to the homeostasis of the body, and the physical changes noted can point to homeostatic imbalance. The skin is also composed of the accessory structures, such as the nails and a number of glands; these are sometimes called the appendages.

The skin has the ability to allow a person to experience pleasure, pain and other stimuli from the external environment.

KEY TERMS

absorption Intake of fluids or other materials by cells of the skin.
apocrine A type of gland found in the skin, apocrine glands in the skin and eyelids are sweat glands.
apoptosis Death of a cell as signalled by the nuclei in a normally functioning cell.
arrector pili A microscopic muscle attached to hair follicles.
cerumen Earwax secreted by ceruminous glands.
collagen A protein that is the main component of connective tissue.
cutaneous Relating to the skin.
cyanosis A bluish discolouration of the skin and mucous membranes.
dermatitis Inflammation of the skin.
enzyme A substance that accelerates chemical reactions.
erythema Redness.
excretion The process of elimination of waste products from the body.
hair A thread-like structure produced by the hair follicles emerging from the dermis.
homeostasis The ability to maintain a constant internal environment.
hyperkeratosis Excess keratins are produced, resulting in thickening of the skin.
innervations Related to the supply of nerves.
integumentary The external covering of the body, relating to the skin.
keratin A tough, insoluble protein found in the hair and nails and other keratinised areas of the body.
keratinisation To convert into keratin.
lanugo Fine, downy hair covering the foetus.
lunula The moon-shaped white area at the base of nails.
malodourous Smelling unpleasant.
melanin Pigment found in some parts of the body; for example, the skin and hair.
nails Hard plates that are mainly composed of keratin.
organ A structure that is composed of two or more kinds of tissue with a specific function and a recognised shape.
papules Small pimples or swelling on the skin, often forming part of a rash.
pathogens Disease-producing microbes.
phagocytosis The act of destroying and ingesting microbes by phagocytes.
pheromones Chemicals that trigger an innate behavioural response in another.
proliferation A rapid and repeated reproduction of new cells.
pruritus Itching.
pustules Small blisters or pimples on the skin containing pus.
sebum An oily substance made of fat and the debris of fat-producing cells produced by the sebaceous glands.
stratum A layer.
tactile Pertaining to touch.
thermoregulation Ability to regulate temperature.
vasoconstriction Reduction in the diameter of blood vessels.
vasodilatation Increase in diameter of blood vessels.

FIND OUT MORE

1. What are the names of the touch receptors?
2. Where does nail growth originate?
3. Describe the anatomical and physiological changes that occur when a person experiences goosebumps.
4. Name three potential complications of body piercing.
5. What procedures can be used to remove tattoos?
6. What is needed to activate vitamin D and why?
7. What is the role and function of the arrector pili?
8. Describe what happens to the skin when vasodilatation occurs.
9. Outline the processes involved as skin repairs itself after being damaged.
10. How does the skin and renal system work together to maintain homeostasis?

CONDITIONS

The following is a list of conditions that are associated with the skin. Take some time and write notes about each of the conditions. You may make the notes taken from textbooks or other resources (e.g. people you work with in a clinical area), or you may make the notes as a result of people you have cared for. If you are making notes about people you have cared for, you must ensure that you adhere to the rules of confidentiality.

Tinea unguium

Skin cancer:
- Malignant melanoma
- Basal cell carcinoma (BCC)
- Squamous cell carcinoma (SCC)

Eczema

Human papillomavirus, types 1, 2, 4, 27 and 57

Burns:
- First degree
- Second degree
- Full thickness

Pressure sores

REFERENCES

AMH (2021) Dermatological drugs — drugs for skin infections. https://amhonline.amh.net.au/chapters/dermatological-drugs/drugs-skin-infections/other-antifungals-skin/terbinafine-skin (accessed 8 February 2021).

Boore, J., Cook, N. and Shepherd, A. (2016) *Essentials of Anatomy and Physiology for Nursing Practice*. London: Sage

Cancer Council Australia (2020) Understanding skin cancer: a guide for people with cancer, their friends and their family. Cancer Council Australia. www.cancer.org.au/assets/pdf/understanding-skin-cancer-booklet (28 January 2021).
Colbert, B.J., Ankney, J. and Lee, K.T. (2012) *Anatomy and Physiology for Health Professionals: An Interactive Journey*, 2nd edn. Upper Saddle River, NJ: Pearson.
eTG complete (2020a) Dermatology: acne. www.tg.org.au (accessed 8 February 2021).
eTG complete (2020b) Dermatology: tinea. www.tg.org.au (accessed 8 February 2021).
Fickertt-Wilson, S. and Foret-Giddens, J. (2017) *Health Assessment for Nursing Practice,* 6th edn. St Louis: Elsevier.
Gawthorpe, D.M. (2018) The principles of medicine administration and pharmacology. In Peate, I. and Wild, K. (eds), *Nursing Practice, Knowledge and Care*, 2nd edn. Oxford: John Wiley & Sons, Ltd; pp. 376–403.
Han, G. and Ceilley, R. (2017) Chronic wound healing: a review of current management and treatments. *Advances in Therapy* 34(3): 599–610.
Hubert, R.J. and Van Meter, K.C. (2018) *Gould's Pathophysiology for the Health Professions*, 6th edn. St Louis Elsevier.
Jenkins, G.W., Kemnitz, C.P. and Tortora, G.J. (2013) *Anatomy and Physiology: From Science to Life*, 3rd edn. Hoboken, NJ: John Wiley & Sons, Inc.
Levett-Jones, T. (2013). *Clinical Reasoning: Learning to Think Like a Nurse.* Pearson Australia.
Lapin, M. (2018) The nursing process. In Peate, I. and Wild, K. (eds), *Nursing Practice, Knowledge and Care*, 2nd edn. Oxford: John Wiley & Sons, Ltd; pp. 111–128.
McLaughlin, M.F. (2018) Integumentary issues. In Stannard, D. and Krenzischek, D.A (2018) *Perianesthesia Nursing Care*, 2nd edn. Burlington: Jones and Bartlett; pp. 83–89.
Nair, M. and Peate, I. (2009) *Fundamentals of Applied Pathophysiology: An Essential Guide for Nursing Students*. Oxford: John Wiley & Sons, Ltd.
Nigam, Y. and Knight, J. (2017) Anatomy and physiology of ageing 11: the skin. *Nursing Times* [online] 113(12): 51–55.
Pullen, R.L., Jr. (2008) Clinical do's and don'ts: administering a transdermal patch. *Nursing 2021* 38(5): 14.
Rizzo, D.C. (2006) *Delmar's Fundamentals of Anatomy and Physiology*, 2nd edn. New York: Thomson.
Shier, D., Butler, J. and Lewis, R. (2016) *Hole's Anatomy and Physiology*, 14th edn. Boston, MA: McGraw-Hill.
Timby, B.K. (2016) *Fundamental Nursing Skills and Concepts*, 11th edn. Philadelphia, PA: Wolters Kluwer Health.
Tortora, G.J. and Derrickson, B.H. (2009) *Principles of Anatomy and Physiology*, 12th edn. Hoboken, NJ: John Wiley & Sons, Inc.
Tortora, G.J. and Derrickson, B. H. (2014) *Principles of Anatomy and Physiology*, 14th edn. Hoboken, NJ: John Wiley & Sons, Inc.
Waugh, A. and Grant, A. (2018) *Ross and Wilson Anatomy and Physiology*, 13th edn. Edinburgh: Elsevier.
World Cancer Research Fund (n.d.) Skin cancer statistics: melanoma of the skin is the 19th most common cancer worldwide. www.wcrf.org/dietandcancer/cancer-trends/skin-cancer-statistics (accessed 2 March 2021).

FURTHER READING

ECZEMA ASSOCIATION OF AUSTRALASIA

www.eczema.org.au

The Eczema Association of Australasia (EAA) supports and educates eczema sufferers, their carers and the wider community, and aims to greatly increase public awareness of eczema.

FIONA WOOD FOUNDATION

www.fionawoodfoundation.com

Fiona Wood Foundation is an Australian charity working to grow the body of knowledge in burns management and recovery.

PSORIASIS AUSTRALIA

www.psoriasisaustralia.org.au

Psoriasis Australia works to help people whose lives are affected by psoriasis and psoriatic arthritis through the provision of up-to-date information and support.

ACKNOWLEDGEMENTS

Photo: © Suzanne Tucker / Shutterstock.com
Photo: © Vizual Studio / Shutterstock.com
Photo: © Dermatology11 / Shutterstock.com
Photo: © Australis Photography / Shutterstock.com
Photo: © bgwalker / Shutterstock.com
Photo: © Alexander Raths / Shutterstock.com
Photo: © Anetlanda / Shutterstock.com
Photo: © Robert Przybysz / Shutterstock.com
Photo: © Anne Webber / Shutterstock.com
Figure 18.2: © World Cancer Research Fund

ANSWERS

Chapter 1 Basic scientific principles of physiology

True or false

1. False — an ion has a net charge and is not therefore electrically neutral.
2. True
3. True
4. True
5. False — lipids are organic molecules.
6. True

Chapter 2 Cells, cellular compartments, transport systems, fluid movement between compartments

True or false

1. False — molecules move from where they are at high concentration to where they are at a lower concentration.
2. True
3. True
4. True
5. False — sodium is the principal extracellular ion.
6. True
7. False — it is a lower than normal sodium level.
8. False — it is an isotonic solution.
9. True

Chemical symbols

Potassium K^+
Sodium Na^+
Bicarbonate HCO_3^-
Chloride Cl^-
Organic phosphate PO_4^{3-}
Sulphate SO_4^{2-}
Calcium Ca^{2+}

Chapter 3 Genetics

True or false

1. True
2. False — the phenotype would be determined by the dominant allele.
3. True
4. False — hydrogen bonds hold the two strands together.
5. True

Chapter 7 The skeletal system

True or false

1. True
2. False — babies have more bones than adults.
3. True
4. False — the ribs protect the organs in the chest cavity.

5. False — red bone marrow produces blood cells.
6. False — male bones tend to be larger and therefore heavier.
7. False — the patella is located between the femur and the tibia.
8. True
9. True
10. False — the appendicular skeleton has many more bones than the axial.

Chapter 10 The digestive system

True or false

1. True
2. False
3. False
4. True
5. True
6. False
7. True
8. False
9. False
10. False

Chapter 17 The immune system

True or false

1. False — phagocytes are white blood cells.
2. True
3. True
4. False — they are descended from multipotent stem cells.
5. False — it is monocytes and tissue macrophages that are included within the family of macrophages.
6. False — it is some of the B-cells that develop into plasma cells.
7. True
8. True
9. True
10. False — sneezing is a mechanical barrier.

NORMAL VALUES

Haematology

Full blood count
Haemoglobin (males) 13.0–18.0 g dL^{-1}
Haemoglobin (females) 11.5–16.5 g dL^{-1}
Haematocrit (males) 0.40–0.52
Haematocrit (females) 0.36–0.47
MCV 80–96 fL
MCH 28–32 pg
MCHC 32–35 g dL^{-1}
White cell count (4–11) × 10^9 L^{-1}

White cell differential

Neutrophils 1.5–7 × 10^9 L^{-1}
Lymphocytes 1.5–4 × 10^9 L^{-1}
Monocytes 0–0.8 × 10^9 L^{-1}
Eosinophils 0.04–0.4 × 10^9 L^{-1}
Basophils 0–0.1 × 10^9 L^{-1}
Platelet count 150–400 × 10^9 L^{-1}
Reticulocyte count (25–85) × 10^9 L^{-1} or 0.5–2.4%

Erythrocyte sedimentation rate

Westergren
Under 50 years:
Males 0–15 mm/1st hour
Females 0–20 mm/1st hour
Over 50 years:
Males 0–20 mm/1st hour
Females 0–30 mm/1st hour

Plasma viscosity 1.50–1.72 mPa s^1 (at 25 °C)

Coagulation screen

Prothrombin time 11.5–15.5 s
International normalised ratio <1.4
Activated partial thromboplastin time 30–40 s
Fibrinogen 1.8–5.4 g L^{-1}
Bleeding time 3–8 min

Coagulation factors

Factors II, V, VII, VIII, IX, X, XI, XII 50–150 IU dL^{-1}
Factor V Leiden Present or not
Von Willebrand factor 45–150 IU dL^{-1}
Von Willebrand factor antigen 50–150 IU dL^{-1}
Protein C 80–135 IU dL^{-1}
Protein S 80–120 IU dL^{-1}
Antithrombin III 80–120 IU dL^{-1}
Activated protein C resistance 2.12–4.0
Fibrin degradation products <100 mg L^{-1}
D-dimer screen <0.5 mg L^{-1}

Haematinics

Serum iron 12–30 μmol L^{-1}
Serum iron-binding capacity 45–75 μmol L^{-1}
Serum ferritin 15–300 μg L^{-1}
Serum transferrin 2.0–4.0 g L^{-1}
Serum B_{12} 160–760 ng L^{-1}
Serum folate 2.0–11.0 μg L^{-1}
Red cell folate 160–640 μg L^{-1}
Serum haptoglobin 0.13–1.63 g L^{-1}

Haemoglobin electrophoresis

Haemoglobin A >95%
Haemoglobin A2 2–3%
Haemoglobin F <2%

Chemistry

Serum sodium 137–144 mmol L^{-1}
Serum potassium 3.5–4.9 mmol L^{-1}
Serum chloride 95–107 mmol L^{-1}
Serum bicarbonate 20–28 mmol L^{-1}
Anion gap 12–16 mmol L^{-1}
Serum urea 2.5–7.5 mmol L^{-1}
Serum creatinine 60–110 μmol L^{-1}
Serum corrected calcium 2.2–2.6 mmol L^{-1}
Serum phosphate 0.8–1.4 mmol L^{-1}
Serum total protein 61–76 g L^{-1}
Serum albumin 37–49 g L^{-1}
Serum total bilirubin 1–22 μmol L^{-1}
Serum conjugated bilirubin 0–3.4 μmol L^{-1}
Serum alanine aminotransferase 5–35 U L^{-1}
Serum aspartate aminotransferase 1–31 U L^{-1}
Serum alkaline phosphatase 45–105 U L^{-1} (over 14 years)
Serum gamma glutamyl transferase 4–35 U L^{-1} (<50 U L^{-1} in males)
Serum lactate dehydrogenase 10–250 U L^{-1}
Serum creatine kinase (males) 24–195 U L^{-1}
Serum creatine kinase (females) 24–170 U L^{-1}
Creatine kinase MB fraction <5%
Serum troponin I 0-0.4 μg L^{-1}
Serum troponin T 0–0.1 μg L^{-1}
Serum copper 12–26 μmol L^{-1}
Serum ceruloplasmin 200–350 mg L^{-1}
Serum aluminium 0-10 μg L^{-1}
Serum magnesium 0.75–1.05 mmol L^{-1}
Serum zinc 6–25 μmol L^{-1}
Serum urate (males) 0.23–0.46 mmol L^{-1}
Serum urate (females) 0.19–0.36 mmol L^{-1}
Plasma lactate 0.6–1.8 mmol L^{-1}
Plasma ammonia 12–55 μmol L^{-1}
Serum angiotensin-converting enzyme 25–82 U L^{-1}
Fasting plasma glucose 3.0–6.0 mmol L^{-1}
Haemoglobin A1 C 3.8–6.4%
Fructosamine <285 μmo L^{-1}
Serum amylase 60–180 U L^{-1}
Plasma osmolality 278–305 mosmol kg^{-1}

Urine

Albumin/creatinine ratio (untimed specimen) <3.5 mg $mmol^{-1}$ (males)
<2.5 mg $mmol^{-1}$ (females)

Lipids and lipoproteins

Target levels will vary depending on the patient's overall cardiovascular risk assessment.
Serum cholesterol <5.2 mmol L^{-1}
Serum LDL cholesterol <3.36 mmol L^{-1}
Serum HDL cholesterol >1.55 mmol L^{-1}
Fasting serum triglyceride 0.45–1.69 mmol L^{-1}

Blood gases (breathing air at sea level)

Blood H+ 35–45 nmol L^{-1}
pH 7.36–7.44
PaO_2 11.3–12.6 kPa
$PaCO_2$ 4.7–6.0 kPa
Base excess ±2 mmol L^{-1}

Carboxyhaemoglobin

Non-smoker <2%
Smoker 3–15%

Immunology/rheumatology

Complement C3 65–190 mg dL^{-1}
Complement C4 15–50 mg dL^{-1}
Total haemolytic (CH50) 150–250 U L^{-1}
Serum C-reactive protein <10 mg L^{-1}

Serum immunoglobulins

IgG 6.0–13.0 g L^{-1}
IgA 0.8–3.0 g L^{-1}
IgM 0.4–2.5 g L^{-1}
IgE <120 kU L^{-1}
Serum β_2-microglobulin <3 mg L^{-1}

Cerebrospinal fluid

Opening pressure 50–180 mmH_2O
Total protein 0.15–0.45 g L^{-1}
Albumin 0.066–0.442 g L^{-1}
Chloride 116–122 mmol L^{-1}
Glucose 3.3–4.4 mmol L^{-1}
Lactate 1–2 mmol L^{-1}
Cell count ≤5 mL^{-1}

Differential

Lymphocytes 60–70%
Monocytes 30–50%
Neutrophils None
IgG/ALB ≤0.26
IgG index ≤0.88

Urine

Glomerular filtration rate 70–140 mL min^{-1}
Total protein <0.2g/24 h
Albumin <30 mg/24 h
Calcium 2.5–7.5 mmol/24 h
Urobilinogen 1.7–5.9 μmol/24 h
Coproporphyrin <300 nmol/24 h
Uroporphyrin 6–24 nmol/24 h
δ-Aminolevulinate 8–53 μmol/24 h
5-Hydroxyindoleacetic acid 10–47 μmol/24h
Osmolality 350–1000 mosmol kg^{-1}

Faeces

Nitrogen 70–140 mmol/24 h
Urobilinogen 50–500 μmol/24 h
Fat (on normal diet) <7 g/24 h

The values listed here are generalisations. Each laboratory will have its own specific reference ranges.

INDEX

12-lead ECG 240
20/20 vision 445

abdominopelvic cavity 92
abduction 179
ABO system 205
Absorption 254, 532, 535–536
accessory muscles 329
accessory organs, of digestive system 268–274
  gall bladder 274
  liver and production of bile 272–273
  pancreas 270–272
  salivary glands 268–270
  teeth 268
acetylcholine (ACh) 133
acetylcholinesterase (AChE) 133
acid 10
acid-base balance 10, 341
acini glands 270
acne 518–519
acquired immune system 498–506
  cell-mediated immunity 498–499
  humoral immunity 500–501
  immunoglobulins 501–503
acquired immunity 488
acromegaly 459
action potential 224, 382–389
  cerebrospinal fluid 388–389
  meninges 387–388
  nerve impulses, simple propagation of 382–383
  neuroglia 386–387
  neurotransmitters 385–386
  refractory period 382–385
  saltatory conduction 382
active immunity 510
active transport 30, 31
acute apinal cord compression 400
acute compartment syndrome 132
acute kidney injury 290–291
acute lymphoblastic leukaemia (ALL) 72–73
adalimumab 497
adduction 179
adenine (A) 49
adenosine diphosphate (ADP) 31, 201
adenosine triphosphate (ATP) 31, 127, 193
adipose tissue 87, 90
adrenal cortex 468–473
  glucocorticoids 470
  mineralocorticoids 468–470
  pancreas 471–473
adrenal gland 467–468
adrenal medulla 467–468
adrenaline 246
adrenocorticotrophic hormone 460–462
aerobic respiration 132, 136–139
afferent fibres. 378
afferent nerve 418
afterload 244–245
age-related macular degeneration (AMD) 439–440
aldosterone 301–302
aldosterone secretion, control of 469
alkali 10
allele 51
allergy 508–509
alveolar minute ventilation 331
Alzheimer's disease 385–386
ampulla 426, 428
amylase 270
anabolic steroids 136
anaerobic 132
anaerobic respiration 136
anaphylaxis 510
anatomical dead space 331
anatomy 2
androgens 353, 357
angiotensin 301–302
angiotensin-converting enzyme inhibitors 291
anion 7
anosmia 416
antagonist 151
anterior 141
anterior pituitary gland 358, 458–462
anterior two-thirds of the tongue 419
antibiotic ear drops 424
antibodies 15, 435
anticoagulants 203
anticodon 54
antidepressants 419–420
antidiuretic hormone (ADH) 302, 392, 457–458
antigen 484
antihypertensives 292
antipsychotics 525–527
anus 254
aorta 326
aortic valve 227
apex 320
apical surface 80
apneustic centres 334
apocrine glands 530
apoptosis 521
appendicitis 267
appendicular skeleton 172–182
arachnoid mater 388
areolar 90
arrector pili 528
arterial blood 236
arterial blood pressure 211–212
arteries, structure and function of 207–209
articulations 159
arytenoid cartilage 321
asthma 324–325, 508–509
astrocytes 387
atelectasis 322
atom 2, 4–6
atomic number 5
atorvastatin 245
atresia 102
atria 227
atrial fibrillation 240–241
atrial natriuretic peptide (ANP) 302
atrioventricular (AV) bundle 237
atrioventricular (AV) node 237
atrioventricular (AV) valves 227
atrophic vaginitis 366
auditory reflex 432
auscultation of heart sounds 229–230
autocrine 453–454
autoimmune diseases 495–496
automaticity 237
autonomic nervous system 246, 379, 401–404, 436
  parasympathetic division 403–404
  sympathetic division 402, 404
autosomal dominant inheritance 63
autosomal recessive disorders 67
autosomal recessive inheritance 63–67
autosomes 51
axial skeleton 172–182
axon 379, 381

B-cell lymphocytes 486, 500–501
bactericidal 489
balanced diet 275–277
ball and socket 179
bariatric surgery 276
baroreceptor 211, 246–247
basal surface 80
base 10, 49
basophils 199, 483
bicuspid (mitral) valve 227
bile 265
  production of 272–273
bile ducts 272
bisphosphonates 162
blood 188
  components of 188–191
    plasma 190–191
    properties of blood 189–190
  functions of 191–206
    blood cells, formation of 192–193
    blood groups 204–206
    haemoglobin 193–197
    haemostasis 200–204
    platelets 200
    red blood cells 193
    white blood cells 197–200
blood cell development 482–483
blood cells 489–490
  formation of 192–193
blood clotting factors 201
blood groups 204–206
blood lipids 15
blood pressure 210–212
blood pressure management 291–293
blood supply 132
  of kidney 290–294
  respiratory system 326
blood transfusion 206
blood vessels 206–212
  arteries and veins, structure and function of 207–209
  blood pressure 210–212

capillaries 209–210
body fluids, composition of 34–36
electrolyte and water balance 34–36
body region 260
bonds 4
bone 91
bone formation 164–165
bone fractures 170–172
bone growth 165–168
bone marrow 483
bone remodelling 168–170
bone shapes 174–178
flat bones 175–177
irregular bones 177
long bones 174–175
sesamoid bones 178
short bones 175–176
botulism 133
Bowman's capsule 296–297
Boyle's law 327, 328
brain 389–395
brainstem 393
cerebellum 393
cerebrum 390–392
diencephalon 392
limbic system and reticular formation 393–395
structures of 391
brainstem 390, 393
respiratory centres of 334
breast, female sex hormones 368–369
breathing
control of 334–335
mechanics of 327–329
work of 329
broad ligaments 364
bronchial arteries 326
bronchial secretions, removal of 321–322
bronchial tree 320, 322–326
bronchial veins 326
bronchiectasis 324
bronchioles 323
bulk transport 33–34
bundle of His 237
burns 39, 86–87
initial management of 98

Caecum 266
calcification 164
calcitriol 467
calcium 466
calcium homeostasis 159
calyces 294
canal 365
cancer 362
canines 268
capacitation/hyperactivation 103
capillaries 209–210
capillary hydrostatic pressures 37, 38
capillary nail bed refill 532
carbamazepine 404
carbohydrates 13, 277, 452
carbon dioxide, transport of 340–341
cardiac catheterisation 233
cardiac cycle 222, 240–248
factors 244
heart rate, regulation of 245–248
stroke volume, regulation of 244–245
afterload 245
force of contraction 245
preload 244–245
cardiac medication 233–234
cardiac muscle 94, 126
cardiac notch 322
cardiac output 222
cardiac region 260
cardiac sphincter 258
cardiac system
cardiac action potential 226–230
endocardium 226
heart chambers 226–230
cardiac cycle 240–248
factors 244
heart rate, regulation of 245–248
stroke volume, regulation of 244–245
electrical pathways of heart 237–240
heart
blood flow through the heart 235–236
blood supply to 230–236
heart, size and location of 222–225
cardioinhibitory centre 246
cardiovascular centre 246
carotid arteries 334
cartilage 87, 90–91, 320, 422
skeletal system, connective tissues associated with 162–163
cartilage strong 163
cartilaginous joints 178
catabolism 277
cataracts 442–443
catecholamines 456
catheter-related bloodstream infections 210
cation 6, 382
cell 24
body fluids, composition of 34–36
cell membrane, structure of 25–26
components of 25
fluid movement 37–40
structure of 25
transport of substances 26–34
active transport 30, 31
bulk transport 33–34
communication 32
energy to power active transport 31–32
facilitated diffusion 30
fluid compartments 32–33
osmosis 28–30
passive transport 27–28
cell body 381
cell cycle 50, 56–60
meiosis 58–60
meiosis I 59–60
meiosis II 60
mitosis 58
cell destruction 499
cell membrane, structure of 25–26
cell-mediated immunity 498–499
cellular anatomical map 46
central adaptation 414
central nervous system 378–379
centromere 50
cephalic phase 262
cerebellum 390, 393
cerebral cortex 390
cerebral hemisphere 388
cerebrospinal fluid (CSF) 334, 387–389
cerebrovascular accident (CVA) 392
cerebrum 390–392
cerumen 530
cervix 366–367
chemical barriers 489
chemical bonds 4
chemical digestion 275
chemical senses 412–416
olfactory receptors 413–416
sense of smell 412–413
chemoreceptors 211, 334
chemotaxis 198
chest drain 322
chest pain 232–233
chief cell 261
cholecystokinin (CCK) 262
cholelithiasis 274
cholesterol 15
choroid 437
chromatids 50
chromosomes 50–52
disorders of 72–73
chronic kidney disease 298, 306–307
chronic obstructive pulmonary disease (COPD) 326, 332–333
chyme 260
cilia 319, 413
ciliary body 437
ciliated simple columnar epithelium 83
circle of Willis 389, 390
circulating hormones 211
circulatory system
blood vessels 206–212
arteries and veins, structure and function of 207–209
blood pressure 210–212
capillaries 209–210
components of blood 188–191
plasma 190–191
properties of blood 189–190
functions of blood 191–206
blood cells, formation of 192–193
blood groups 204–206
haemoglobin 193–197
haemostasis 200–204
platelets 200
red blood cells 193
white blood cells 197–200
circumvallate 417
clavicle 320
clotting disorders 202–203
clotting process, stages of 202
clotting system 494
clusters of definition (CDs) 498
coagulation 201–204
cochlea 431
codon 54
coenzymes 278
collagen 160, 527
collecting ducts 298–299
Colles' fracture 171–172

colostrum 114
compartments 25, 214
compounds 6
conceptus 105
concussion 393
conduction region 318
conduction system of heart 237
condyloid joints 179
cones 438–439
congenital genetic defects 71–72
conjunctivitis 435
connective tissue 80, 87–94, 353
  bone 91
  cartilage 90–91
  connective tissue proper 89–90
  constituents of 89
  fibre 88–89
  ground substance 88
  liquid connective tissue 91–92
  membranes 92–94
  with skeletal system 162–172
    bone formation 164–165
    bone fractures 170–172
    bone growth 165–168
    bone remodelling 168–170
    cartilage 162–163
    ligaments 163
    tendons 163–164
connective tissue proper 89–90
contraception 362–363
convergence 414
corniculate cartilage 321
coronary arteries 230, 231
corpus albicans 362
corpus luteum (CL) 103, 362
corticosteroid therapy 326
covalent bonding 6
cranial nerves 393, 395–397
  functions of 396
creatine phosphate 136
creon 271
cricoid cartilage 320
cricothyroid ligament 320
Crohn's disease 271–272
cryptorchidism 354–355
cuboidal epithelial tissue 85
cuneiform cartilage 321
Cushing's disease 460–461
cutaneous membranes 92
cutaneous sensations 532
cyanosis 537
cytoplasm 198, 470
cytosine (C) 49
cytotoxicity 489–490, 493, 499

deglutition 255–258
dehydration 38, 535
dendrites 379–381
dense connective tissue 90
deoxyribonucleic acid (DNA) 46–48
deoxyribose 49
depolarisation 240
depression 400
dermatitis 524
dermis 527
desmosomes 224
diabetes mellitus 96–97, 471–472
diabetic foot ulcers 96–97
diabetic gastroparesis 262
diaphragm 320
diaphysis 175
diarrhoea 293–294
diastole 241
diclofenac 181
dicrotic notch 242
diencephalon 390, 392
diffusion 27, 28, 81, 209
digestion 254
digestive hormones 274–275
  chemical digestion 275
  role 274
digestive system 254
  accessory organs of 268–274
    gall bladder 274
    liver and production of bile 272–273
    pancreas 270–272
    salivary glands 268–270
    teeth 268
  activity of 254–267
    mouth 255–256
    oesophagus 258–259
    organisation of 255
    pharynx 256–258
    structure of 259–267
  balanced diet 275–277
  body map 253
  digestive hormones 274–275
    chemical digestion 275
    role 274
  nutrient groups 277–282
  nutrients 275
digestive tract 83
digoxin 31, 238
distal convoluted tubule (DCT) 298
dominant allele 52
dominant follicle 102
Down syndrome, hypothyroidism in 465–466
downregulation 455
dropsy *See* oedema
duodenum 258
dura mater 388
dysphagia 257–258

ear care 422–423
ear damage 433–434
ear drops, instillation of 424
ear, structure of 421–426
  external ear 421–425
  inner ear 426–427
  middle ear 425–426
eccrine glands 529
ECG 239–240
ectoderm 109
ectopic pregnancy 116, 370–371
effacement 114
effector 379
efferent fibres 379, 414
ejaculatory duct 356
elastic cartilage 90, 163
electrical pathways, of heart 237–240
electrocardiogram 243
electroencephalogram (EEG) 385
electrolyte 9–10, 34–36, 188, 468
electromyography (EMG) 135
electrons 4
elements 4
elongation 54
emboli 210
embolism 338
embryology 102
  complications of pregnancy
    ectopic pregnancies 116
    pregnancy loss/miscarriage and stillbirth 116–120
  implantation 106–108
    early placental formation 106–108
  oocyte and sperm, final maturation of 102–105
    fertilisation 104–105
    oocyte maturation and ovulation 102–103
    sperm maturation 103–104
  post-implantation embryonic development 109–115
    embryonic/germ layers, differentiation of 109–110
    late gestation and birth 113–115
    week 4 111
    week 5 111
    week 6 111
    week 7 and 8 111–113
  pre-implantation development 105
enamel 268
end diastolic pressure 242
end diastolic volume (EDV) 242
endocardium 226
endochondral ossification of the tibia 165
endocrine 453–454
endocrine glands 85–87
endocrine system
  body map 451
  hormone release control 456–473
    adrenal cortex 468–473
    physiology 456–462
    thyroid gland 462–468
  hormones 453–455
    effects of 455
    transportation of 455
  insulin 473–475, 477
    glucagon 475–476
    somatostatin 476–477
  organs 452–454
endocytosis 33
endoderm 109
endolymph 426
endometriosis 364
endometrium 103, 360
endomysium 128
enteral feeding 262
enzyme 15, 435, 533
eosinophil 199
eosinophils 483
ependymal cells 387
epidermis 519–523
  layers of 523–527
    stratum basale 525–527
    stratum corneum 524–525
    stratum granulosum 525
    stratum lucidum 525
    stratum spinosum 525
  types of cells 520

epididymis 103, 355
epiglottis 256, 320
epilepsy 384–385
epimysium 128
epithalamus 390, 392
epithelial tissue 80–87
  glandular epithelia 85–87
  simple epithelium 81–84
  stratified epithelium 84–85
epithelium 226
epitopes 503, 504
Epstein-Barr virus (EBV) 486
equator of the cell 59
equilibrium 412, 426–430
  equilibrium sensations, pathways for 428–430
equilibrium sensations, pathways for 428–430
erectile dysfunction 357
erythema 526
erythrocytes *See* red blood cells
erythropoiesis, negative feedback for 196
erythropoietin 288
ethmoid bone 319, 414
excretion 3, 288, 300, 532, 535–536
exocrine 453–454
exocrine glands 85, 86
exocytosis 33–34, 199
expectorate 321
expiration, movements of 329
expiratory reserve volume (ERV) 331
external ear 421–425
external genitalia 367–368
external os 366
external respiration 318, 335–338
  factors 335–337
  gaseous exchange 335
  ventilation and perfusion 338
external structures, kidney 289–290
extracellular compartments 29
extracellular fluid 34, 189
extracellular matrix 80
eye 434–438
  accessory structures of 434
  anatomy of 436
  chambers of 437–438
  lacrimal apparatus 435
  main eye structures 435–438
  structure of 434–438
eye drops 438

facilitated diffusion 30
faeces 254
Fallopian tube 83, 102, 364–365
fast glycolytic fibres 132
fast oxidative-glycolytic fibres 132
fats 13–15, 265, 277–278
fatty acids 13–14, 473
fauces 319
female reproductive system 359–362
  corpus luteum 362
  oogenesis and follicular development 360
  ovaries 359
female sex hormones 362–369
  breast 368–369
  external genitalia 367–368
  internal organs 363–367
    cervix 366–367
    Fallopian tubes 364–365
    uterus 363–364
    vagina 365–366
female urethra 311–312
fertilisation 102, 104–105
fibre 88–89
fibroblasts 96
fibrocartilage 90, 163
fibromyalgia 137–139
fibrous joints 178
fibrous pericardium 223
fibrous tunic 435
Fick's law 335–336
filiform 417
filtration 288, 299–302
  selective reabsorption 299–300
  tubular reabsorption and secretion, hormonal control of 301–302
fimbriae 364
fingernails 530
flat bones 175–177
flexion 179
flixonase 413–414
fluid balance 291
fluid compartments 32–33
fluid movement 37–40
foetal alcohol spectrum disorder (FASD) 112–113
foetal wellbeing 119
foetus 350
foliate 417
follicle 359
follicle-stimulating hormone (FSH) 102, 359, 459
follicular development 360
food 3
food pyramid 276
fovea 438
fractures 160
free T_4 455
frenulum 255
fundus 260
fungiform 417

gall bladder 274
gamete 47, 102, 350
ganglion 441, 467
gap junctions 224
gas laws 327
gastric glands 261
gastric juice secretion, phases of 263
gastric phase 262
gastrulation 109
gene crossover 60
gene expression 52–56
  DNA, RNA and protein 56
  protein synthesis 52–56
gene replacement therapy 65
genetic counselling 65–66
genetics
  cell cycle 50, 56–60
    meiosis 58–60
    mitosis 58
  cellular anatomical map 46
  deoxyribonucleic acid and ribonucleic acid 46–48
  DNA double helix 49–52
    chromosomes 50–52
  gene expression 52–56
    DNA, RNA and protein 56
    protein synthesis 52–56
  inheritance
    autosomal dominant inheritance 63
    dominant *versus* recessive disorders, morbidity and mortality of 67
    x-linked recessive disorders 67–69
  non-Mendelian (complex) inheritance 69–73
    disorders of chromosomes 72–73
    spontaneous mutation 70–72
genotype 52
gestational diabetes 117–118
gigantism 459
glands 452
glandular epithelia 85–87
Glasgow coma scale (GCS) 395
glaucoma 437
gliding 180
glomeruli 288, 414
glossopharyngeal nerve 334
glucagon 475–476
glucocorticoid steroids 470
glucocorticoids 470
gluconeogenesis 277, 475
glycogen 132, 470
glycogenolysis 467
glycolysis 277
glycoproteins 80
goblet cells 265, 319
goitre 464
gonadotrophin-releasing hormone (GnRH) 358
gonadotrophins 459
gonads 350
gout 159–160
Graafian follicle 360
granulation 96
granulocytes 483
ground substance 88
growth 3
growth hormone 459
guanine (G) 49
gustatory 418
gustatory pathway 419–421
Guthrie test 71

haemoglobin 193–197
  red blood cells
    formation of 194–196
    life cycle of 196–197
  respiratory gases, transport of 197
haemophilia 203–204
haemopoiesis 159
haemostasis 200–204, 534
  coagulation 201–204
  platelet aggregation 201
  vasoconstriction 200–201
hair 519, 528
hair cells 429
handwashing 507
haploid 354

haustrum 267
head and neck, muscles of 140, 143
hearing aids 425
hearing perception 430–434
  hearing process 432
  hearing reflex 432–434
hearing process 432
hearing reflex 432–434
heart
  blood supply to 230–236
    blood flow through the heart 235–236
  electrical pathways of 237–240
  size and location of 222–225
    structures 223–225
heart chambers 226–230
heart defect 228–229
heart rate, regulation of 245–248
heart wall 223–225
heparin 203
hepatic portal vein 265
hepatocytes 272
hepatopancreatic sphincter 274
hereditary transmission 47
heterologous 50
heterozygous 52
hilum 289
histone protein 47
HIV/AIDS 498–499
Hodgkin lymphoma, ABVD and chemotherapy treatments for 217
homeostasis 15–20, 452, 533
  SI units 17, 18
  units of measurement 17–20
homologous 50
homozygous 51
hormonal control, of male reproductive system 357–358
hormonal stimulation 456
hormone 85, 237, 350, 453–455
  effects of 455
  of menstrual cycle 103
  transportation of 455
hormone activity 246–248
hormone release control 456–473
  adrenal cortex 468–473
    glucocorticoids 470
    mineralocorticoids 468–470
    pancreas 471–473
  physiology 456–462
    anterior pituitary gland 458–462
    hypothalamus and pituitary gland 456–458
  thyroid gland 462–468
    adrenal gland 467–468
    adrenal medulla 467–468
    parathyroid glands 466–467
human chorionic gonadotropin (hCG) 106
humoral immunity 500–501
humoral stimulation 456
hyaline cartilage 90, 162
hydrochloric acid 258
hydrolysis 277
hydrophilic 26
hydrophobic 26
hyoid bone 255
hypercholesterolemia 245
hyperglycaemia 471
hyperkeratosis 519
hyperopia 444–447
hypersensitivity 509–510
hypertension 211–212
hyperthyroidism 464
hypertonic 36, 189
hypertropic cardiomyopathy 225
hypochondriac region 272
hypoglycaemia 468, 475
hyponatraemia 36
hypothalamus 211, 335, 392, 456–458
hypothermia 87
hypothyroidism 464
  in Down syndrome 465–466
hypotonic 189
hypoventilates 338
hypovolaemia 191, 468
hypoxaemia 340
hypoxia 321, 340

immune system 489
  acquired immune system 498–506
    cell-mediated immunity 498–499
    humoral immunity 500–501
    immunoglobulins 501–503
    natural killer cells 506
  blood cell development 482–483
  body map 481
  control of 499
  infection
    anaphylaxis 510
    hypersensitivity 509–510
    immunisations 510–511
    primary and secondary response to 506–511
    primary immune response 506–507
    secondary immune response 507–509
  organs of 483–490
    blood cells 489–490
    immunity, types of 488
    innate immune system 489
    lymphatic system 484–488
    lymphoid tissue 488
    thymus 483–484
  phagocytosis 489–497
    cytotoxicity 493
    inflammation 493–497
immunisations 510–511
immunity 488
  types of 488
immunoglobulin D 503
immunoglobulin E 502–503
immunoglobulin G 501–502
immunoglobulin M 502
immunoglobulin therapy 504–505
immunoglobulins 490, 501–503
  immunoglobulin A 502
  immunoglobulin D 503
  immunoglobulin E 502–503
  immunoglobulin G 501–502
  immunoglobulin M 502
  role of 503–506
implantation 103, 106–108
incisors 268
infection
  anaphylaxis 510
  hypersensitivity 509–510
  immunisations 510–511
  primary and secondary response to 506–511
  primary immune response 506–507
  secondary immune response 507–509
inferior vena cava 227
inflammation 490, 493–497, 534
inflammatory diseases 470
ingestion 254
inguinal canal 352
inheritance 60–69
  autosomal dominant inheritance 63
  autosomal recessive inheritance 63–67
  dominant *versus* recessive disorders, morbidity and mortality of 67
  Mendelian inheritance 61–62
  x-linked recessive disorders 67–69
initiation 54
innate immune system 488–489
inner ear 426–427
innervated 80
innervations 519
inorganic substances 12
inspiration, movements of 329
inspiratory reserve volume (IRV) 331
insulin 473–475, 477
  glucagon 475–476
  somatostatin 476–477
integumentary 518
interatrial septum 227
intercostal nerves 334
intercostal spaces 328
internal organs, female sex hormones 363–367
  cervix 366–367
  Fallopian tubes 364–365
  uterus 363–364
  vagina 365–366
internal os 366
internal respiration 318, 341–342
internal structures, kidney 294–295
interphase 57
interstitial compartments 32
interstitial fluid 88, 193
intestinal crypts 275
intestinal phase 262
intracellular compartment 32
intracellular fluid (ICF) 29, 34
intramuscular (IM) injection 128–129
intravenous cannula 209–210
intravenous fluids, administration of 40
  intravenous fluid therapy 191–192
intrinsic factor 261
in utero 164, 352
ionic bonds 6–8
ions 6, 7
iron deficiency anaemia 194
irregular bones 177
isovolumetric contraction phase 242
isthmus 363

joints, skeletal system 178–182
  cartilaginous joints 178

fibrous joints 178
six types of 179
synovial joints 178–182

keratin 84, 519
keratinisation 525
keratinocytes 519
kidney 288
blood supply of 290–294
external structures 289–290
functions of 288–289
internal structures 294–295
kidney disease 306
kinin 494
kinin system 494
knee reconstruction 164
Kupffer cells 272

lacrimal apparatus 435
lacrimal caruncle 434
lacteal 275
lactulose 267
lamellar arrangement 171
lamina propria 259, 412
Langerhans cells 523
lanugo 528
large intestine 266–267
large lymph vessels 214–215
laryngopharynx 256, 319
larynx 318, 320–321
lateral 364
lateral end 425
levothyroxine 466
Leydig cells 353
ligament 142, 359, 426
skeletal system, connective tissues associated with 163
limbic system 335, 393–395, 414
lingual tonsils 319
lipase 275
lipid-rich substance 412
liquid connective tissue 91–92
liver 272–273
liver lobule 273
liver sinusoids 272
lobes 322, 390
lobule 323
locus 51
long bones 174–175
loop of Henle 297
loose connective tissue 90
loss of the sense of smell 416
lower limbs, muscles of 142, 147
lower oesophageal sphincter 258
lower respiratory tract 318, 320–326
larynx 320–321
trachea 321–322
lumbar puncture 389
lung cancer 333
lung compliance 330
lunula 530
luteinising hormone (LH) 102, 358, 459
lymph 188, 212, 483
lymph capillaries 214–215
lymph node 214–217, 320, 483, 486–488
lymph vessels 323, 484
lymphatic circulation 215
lymphatic organs 217–218
lymphatic system 212–218, 483–488
lymph 212
lymph capillaries and large lymph vessels 214–215
lymph nodes 214–217, 486–488
lymphatic organs 217–218
lymphocyte 200
lymphoid tissue 488
lysozyme 269

Macronutrients 275
macrophages 87, 483
macular degeneration 440–441
magnetic resonance imaging (MRI) 6
male reproductive system 350–357
epididymis 355
hormonal control of 357–358
penis 356–357
scrotum 351–352
seminal vesicles and prostate gland 356
sperm 355
spermatogenesis 353–355
testes 351–353
vas deferens, spermatic cord and ejaculatory duct 356
male urethra 311
malodorous 530
marrow 158
mast cell degranulation 494
mastication 255
meatuses 319, 359
mechanical barriers 489
medial 434
medulla 456, 487
medulla oblongata 246, 334, 390, 393, 428
meiosis 57–60, 354
meiosis I 59–60
meiosis II 60
Meissner's plexus 259
melanin 519
melanocytes 519–523
membrane 80, 92–94
memory 499
Mendelian genetics 61
Mendelian inheritance 61–62
Mendel's law of independent assortment 61
Mendel's law of segregation 61
meninges 387–388
meningitis 388
menopause 359
menstrual cycle, hormones of 103
mental illness 232–233
Merkel cells 523
mesenchyme 164
mesoderm 109
metabolism 254
metaphysis 175
microglia 387
micronutrients 275
microvilli 259, 418
micturition 312–313
midazolam 393–394
midbrain 390, 393
middle ear 425–426
mineral salts 269
mineralocorticoids 468–470
minerals 278–282
minute volume 331
miscarriage 111, 116–120
mitosis 57–58, 96
mitral valve 228
molars 268
molecules 3
monocytes 199
monozygotic twins 64
motor (efferent) nerves 379, 382
motor area 390
motor unit 132, 133
mouth 255–256
mouth care 270
movement 3
mucosa 258
mucous membranes 92
mucous neck cells 261
multiple sclerosis (MS) 381, 496–497
muscle contraction, energy sources for 136–139
aerobic respiration 136–139
ATP sources 137
muscle cramping 128
muscle fatigue 137–139
muscle fibres, types of 132
muscle tissue 94–95
skeletal muscle contraction and relaxation 132–136
types of 126–132
cardiac 126
composition of 127–128
functions of 126–127
skeletal 126
skeletal muscle fibre, microanatomy of 129–132
skeletal muscles, gross anatomy of 128–129
smooth/visceral muscle 126
muscular dystrophy 131–132
muscular system
muscle contraction, energy sources for 136–139
aerobic respiration 136–139
ATP sources 137
muscle tissue, types of 126–132
cardiac 126
composition of 127–128
functions of 126–127
skeletal 126
skeletal muscle fibre, microanatomy of 129–132
skeletal muscles, gross anatomy of 128–129
smooth/visceral muscle 126
skeletal muscle contraction and relaxation 132–136
skeletal muscular system organisation of 139–152
muscularis 259
muscularis mucosa 259
musculoskeletal injury 163–164
myasthenia gravis 134
myelin sheath 381
myenteric plexus 259

myocardial infarction 234–235
myocardium 224–225
myocytes 224
myofibrils 130
myometrium 363
myopia 444–447

Na^+/K^+ pump 30
nail 530–532
nasal cavity 319
nasal conchae 319
nasal septum 319
nasogastric tube 262
nasojejunal tube 262
nasopharynx 319, 425
natural killer cell 506
negative feedback control, of thyroid hormone production 463
negative feedback system 358, 456
negative feedback, for erythropoiesis 196
nematode therapy 503
nephron 294, 296–299
  Bowman's capsule 296–297
  collecting ducts 298–299
  distal convoluted tubule 298
  loop of Henle 297
  proximal convoluted tubule 297
nephrotoxic drugs 298–299
nerve conduction studies 135
nerve impulses, simple propagation of 382–383
nervous system 378, 452
  action potential 382–389
    cerebrospinal fluid 388–389
    meninges 387–388
    nerve impulses, simple propagation of 382–383
    neuroglia 386–387
    neurotransmitters 385–386
    refractory period 382–385
    saltatory conduction 382
  body map 377
  organisation of 378–382
    central nervous system 379
    peripheral nervous system *See* (peripheral nervous system)
nervous tissue 94–96
neural stimulation 456
neural tunic 437
neuroglia 94, 386–387
neurological assessment 394–395
neuromuscular junction 385
neurone 80, 94, 379–380, 412
neurotransmitters 385–386
neurulation 109, 110
neutral 4
neutrons 4
neutropenia 198, 490–492
neutrophil 198, 483
NK cells 506
nodal cells 238–239
noise exposure 433–434
non-ciliated columnar epithelium 83
non-keratinised stratified squamous epithelial tissue 84, 319
non-Mendelian (complex) inheritance 69–73
  disorders of chromosomes 72–73
  spontaneous mutation 70–72
nucleic acid 47
nucleosome 50
nucleotides 49
null cells 506
nursing practice 97
nutrient 254, 275
nutrient groups 277–282
  carbohydrates 277
  fats 277–278
  minerals 278–282
  proteins 278
  vitamins 278
  water 277
nutrition 3

obesity 280–281
obstetric ultrasound 118–119
occupational dermatitis 534–535
oedema 215, 493
oesophageal phase 256
oesophagus 258–259, 320
oestrogen 102, 359
olfactory 412, 412–413
olfactory discrimination 414–416
olfactory dysfunction 416
olfactory epithelium 412
olfactory pathway 414–415
olfactory receptors 319, 413–416
  olfactory discrimination 414–416
  olfactory pathway 414–415
oligodendrocytes 387
omeprazole 258–259
ondansetron 264
oocyte maturation 102–103
oocytes 83
oogenesis 360
opsin 438–439
opsonins — complement factors 492
oral cavity 255–256
organ 518
organ of Corti 432
organelles 24, 193
organic molecules 12–15
  carbohydrates 13
  fats 13–15
  proteins 15
organic substances 12
oropharynx 256, 319
osmolality 457
osmosis 28–30, 190
osmotic pressure 29, 37, 38, 189
osseous callus 171
ossification 164
osteoarthritis 180–181
osteoblasts 160–161
osteoclasts 160, 464
osteocytes 160–162
osteomyelitis 169–170
osteophytes 181
otolith 429
ototoxicity 433
ova 47
ovarian cycles 370
ovarian follicles 359
ovaries 350, 359
ovulation 102–103, 359
ovum 350
oxygen 3, 337
  transport of 338–340
oxygen debt 136
oxyhaemoglobin dissociation curve 339
oxytocin 457

pacemaker 239
paediatric urinary tract infection 309–310
pain relief 114–115
palate 256
palatine tonsils 319
pancreas 270–272, 471–473
pancreatic duct 270
paneth cells 265
panic attack 401
papillae 255
papules 518
paracetamol 401
paracrine 453–454
paramedic practice 97–98
parasympathetic fibres 269
parasympathetic nervous system 403–404, 436
parathyroid glands 462, 466–467
parenchyma 96
parietal cells 258
parietal pericardium 223
parietal pleura 322
parotid glands 268
passive immunisation 510
passive immunity 502
passive transport 27–28, 193
pathogens 435, 518
peak flow 333–334
pedigree 66–67
penis 350, 356–357
pepsin 261
pepsinogen 261
peptidyl transferase 54
percutaneous coronary intervention (PCI) 234
percutaneous endoscopic gastrostomy (PEG) tube 262
percutaneous endoscopic jejunostomy (PEJ) tube 262
perfusion, external respiration 338
pericardial fluid 224
pericarditis 223–224
pericardium 223–224
perilymph 426
perimetrium 363
perimysium 128
periosteum 158
peripheral intravenous cannula 209–210
peripheral nervous system 378, 395–401
  cranial nerves 395–397
  motor division of 379–382
    autonomic nervous system 379
    axons 381
    cell body 381
    dendrites 379–381
    motor (efferent) nerves 382
    myelin sheath 381

neurones 379
sensory (afferent) nerves 381–382
somatic nervous system 379
sensory division of 378
spinal cord 397
spinal nerve 398–401
peristalsis 256–257
peritoneum 260
peritonitis 93
personal hygiene 524
Perthes disease 168–169
Peyer's patches 265
pH 10, 356
phagocytes 487
phagocytosis 33, 353, 489–497, 523
cytotoxicity 493
inflammation 493–497
pharyngeal phase 256
pharyngeal tonsil 319
pharynx 256–258, 319
phenylketonuria (PKU) 69
phenytoin 394
pheromones 530
Philadelphia abnormality 72
phlebitis 210
phosphate 49
phospholipids 15–16
photoreceptors 412
phototransduction 438
phrenic nerve 334
physical barriers 489
physiology 2
acids and bases 10–12
blood and pH values 11
chemical equations 11–12
characteristics of life 3–4
homeostasis 15–20
levels of organisation 2–3
life at chemical level 4–10
chemical reactions and chemical bonds 6–10
elements 4
smallest unit of matter 4–6
organic molecules 12–15
carbohydrates 13
fats 13–15
proteins 15
pia mater 388
pilosebaceous unit 529
pineal gland 392
pinocytosis 33
pituitary gland 392, 456–458
pivot 179
placenta 106–108, 363
plasma 188, 190–191
plasma cells 483
plasma membrane 25, 193
plasma osmolality 189–190
platelet 200, 483
platelet aggregation 201
pleural space 322
plicae circulars 275
pneumonia 330
pneumotaxic centre 334
pneumothorax 93–94
polar bonds 7
polar molecules 9
poles 58
polypharmacy 302
pons 334, 390, 393, 428
portal fissure 272
portal triad 272
posterior surface 141
post-implantation embryonic development 109–115
embryonic/germ layers,differentiation of 109–110
late gestation and birth 113–115
week 4 111
week 5 111
week 6 111
week 7 and 8 111–113
posterior third of the tongue 419
pre-eclampsia 116
pre-implantation development, embryology 105
pre-term birth 113
pregnancy loss 116–120
pregnancy tests 108
preload 244–245
premature myocardial infarction 235
premolars 268
prenatal monitoring 114
presbyopia 444–447
primary immune response 506–507
products 11
progesterone 103, 359
prolactin 368, 459
proliferation 534
propulsion 254
prostaglandins 494
prostate gland 356
prostatic hyperplasia 310
protection 534–535
protein 15, 261, 278
protein synthesis 52–56
structural differences 52
transcription 52–53
translation 53–56
protons 4
proximal convoluted tubule 297
pruritus 528
pseudopodia 492
pseudostratified ciliated columnar epithelium 84, 319
pulmonary arteries 326
pulmonary circulation 222
pulmonary valve 227
pulmonary veins 227, 326
pulmonary ventilation 318, 327–334
breathing, work of 329
mechanics of breathing 327–329
volumes and capacities 331–334
pulp cavity 268
pulse oximeters 340
Punnet squares 63
pupil 436
pupillary constrictor muscles 436
pupillary dilator muscles 436
purines 49
Purkinje fibres system 237
pustules 518
pyloric canal 260
pyloric region 260
pyloric sphincter 260
pyrexia 335
pyridostigmine 134–135
pyrimidines 49

reactants 11
receptors 378
recessive allele 52
rectum 266
red blood cells 193, 483
destruction of 197
formation of 194–196
life cycle of 196–197
refraction 441–444
refractory period 382–385
remodelling 534
renal arteries 288
renal cortex 294
renal medulla 294
renal pelvis 294
renal pyramids 294
renal system
body map 287
filtration 288, 299–302
selective reabsorption 299–300
tubular reabsorption and secretion, hormonal control of 301–302
kidney
blood supply of 290–294
external structures 289–290
functions of 288–289
internal structures 294–295
nephron 294, 296–299, 301
Bowman's capsule 296–297
collecting ducts 298–299
distal convoluted tubule 298
loop of Henle 297
proximal convoluted tubule 297
organs of 288
urine, composition of 303–313
characteristics of 303–307
micturition 312–313
ureter 307–308
urethra 310–312
urinary bladder 308–310
renal veins 289
renin 211, 288
reproduction 3
reproductive systems
body map 349–350
female reproductive system 359–362
corpus luteum 362
oogenesis and follicular development 360
ovaries 359
female sex hormones 362–369
breast 368–369
external genitalia 367–368
internal organs 363–367
female sex hormones, role of 362–369
male reproductive system 350–357
epididymis 355
hormonal control of 357–358
penis 356–357
scrotum 351–352
seminal vesicles and prostate gland 356
sperm 355
spermatogenesis 353–355

testes 351–353
vas deferens, spermatic cord and ejaculatory duct 356
residual volume (RV) 331
resorption 161
respiration 3, 327
respiratory gases, transport of 197
respiratory rate 335
respiratory regions 318
respiratory system
body map 317
breathing, control of 334–335
external respiration 335–338
factors 335–337
gaseous exchange 335
ventilation and perfusion 338
organisation of 318–327
blood supply 326
lower respiratory tract 320–326
respiration 327
upper respiratory tract 319–320
pulmonary ventilation 318, 327–334
breathing, work of 329
mechanics of breathing 327–329
volumes and capacities 331–334
transport of gases 338–342
acid-base balance 341
internal respiration 341–342
transport of carbon dioxide 340–341
transport of oxygen 338–340
rete 355
reticular formation 393–395
reticular tissue 90
retina 439
focusing images onto 441–447
myopia, hyperopia and presbyopia 444–447
refraction 441–444
organisation of 438–441
rhabdomyolysis 127–128
rheumatic heart disease 227–228
rheumatoid disease 495
rhodopsin 438
ribonucleic acid (RNA) 46–48
rickets 160
right cerebral hemisphere 391
RNA polymerase 52
rods 438

saddle 180
salbutamol 325
salivary amylase 269
salivary glands 268–270
saltatory conduction 382
sarcolemma 130, 224
sarcomeres 130–132
sarcopenia 139
sarcoplasm 130
satellite cells 387
schizophrenia 70
Schwann cells 387
scrotum 351–352
sebum 518
secondary immune response 507–509
secondary immunodeficiencies 487–488
secretin 262
segmentation 266
selective reabsorption 299–300
semen 351
seminal vesicles 356
seminiferous tubules 353
sensation 532–534
sense 412
chemical senses 412–416
olfactory receptors 413–416
sense of smell 412–413
equilibrium 426–430
equilibrium sensations, pathways for 428–430
eye 434–438
accessory structures of 434
anatomy of 436
chambers of 437–438
lacrimal apparatus 435
main eye structures 435–438
structure of 434–438
hearing perception 430–434
hearing process 432
hearing reflex 432–434
retina 439
myopia, hyperopia and presbyopia 444–447
organisation of 438–441
refraction 441–444
sense of hearing and sense of balance 421–426
external ear 421–425
inner ear 426–427
middle ear 425–426
sense of taste 416–421
gustatory pathway 419–421
taste receptor 418–419
tastebud 418
sense of balance 421–426
sense of hearing 421–426
sense of smell 412–413
sensitivity 3
sensory (afferent) nerves 381–382
sensory area 391
sensory nerve fibres 378
sepsis 495
serosa 260
serous membranes 92
serous pericardium 223
sesamoid bones 178
sexual health 367–368
shells 5
short bones 175–176
simple epithelium 81–84
sinoatrial (SA) node 237
skeletal muscle 94, 126
contraction and relaxation 132–136
gross anatomy of 128–129
skeletal muscle fibre, microanatomy of 129–132
skeletal muscle movement 150–152
skeletal muscular system
organisation of 139–152
ageing, effects of 152
skeletal muscle movement 150–152
skeletal system
axial and appendicular skeleton 172–182
bone shapes *See* (bone shapes)
joints 178–182
bone as tissue 160–162
osteoblasts 161
osteoclasts 161
osteocytes 161–162
connective tissues associated with 162–172
bone formation 164–165
bone fractures 170–172
bone growth 165–168
bone remodelling 168–170
cartilage 162–163
ligaments 163
tendons 163–164
functions of 158–160
skin
accessory skin structures 528–532
hair 528
nail 530–532
sweat gland 529–530
body map 517
functions of 532–537
excretion and absorption 535–536
protection 534–535
sensation 532–534
vitamin D, synthesis of 536–537
layers of 527
structure of 519–528
dermis 527
epidermis 519–523
keratinocytes 519
melanocytes 519–523
papillary and reticular aspects 527–528
types of cells 520
skin biopsy 522
skin cancer 520–522
slow oxidative fibres 132
small intestine 264–266
smooth/visceral muscle 94, 126
snake antivenom 506
Snellen chart 445
solute 29
somatic nervous system 379
somatostatin 476–477
sperm 355
sperm maturation 103–104
spermatic cord 356
spermatogenesis 353–355
spermatozoon 47, 104
sphincter 308
spinal cord 390, 397
functions of 398
spinal nerve 395, 398–401
spirometry 333–334
spleen 217, 483, 488
spongy (cancellous) bone 158, 175
spontaneous mutation 70–72
sprained ankle 151–152
Sputum 336–337
stercobilin 267
steroids 15
stillbirth 116–120
stomach 260–264
strands 49
stratified epithelium 84–85
stratum basale 525–527

stratum corneum 524–525
stratum granulosum 525
stratum lucidum 525
stratum spinosum 525
stress 471
stroke 392
stroke volume
  regulation of 244–245
    afterload 245
    force of contraction 245
    preload 244–245
stroma 90
subcutaneous 87
sublingual glands 268
submandibular glands 268
submucosa 259
substrates 452
sun exposure 525–527
sunlight 3–4
superior mesenteric artery 265
superior mesenteric vein 265
superior vena cava 227
surface mucous cells 261
surfactant 330
swallowing 256–258
sweat gland 529–530
sympathetic nervous system 402, 404, 436
synapse 412
syndrome of inappropriate ADH secretion (SIADH) 458
synovial cavity 178
synovial joints 178–182, 426
synovial membranes 92–94
systemic circulation 222
systole 241

T tubules 129
T-cell lymphocyte 484, 498–499
tactile 523
taeniae coli 267
taste disorders 421
taste receptor 418–419
tastebud 418
Teeth 268
tendons 127
  skeletal system, connective tissues associated with 163–164
termination 55
termination codon 55
testes 350–353
testicular torsion 352
testosterone 353
thalamus 390, 392, 412
thalassaemia 195–196
thermoregulation 528, 533
thoracic cage 320
thorax 320
three-parent babies 56
thrombin 201
thrombolysis 234
thromboplastin 201
thromboplastinogenase 201
thymine (T) 49
thymus 483–484
thymus gland 217–218
thyroid cartilage 320
thyroid gland 462–468
  adrenal gland 467–468
  adrenal medulla 467–468
  parathyroid glands 466–467
thyroid hormone production, negative feedback control of 463
thyroid-stimulating hormone (TSH) 459–460
thyroxine 246–248
tidal volume (V_T) 331
tinea 531
tissue
  connective tissue 87–94
    bone 91
    cartilage 90–91
    connective tissue proper 89–90
    constituents of 89
    fibre 88–89
    ground substance 88
    liquid connective tissue 91–92
    membranes 92–94
  epithelial tissue 80–87
    glandular epithelia 85–87
    simple epithelium 81–84
    stratified epithelium 84–85
  muscle tissue 94–95
  nervous tissue 94–96
  tissue repair 94–98
  types of 80
tongue 255–256, 417
tonometry 437
tonsils 319, 483
topical steroids 535–536
total lung capacity (TLC) 331
trabeculae 486
trachea 84, 321–322
tracheostomy 320
transcription 50, 52–53
transdermal patches 533–534
translation 53–56
transparent 436
transport of gases 318
transport proteins 26
transverse tubules 130
triacylglycerols 14–15
tricuspid valve 227
triglycerides 14–15, 473
triplets 54
tRNA 54
trunk, muscles of 142
tunica externa 207
tunica interna 207
tunica media 207
Turner syndrome 47–48
type 1 diabetes 474
type 2 diabetes 472

ultrasound 118–119
umami 417
unplanned out-of-hospital births 119–120
upper limbs, muscles of 141, 144
upper oesophageal sphincter 258
upper respiratory tract 318–320
upregulation 455
ureter 288, 307–308
urethra 288, 310–312
  female 311–312
  male 311
urinary bladder 308–310
urinary tract infection (UTI) 309
uterine cycle 369–371
uterus 350, 363–364

vagina 350, 365–366
vaginal swab 366–367
vagus nerve 334
valency 8
valve stenosis 229
valvular incompetence 229
vas deferens 351, 356
vascular tunic 436
vasoconstriction 200–201, 533
vasodilatation 533
vasomotor centre 246
veins, structure and function of 207–209
venous 236
venous blood 236
ventilation V_A 338
ventilation, external respiration 338
ventricles 225, 227–230, 387, 389
vermiform appendix 266
vertebrae 90
vertigo 430
vestibule 319
villi 275
visceral pericardium 223
visceral peritoneum 260
visceral pleura 322
visual information
  central processing of 446–447
  processing of 446
vital capacity 331
vitamin 278
vitamin B{12} 261
vitamin B{12} 261
vitamin D, synthesis of 536–537
voluntary phase 256
vomer 319
vomiting 293–294
vulva 350

warfarin 203
water 3
  in plasma 191
water balance 34–36
white blood cells 197–200
  basophils 199
  lymphocyte 200
  monocytes 199
  neutrophil 198
white matter 381
wound healing 534

x-linked recessive disorders 67–69
xeroderma pigmentosum 69

zona pellucida 104
zygote 102